# Advance praise for *Bouncebacks! Medical and Legal*

"No matter where you are in your medical career, Bouncebacks! is for you! I am a huge fan of this series; it has truly made me a better physician. Every book is an amazing educational resource and entertaining read; I learn from every case in the series! What better place to start than the anniversary edition with updates and multiple brand-new chapters?"

**Brit Long, MD**
Associate Professor, Emergency Medicine
San Antonio, TX
Editor-in-chief of clinical content for emDocs.net

AF894464

What impresses me with this book is how conversational the tone is - which is welcome given the seriousness of the topics. I can imagine having coffee (or another beverage of choice) and discussing these cases at a round table. There are few books that have the ability to revolutionize your practice, and every Bouncebacks! book is on that short list. This book belongs on your bookshelf, or better yet, on your nightstand!

**Benjamin Cooper, MD, MEd, FACEP**
Associate Professor of Emergency Medicine | McGovern Medical School at UTHealth Houston
Lead Author of ECG Stampede

"Wow! 13 years since Bouncebacks version 1.0. We've made it through a pandemic and seen the world change is so many ways. What hasn't changed? Malpractice lawsuits and the fear of litigation. There are two types of clinicians: those who've been sued and those who haven't been sued – yet. Whichever one you are, Bouncebacks offers practical, case based wisdom to quell our fears and practice with more peace-of-mind by arming us with the essentials for what we need to know to keep both ourselves and our patients out of hot water."

**Joshua W. Russell, MD, MSc, ELS, FCUCM, FACEP**
Emergency & Urgent Care Medicine
Editor-in-Chief, Journal of Urgent Care Medicine (JUCM)
Senior Editor, UCMax Podcast, EM:RAP
Board of Directors, College of Urgent Care Medicine (CUCM)
Clinical Educator, University of Chicago Pritzker School of Medicine

Read it or BE it!
The Bouncebacks teaching method is a cornerstone of how Emergency Medicine should be taught! It frames our thought process and common pitfalls we can avoid in real world stories and lessons. By emphasizing the fundamentals and giving us a framework, we can internalize and utilize the lessons that will make us better clinicians and give our patients better and safer outcomes. I love to read Bouncebacks so I can avoid being a cautionary tale in the next edition!

**Jaime Hope, MD**
Medical Director, Corewell Health Livonia
Assistant Professor, Oakland University William Beaumont School of Medicine

Mike Weinstock and his team have done it again! The 13th-anniversary edition of Bouncebacks! Medical and Legal is another valuable resource to the practice of emergency medicine. Whether you're an experienced clinician or new to the specialty, there will be pearls for all to learn. The case-based format presents cases of emergency department patients with unscheduled return visits, the risk management pearls, and the legal perspectives from the defense and plaintiff as the case goes to trial. New chapters also include topics on the litigation process. Be sure to review this book before your next "bounceback" case!

**Fred Wu, MHS, PA-C**
Program Director, Emergency Medicine PA Residency
Lead APP, Department of Emergency Medicine
University of California San Francisco - Fresno

I've always been proponent of Eleanor Roosevelt's quote: "Learn from the mistakes of others. You can't live long enough to make them all yourself." This book epitomizes how much there is to learn from others' mistakes in our high-risk practice environment of the emergency department. The case-based, walk-through discussion of each scenario immediately transports the reader into the emergency clinician's clogs. What happened, why were things overlooked, and what could have been done better? This is an essential read for all who practice in the emergency department.

**Michelle Lin, MD**
UCSF Professor of Emergency Medicine
San Francisco General Hospital
Founder ALiEM

"Bouncebacks! Medical and Legal" demystifies the lived experience of the physician. We are fallible creatures capable of great learning and this series continues to offer us the opportunity to grow in our practices. Sharing these cases and escorting us through the oft confusing and terrifying space of case litigation helps us to know that we are not alone in these journeys. Learning to recognize the pitfalls in practice and remain well in a continually more challenging place of practice, these books truly open a door into spaces Emergency Physicians dread. Well worth the read!!

**Carissa J. Tyo, MD**
Assistant Professor, Depts of
Internal and Emergency Medicine
University of Illinois at Chicago
Medical Director-Clinical Decision Unit (CDU)
Medical Director-Care Management and Physician Advisors

"Bouncebacks! Medical and Legal" is a tour de force in educating emergency clinicians about how to provide great patient care and, in the process, substantially reduce their risk of a lawsuit. The authors are the real McCoy -- they know their stuff and have been engaged in the legal aspects of emergency medicine for decades. I can recommend this book without reservations -- assimilate its spot-on recommendations and do yourself and your patients a tremendous favor.

**W. Richard Bukata, MD**
Host, Risk Management Monthly, Emergency Medicine
Medical Director, The Center for Medical Education

Dr. Weinstock and team have done it again! Bringing to light the dreaded "patient that you saw yesterday" into an educational experience that you will remember and use to improve care for your next patient!!

**Ann M Dietrich, MD, FAAP, FACEP**
Division Chief Pediatric Emergency Medicine
Department of Emergency Medicine, Prisma Health
Professor of Pediatrics and Emergency Medicine
University of South Carolina School of Medicine

"Bouncebacks! Medical and Legal" is one of those rare books that takes a difficult but important topic and presents the information in a format we can all easily learn from. The use of real cases taking the reader all the way from the initial chief complaint to the eventual outcome including depositions and critical learning points along the way is not only innovative, but also highly engaging and effective. One of the things I like best about the book is that it does not promote the practice of defensive medicine, but rather emphasizes simply practicing good medicine and documenting what you have done in a way that is defensible. These authors are simply the best minds in the game, and this book is a must read.
**Sanjay Arora MD**
Professor of Clinical Emergency Medicine
Vice Chair for Academic Affairs
Keck School of Medicine of USC

The first medical textbook I ever read cover to cover was the original Bouncebacks, and I followed that in short order by reading the original addition of "Bouncebacks! Medical and Legal" in its entirety. These books were profoundly important in shaping my understanding and practice of emergency medicine. I have always been uncomfortable shaping medical education around the legal system. I have never liked the "retrospectoscope" that we apply in M&M conferences. It might therefore seem like an odd fit, but the Bouncebacks series are the best medical textbooks I have read, pulling you into cases, and presenting patients as we actually see them, allowing you to learn as you work. They delve into important topics of meta-cognition that we need to master to become expert physicians. They are full of clinical pearls. I loved these books, and I am certain you will too.
**Justin Morgenstern, MD**
Associate professor, University of Toronto
Creator/ Founder First10EM

The Bouncebacks! books have been a staple series for my reading as a new attending and education fellow, and the Medical and Legal book has already been helping me reap benefits. This book is massive for quelling the anxiety I have about being a new attending and is giving me lessons that are helping my career, teaching my residents, and improving my patient care. I am forever grateful of the time Dr. Weinstock and his team took to put these together, and I'm sure my patients are too!
**Mackenzie Brown, MD**
Fellow of Medical Education
Emergency Medicine Physician
John Peter Smith Hospital

Once again, "Bouncebacks!" is elevating my care! Between breaking down common medical-legal processes, snapshots of courtroom proceedings and relatable physician anecdotes, this latest "Bouncebacks!" edition keeps finding ways to be an incredible resource. Whether you're a recent residency graduate or a seasoned EM physician, this is a must read to improve patient care and avoid the minefield.
**Masood R. Mohammed, DO MS**
Associate Director of Education
Department of Emergency Medicine
Abrazo Health System
Founder of Med School Moose

“This is such a resourceful book! Giving concrete information in the context of cases is critical for clinicians and learners alike. It is easy to fear the legal aspects of medicine but understanding it and practicing smart medicine using the tips in this book is transformative. A must read for everyone!”
**Lindsey E. Fish, M.D.**
Medical Director, Federico F. Peña Southwest Urgent Care Clinic
Denver Health and Hospital
Associate Professor of Medicine, Division of General Internal Medicine
University of Colorado School of Medicine
Member, Board of Directors, College of Urgent Care Medicine

Mike Weinstock continues to curate an exceptional roster of contributors, fascinating medical cases with unexpected outcomes, and medicolegal implications that humble us all. These are the patients you could see on your next shift! Rooted in evidence-based medicine, Bouncebacks! transcends traditional medical education. Mike takes you into the mind of the clinician, the experience of the patient, and recruits top defense experts to offer their legal perspective. Another win for medical education!
**Cameron Powell, MPAS, PA-C**
Chair, Health Science Division
Program Director and Assistant Professor, PA Studies
Ohio Dominican University

# BOUNCEBACKS!
# MEDICAL AND LEGAL

*13th Anniversary Edition*

**Michael B. Weinstock, MD**
**Kevin M. Klauer, DO**
**T. Marc Calvert, JD**

**Foreword by: Mel Herbert, MD**

Designed and illustrated by:
**Shannon Lynch**
(Hudson Meredith & Alyssa Klauer: First Edition)

Anadem
Publishing

**Anadem, Inc.**

## INTELLECTUAL PROPERTY RIGHTS



## USING THIS BOOK

***Bouncebacks! Medical and Legal does not provide medical advice for specific patients:***
The text, information, graphics, images, and other material ("Content") contained in *Bouncebacks! Medical and Legal* is for informational purposes only. The Content is not intended to replace or be a substitute for professional medical advice, diagnosis, or treatment. Readers of *Bouncebacks! Medical and Legal* are cautioned to use their own judgment in making clinical decisions and, when appropriate, consult and compare information from other sources.

All information and recommendations are meant to aid in general patient care and are not meant to apply to specific patients or patient care scenarios. Anadem, Inc., its employees, contractors enlisted to assist Anadem, Inc. in preparing this book for publication, or authors, contributors, editors or reviewers do not accept responsibility for the application of the Content in direct or indirect patient care. It is the responsibility of the healthcare provider to ensure that treatment recommendations are appropriate for an individual patient-care situation.

*Bouncebacks! Medical and Legal* Content consists of medical cases and contains the opinions and recommendations of authors, commentators, contributors and editors who are medical providers. Their opinions and recommendations expressed in this book are beyond the scope of knowledge or understanding of Anadem, Inc., its employees or contractors. The opinions and recommendations of the authors, contributors, editors and reviewers are their own and do not necessarily reflect any position, policy or recommendation of Anadem, Inc., its employees or contractors.

If you are a consumer, you access *Bouncebacks! Medical and Legal* at your own risk. Do not rely on *Bouncebacks! Medical and Legal* as a substitute for professional medical advice or a relationship with a physician or other qualified healthcare professional.

Anadem, Inc.
www.anadem.com
anadem@anadem.com
614-262-2539
BOUNCEBACKS MEDICAL AND LEGAL ISBN: 978-1-890018-88-7

## DEDICATION

This book is dedicated to Eli Weinstock;
son, brother, and the sweetest, most creative and original boy in the world.

# FOREWORD—MEL HERBERT

***We must not say every mistake is a foolish one.***
***Cicero 106-43 BC***

"Remember that patient you saw yesterday?" Rarely is this question followed by "Good job! They did great!" Is there any other statement in the practice of Emergency Medicine that creates such a swirling pit of angst? You are left to wonder how bad the return visit was, did the patient live or die, and whether or not you are going to be sued. Bouncebacks confronts these dark encounters and drags them into the light.

It was Greg Henry that first taught me, "nothing focuses the mind like someone else's screw-up!" This is the essence of Bouncebacks. It is hard to believe that it's been 13 years since the last revision and 16 years since the first Bouncebacks! book graced our lives. Not only one of the most innovative and successful textbooks in Emergency Medicine of the last few decades, Bouncebacks has also become a "radio show" and a live event at some of Emergency Medicine's most prestigious CME meetings.

Using real cases and expert commentary by some of the most well-known and influential educators in the field, Drs. Weinstock and a host of expert colleagues, have spared no effort in creating a unique and exceptionally educational textbook. The cases are compelling, common and "real world." The reader has that sinking feeling in the stomach; "Hell! I would have sent that patient home too!" This expanded edition with six new chapters contains actual legal testimony, almost impossible to find elsewhere. This is simply a remarkable resource for the Emergency Medicine community; there is just nothing like it.

Bouncebacks should be required reading for all residents, mid-levels and attending physicians. Anyone can look after the "clearly sick" patient, but more importantly, it is the clinician's approach to the "not obviously sick" that sorts the wheat from the chaff. Learn from others' "mistakes" and absorb the educational pearls from the expert faculty. Read actual courtroom testimony, hear from the legal experts, muse and ponder. Immerse yourself in other peoples' "bouncebacks," and spare yourself the same fate. This book is a treasure—an absolute must read for every clinician!

Mel Herbert, MD

# PREFACE

The format of *Bouncebacks: Medical and Legal* is modeled on the TV show Law and Order; each case starts with a patient's story… then progresses to the attorney's desk. This book is not bathroom reading; 15 cases (plus a bonus case from the Bouncebacks! Critical Care book) formatted to suck you into the personal experience of both the patient and the clinician. As a lengthy medical and litigation process is compressed into a single chapter, we want you to feel empathetic, indignant, enlightened and humbled.

All of these stories are true; from the 15-year-old girl who presented with a headache hours after the World Trade Centers were hit on September 11, 2001, to the 42-year-old fireman whose symptoms began after walking out of an estate-planning meeting, to the playwright who collapsed on opening night to the PA and physician who were unaware of a concerning radiology read hours after they completed a night shift. These cases not only impacted the patients and their families, but also their physicians and attorneys; many were a defining time in the career of the clinician, and the counselor; even years later, my call prompted memories of the most-minute details. One attorney told me he thinks about his experience "at least once a week," and one physician thinks about his patient daily.

How did we get these cases? Well, that's a long and painful story. I spent the first six months in a futile search—it seems no one knows for sure where patient confidentiality ends and medical education begins. I begged insurance companies ("You are doing a good thing, but we don't want to be a HIPAA test case") and searched the net. Finally, I was handed a few appeals decisions by the old lead guitar player in my blues band (also an attorney). Reading through these decisions, it became obvious these were not only intricate medical cases, but they were also amazing stories. Unfortunately, it turns out that complete records are not available on the web; without the actual ED chart and trial testimony, there is no teaching value, and without the deposition and trial testimony, this was another summary of a case study in a medical journal … another seeming dead end.

I eventually realized that I was focusing on the wrong section of the appeals summary, not noticing the answer was right in front of me; the appeals decision began with a listing of the attorneys who had tried the case. On a whim, I cold called one of the plaintiff's attorneys, Dwight Brannon, and had the strangest experience. He was enthusiastic about the project and told me he was happy to help. A few weeks later, he drove to Columbus and filled my car with boxes and boxes of hospital records, depositions, 4 × 6 foot posters, and 5,000 pages of trial testimony. Finally, some success ... but could it be duplicated?

I called more attorneys, some had heard of Bouncebacks! and many had heard of Greg Henry, past president of ACEP and an expert in hundreds of malpractice cases. Most said they were happy to help. In a unique situation, I received the emergency department chart from one, the depositions from another and the trial testimony from a third. Mr. Brannon even flew to San Francisco to re-try his case in front of hundreds of doctors and a true "jury of our peers" at Mel Herbert's Essentials of *Emergency Medicine* conference.

Compiling each case took about a month, depending on the complexity of the legal process. I read thousands of pages of depositions and trial testimony, sorted through hundreds of folders filled with income estimation, witness statements and sadly, family photos. Some cases required releases from a hospital, others from patients, and some from the State. We include cases in which the patient was initially seen by a mid-level provider (MLP), a resident in an academic center, or a community emergency physician—all deceived by well-appearing patients who were, in fact, mortally ill. Each chapter has discussion of the presenting medical complaint and final diagnosis by nationally recognized experts in emergency medicine, as well as a legal review by plaintiff and defense attorneys, some who were involved in trying the case. Most names have been altered, some abbreviations have been expanded, and lengthy testimony has been compressed; though much of the full testimony is available on my website www.embouncebacks.com.

Since the first edition of the original Bouncebacks! book in 2006, we have expanded the Bouncebacks! series to include a total of 4 books with this updated version of Bouncebacks! Medical and Legal (originally published 2011), a new edition of the original Bouncebacks!, plus Bouncebacks! Pediatrics and Bouncebacks! Critical Care where we focus on the return visit and decision points during the resuscitation. We have conducted numerous mock trials based on these cases (links on the website) and have discussed these cases on numerous podcasts including EM RAP, UC MAX, EM CRIT, Risk Management Monthly, and UC RAP.

One final consideration when reading these engaging… but scary cases. We don't want you to practice defensive medicine, but to evaluate and document in a way that is defensible. This will be the best way to use legal outcomes to make patients safer. That will be the best way to move from standard of care to excellence in care.

**Michael Weinstock**
**Kevin Klauer**
**T. Marc Calvert**
May, 2024

# ABOUT THE AUTHORS

**Michael B. Weinstock, MD**

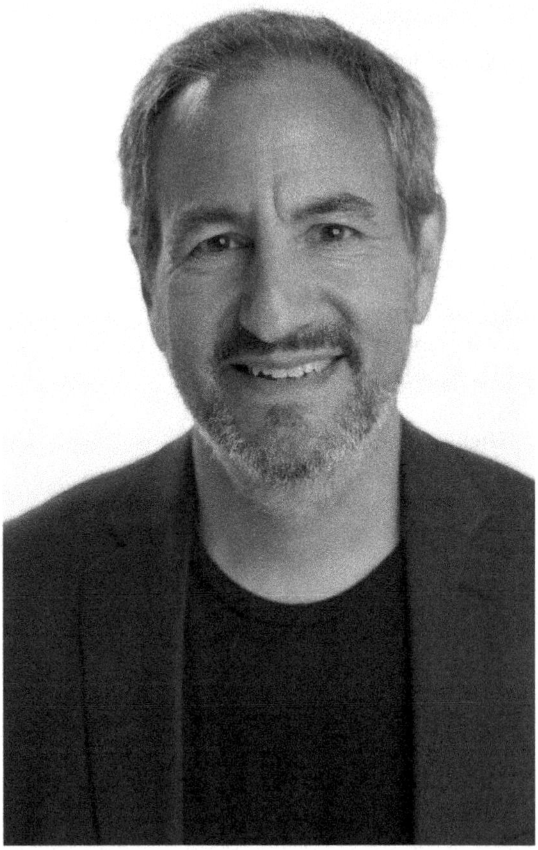

Mike is an emergency medicine physician as well as the Director of Research at the Adena Medical Center and Professor of Emergency Medicine, Adjunct at the Wexner Medical Center at The Ohio State University. He is the risk management section editor for EM RAP, and the executive editor for the new podcast UC MAX (part of the EM RAP family of products) and has contributed to ERCast, EmCrit, and Risk Management Monthly. He has been the principal investigator for original research published in JAMA IM and Annals of Emergency Medicine and is the risk management section editor for CorePendium and chapter author of chest pain evaluation and EM documentation. He is the senior editor for clinical content for The Journal of Urgent Care Medicine (JUCM). He is the medical director for the Ohio Dominical University PA studies program. Michael has practiced medicine nationally and internationally including volunteer work in Papua New Guinea, Nepal, and the West Indies. Research interests include ED evaluation and management of chest pain, patient safety, EM medical education, and of course, Bouncebacks! He is married to family physician Beth Weinstock, with children Olivia, Eli, Theo and Annie. He is the leader of The Big Rockin' Blues Band.

# ABOUT THE AUTHORS

**Kevin M. Klauer, DO**

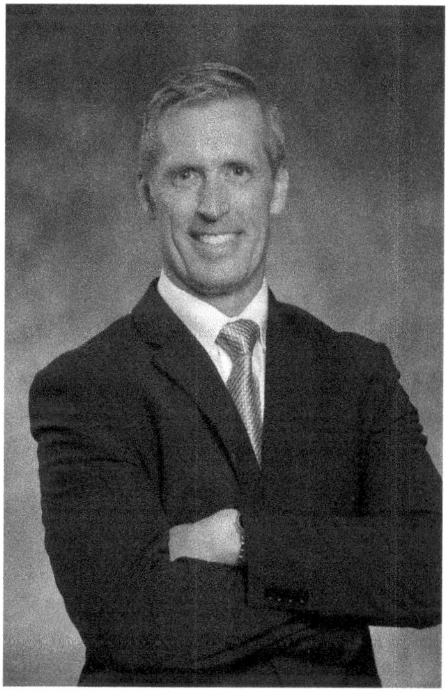

Dr. Klauer is the CEO of the American Health Information Management Association, serving the health information management community of more 90,000 professionals. He formerly served as System Chief Medical Officer for HCA Florida Ocala and West Marion Hospitals, and the CEO of the American Osteopathic Association. Dr. Klauer served as the Chief Medical Officer, Hospital Based Services, Enterprise Chief Risk Officer, and Executive Director of the Patient Safety Organization for TeamHealth. He holds the following faculty appointments: Assistant Clinical Professor at Michigan State University College of Osteopathic Medicine and Clinical Assistant Professor, Ohio University Heritage College of Osteopathic Medicine. He received his Doctor of Osteopathic Medicine degree from Des Moines University College of Osteopathic Medicine and completed his residency training in Emergency Medicine at LSU Health Sciences Center, Charity Hospital New Orleans, where he served as Chief Resident. Dr. Klauer earned his Executive JD, with honors, from Purdue Global Law School in 2011.

He has served as the Medical Editor-in-Chief for ACEP Now as former Editor-in-Chief for Emergency Physicians Monthly publication. He has received the Emergency Medicine Residents' Association (EMRA) Robert Dougherty ACEP/EMF Teaching Fellowship and the ACEP National Faculty Teaching Award. In 2016, he was honored with the ACEP Outstanding Speaker of the Year Award, as well as EMRA's highest honor, the Joseph F. Waeckerle award. In 2018, Dr. Klauer received the Janice A. Wachtler Educator of the Year Award by the American College of Osteopathic Emergency Physicians. In 2021, he was recognized by Modern Healthcare as one of the nation's "Top 150 Most Influential Clinical Executives."

# ABOUT THE AUTHORS

**T. Marc Calvert, JD**

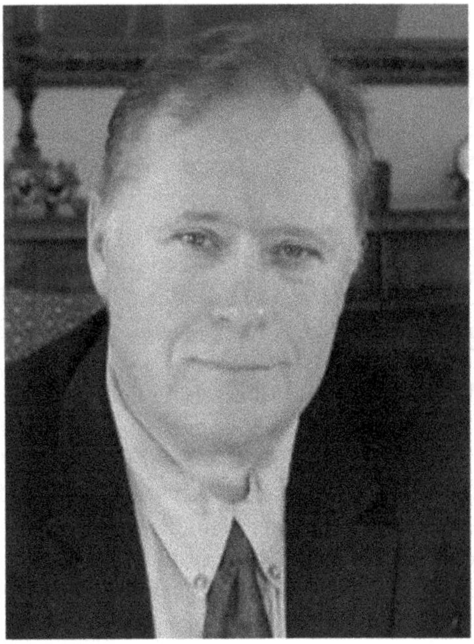

T. Marc Calvert graduated from the University of Texas law school in 1987 and has defended healthcare providers ever since. He became board certified in personal injury trial law in 1994 and established a law firm in 1996. Calvert, Leever, & Ostler defends lawsuits, board matters, peer reviews, and other claims involving healthcare providers. He has been a frequent presenter to students, residents, providers, and to risk management professionals. His true treasure is his family, marrying his high school sweetheart Suzanne in 1982, and being blessed with 4 children and 12 grandchildren.

# TABLE OF CONTENTS

# TABLE OF CONTENTS

# Introduction

## How to Spot the Well-Appearing Patient Who Will Soon be Dead

Michael Weinstock

## I. Deceptively Well Patients

Who is the scariest patient? Not the 80 year-old with an acute MI, the septic dialysis patient or the patient in full cardiac arrest. Contrary to what I feared as a medical student, the sick, well-appearing patient is the most frightening: the 22 year-old woman with a cough and blood tinged sputum in the middle of cold and flu season, the 38 year-old with recurrent headaches and pressure from the staff to "treat and street," the multiple-complaint patient with fibromyalgia who says "everything hurts … and my pain doctor is in prison!"

We can simplify and assign three categories of ED patients:

1. **The straightforward** patient: Our easiest and least-satisfying encounter—an easy diagnosis in a healthy patient (ankle strains and corneal abrasions). It is unlikely we will miss serious illness, but this is not why we chose emergency medicine.
2. **The sick** patient: Our ***raison d'être***, the critically-ill patient who can actually be helped. We act quickly, perform procedures and affect lives in a positive manner; it is the patient with a ruptured AAA that makes it to the ED alive, the crashing MVA victim with a tension pneumothorax, the hypotensive STEMI patient.
3. **The patient with diagnostic uncertainty** and a potentially life-ending complaint: The most difficult, frustrating and riskiest; a cadre of unclear diagnoses in patients with poor access to the medical system. The worried-well who tell you the diagnosis, as well as the therapy. The "frequent flier" who wrote a complaint at the last visit. These dispositions can be influenced by bias, "He's back ***again***?"

Clearly, this last patient will be our focus. While dissecting each of the following 16 cases, we concentrate on two of the most risk-fraught areas of emergency medicine: diagnosis and documentation. Both are important for our patients, while the latter is the cornerstone of our defense when something goes wrong.

Ours is a strange profession, where we are subject to litigation when an adverse outcome occurs. With a sick ED population, often underserved, and previously unknown to us, it's surprising that things don't go wrong more often!

As human beings, we are comfortable recognizing patterns. As ED physicians, the ability to rapidly categorize ***life-threatening*** patterns, such as respiratory distress or toxidromes, enables us to provide emergent life-saving interventions. However, these very skills, which normally serve us well, can also fool us easily in healthy-appearing patients with serious illness. We find ourselves swimming in a sea of the worried-well, which paradoxically causes us to worry ***less***.

Is there a way to create a recognition pattern for this "time bomb" subset? Examination of the bounceback data and ED litigation analysis provides some clues.

## II. Bounceback Literature Review

**A. What is the incidence of ED bouncebacks?**

- Using the commonly-accepted time frame of an ED return within 72 hours, The incidence is about 3%.[1-3]
- Gabayan, et al.[4] extended the time frame to 7 days in over 5 million patient visits, finding a rate of 2.6%
- For an average provider, this is approximately one patient per shift

**B. What is the incidence of patients who bounce back and are admitted?**

- Answer: About 0.6%[5, 6]
- High-risk features for readmission include: age over 65, mental disorders, alcohol-related complaints and abdominal and chest pain

**C. What is the incidence of bouncebacks due to medical errors?**

- Answer: 18–30% (over 30,000 patients studied)[7]

**D. What percentage of patients die with one week of ED discharge?**

- Kefer found an incidence of 9/100,000 visits[8] and Sklar found 30/100,000 visits,[9] both using a time frame of death within seven days of initial ED visit
- Sklar's study is likely more accurate due to examination of over 387,000 ED visits to the University of New Mexico Health Sciences Center over a 10-year time span, providing a unique geographic analysis as the only level I trauma center for the state and the only public hospital in two counties, likely best able to capture almost all return visits
- Possible error cases comprised about 30% of the total deaths (for Sklar's patients, this is nine possible error deaths per 100,000 visits)
- Gabayan found a rate of 50/100,000[10]
  - Discharge diagnoses:
    1. Noninfectious lung disease
    2. Renal disease
    3. Ischemic heart disease
    4. Neoplasm
    5. Disease of the blood
  - Causes of death:
    1. Malignancy (20%)
    2. Ischemic heart disease (17%)
    3. Nonatherosclerotic heart disease (11%) inc. pericarditis, endocarditis, myocarditis, cardiomyopathy, dysrhythmia

**E. Sklar found four main themes in the possible error cases:[11]**

1. Atypical presentation of an unusual problem
2. Chronic disease with decompensation (e.g., CHF)
3. Mental disability, psychiatric problem or substance abuse (making the history and ability to follow-up less reliable)

4. Abnormal vital signs
   - 71% had tachycardia on ED discharge
   - 83% had abnormal vital signs on ED discharge
     (See preface by Dr. Sklar titled: Avoiding Catastrophic Failures)

**F. Bringing it home (to *your* home)**

- If you see three patients per hour and practice 35 hours per week for 35 years, you will see 190,000 patients in your career
- ***During this time, you will send home 17 patients who will die an avoidable death within seven days of ED discharge***

## III. Law and Order

**A. There are several important points to be made up front regarding the legal aspect of work in the ED:**

- Just because you didn't get sued, doesn't mean an error did not occur. Of the 35 "possible error" cases in Sklar's study, none resulted in a lawsuit—despite the fact that all the patients died.[11]
- Our goal is not to merely avoid being sued, but to make patients safer—can awareness of potential litigation improve patient care? How can we move from "standard of care" to "excellence in care?"

**B. Consider these numbers gleaned from a study by Brown, et al., An Epidemiologic Study of Closed Emergency Department Malpractice Claims in a National Database of Physician Malpractice Insurers:**[12]

- The authors analyzed data from the Physician Insurers Association of America (PIAA) databank, a trade association whose participating malpractice carriers insure over 60% of physicians in the U.S. They reviewed 11,529 claims. ED physicians were the principal defendants in about 2,000 of the total.
- The number one source of suit was error in diagnosis (failure to diagnose and/or incorrect diagnosis), representing 37% of the cases.
- The three most common conditions misdiagnosed were fracture, including vertebral/cervical fractures (6%), acute MI (5%) and appendicitis (2%). Others included symptoms involving the abdomen and pelvis, injury to multiple body parts, aortic aneurysm and pulmonary embolism.
- Acute MI (AMI) was associated with the highest ratio of payments (42%) and the highest average indemnity ($317,000), with the majority being error in diagnosis. AMI was the most common claim involving a patient who died.
- 80% of the total indemnity was associated with severe injury, including loss of sight, amputation, quadriplegia, brain damage, and death.
- Of the total number of claims:
  - 70% closed without payment to the claimant.
  - Only 7% went to jury verdict—of these 85% found for the defendant ED physician.

**C. Kachalia, et al., examined the causes of missed and delayed diagnosis** and found multiple breakdowns in the system including failure to order an appropriate diagnostic test (58% of errors), failure to perform an adequate H&P (42%), incorrect interpretation of a diagnostic test (37%) and failure to order an appropriate consultation (33%).[13]

**D. Wong, et al. examined 6,779 closed claims, finding**

- 65.9% were dropped, withdrawn, or dismissed
- 22.8% settled for an average indemnity of $297,709
- 7.6% went to trial
    - Juries returned a verdict for the defendant in 92.6% of cases
    - Of the remaining cases (7.4%) where the jury returned a verdict for the plaintiff, the average indemnity was $816,909
- The most common medical condition in paid claims was cardiac or cardiorespiratory arrest (10.4%)

The most common allegation was "Error in diagnosis" [14]

## IV. Is There a Way to Improve Patient Safety and Decrease Legal Risk?

If you are sued, one approach is just to ***stick it out***; if you can make it to a jury verdict, you have a very high chance of winning. (over 90% per Wong, et al. above). However, we do not recommend this approach; as Greg Henry has often said, "In a lawsuit there are two losers: one loser, and a bigger loser."

Short of investing four to five years of your life to await the "probable" jury verdict, not getting sued in the first place is our recommended policy. If you want to put the book down and stop reading now, here is a little secret: the easiest way to avoid a lawsuit is to just "be a nice person." Seriously. Just don't be a jerk! There are a lot of mistakes we have all made, surely too many to fill the pages of thousands of these books, and we all have stories of an avoidable error we have committed:

"Remember that patient you saw last night? Well, he bounced back this morning ...horizontal." Most "malpractice" does not result in a legal action.

For those who already are kind, compassionate doctors and still want to avoid misdiagnosis ... ***is there a way to use the results of bounceback studies and malpractice numbers to improve patient safety?*** Are we able to recognize the well-appearing patient who will soon be dead?

- Martin-Gill (bounceback admissions study above) wrote, "by identifying high risk patients prospectively, physicians will be better able to make informed decisions when considering the depth of evaluation, timing of discharge decisions, and extent of follow up care."[6]
- Sklar (bounceback death study above) wrote, "Recognition of the presence of abnormal vital signs and a cautious assessment of these patients offer an opportunity to prevent bad outcomes."[9]

At an M&M conference, where 50 people are focused on diagnosing one patient they know had a bad outcome, it does seem primary. But during a busy shift, where you are being assaulted by 15–17 patients at a time and reinforcements are not arriving for three hours, a father of the three year-old with otitis media is standing at the door tapping on his watch while the squad-bay doors open with paramedics bagging a trach patient, the subtleties of these deceptive patients can easily slip through your fingers.

**Hard stop your MDM!**

Will you be able to convince a jury ("hard-stopping" your MDM)?
Consider this: Would you be comfortable defending your documentation and evaluation at your department's M&M conference or from the witness stand?

As you proceed through the following cases, consider if the evaluation would have changed by using these two simple rules. Then, as you report for your next shift, consider whether your thought process can be extrapolated from your documentation and if patients with concerning stories or vitals have been evaluated for the worst-case scenario. Our patients give us a lot of slack; most elderly with back pain do not have a ruptured AAA, most headache patients with fever do not have meningitis. But just because the patient didn't die, doesn't mean you did a great job ...

## V. The Two-Step Approach

Our approach is straightforward and is being done almost all the time already.

1. Identify "high risk" patients who are being discharged.
2. Review their ED evaluation before they leave including the 3 R's: revisit, record, recruit.

The approach seems so simple as to be obvious, but the charts of litigious patients with poor outcomes are rife with inconsistencies, poor correlation of assessment with the chief complaint, abnormal vital signs, inadequate/poor documentation, and poor medical decision making.

The two-step approach encourages a "second look" at patients who have an increased risk of bouncing back or dying within seven days of initial ED evaluation; a second look before they leave the ED and end up in peer review or the courtroom!

**Rule #1: Recognition: Recognize patients at high risk for bouncing back with a poor outcome.**

A. The patient is tachycardic (or has unstable or worsening vital signs):

- Tachycardia
- Tachypnea
- Hypotension
- Repeated vital signs which are not improving

B. You are tachycardic (or should be):

- Diagnostic uncertainty with high-risk complaints (i.e., cp, sob, abd. p., HA and fever)
- Difficulty in obtaining an adequate history or multiple-complaint patients
- Elderly patients
- Chronic medical problems with high likelihood of deterioration
- Discrepancy between the physician and nurse notes

So basically, any patient you would worry about on the drive home. When these patients are identified, what should be done?

**Rule #2: Re-evaluation: Revisit, record, recruit.**

**1. Revisit:** Re-evaluate the patient at the bedside:

- Ensure all documented complaints have been addressed.
- Confirm the history is accurate and complete.
- Gather new information from family members or friends who arrived after the initial assessment.
- Reassess patient and consider a focused re-examination of presenting complaint (ex. a repeat abdominal exam, reassessment of the mental status/neuro exam, or watching the patient walk).

**2. Record:** Document a medical decision making (MDM) note:

- The MDM should be your "closing argument" why you have made a certain diagnosis, initiated a specific management strategy, chose a disposition strategy, and why the most serious diagnoses are not occurring.
- The MDM should be a "hard stop"—use the concept of metacognition,[15, 16] the highest level of cognitive functioning, where we monitor our own thought-making processes, to objectively assess whether our evaluation and management makes sense. Ask the question: "If I can't even convince myself that my care was excellent, how will convince a parent, sibling, child, spouse… how will I convince a jury?"
- The MDM is not a place just to restate (copy and paste) the HPI. It is the medical decision-making note—an opportunity to use plain language to explain why you decided to proceed down a certain pathway.

**3. Recruit:**

- Why not use all the resources we have available as a last line of defense?
- If the patient is being sent home, how about using a 24-hour home nurse (i.e., the family member or friend) to monitor for the onset or progression of specific symptoms. Informing of diagnostic uncertainty is not a stain upon the expertise of the emergency provider, rather an honest assessment that the data available at the time suggests that the management plan is reasonable but leaving open the possibility for alterations if the patient's symptoms change or progress. The last thing we want is for the patient to say (as occurs at trial), "there was no point in going back to the ED because they told me everything was fine"—this is when a bounceback is good. In the words of Steve Colucciello (Co-author of Chapter 9), this is a patient "giving us a second chance."
- Aftercare instructions should be focused and action and time specific. A little trick, duplicate the discharge discussion in the MDM section. (i.e., When editing the discharge instructions, say something like "As we discussed, return if…."). This provides additional documentation that the conversation occurred and the patient was engaged in their own decision-making.

## VI. A Two-Minute Legal Primer

We all fear malpractice litigation, and emergency medicine is one of the highest litigation specialties. What a bizarre field we inhabit, where a seemingly routine evaluation today can morph into a four-year legal ordeal regarding a patient we don't even remember! Can you imagine a schoolteacher enduring a multi-year lawsuit because a student did not graduate or get a good job? How about a dog trainer who goes through years of interrogatories, depositions and court proceedings because his "pupil" bit the mailman years after graduation?

Can the threat of a lawsuit make patients safer? This seems counterintuitive, but the threat of legal action often results in a more cautious clinician, sometimes over testing, but also with better documentation and a more thorough evaluation. The trick is to walk the tightrope between fear and concern while maintaining a balance between speed and vigilance. ***Don't practice defensive medicine, but evaluate patients and document in a way which is defensible.***

May we all be blessed with grateful patients who present with textbook symptoms. For all the rest, the following legal terms are defined when bedside care progresses to the courtroom.

**Burden of proof:** The plaintiff must prove by the greater weight of the evidence that the defendant was negligent, that the defendant's negligence was a direct and proximate cause of the plaintiff's injuries and that the plaintiff was damaged by the defendant's negligence.

**Standard of care:** The standard of care is to do those things which a reasonably careful physician would do and to refrain from doing those things which a reasonably careful physician would not do.

**Proximate cause:** To prevail, the plaintiff must not only prove that the physician fell below the standard of care and was therefore negligent, but that the negligence was a direct and proximate cause of injury to the plaintiff. This includes failure to provide therapy (or provide it in a timely manner) which may have proximately improved the patient's symptoms.

As the 16 cases in this book unfold, it will become apparent there is a highly subjective interpretation of the above terms. For example, the First Amendment to the Constitution of the United States is only two sentences long, but the Supreme Court often splits 5–4 in its application. So it is not surprising that standard of care and proximate cause can mean different things to different people, especially if they don't have prior medical training … or couldn't get out of jury duty.

## VII. Approach to the Bounceback Patient

Are bounceback patients annoying or are they giving us a second chance? Is there a way to approach these high-risk patients which improves patient safety?

**Top 10 list for handling bounceback patients:**

1. Thank the patient for returning
2. ***Sit down*** when taking history
3. Specifically ask the ***main reason*** for the return visit
4. After history is taken, verbally repeat a summary back to the patient
5. Ensure all documented complaints are evaluated (including nurse/triage notes)
6. Review the documentation from the ***previous visit***, looking for:
    a. Symptoms that were not evaluated
    b. Abnormal findings or abnormal vital signs not addressed
    c. Accuracy of initial diagnosis
    d. Appropriateness of treatment
    e. Life-threatening conditions which were not considered
7. Document a progress note explaining the medical decision-making process
8. Address concerns with family members
9. Inform patients of ***diagnostic uncertainty*** and ensure the patient understands the diagnosis which has not been excluded and ensure they understand they are welcome to return if the symptoms progress, change, or do not resolve
10. Provide action- and time-specific aftercare instructions
    a. Recommend defined follow up with the primary care provider (PCP) or a specialist
    b. Give the patient focused instructions, including specific reasons to return Summary: Perform a fresh evaluation with each visit—do not be misled by ***diagnosis momentum***. [15]

## VIII. Conclusion

As we proceed through our careers, sometimes tired, sometimes cynical, our challenge is to maintain a high vigilance for the patients who appear well but are soon to decompensate. Like an airport screener, we can become inoculated by the "narcotizing effect of obvious,"[17] but approaching each presentation with a thorough evaluation and defensible documentation will not only be legally protective, but also medically protective, due to improved patient safety, the most important goal of this book.

The following cases are all real. The documentation has not been changed except to streamline for the purposes of readability and focus for teaching points; some names have been changed, a few medications have been updated, extraneous and redundant EMR documentation has been eliminated. These cases reflect the pulse of life-in-the-ER. We have included the actual documentation of the provider, deposition testimony from families and physicians, attorney opening and closing statements, direct and cross-examination of expert witnesses, physician testimony, the judge's instructions to the jury and, at the end of each section, the verdict.

One final question before embarking on this journey; what's the best way to learn from case studies?[18] It's easy to look back at a case that has gone bad and to find areas to criticize and to imagine that we would have done things differently. But this strategy may be backward.

Wears and Nemeth suggest the opposite approach: **[As quoted directly from the article]:** "Questions such as 'How could they not have noticed?' and 'How could they not have known?' often arise in retrospective examinations of adverse events. These questions arise not because people were behaving bizarrely but rather because we (the reviewers) have chosen the wrong frame of reference to understand their behavior. We do not learn much by asking why the way a practitioner framed a problem turned out to be wrong. We do learn when we discover why that framing seemed so reasonable at the time."[19]

Enough said! It's time to report for your next shift, put on your white coat, hang a stethoscope over your shoulders, walk through those double doors, turn the page and get ready to see a bunch of seemingly well-appearing patients.

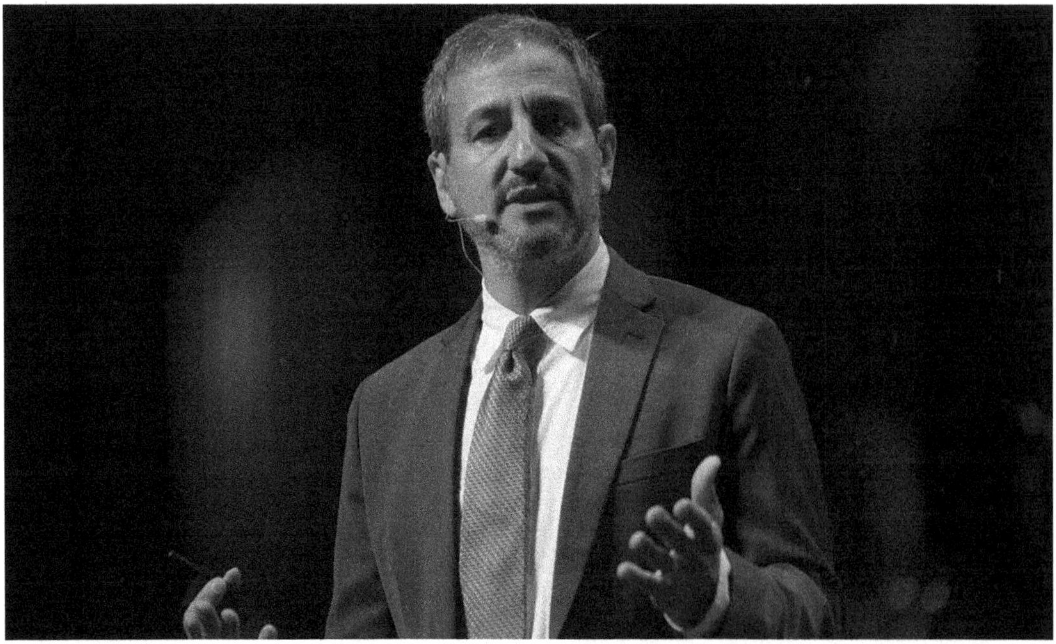

## References


1. Wilkins PS, Beckett MW. Audit of unexpected return visits to an accident and emergency department. Arch Emerg Med 1992;9(4):352-6.
2. O'Dwyer F, Bodiwala GG. Unscheduled return visits by patients to the accident and emergency department. Arch Emerg Med 1991;8(3):196-200.
3. Pierce JM, Kellermann AL, Oster C. "Bounces": An analysis of short-term return visits to a public hospital emergency department. Ann Emerg Med 1990;19(7):752-7. (over 30,000 patients studied)
4. Gabayan GZ, Asch SM, Hsia RY, et al. Factors associated with short-term bounce-back admissions after emergency department discharge. Ann Emerg Med 2013;62(2):136-144.e.1.
5. Gordon JA, An LC, Hayward RA, et al. Initial emergency department diagnosis and return visits: risk versus perception. Ann Emerg Med 1998;32(5):569-73.
6. Martin-Gill C, Reiser RC. Risk factors for 72-hour admission to the ED. Am J Emerg Med 2004;22(6):448-53. (almost 200,000 patients studied)
7. Nunez S, Hexdall A, Aguirre-Jaime A. Unscheduled returns to the emergency department: An outcome of medical errors? Qual Saf Health Care 2006;15(2):102-8. (over 30,000 patients)
8. Kefer MP, Hargarten SW, Jentzen J. Death after discharge from the emergency department. Ann Emerg Med 1994;24:1102-7.
9. Sklar DP, Crandall CS, Loeliger E, et al. Unanticipated death after discharge home from the emergency department. Ann Emerg Med 2007; 49(6):735-45.
10. Gabayan GZ, Derose FS, Asch SM, et al. Patterns and predictors of short-term death after emergency department discharge. Ann Emerg Med 2011(6);58:551-58.
11. Sklar DP. Personal communication, 2010.
12. Brown TW, McCarthy ML, Kelen GD, et al. An epidemiologic study of closed emergency department malpractice claims in a national database of physician malpractice insurers. Acad Emerg Med 2010;17(5):553-60.
13. Kachalia A, Gandhi TK, Puopolo AL, et al. Missed and delayed diagnoses in the emergency department: A study of closed malpractice claims from 4 liability insurers. Ann Emerg Med 2007;49(2):196-05.
14. Wong KE, Parikh PD, Miller KC, el al. Emergency department and urgent care medical malpractice claims 2001–15. West J Emerg Med 2021;22(2):333-38.
15. Croskerry P. Achieving quality in clinical decision making: Cognitive strategies and detection of bias. Acad Emerg Med 2002;9(11):1184-04. doi:10.1111/j.1553-2712.2002.tb01574.x
16. Croskerry P. The theory and practice of clinical decision-making. Can J Anesth 2005;52(6) (Suppl 1), R1-R8. https://doi.org/10.1007/BF03023077.
17. Hellstern R. Bouncebacks! testimonial, 2006.
18. Weinstock MB, How we learn from cases. Emergency Medicine Reviews and Perspectives (EMRAP) podcast: Segment 10;Feb 2023.
19. Wears RL, Nemeth CP. Replacing hindsight with insight: Toward better understanding of diagnostic failures. Ann Emerg Med 2007;49(2):206-9.

# Help! I Am Being Sued

**Kevin Klauer**

## I. The Complaint

Returning home after a busy shift, a certified letter from Harkin, Smith, Rose, and Jabberwocky greets you at the door. Your heart skips a beat as you remember the great save of a 44 year-old woman with breast cancer and a PE, intubated and stabilized, several hours earlier. Scanning down the page, there is no memory of the patient's name. The letter is concise: This document hereby serves as notification of a formal complaint regarding the care you rendered to Bruce Britt, on September 10th. You contemplate the next 4 years of your life…

Lawsuits begin with the legal complaint, much different than a patient dissatisfaction complaint. Depending on individual circumstances, a risk management incident report should be generated to track for the potential of formal legal action. Some providers are reluctant to do so, as they may feel that they are admitting to error or highlighting their inadequacy as a provider. However, a complaint that flies under the radar handicaps the risk manager's ability to mitigate risk, reduce financial liability, and to begin planning for a future defense. In addition to the certified letter, other reasons to file a report include:

- Cases with known bad outcomes (regardless of fault or whether an error occurred)
- Complaints in which the patient or family mention potential litigation
- Cases with a known treatment complication
- Discharged patients who return with a previously missed diagnosis

Filing an incident report will allow the risk manager to assess the level of risk and determine whether the complaint can be resolved without legal intervention, notify the insurer of a potential claim, and begin accumulating necessary documents. As in some of the cases in this book, certain pieces of the chart may turn up missing, interpreted as sloppy medical care. If there is a fact in dispute there is no doubt that the plaintiff's attorney will imply that the "mystery document" vanished into thin air to benefit the defense.

## II. A Case of Failure to Report

An emergency physician who was a hospital employee evaluated a 55 year-old man with chest pain. Despite minimal risk factors and atypical, reproducible pain, he suffered an acute myocardial infarction and died. A claim was filed which progressed to lawsuit. In addition to being unfortunate for the patient, it was also unfortunate for the physician upon discovering that his policy did not cover this act.

Why? Thirteen months prior, the hospital became self-insured and advised the employed medical staff members that all suspicious cases should be submitted to the risk manager so that these "prior acts" could be covered by the former policy. Despite the fact that the physician knew of the bad outcome two weeks after it occurred, he failed to report. The prior policy was a "claims-made" policy, covering claims identified during the policy period. (This is distinct from an "occurrence policy," which covers all claims filed during or subsequent to the policy period). Thus, a "claims-made" policy requires tail coverage to cover claims received beyond the policy period for events that took place during the policy period. In this situation, in order to save cost, the hospital elected to provide "prior acts" or "nose coverage" to cover claims during the transition period instead of purchasing tail coverage. When this claim was received, it was not covered by the previous claims made policy, and since the physician ignored the request to report potential claims, the hospital refused his coverage for this "prior act" under their new captive.

## III. The Complaint is Filed with the Court

Complaints are usually filed with the court simultaneously with the summons, advising the defendant that they are being sued. For malpractice lawsuits, delivery may be by a court courier, Sheriff's deputy, or sent by certified mail.

A summons requires a response within a proscribed period of time. The response usually consists of an answer and should address each allegation, though it is acceptable for a defendant to state that they don't possess sufficient information to confirm or deny the allegations. One possibility is to file a motion of dismissal if there is a clear and compelling reason why the suit should not be allowed to continue, for example, if an emergency physician not involved in the care was erroneously named in a lawsuit. If such a motion is filed, the plaintiff must then respond. Do not respond to any questions without the oversight of your attorney.

In some states, additional documentation is required. For instance, in Pennsylvania, a certificate of merit must be filed within 60 days of filing a lawsuit. The certificate must confirm that a licensed physician has reviewed the case and feels that with reasonable probability, the care rendered fell below the standard of care.

What should you do when you receive a summons or notice of intent to sue? An all too common tale is to bury your head in the sand, but like an abscess, it only gets worse until the I&D. Regardless of merit, failure to respond is a big mistake. The doctor is in control in the ED, but with a legal proceeding, everyone needs to follow the legal rules of engagement, known as civil procedure. In many jurisdictions, if no response is received, the default is summary judgment for the plaintiff. If your head is buried in the sand, what is the most visible anatomical part? Feel free to take this analogy to its appropriate conclusion

## IV. The Complaint Moves to Discovery

Discovery is a data-gathering period, providing an opportunity for the plaintiff and defendant to get the flavor of the case the other side will present. Certain disclosures are mandatory, such as hospital documents and witnesses that will be deposed or called to testify. If any items are discovered without disclosure, they will likely be perceived as an attempt to intentionally withhold them.

Several mechanisms are available to solicit and obtain information during discovery.

- Documents – Medical records and hospital policies
- Interrogatories – Written questions requiring a response under oath
- Depositions – Almost universally utilized in medical malpractice cases
- Admissions – Narrowly focused questions that the opposing side must deny or admit to. Such questions help to clarify if a party is uncertain of a fact or what position the other side will take

## V. Attorney Client Privilege and Discoverable Conversations

The communication known as client-attorney privilege is granted the greatest power of any professional-client relationship. However, it is human nature to vent and seek validation by asking the opinion of others we trust. Unfortunately, casual conversations with colleagues are open to discovery. One of the first questions asked in a deposition is whether you have spoken to anyone about the case… and guess who gets deposed next week? One exception is spousal privilege; however, if the spouse speaks with others, it is non-privileged and discoverable.

## VI. Preparation of A Defense—Necessary Elements of a Lawsuit (Tort of Negligence)

- Duty to Treat
- Breach of the Standard of Care (SOC)
- Causation (Direct and Proximate)
- Damages

**A. Duty** – The element of duty is critical but is rarely a factor in medical malpractice claims involving hospitals or when a physician-patient relationship clearly exists. The nature of our work and EMTALA establish a duty owed by the emergency physician to anyone and everyone who presents to the ED. There are some circumstances in which a duty does not exist, such as with "Good Samaritans," but be careful. Even if you render care voluntarily, such as the syncope patient on a flight, if you receive any compensation, it can be deemed that a duty is now owed and the "Good Samaritan" protection may disappear. Though appealing, decline the bottle of champagne offered by the patient's family or the first-class upgrade from the airline.

**B. Standard of care** – The standard of care in medical practice is almost always a national standard, defined as what a reasonable provider with similar training under similar circumstances would do. If the provider's actions are deemed to have fallen below the standard of care, negligence will be found, if not then no liability is assigned

**C. Causation** – Many cases pivot on the merits of causation, another very common defense strategy. To prove causation, the plaintiff's injury (damages) must be the direct cause of the defendant physician's negligence. However, the defendant's negligence must also be the proximate cause of the injury. Proximate cause requires no disruption in the chain of causation between the negligent act and the injury to the plaintiff. There can be no superseding or intervening events that break the chain of causation. If some other event occurred after the defendant's negligence that may have resulted in the plaintiff's injury or damages, this may relieve the defendant of their liability.

For example, if a patient is seen at Blue Hospital's Emergency Department for abdominal pain due to an undetected abdominal aortic aneurysm (AAA) and is inappropriately discharged and dies, Blue Hospital and its providers will likely be found negligent, a duty to treat was owed the patient, the care was below the standard of care and their negligence was the direct and proximate cause of the patient's death.

Let's throw a causation twist into this scenario. What if the patient had a CT of the abdomen and pelvis that was misinterpreted as normal, missing the AAA? Of course, the hospital and radiologist will have substantial exposure. However, the emergency physician's alleged negligent act of discharging the patient is defensible under the theory of causation and standard of care. The misinterpreted CT was the superseding act that relieves the emergency physician of his or her liability. Furthermore, it would be argued that discharging the patient with a normal CT was not a violation of the standard of care.

**D. Damages** – Without damages, negligence carries no liability and there are no grounds for a lawsuit. While standard of care and causation are the cornerstones of any defense, damages are what strengthen a plaintiff's case. The more injured a plaintiff, the greater a jury's sympathy and the more likely for a large verdict.

## VII. Preparation of a Defense—The Initial Review of a Claim

The initial review will often provide a good sense of the cause of action, and what acts, either of commission or omission, constitute the plaintiff's claim. Review of the medical care can be accomplished by an expert panel or commissioned experts. Discussions need to remain confidential and as a work product of the attorney-client privilege, a more powerful protection than afforded under peer review protection statutes. The summary should identify strengths and weaknesses of the care focusing on standard of care and causation issues, damages and potential defense strategies.

The primary documents utilized are the defendant's own words as documented in the medical record. The medical record is usually taken at face value unless there is documentation to cast doubt about its accuracy. For instance, if the nurse documents that the patient had syncope and the physician stated the patient didn't, such discrepancies may lead to a weakness in a case if left unaddressed. (This also emphasizes how important it is to read the nurses' notes.)

Unfortunately, many cases focus on undocumented provider claims such as:

- "I told the patient about the possibility of appendicitis."
- "I offered admission but they refused."
- "I re-examined the abdomen twice."

Plaintiff's attorney:

- "Would you consider these items important to the care of a patient with abdominal pain?" (The obvious answer would have to be yes. Otherwise, the physician wouldn't be claiming that they did them.)
- "If they are that important, why didn't you document them? You took the time to document the social history. Did you really reexamine the abdomen twice or just wish you had?"

It is easy to see how this will play out.

## VIII. Preparation of a Defense—Assessment of Damages

The next step is to assess the alleged damages, which helps to set reserves for the case. Reserves are an estimate of the potential judgment should an adverse verdict be rendered, set aside by the insurer to cover the worst-case scenario. If the case is settled or the judgment is less than expected, the excess reserves will be returned to the insurer's general funds.

## IX. Multiple Defendants

The strengths and weaknesses of a given case may be viewed differently by co-defendants. Although "we are all in this together," each may not have the same exposure or share the same goals and defense strategy. It is important to assess the defense provided by your insurer and any conflicts of interest.

For instance, if you and the hospital are co-defendants, insured by the same company, this may create an inequity in the defense. The hospital may have a large amount of exposure and you may have very little. However, if the hospital's strategy is to avoid an excess limits judgment, they may be willing to settle and take you along for the ride, even if your exposure is disproportionately small. In such circumstances, it may be worthwhile to consider obtaining independent counsel. This will often be at your own expense, but in the right circumstances, money well spent.

## X. Preparing a Witness

Once the case has been assessed, reserves have been set, and a defense strategy initiated, the defendant(s) must be prepared to be a witness. This can be a long and painful process, as the average lawsuit will take 45 months to resolve. Many a physician-defendant is lulled into complacency in the preparation phase, with the thought that no attorney could possibly triumph when debating medicine. This is a critical error, and one that the plaintiff's attorney hopes you'll make. They'll never debate the medicine; they'll let their experts do that. They will use language and the subtleties of law to spin the facts to their advantage, while using your own words, documented or spoken, to discredit you.

This journey isn't about finding the truth; it's about winning. This assessment may seem harsh, but these are the ground rules. Therefore, every defendant needs to be trained in their conduct during a deposition and courtroom proceedings. This is foreign to most of us. Your best foot must be forward from the beginning of the case, not just for your courtroom appearance. If you make a good showing as a credible defendant during the deposition, the plaintiff will be more apt to move toward settlement or even dismiss you altogether. It is important to be vigilant about appearance, mannerisms, attire and attitude. These subtle nuances can turn a jury off and escalate a plaintiff's attorney's interest in proceeding with the case. Although unfair, these are the harsh realities that every defendant will face.

Emotional support is necessary but infrequently provided. This process causes us to question the core of our existence as healthcare providers. Ensure social, emotional and even mental health resources are available.

## XI. The Trial

The decision to go to trial is a complex one, based on the merits as well as the economics. To the physician, this is personal; our pride and professional credibility are at stake. Should an inappropriate lawsuit without negligence be fought to deter subsequent cases? The answer: yes, and maybe.

We all have a responsibility to fight frivolous lawsuits and the defendant should always be consulted about a decision to settle, however, when the damages are potentially high and the defense weak, settlement is a reasonable consideration. Losses can be minimized, expenses reduced and the defendant spared the emotional, personal and professional hardship of enduring a lengthy adjudication process.

What if the insurance company wants to settle and you don't? Well, your goals are pride and justice whereas theirs are largely economic. Most insurers will align your goals and reassess your position. In other words, if they can settle the case for $100,000, but could be at risk for a $500,000 jury verdict, they won't be too excited about taking this risk to protect your honor or to ensure justice is served. If the insurer requires your consent to settle, they will ask you to sign a "bad faith letter" if you are unwilling to give your consent, and you'll be responsible for paying the portion of a jury verdict that could have been avoided by the proposed settlement. In this scenario, the defendant would be personally responsible for $400,000. Oftentimes, when the defendant has to consider the true economic risk of the case, they agree that settlement is the best option.

All is not lost. "Bad faith" claims cut both ways. There are many instances in which a defendant just wants out, preferring to avoid the emotional strain of a lengthy legal battle. They don't want to testify in court or they feel the settlement offer is just compensation for the patient's injury. Consider that a settlement offer for $600,000 is received, but the insurer wants to try the case to avoid any and all indemnity loss. A "bad faith letter" should be sent to the insurer, protecting the defendant against an excess limits judgment. If the case is eventually lost for excess of policy limits, let's say $1.5 million, the defendant would have grounds for a bad faith claim against the insurer and would not be responsible for the portion outside the policy limits.

Medical malpractice trials typically take a week or two, though can last longer; The Fireman's trial in Chapter 2 lasted four weeks. The good news is that if the decision is made to take a case to trial, the majority of cases result in a defense verdict.

## XII. Appeals

Although appeals are often more publicized in criminal cases, they may be filed in tort cases as well. The grounds for an appeal are to argue a procedural error, not to retry the facts of the case. For example:

- The Judge gave the Jury an inappropriate instruction
- The court abused its power in disallowing a critical defense expert to testify

Appeals can take years to complete. Filing an appellate motion without proper grounds is time consuming, costly, and ultimately futile.

# Avoiding Catastrophic Failures

**David Sklar, MD**
Emergency Medicine Physician
Senior Advisor to the Provost
Professor College of Health Solutions
Arizona State University

Dr. Sklar is the principal investigator of the study *Unanticipated death after discharge from the emergency department* published in Annals of Emergency Medicine

Most catastrophic medical cases arrive with the patient already showing signs of a life-threatening emergency; the vitals are seriously abnormal, often demonstrating shock or altered mental status or both. The challenge is to determine the specific cause quickly and begin an intervention that will interrupt the progression toward death. These are the patients with rupturing abdominal aortic aneurysms, third degree heart block, septic shock, stroke and severe asthma. These are not the patients who will be discharged only to bounce back or die at home. While these patients present many challenges sometimes resulting in a misdiagnosis or delay in care, these are not the catastrophic cases I will discuss in this chapter.

No, it's the patient who is talking to us, who "looks good," whose pain seems to be going away, whose vomiting seems to be responding, whose blood pressure improves with a liter of saline, and who wakes up and wants to go home; these are the patients who are our nightmares. We give them diagnoses of abdominal pain, viral syndrome, gastroenteritis, pulled muscle, vasovagal episode, alcoholic gastritis, or chest contusion and convince ourselves that whatever is causing the problem, it is self-limited and will improve over time. However, hidden within this group of benign, self-limited illness are the patients who decompensate because there is a critical process evolving: Bacteria may be quietly spreading, a blood clot may be about to break loose from a pelvic vein, or an artery may be about to burst. Unfortunately, the tests we've ordered don't give us the answer, and the symptoms go through peaks and valleys that reassure us that whatever is going on is not serious. Alternatively, we're in a hurry and we're looking for a clear constant trajectory of illness, and we can't see one. So, we scratch our head, write the discharge orders and wonder what we might have missed, and move on to the next patient. Yet there are often clues which have eluded our assessment.

In general, we know the problems that lead to catastrophic failure, malpractice cases, and Morbidity and Mortality conferences. They are also the cases that make up many of our 72-hour returns. The list of diagnoses has not changed much over the years, though some high-risk problems have been reduced due to changes in technology that have improved diagnosis or preventive strategies. Vaccination for H-influenza has reduced the risk of epiglottitis in children, and ultrasound availability and rapid pregnancy testing have reduced the risk of ectopic pregnancy, which were two of the diagnoses that were often initially missed. Emergency medicine residency training has replaced on the job training and standardized our diagnostic approaches.

Nonetheless, diagnostic errors that lead to death still occur. The list of catastrophic conditions includes abdominal aortic aneurysm and thoracic aortic dissection, strokes of various types including aneurysms, dissections, hemorrhages, and vascular occlusions. There are cases of pulmonary emboli, septic shock, and myocardial infarction,[1] among the most common causes of malpractice litigation.[2,3] Also, there are less common catastrophic conditions like necrotizing fasciitis and airway emergencies that can initially appear to be benign, but rapidly transform into life-threatening catastrophes. The most common causes of pediatric litigation are appendicitis, diseases of the male and female genital organs (such as testicular and ovarian torsion), meningitis and cardiac conditions.[4,5] How can knowledge of the catastrophic conditions and the reasons for missing them help us avoid an incorrect or delayed diagnosis?

Unfortunately, research on emergency medicine errors is limited because misdiagnoses are only evident in retrospect; if someone gets better after inadequate history or testing, as most people do, we may never recognize the errors in diagnosis or testing.

Further, if patients get worse and die in spite of excellent care, in retrospect, someone may still find an element in the history or exam that might have made a difference, and the case may still end up in peer review or subject to legal action. Outcomes do not provide proof of the quality of care or the absence of errors. While we might expect that if a patient did not get better, he or she would return to the ED for more testing and care, that is also not always the case. Some people do not want to return or are unable to return despite worsening illness. It is important to identify such cases in research on diagnostic errors, but this is not always done due to complexities of data linkage. Optimally, we would be able to track down all the patients who visited the ED and link them to the vital records or the medical investigator/ coroner records.[6]

I reviewed cases with colleagues that ended in death after an emergency department visit.[6] What we found was surprising and important. First of all, the number of patients who were seen in our emergency department and who were sent home and died within seven days was small, 30 patients per 100,000 discharges. Only half of them were unexpected and related to the visit; many patients die of totally unrelated causes. For example, a patient who was seen with chest pain was shot in an altercation two days after visiting the ED. Sometimes deaths are expected, like a cancer patient seeking pain medicine during the last few days of a long illness. However, in our study, there were 9 cases per 100,000 discharges (approximately .01 %) which is 1/10,000 patients that died of a problem related to the visit where the death was unexpected and was likely related to an error. These rare cases were the cases we were most interested in, and we reviewed each of them carefully and tried to see what common themes might have been present.

What we found was that abnormal vital signs in these patients were quite common (present in 85%), and usually there was no explanation in the chart. While some of the abnormal vital signs, such as tachycardia (present in 71%) were nonspecific and occurred commonly, others like tachypnea are not so common and have been recognized as significant risks in other studies of ED patients who were discharged and later died of an unexpected and related problem. While abnormal vital signs are generally nonspecific, they should be a clue that some process may be occurring that is eliciting a physical stress reaction in the body. For example, tachypnea could be a response to hypovolemia from loss of blood, pulmonary infection or hypoxia from pulmonary edema. Fever could be a response to a serious bacterial infection, a reaction to a medication, or a sign of thyrotoxicosis. Unexplained tachycardia could be a sign of myocarditis, thoracic aortic dissection, toxic ingestion, diabetic ketoacidosis (DKA), or sepsis. An explanation for the vital sign abnormality should be identified before the patient is discharged and if no explanation can be found, further data gathering (repeat history and exam) and close follow up should be arranged.

Another theme in our study was the presence of cases that were relatively rare like abdominal aortic aneurysm that presented with atypical symptoms. We see this in the case of Jonathan Larson in Chapter 4 of Bouncebacks! Medical & Legal who had an aortic dissection but did not have the typical presentation of intense tearing chest and back pain. When rare conditions occur and present with atypical symptoms, the chances that they will be misdiagnosed are great because the information that would increase the probability of the disease to a level of concern that would justify invasive and expensive tests like a CT arteriogram may be absent. There are certain clues that I use when determining how aggressive to be when initial tests are negative. If the patient has been relatively healthy previously, yet the problem is severe enough to send the patient to the ED, my concern is heightened. Such was the profile of Mr. Larson and was similar to a recent case of a soccer reporter Grant Wahl who was misdiagnosed and died at the World Cup soccer championships likely of an ascending rupture of the aorta and hemopericardium. He described symptoms of a "cold" for 10 days, little sleep, high stress and later tightness and chest pressure.

He wrote, "I went into the medical clinic at the main media center today, and they said I probably have bronchitis. They gave me a course of antibiotics and some heavy-duty cough syrup, and I'm already feeling a bit better just a few hours later." He soon after suffered a catastrophic aortic rupture.

Following are some approaches to avoid catastrophic failures:

1. **Abnormal vital signs** – Recently published a study similar to ours and also found that abnormal vital signs occurred commonly in patients who were discharged from the ED and died subsequently[7] [Hoang, et al.]. Anxious people can become tachycardic but over time they usually calm down and their heart rate returns to normal. They will also usually slow their rapid breathing over time with reassurance. It is important to examine all sets of vitals. Nurses may not communicate that the blood pressure dropped just prior to discharge because they think that the physician had checked the nursing notes. An altered mental status should be considered similar to an abnormal vital sign; if the brain is not receiving crucial nutrients or is impaired by toxins there will often be an alteration of the thought processes. In the study by Obermeyer, et al., altered mental status was the leading diagnosis for patients who left the ED and later died.[6] Such a finding should give pause to the consideration that a catastrophic process may be developing.

2. **Something's changed** – It is important to understand the patient's baseline. Are they chronically short of breath, in pain, or confused, or is there something new that might indicate decompensation of a chronic condition. For many patients who live within a narrow physiological balance, the added stress of a viral infection, a change in medication, or a minor trauma can lead to catastrophic decompensation. This theme of decompensation of a chronic disease was a finding in our study. If the patient's baseline is a cardiac ejection fraction of 15%, even an additional loss of 1% could lead to a fatal outcome. There are rarely clear guidelines, and the current shortages in hospital beds have made admission decisions more difficult. Patients are often able to judge if they can handle their worsening symptoms at home. An observation unit may be a reasonable alternative to discharge or admission.

3. **Communication difficulties** – Another group that presents serious challenges are the patients with communication difficulties due to mental illness, drug abuse or non-English proficiency without access to interpreters. These patients may not be able to convey their symptoms due to their impaired consciousness, delusions, poor health literacy or unfamiliar language. While emergency

departments are required to offer medical interpreter services, the increasing presence of patients from every corner of the globe can overwhelm interpreter resources. Such patients may not be able to understand instructions to return if symptoms worsen.

4. **Patients unable to walk out of the ED on their own** – Finally, there are some patients who refuse to go home. Sometimes that may be due to pain or subtle neurological deficits that only become evident when the patient is unable to walk to the car; a patient newly unable to walk or talk should not be discharged. I can recall several patients with spinal cord compression that were only diagnosed because on discharge they could not walk out on their own. Sometimes patients refuse to leave because they are fearful of deteriorating at home; such fears should be taken seriously. Patients usually know when their condition is too fragile to be able to do well at home, and for many patients a discharge to home means that there will be no one to prepare food, shelter medical treatments or assist with use of the bathroom. Sometimes, the patient has already gone home and now returns feeling worse. Because illnesses evolve over time, admission to the hospital or observation unit may provide more time to evaluate an inapparent infection or other process. While many of the cases in Bouncebacks! resulted in a malpractice lawsuit that produced expert testimony that seems to be clear and convincing, it is important to recognize that there are differences in how the legal system and the medical system try to arrive at an understanding of truth. What seems to be clear for legal experts may be an illusion.

At a trial, juries listen to testimony of witnesses and experts and opinions of lawyers who try to build a case for innocence or guilt. Experts often guide the jury in understanding the standard of care with differing opinions as to whether the standard of care was met. There are often two opposing views about meeting the standard of care, and the jury attempts to decide which argument is most convincing. The approach to truth is often adversarial.

Alternatively, in medicine, there is a recognition of the uncertainty accompanying many diagnostic decisions. Efforts are made to understand what happened in a difficult environment using evidence and consensus building. In medicine, there is also a recognition that errors in diagnostic decision making are inevitable, just as they are in other human endeavors, and that we should build in safety procedures so that errors do not harm patients. The medical approach is usually cooperative and scientific.

Even the best baseball players only get a hit one third of the time. Basketball players miss foul shots at least ten percent of the time. Football players drop passes. That is because these are difficult tasks that present new challenges in a changing landscape.

Like athletes, emergency physicians face an array of unique problems, and systems must be built so that when errors occur, they are identified through system design and redundancy and do not harm patients. Medical malpractice is harmful to both health professionals and patients, while adding to the expense of healthcare. Caution must be employed to avoid the temptation to use expert testimony to suggest certainty when the reality of medicine is gradations of uncertainty. It is too easy to look back in the quiet light of day and examine a decision made in darkness, in the middle of a storm, and express clarity and certainty that did not and could not exist at the time.

Our time and effort in improving diagnostic decision making are best spent creating a safer health system with consistent teams of health professionals, information when we need it, and efficient access to specialty care.

## References


1. Newman-Toker DE, Peterson SM, Badihian S, et al. Diagnostic errors in the emergency department: A systematic review. Comparative Effectiveness Review No. 258. (Prepared by the Johns Hopkins University Evidence-based Practice Center under Contract No. 75Q80120D00003.) AHRQ Publication No. 22(23)-EHC043. Rockville, MD: Agency for Healthcare Research and Quality; December 2022. DOI: 10.23970/AHRQEPCCER258.
2. Wong KE, Parikh PD, Miller KC, et al. Emergency department and urgent care medical malpractice claims 2001–15. West J Emerg Med 2021;22(2):333-38. doi: 10.5811/westjem.2020.9.48845. PMID: 33856320; PMCID: PMC7972370.
3. Brown TW, McCarthy ML, Kelen GD, et al. An epidemiologic study of closed emergency department malpractice claims in a national database of physician malpractice insurers. Acad Emerg Med 2010;17(5):553-60.
4. Glerum KM, Selbst SM, Parikh PD, et al. Pediatric malpractice claims in the emergency department and urgent care settings from 2001 to 2015. Pediatr Emerg Care 2021;37(7):e376-e379. doi: 10.1097/PEC.0000000000001602. PMID: 30211835.
5. Weinstock MB, Jolliff H. High-risk medicolegal conditions in pediatric emergency medicine. Emerg Med Clin North Am 2021;39(3):479-91. doi: 10.1016/j.emc.2021.04.001. Epub 2021 Jun 9. PMID: 34215398.
6. Sklar DP, Crandall CS, Loeliger E, et al. Unanticipated death after discharge from the emergency department. Ann Emerg Med 2007;49(6):735-45.
7. Hoang R, Sampsel K, Willmore A, et al. Remember that patient you saw last week: Characteristics and frequency of patients experiencing anticipated and unanticipated death following ED discharge. Can J Emerg Med 2021;23(6):767-71.
8. Obermeyer Z, Cohn B, Wilson M, et al. Early Death after discharge from emergency departments analysis of national US insurance claims data. BMJ 2017;356:j239.

# Litigation Stress: A Personal Story

**Gita Pensa**
Adjunct Associate Professor
Brown University, Warren Alpert School of Medicine
Department of Emergency Medicine
Providence, Rhode Island
Co-host UC MAX podcast

I was an emergency medicine nocturnist in a community hospital back in 2006, the only doctor in the hospital after midnight. I'd often had to leave the ED to intubate patients or run codes on the floor, or to deliver a baby while waiting for the obstetrician to make their way in. Those excursions always made me uneasy; high-pressure procedures in unfamiliar environments, leaving my own department unattended for long periods of time, seemed fraught with risk. Yet, the most singular career-altering case I had in those years presented as a regular ED patient with only a slightly puzzling complaint.

The patient was a 30-year-old woman who complained of pain, photophobia, and blurred vision in her right eye. She had had an anterior cervical discectomy recently but had recovered well and had no other significant medical history. I examined her with the slit lamp, performed a fundoscopic exam and tonometry, and all were normal, even including a neurological exam. I sent her for a non-contrast CT scan of the brain, which was normal. Over a few hours her symptoms dissipated, and she was pacing around the department, asking to be released so she could go home and go to sleep. I spoke with an ophthalmologist who agreed to see her in their office at 9 am that morning, and I subsequently discharged her.

At home, an hour later, she suddenly had ataxia, dysarthria, dysphagia, vertigo, and weakness. She was taken to a tertiary care center, and a repeat non-contrast head CT showed a new cerebellar infarct. Eventually she had an MRI/MRA of the brain and neck and was diagnosed with a vertebral artery dissection, which they surmised had come from her previous discectomy.

## The Letter Arrives in the Mail

I had no idea any of this had occurred until I was named in a lawsuit several months later, causing my whole world to shift on its axis. Before that, I had thought I was a good doctor, capable of running a whole hospital herself at night! And now? Now I was a bad doctor who had missed something huge, even though I'd been trying my hardest to pay attention. Many years later, I allow myself some grace for missing a rare event that presented in a highly atypical fashion, in an age when CT angiograms of the brain and neck weren't possible at my institution. But not then.

In the end, the litigation surrounding this case lasted twelve years and two lengthy jury trials. I was the sole physician defendant in a case with an initial demand of 28 million dollars. And the odyssey taught me a great deal about litigation and litigation stress, what it means to be a human being coping with it all, and the disservice we do our students and trainees by not talking about it more openly.

## Litigation Stress and Malpractice Stress Syndrome

Although malpractice litigation is very common, with estimates that 75% to 99% of all physicians will be sued for malpractice at least once by age 65, many physicians are fearful of litigation and are greatly impacted when personally named. The traumatic effects of litigation on the provider start at the very beginning, with the adverse event itself or with receiving notice. The accusation of malpractice, whether or not substandard care was rendered, creates a cascade of responses in the defendant that may have significant psychological, cognitive, spiritual, and physical effects, known collectively as "litigation stress."

Litigation stress among physicians was first researched by Sara Charles, MD, a psychiatrist who was sued for malpractice in federal court in the 1970s. She was so affected by the experience that she felt compelled to investigate the topic further, at a time when few physicians would even whisper that they were being sued. The book "Defendant" describes her experiences in court, and she later published "Adverse Events, Stress and Litigation," detailing her subsequent work and research in this area.

Physicians undergo a range of reactions, from feeling minor annoyance to frank depression and suicidality. More significant stress reactions and the resultant personal, professional, or social dysfunction are termed "medical malpractice stress syndrome," sometimes used interchangeably with "litigation stress."

In general, litigation stress is a normal human reaction to an outsized and long-lasting stressor. Whether or not error occurred, litigation can feel like an assault on your identity, and leave you questioning the sacrifices you made to become a physician: The years of school and training, thousands of dollars of debt, missed holidays, birthdays, anniversaries and first steps, as well as the emotional burdens of living a life in medicine. It can feel like all of it was for nothing, as the sum of your career becomes encapsulated in that legal complaint.

Although it varies from physician to physician, there are some common themes:

**Emotional/psychological**
- Depression, anxiety, isolation, shame, anger, betrayal, disillusionment, shock, overwhelm, apathy

**Cognitive**
- Difficulty with attention and concentration, low frustration tolerance, difficulty making decisions, "analysis paralysis"

**Physical**
- Insomnia, palpitations, gastrointestinal upset, headaches, shakiness

**Interpersonal**
- Withdrawal from, or conflict with, significant other, children, or other key relationships
- Decline in desire to participate in social activities

**Spiritual**
- Loss of faith, withdrawal from spiritual community, loss of sense of purpose, loss of the feeling of the "calling" of medicine

Many physicians find it difficult to see patients with similar complaints, or to perform a procedure that was involved in the complaint. Post-traumatic symptoms of flashbacks, rumination, and panic physiology is common – and quite understandable.

The usual admonition to "not talk about it" is both misguided and unhealthy. It is important to discern the difference between discussing the specific events of a case (the presentation, documentation, testing, management) from the emotional toll it takes on the provider. Peer support, therapy, coaching, talking with trusted friends, family, and colleagues can be therapeutic and a healthy way to process the trauma associated with adverse events and litigation. Isolation and shame unfortunately can compound stress and depressive symptoms.

Medical malpractice stress syndrome exists on a continuum with litigation stress, with more significant symptoms of depression, anxiety, or stress-related physical symptoms. Physicians may struggle with work or interpersonal relationships. This is a high-risk time for substance abuse or relapse. Unfortunately, there is an association between litigation and physician suicide.

## Mitigating Litigation Stress

Litigation can last for years, but it does not need to exact the toll on physicians that it has historically. Openly discussing litigation in medical culture can help destigmatize this exceedingly common event, lessening the shame and isolation that inherently worsen the experience. The creation of more robust peer support programs and initiatives that protect the privacy of physicians seeking mental health care are gaining ground. Here are some additional suggestions:

**A. Wellness and self-care**

- Look at litigation as a difficult event that gives you permission to make changes that support your overall well-being
- Attend to exercise, nutrition, and sleep as best you can
- Nurture personal relationships
- Deliberately schedule time off from work for non-work-related, enjoyable activities
- Consider an hours reduction or leave of absence if work presents a significant stressor or you are feeling overwhelmed
- Be cautious with the use of alcohol, other drugs, or sleep aids
- Do not let rumination over litigation consume your life. You may find it helpful to block out specific time to think, worry, and learn about litigation, and to use positive distractions at other times to prevent rumination and catastrophizing

**B. Develop your litigation skill set**

- Read books on malpractice litigation and how to perform as a defendant
- Follow your attorney's counsel
- Consult professional society resources
- Attend lectures and listen to podcasts
- A prepared defendant is a more effective and confident defendant
- Know-how and practice can be antidotes to anxiety

**C. Investigate support resources**

- Sara Charles Physician Litigation Stress Resource Center
- American College of Emergency Physicians (ACEP) List of Resources
- Consult professional society resources
- Seek out peer support, therapy, or coaching
- Speaking with physicians who have previously been sued
- Learn about research-based coping and resilience strategies such as

    - ◊ Cognitive behavioral therapy techniques
    - ◊ Acceptance commitment therapy techniques
    - ◊ Work with a therapist or coach to implement these
- Professional intervention is recommended for physicians with severe symptoms of malpractice stress syndrome

**D. Reframe how you think about the litigation process**

- Consider it an occupational hazard rather than a sign that you are a bad doctor ( most physicians are sued at some point)
- You will be purposefully made to feel like a bad person and bad physician: recognize this as a deliberate plaintiff's attorney strategy, and do not internalize it
- Seek support from family, friends, and peers
- Some institutions have formal peer-support networks

**Red Flags**

Sometimes physicians have a hard time recognizing when their stress is becoming severe; we can recognize these signs in patients, but not in ourselves, and feel as though we "should be able to handle it." In truth, distress from litigation is exceedingly common; we just historically haven't talked about it. Suicidal thoughts, overdrinking or substance use, social withdrawal and isolation, or emotional outbursts are all signs that professional help and perhaps time away from work are indicated. If a colleague, family member, or friend expresses concern about your behavior, do your best to see this as a reason to accept help.

**Conclusion**

Although now I understand that the overwhelming stress I felt during litigation has a name, and that I was in good company, for many years I allowed my psychological distress to dominate my professional and personal life. I kept myself isolated, lived deeply in depression and anxiety, and didn't understand why I wasn't able to "handle it." It took almost eight years before I finally accepted that I might need help and began the journey that eventually led to a much better place for myself, my family, and my career satisfaction. If you are being sued, know that there are resources out there to help you, and arming yourself with knowledge and support is the first step.

# How Does the Lawsuit End?

**T. Marc Calvert, JD**
Medical malpractice defense attorney
Calvert, Leever, Ostler
Cypress, Texas

The best way for a lawsuit to end… is for it to never begin.

A great benefit of the Bouncebacks format is using it to learn from the patient encounters and, perhaps, the mistakes of others. A solid bedside manner, a well-honed antenna for red-flag symptoms and signs, excellent clinical judgment, and reliable records are proven ways to minimize or avoid lawsuits.

But after the litigation is initiated, what is the exit strategy? There are four basic ways that lawsuits end:

**1. Voluntarily Dismissed**

The easiest way for a case to end is if it is simply dismissed by the plaintiff. This may occur if you were named in a wide net of clinicians who had contact with the patient and with further inspection, the plaintiff's attorney determines that you did not impact the patient's outcome. Or as the evidence unfolds, it becomes apparent that you did not breach the standard of care. Or they may find that the cost of litigation is not worth their time either because the potential judgment would be too low or the chances of winning too remote.

It is sometimes worthwhile for counsel to approach the other side early on and have a frank discussion. It may show the opponent the reasons the case should be dismissed, and though there are no guarantees, it may succeed. Over the years we have persuaded some plaintiff's lawyers to drop our clients.

**2. Dismissed by the Court**

A second possible path is based on the action of the court; the defense counsel files a motion, and the court issues a favorable ruling. This is somewhat rare, mainly because having a genuine issue of material fact is not that hard to show and that may be all the judge needs to deny the motion. Here are some examples of the types of motions which can result in your exit from the lawsuit (depending on the state):

- Motion for Summary Judgment (MSJ)
  - ◊ This motion argues to the court that there is no genuine dispute as to any material fact and that you are entitled to judgment as a matter of law. For example, if the opposing expert concedes that he cannot opine that the patient would have had a different outcome if you had done a specific test, then a MSJ could be filed on your behalf because the plaintiff's ability to support the element of causation is legally compromised by their own expert.

- Daubert Challenge (to the reliability of the scientific evidence against you)
  - ◊ This is a motion which challenges the reliability of the evidence against you, typically from the view of the scientific data. For example, if the expert maintains that the outcome would have been different if the test in question had been timely done, he should be challenged as to what scientific principles or data support such an opinion. Imagine he then says in his deposition "I do not have anything to cite for you, but it is simply my belief that the patient would not have died and that is based on my education, training, and experience." A Daubert motion which challenges this speculative guess could be pursued. That is just because an expert says it is so, does not make it so—ipse dixit—is one of the pillars of the Daubert arena. A motion requesting that the trial judge evaluate the evidence in detail can result in your exit from the lawsuit.
- Motion to Dismiss
  - ◊ This is state dependent, but in Texas we have requirements for initial expert reports. If the plaintiff does not meet those requirements, a motion to dismiss can be pursued.
- Motion for Directed Verdict (after plaintiff has put on their evidence)
  - ◊ If the case goes to trial, the plaintiff puts on their evidence first and then rests their case. Before the defense puts on evidence, they may want to pursue a motion which asks the trial judge to halt the trial and render a verdict in favor of the defendant. The basis would be that the evidence of proof on the central issues of negligence, causation, or damages has been inadequate to sustain a finding against the defendant by the jury.

Because there are often decent arguments on both sides of these motions, most trial courts are reluctant to dismiss a defendant, even if they have some fairly serious questions about the strength of the case. It is often easier for the trial judge to just allow the case to keep going rather than to intervene and grant a motion for summary judgment, or some type of motion to dismiss, only to be reversed on appeal. Sad but true.

### 3. Settlement

The classic fork in the road often comes down to settlement versus trial. If beauty is in the eye of the beholder, certainly the decision to settle a case versus going to trial is equally subjective and individualized. Laden with many different factors, both have some perceived advantages as well as disadvantages. Before weighing the pros and cons, it is worth considering some of the variables that can come into play:

- What is your insurance coverage? For example, it you have a policy of $100,000 and the potential damages are much higher than that, this is a disparity to be considered. Additionally, is your policy an eroding policy (i.e. where fees and expenses are paid in a way which reduces your coverage for potential liability)? Does settlement require your consent?
- Are you at risk for an excess judgment (i.e. is there risk that your personal assets are at risk because the realistic potential damages are greater than the available insurance coverage?) This is something to discuss with your defense counsel on a periodic basis throughout the case.
- What is the stage of your career? Are you 32 years old and worried about being able to get hospital privileges and malpractice insurance in the future -or- are you 66 years-old and getting ready to retire and just want the case to be over?
- Is this your first lawsuit or your 20th? If this is a new frontier for you, it can be helpful to check with respected colleagues about the path forward. Regular conferences with your

attorney are necessary, as they will do their best to steer the case to the end game that you desire.

- In your heart of hearts, do you feel that you can defend your care in a deposition or at trial? Can you exude competence, display compassion, and offer a plausible and reasonable explanation for your care, with clarification of any hiccups in your notes?
- Are you able to devote the time and energy needed to prepare, attend, and present at trial?
- What will be the psychologic impact of a protracted legal proceeding (which could last 4 years or longer)?

### A. <u>Potential Advantages to Settling</u>

First, it is impossible to predict what a jury will do; a handful of citizens will be "voting" at the end of the case and you are trying to anticipate how they will vote.

Think about the New York Times predicting, shortly before the 2016 election, that Hillary Clinton had an 87.5% chance of winning; no amount of expertise allows one to predict with certainty how a human being will vote. The human mind and heart can change on a dime. Thus, a prominent reason for settling a case is that it removes the risk of a jury returning an adverse verdict, and potentially an excess verdict which could expose your personal assets.

As part of most settlements, there is an agreement that the plaintiff will not publicly divulge details of the case and settlement, nor disparage the provider on social media platforms. The term "buy your peace" is pretty accurate, and it can be a benefit.

Another advantage is that trial is a time-consuming venture. Most healthcare providers are busy, and if they are going to carve out two weeks, they would rather be at a lake house versus prepping their testimony and sitting through a brutal battle. This amount of time not working can also have a significant impact on income, as well as inflicting a level of stress that is typically not experienced, even at the bedside of a busy ED!

Another possible advantage is to view settling as a pragmatic business move. If your insurance company spends $250,000 to prevail on a case that you could have settled for $65,000, you should not be terribly surprised when you receive the non-renewal notice a few weeks after the jury has found in your favor. I have had insurance professionals tell me "I had to spend four times more to take the case to trial when a nominal settlement was indicated. This guy just did not have the judgment to see that that was a more discrete and preferred path, and the company felt like he wasn't someone they wanted to insure anymore." This is largely dependent on the insurance company. Some take a position to try almost all cases, and other companies are more prone to settle. It is best to have an early discussion with the company and your attorney regarding your preference and if this impacts the ultimate decision of the insurance company.

### B. <u>Potential Disadvantages to Settling</u>

Over the years, I have had doctors tell me that they have regretted settling a case; when a physician feels they gave good care, the buyer's remorse of settling that case can be hard to shake. This feeling varies from person to person, but it can be a factor and should be weighed.

Having a perceived "mark" on the record is another con. A settlement is reported to the National Practitioners Databank (NPDB), which is not open to the public but which can be accessed by some in the industry. Though we can debate about that impact, some healthcare providers feel that it is a negative mark that should be avoided at all costs. But it is important to note, that one report to the NPDB for a random, reasonable settlement, is often simply viewed as the cost of doing business. It's the monster-sized settlements, or a pattern of settlements, that give pause to those who can access the NPDB.

In all likelihood, the settlement will be a public record, and it is frequently mandated that simply being named a defendant in a lawsuit must also be reported to licensing boards, facilities, and insurance companies.

I encourage my clients to understand that being sued, giving depositions, or having a report filed with the NPDB—all are eventually part of the job. Even the famed heart surgeon Michael DeBakey, viewed by some as the greatest surgeon of all time, was involved in a few lawsuits, and one went to trial where I defended a colleague of his. I watched from the counsel table as he testified at trial. I was struck by his good humor and impressed with his graceful acceptance of his situation. I would venture a guess that Dr. DeBakey settled many cases over the years, and that he had more than a few reports to the Texas Medical Board and the NPDB. He picked his battles, worked out some settlements, and went to trial when it was indicated.

### 4. Trial: Pros and Cons

The advantages of going to trial include being able to defend your care. No regrets for paying a settlement. No negative mark for making a settlement.

Additionally, prevailing in a trial can be exhilarating, validating, and just the type of principled stand that you always envisioned making. The barbarians were at the gate, and you beat them. It can feel so good!

On the other hand, I have had a fair number of doctors who won their trials, and soon after "winning," they quietly told me that they would never go through that experience again. For it is not just the time commitment and the stress, but also the dehumanizing experience. They were discouraged by the system and the lack of respect with the repeated drumbeat of being disparaged throughout the trial. In retrospect, the "win" was just not that enriching, and was not worth it. It reminded me of the quote from the Duke of Wellington: "Nothing except a battle lost can be half so melancholy as a battle won." While the statistics may favor doctors in winning at trial, I believe that people (meaning those sitting on juries) today are more willing to go against a doctor at trial than in years past and are more interested in returning bigger dollars in damages than before. That shift should be considered, and respected.

Losing at trial stings. The loss is a gut punch. It can also result in adverse press reports in the local newspaper or on the TV news, and a public record of the loss which can be accessed by anyone. This needs to be weighed in the consideration of whether to settle.

## 5. The Bottom Line

Understanding how the "nightmare" may end is important. There are many factors beyond your control; but deciding on settling vs. defending a case can have major implications. It is not a simple analysis, as different clinicians will make reasonable choices based upon their individual circumstance; the variables and factors involved are endless. Obtain advice from your attorney, and perhaps from some colleagues who have been in a similar situation. Sometimes, there are two bad outcomes, and you need to pick the lesser of two evils.

Remember the words of Cicero: "If you want peace, prepare for war." This means analyzing the specifics of the case, considering the documentation, factoring how you, the defendant, will come across to a jury, how much the literature supports your case, and securing strong experts. Building a strong defense allows you to have the leverage to later choose the path—settlement or trial—which is in your best interest.

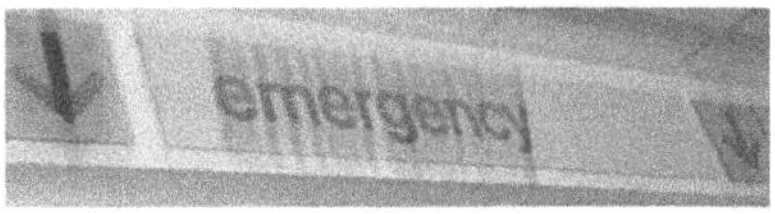


# Case 1

## A 39 Year-old Woman with Multiple Complaints: Coughing During Cold & Flu Season

Primary case authors:
Leen Alblaihed
Emilie Cobert
Amal Mattu

### PART 1—MEDICAL



### PART 2—LEGAL

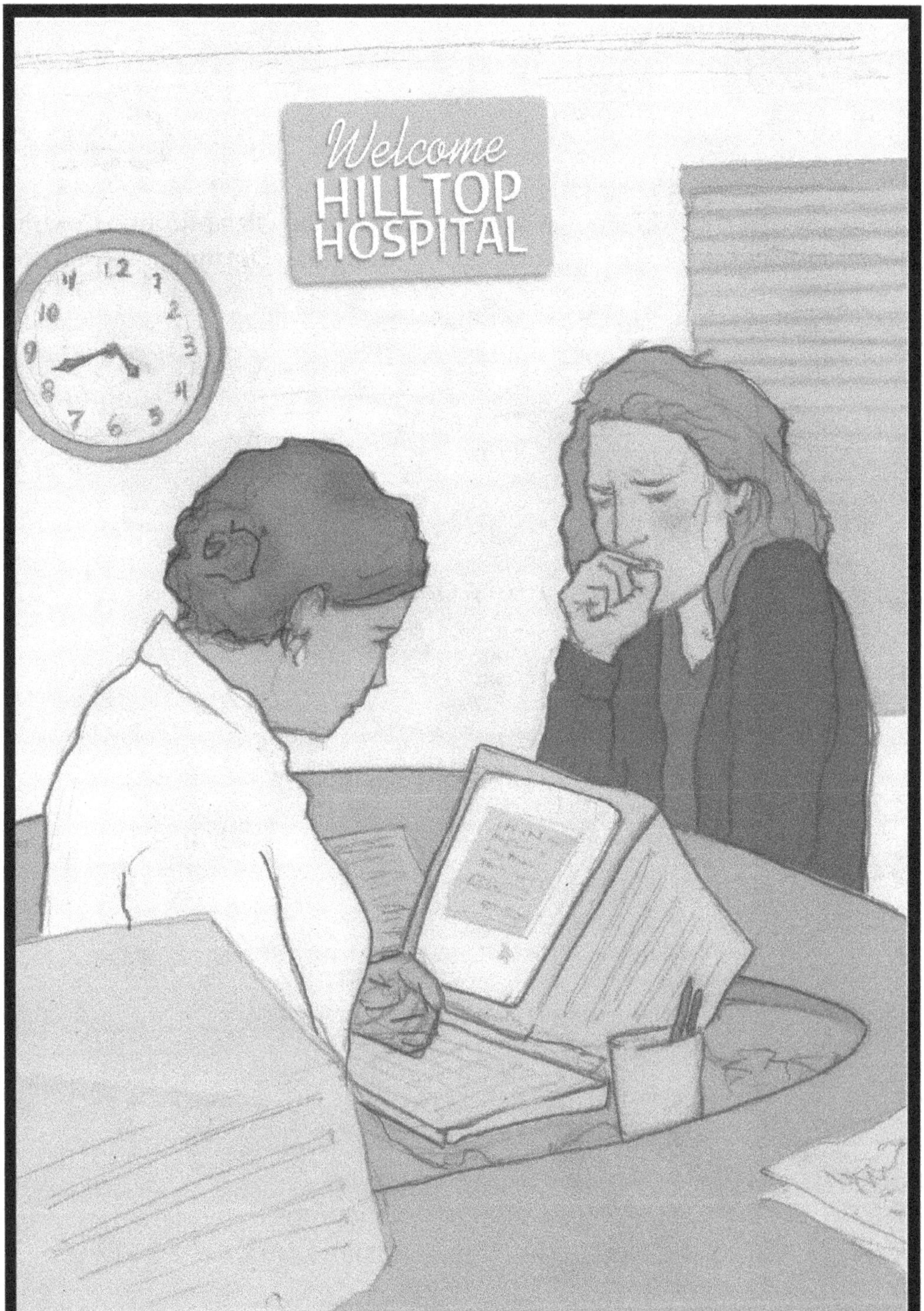
Welcome
HILLTOP
HOSPITAL

# Case 1

## A 39 Year-old Woman with Multiple Complaints: Coughing During Cold & Flu Season

Why do so many bounceback patients with poor outcomes have an initial diagnosis of bronchitis or gastroenteritis or receive a prescription for a Z-pack? It is a coincidence...right?

***Deep thoughts:***

1. *How do we balance the risk of missing serious disease with the risk of over-testing?*
2. *Who wins when the nurse and doctor disagree on the chief complaint?*
3. *How should we approach the "positive review of systems" patient?*
4. *Does our "index of suspicion" decrease in the early morning hours of a night shift?*

**PART 1—MEDICAL**

## I. The Patient's Story

In 1979, at the age of 16, Anna marries her high school sweetheart, Mike. Through the years, they raise three boys, always making time for baseball games, despite each working full-time.

As a family, they do not have much. Mike works on an hourly basis for Nebraska Milling, and Anna works at "Barb's Burgers and Such," a low priced restaurant off the highway. For her, it is not just another job; she has established a first-name relationship with her customers, working as waitress and cashier. She is a warm and inviting person. Neither have health insurance.

For the last 10 years Mike has been the little league coach. This year marked a special occasion for the Kamianka family; after years of watching their kids play baseball, Coach Mike takes the little leaguers to play a tournament game at Jacobs field. Anna has never been to a professional baseball stadium, she has never seen the Cleveland Indians play. She poses for a picture in the dugout with a player on each side.

Anna is generally healthy, but moderately overweight. She is a smoker who has unsuccessfully struggled to quit on several occasions. On September 5, she is at work and doesn't feel well. She calls her primary care physician, Dr. Brian Rembrandt, for a "sick visit" appointment and is told that if she can make a payment on the balance of her bills, she will be seen. The bill is paid and she arrives at 3:00 in the afternoon. The exam is routine, a CXR is normal, she is diagnosed with bronchitis and she is prescribed antibiotics. A later review of the records shows that this is not a unique occurrence; she has been treated each of the last six years for upper respiratory infections.

Anna is not the type to complain. Despite feeling bad, she does not miss a day of work. After taking her medication, her symptoms are improved, and she is well until the morning of November 6, when she is awakened by a pain between her shoulder blades. The pain is so bad, she throws up. She takes two ibuprofen, without improvement. Mike wakes up to see his wife up and putting her coat on.

She says, "I'm going to the hospital."

"Do you want me to take you?"

"No, you stay here and get the kids to school."

"All right, but I'm going to wait for you; I won't go to work until you get home."

At 4:42 AM, Anna Kamianka walks into the emergency department at Hilltop Hospital

## II. The Doctor's Version (the following is the actual documentation of the provider)

**Chief Complaint per RN (05:05):** "Back pain, chest pain, vomit, arm pain"

**Date:** November 6

Vital Signs

| Time | Temp(F) | Pulse | Resp | Syst | Diast | Pain Scale |
|---|---|---|---|---|---|---|
| 05:07 | 97.4° F | 72 | 18 | 138 | 93 | 8/10 |

**Triage (05:05):**
Woke from sound sleep with above symptoms. Took 2 motrin without relief. Most pain between shoulder blades radiating down right arm. No numbness/tingling. Chest midsternal pressure. No SOB. No nausea. Vomiting × 1

**Chief Complaint (physician):** Chest pain, coughing, and vomiting

**History of Present Illness:** The patient is a 39 year-old female who approximately one month ago started developing a cough and congestion. She was seen [by her PCP] and started on an antibiotic. She started improving, but after going off the antibiotics, the cough came back and she has been coughing up yellowish sputum. She had post-tussive vomiting today. She indicates that when she coughs, she gets very sharp pain both in the front of the chest and the back. Those are the symptoms that she has been having. She denies any fever or SOB.

**Past Medical History:**
**Allergies:** NKDA
**Meds:** Birth control pills
**PMH/PSH:** Negative
**SH:** Smoker 1 1/2 PPD. Drinks 6 pack daily

**Physical Examination:**
**Constitutional:** She is alert. She does not appear to be in any distress at this point
**HEENT:** Mouth and pharynx are clear
**Neck:** Supple; no adenopathy of JVD
**Lungs:** Some wheezing in both bases but otherwise clear
**Chest:** She is tender over the anterior chest wall
**Card:** Regular rate and rhythm, nl. S1 S2
**Back:** Non-tender
**Ext:** No cyanosis, edema, swelling

**Emergency Department Course:**
**05:20:** Pt. ambulatory to XR. CXR results: Interpreted by myself is normal without infiltrate or edema. Heart size is normal. [The reading is later confirmed by radiology over-read.]
**05:45:** Pt. medicated with acetaminophen 975mg PO. Albuterol aerosol
**06:15:** Pt. reports pain decreased to 5/10

**Progress Note:** The patient felt much better after the aerosol. Her lungs are completely clear
**Diagnosis:** Acute bronchitis.

**Disposition (06:35):** Azithromycin for 10 days. Follow-up with Dr.Rembran

*Timothy Madison, MD*

## III. Risk Management/Patient Safety Opportunities (Weinstock)

**Author comments (Weinstock):** What could possibly be wrong? Our patient gets bronchitis every fall, and this year is no exception. After two months of being asymptomatic, was this a new infection, an incompletely treated infection, or perhaps something else?

**Risk Management/Patient Safety Opportunity #1:**

**Opportunity:** Poor correlation between doctor and nurse notes.
**Discussion:** Buckle up for the ride, this is going to be a broken record alert: The chief complaint needs to be addressed. It is not a coincidence that this is the first Risk management/patient safety opportunity of the first chapter in this book... it is a frequent theme in medical legal cases. In this case the "chief complaint" for the nurse starts with back pain and for the doctor starts with chest pain. The patient's presentation is a question: Do I have a life-threatening problem? Could the chest pain and back pain be related?
Of course! All of the "big three" causes of life-threatening chest pain are still in play: Acute coronary syndrome (ACS), pulmonary embolism (PE) and thoracic aortic dissection (TAD).
✔ **Teaching point:** Though time-consuming, all chief complaints documented need to be addressed.

**Risk Management/Patient Safety Opportunity #2:**

**Opportunity:** Inadequate history of chest pain.
**Discussion:** Here is the history recorded for chest pain: She indicates that when she coughs, she gets very sharp pain both in the front of the chest and the back. No one is recommending a cardiac cath with this presentation, but how about asking some basic questions such as:

• Is it worse with exertion?
• Is there radiation (including specifically to the back)?
• Is this the first time you had it or has this been ongoing?
• Do you have any chest pain when you are not coughing?
• Is there associated diaphoresis?
• Is the pain pleuritic?
✔ **Teaching point:** All evaluations begin with a good history.

**Risk Management/Patient Safety Opportunity #3:**

**Opportunity:** Poor explanation for back pain.
**Discussion:** Why did she have back pain? Was it because of a muscular strain from the coughing and vomiting, was it worse with movement? There was no back pain to touch. However, her chest did hurt with palpation. Did the chest pain radiate to the back? If her chest was strained from the vomiting, maybe she strained her back also; but it didn't hurt with palpation? Could this be a PE? How about Boerhaave's syndrome? Could a patient living in Cleveland have an aortic dissection and concomitant URI?
✔ **Teaching point:** When multiple complaints are present, a viable explanation for each should be documented.

**Risk Management/Patient Safety Opportunity #4:**

**Opportunity:** Not exploring cardiac risk factors.
**Discussion:** I have mixed feelings about this one. When a 17 year-old presents with a sudden onset of reproducible chest pain after lifting a refrigerator, I don't want to know that his grandmother had an MI at the age of 25. However, how firm is the diagnosis in our patient? The doctor's chart as a "stand-alone" seems quite convincing; a productive cough with sharp chest pain when coughing sounds like bronchitis. But read the nurse's notes and a different story emerges; chest pressure with radiation down the right arm with associated vomiting severe enough to wake her from sleep and prompt a 5 AM visit to the ED. Risk factors? If Anna would have been asked about her family history, she would have relayed that her brother died at the age of 32 from an MI. Coupled with smoking, use of oral contraceptives and moderate obesity, this could paint the picture of acute coronary syndrome (ACS) or PE.
✔ **Teaching point:** Sometimes, risk factors matter ...

**Risk Management/Patient Safety Opportunity #5:**

**Opportunity:** Not getting an ECG.
**Discussion:** Though the nursing protocol at Hilltop Hospital required an ECG be performed on all chest pain patients (this was brought out during the legal proceedings), I do have an issue with this. The true cost of the test to society is really only the electricity used and the ink and paper it is printed on. But is there a greater cost? If she would have had flipped "T-waves" in II, III and aVF, she would have been admitted, contracted a hospital-acquired infection and died. OK. Probably not. But, there is certainly a cost to a false positive result in an uninsured patient struggling to buy her kids Christmas presents, especially when you won't believe the results ... or would you?
✔ **Teaching point:** An ECG is a simple, inexpensive test, which can be helpful when excluding heart disease.

**Risk Management/Patient Safety Opportunity #6:**

**Error:** What's the deal with Azithromycin?
**Discussion:** This patient didn't just get one Z-pack; the doctor "doubled-down" and gave her two! This reminds me of the Monty Python skit where the King built his castle on a swamp. It sank, but he would not be deterred and built another and another. Though the Z-pack is a great virus-killer, thrombolytic and aortic sleeve (haha), it still was not indicated for this patient.
✔ **Teaching point:** Azithromycin does nothing for viral bronchitis.

## IV. The Bounceback

Anna arrives home between 7:00 and 7:30 and tells her husband, "Mike, I've got bronchitis. I'm going to lie down." Mike is relieved his wife is OK; he leaves for work and Anna spends most of the day laying around. When he arrives home at 4PM he asks his wife how she is doing. "So-so. I still feel rotten like I did in the morning. The medicine hasn't helped."

One hour later, the boys have eaten, and Anna has fixed dinner for her husband. After they eat, she picks up a glass of water and walks into the kitchen, but Mike is startled to hear her fall to the ground, water glass crashing to the floor. He and his sons rush in to find her unresponsive on the floor. One son calls 911, and Mike does what he can to revive her.

Per Cleveland EMS:

**17:17** – 911 call is received; nature of call from dispatch: "choking"
**17:21** – EMS arrive on the scene to find pt. "lying supine on the floor, unresponsive." They record: "Husband states she choked on food."
**17:23** – Asystole. CPR is initiated. Pt. is intubated
**17:38** – Pulse -0-, resp -0-, BP -0-
**17:40** – Monitor confirms coarse v-fib Æ shock 200–300–360 without improvement
**18:01** – Arrival at Hilltop Hospital: (documentation per physician)
• **Chief complaint:** Full arrest
• **HPI:** 39 year-old female intubated with CPR in progress. [EMS] have given several rounds of epinephrine and electrically cardioverted for a run of ventricular fibrillation. I talked with the husband and he states she had been seen this morning around 5 AM. She had a cough and in general, complained of not feeling well. She had gotten a piece of cube chicken and was eating that when they heard her hit the floor.
• **ED course:** ET tube is pulled back slightly to account for right main stem intubation and now there are bilaterally equal breath sounds.
**18:09** – Code called. The patient is pronounced at 1809 hours. The case is discussed with her husband in the presence of Father Patrick. A call will be placed to the PCP, Dr. Rembrandt and to the coroner.

**Emergency Department Diagnosis:** Cardiopulmonary arrest, questionable etiology

**Author comments (Weinstock):** What was the etiology of the arrest? The husband thinks she choked on chicken, but just because she was eating it when she collapsed does not prove cause and effect. Similarly, just because she had a cough earlier in the day does not mean her two previous diagnoses were necessarily from a URI. Is there a way to know if she really had a URI on September 5th? Enter the coroner...

**Autopsy Diagnosis:**
The coronary arteries are patent except for a focal area of the LAD which shows 99% luminal narrowing by gray-tan material. There is focal grey scar tissue in the interventricular septum.
Aorta shows mild atheromatous streaks and plaques.
Coronary atherosclerotic heart disease:

- Acute thrombosis in left anterior descending coronary artery
- Intramyocardial arteriosclerosis
- Remote, organizing and acute myocardial infarcts

**Final Diagnosis:** Acute myocardial infarction

**Author comments (Weinstock):** So now the diagnosis is clear. No PE. No aspiration. No pneumonia. No dissection. The patient had a small septal MI in September. She didn't improve *because* of antibiotics, but improved coincidental with the prescription of antibiotics. She then awoke around 4AM with symptoms of her acute MI (AMI), including chest and back pain from an acute thrombus in the LAD, the "widow maker." At her first ED visit, an ECG would likely have shown STEMI and there was plenty of time for revascularization or thrombolysis.

This was not an easy diagnosis. She did have symptoms typically seen with bronchitis and associated chest-wall strain reproducible with palpation. But some aspects of the evaluation did not make sense for URI. A previously well person who had never missed a day of work woke up on a cold November morning at 4AM, left her husband and children at home and drove herself to the ED for chest pain, back pain, vomiting, arm pain and cough. That must have been some URI ... Would you have done an ECG? Should the nurse have automatically done an ECG per the hospital protocol? Does a complaint of chest pain require at least a few questions as to exacerbation (exertion) or associated symptoms (diaphoresis)?

The doctor was aware of the chest pain and did mention that in the HPI, but his impression was certainly different than the nurse's. His documentation suggested a musculoskeletal etiology. This was a tough diagnosis. Did the lawyers agree? What did they think of the doctor's evaluation?

## PART 2—LEGAL

## I. The Accusation/Cause of Action

The accusation here is pretty clear: failure to diagnose. For a legal action to be successful, the plaintiff must also prove "causation;" in other words, that the alleged negligence—failure to diagnose—actually caused the patient's injuries. The actual trial involved two defendants, the emergency physician and the primary care doctor who initially diagnosed bronchitis on September 5th. The autopsy suggests an initially missed septal infarct at the PCP visit and a fatal MI with thrombosis to the LAD on November 6th. We will just focus on the action against the EP; the diagnosis is clear and uncontested. The question here is if this was a "diagnose-able" condition when Anna presented at 4:42AM on the sixth. To answer that question, eight non-physicians were chosen; the courts call it a jury ...

## II. What Would Greg Do (WWGD)?

**Greg Henry, MD**
Past president of The American College of Emergency Physicians (ACEP)
Past Professor of Emergency Medicine at the University of Michigan

Greg opines on evaluation of chest pain, defense and plaintiff strategy, and if he would settle.

**"If I sit back and state only the pertinent parts of any case, no one will miss this diagnosis—But that's not how patients present."**

Chest pain is still our biggest pain. When I first started to do medical legal cases in 1976, misdiagnosis of chest pain accounted for between 35% and 40% of cases. Guess what? Chest pain is still a lot of the cases. The reason is simple. Most people with chest pain don't have something bad. When they do have something bad, it can be deadly.

The public at large is inundated with TV advertisements and dramatic scenarios of chest pain; every layperson can give you the differential diagnosis. The problem is we have a high signal-to-noise ratio. If I sit back and state only the pertinent parts of any case, no one will miss this diagnosis, but that's not how patients present. They have strange stories that go up and down and around. They ascribe their symptoms to factors having nothing to do with their actual disease. Just because you cough doesn't mean it's bronchitis. There's certainly no evidence to suggest that viral bronchitis is made better with a Z-Pack, but don't try telling that to my friends. The complex interaction between scientific medicine and patient satisfaction drives every emergency physician crazy.

What is difficult to avoid in this case is that a 39 year-old woman was awoken from sleep with severe pain between her shoulder blades. This is compounded with the history of a brother who died at age 32 of some medical condition—no matter how you cut it, the brother probably had cardiovascular disease. She smokes 1 1⁄2 packs per day, is on birth control pills and has chest pain radiating down to her right arm. That is a very difficult scenario to ignore. But I've dissected the facts after knowing the outcome ...

The problem with settlement is that there are huge potential financial loses; this case is not going to settle for a small amount of money. If you tried this case in front of a reasonable jury, you would win 7 out of 10 times. She does have confusing history and improved after leaving the ED.

The defense will have to concentrate on the complexity of the problem, her history of bronchitis and the fact that she felt improved with respiratory treatment. Defense revolves around the fact that 39 year-old women, in general, don't drop dead of heart attacks. The great danger in this case is jury sympathy.

The plaintiff's strategy is simple—heart disease is still as much a common killer of women as it is of men. The fact that she had chest pain running into arms is one of the symptoms taught by the American Heart Association (AHA). As plaintiff, I would bring in posters showing the warning symptoms of heart attack; a simple story and qualified experts could make a substantial impact on the jury.

Would I settle? It's a toss-up. Knowing that we would win this case in 7 out of 10 times, if I could get a settlement for under $200K, I would definitely do it. If not, let's go to trial!

## III. The Trial—Monday September 26th (almost 3 years after the patient was seen in the ED)

**Author comments (Weinstock):** This was a tough trial and a tough case. We all feel for the family and this devoted couple, high school sweethearts who have worked hard and struggled to provide for their family. But who else works in a profession where you can be forced to go to court to defend your actions if there is a poor outcome? Still... would we be happy if Anna was our family member?

**The following is the actual trial transcript.** The court's instructions and both opening statements have been significantly shortened. All names have been changed except Mark Jones, who was the actual defense attorney for the case. All other trial testimony is exactly reproduced, but may be shortened and syntax minimally changed to enhance readability. In Chapter one, we reproduce a shortened version of the opening statements and in Chapter two we focus on the closing statements.
**Additional trial testimony is available at:**
**https://www.embouncebacks.com/bouncebacks-medical-and-legal**

Cast of characters (names changed, except as noted):
**The patient:** Anna Kamianka
**ED physician defendant:** Timothy Madison
**Plaintiff's attorney:** Albert August
**Plaintiff's expert witness:** Drew Florra (board certified emergency medicine)
**Defense attorney:** Mark Jones (actual attorney)

**Judge's instructions to jury:** Before we hear the opening statements of counsel and begin to take evidence, it will be helpful if you have some preliminary instructions to follow. Later, after you have heard all the evidence, I will give further instructions covering additional [issues of] law. It is the duty of the judge to instruct you in the law and your duty to follow the law.

First of all, it is your exclusive duty to decide all questions of fact submitted to you. In connection with this duty, you must determine the effect and value of the evidence. You must not be influenced in your decision by sympathy, prejudice or passion towards any party, witness or attorney in the case.

The attorneys will have active roles in the trial. They will make opening statements to you, question witnesses and make objections. And finally, they will argue the case as a last step before you hear my final instructions and commence with deliberations. Remember that attorneys are not witnesses. Since it is your duty to decide the case solely on the evidence which you hear in the case, you must not consider as evidence any statement of any attorney made during the trial, [with the exception being] if the attorneys agree to any facts.

The burden of proof is upon the plaintiff to prove the facts necessary to his case by a preponderance of the evidence. Preponderance is the "greater weight of the evidence," that is the evidence that you believe because it outweighs or overbalances in your minds the evidence opposed to it. As jurors, you have the sole and exclusive duty to decide the credibility of witnesses who will testify in the case. As you are all aware, two persons who are witnesses to an incident may often see or hear it differently.

Any fact in this case may be proven by direct or circumstantial evidence. Direct evidence directly proves a fact without having to infer the fact from some other fact. It includes the witnesses who have seen or heard the facts in a case and also includes the exhibits admitted as evidence. Circumstantial evidence, on the other hand, is the proof of facts from direct evidence from which you may reasonably infer a fact in question. For example, if the question in a case is whether Johnny ate a piece of cherry pie, direct evidence is a witness who says she saw Johnny put a piece of pie in his mouth and eat it. Circumstantial evidence is a witness who testifies that she arrived in the kitchen to see Johnny standing there with an empty pie tin and cherry pie on his face.

So with those definitions ... Mr. August, [for the plaintiff], are you prepared with your opening statement?

**Opening statement, plaintiff's attorney, Mr. August:** Good morning ladies and gentlemen. May it please the court? This is our chance to give you an overview. Please relax. I wouldn't be surprised if you're a little nervous. I'm a little nervous. I know Mike (her husband) is a little nervous. I think it's appropriate we're all a little nervous.

This is a very, very important matter. It involves the destruction of a life and the destruction of a family because of the negligence of two different doctors at two different times. And as the evidence unfolds in this case, you will see that this was truly a preventable tragedy.

Anna Kamianka was a working housewife and mother of three sons. Her contribution to the family was immeasurable. She was the center of the family. She was the glue that held them together. She was the motivating force that got things done. The family relied on her.

Dr. Madison [the ED physician] latched onto the prior diagnosis of bronchitis and in the end, that's exactly what he came up with as a conclusion for what was wrong with her. You will not find anything in this record to even suggest that he asked about family history. He didn't know. He didn't ask. If he had, she would have told him. Why is that important? Well, you got chest pain. You have radiation. The possibility of it being cardiac is clearly there. Chest pressure, chest tightness, suspicious for cardiac problems, but he didn't ask. Had he asked, he would have discovered that she had 5 risk factors for cardiac disease. Dr Madison didn't even take an ECG. No enzymes. No cardiac work-up. Sent home with a prescription for an antibiotic. She was flashing red lights about a heart problem, and no tests were done.

Anna didn't have to suffer a heart attack. She didn't have to die. I can't speak for you, but I have seen several TV commercials telling people that if they have chest pain, get to an ER. That's just what Anna did on November 6th. The problem is that Anna did what she was supposed to do. These two doctors did not. And, unfortunately Anna is not here today as a result. And that's what I said at the onset, Ladies and Gentlemen, that this was truly a preventable tragedy.

**Opening statement, defense attorney, Mr. Jones:** Good morning, folks. I represent Dr. Timothy Madison. We're not going to be discussing Dr. Madison's personal and family life like we will Mrs. Kamianka's, so in a sense you won't get the same sense for him as a person, but you will get a very clear picture of Dr. Madison as a physician. You will hear from him twice in this case, first when he is called by Mr. August for cross-examination and again later in the case when I call him to testify in his own defense. You will learn that he is an intelligent, conscientious, and thorough physician. He's board certified in emergency medicine. He has seen thousands and thousands of patients.

Among those thousands of patients, it is not unusual that several times a day he will see somebody with chest pain and somebody with respiratory problems like bronchitis. These are not unusual problems for patients in an emergency department. And it is not unusual that a doctor orders an ECG, not just for chest pain, but for any number of complaints.

You will see records of Dr. Madison's dictated note; a thorough history, exam and what he thought was going on with the patient. He [documents] that she was having pain in her back with a cough. Oh, that hurts. Had the cough bad enough to throw up. She strained herself. Oh, man that hurts here; it's radiating down my right arm.

So what's this case all about? [Mrs. Kamianka] has a cough—she's coughing up yellow sputum. Dr. Madison pushed on her chest and it was sore—that's what we call reproducible pain. The first thing you [the jury] will have to decide is whether Dr. Madison deviated from the accepted standard of care. We believe he did act appropriately. We are confident that when you have [looked at the evidence] you will walk back into this courtroom and give Dr. Madison his defense verdict.

**Author comments (Weinstock):** So now the allegations are better defined. It is indisputable that she had chest pain, but the doctor is relying on his history and evaluation and thinks she has an infectious cause. How will he defend himself on the stand? How would you defend yourself on the stand? Let's see …

**Cross-examination of defendant ED physician, Dr. Timothy Madison, by plaintiff's attorney Mr. August:**

### A. The importance of data gathering (history):

**Q.** Mr. August (plaintiff 's counsel): Would you agree with me that potential cardiac symptoms include back pain, chest pain, vomiting, and arm pain?
**A.** Dr. Timothy Madison (defendant): They are potential symptoms, that's correct.

**Q.** Now, when you are interested in trying to determine if a patient has myocardial ischemia, what do you do?
**A.** Initially I would try and elicit a history. I would look at notes and vital signs that the nurse has taken. And then I would examine the patient and make a determination if further testing needs to be done.

**Q.**Well, I was talking about a patient where you suspected cardiac ischemia, all right?
**A.** Yes.

**Q.** So it is true that after the history and physical is taken in a patient with potential cardiac ischemia, you would order an ECG?
**A.** That is a possibility.

**Q.** And you would probably order blood work, cardiac enzymes?
**A.** That's a possibility also.

**Q.** Part of what you're doing when you're talking to the patient and getting this history is also to assess risk factors, right?
**A.** In relation to presenting with cardiac symptoms?

**Q.** Right, yes.
**A.** That's correct.

**Author comments (Weinstock):** The defendant cannot really answer any other way to these questions, but what he wants to say is, "I did not think this patient had cardiac ischemia. So, of course I didn't get an ECG." This part of the trial is not damning, just a few statements of fact. It is also by the plaintiff's attorney and there will be plenty of time for Dr. Madison to defend himself when he is called back to the stand by his defense attorney.

The ECG is a simple test, inexpensive, noninvasive and could almost certainly have diagnosed the MI. There are false positives; for example, a chronically flipped T wave without an old ECG for comparison could prompt an unnecessary admission, but a STEMI is very specific. Does that mean all chest-pain patients require an ECG? Absolutely not.

However, if a patient has chest pain, the onus is to prove that the pain is not from ischemia, just as a young woman with pelvic pain and a positive pregnancy test has an ectopic until proven otherwise. An alternative explanation for her symptoms, such as a productive cough suggesting bronchitis, goes a long way toward excluding ACS/MI. But just as important as proving a likely diagnosis is excluding the more life-threatening diagnoses per our mantra, "Think Worst First."

The doctor continues with a plausible explanation of deciding not to order an ECG. It seems reasonable and well thought out. It seems like something many of us would do. But how does he answer the questions in front of a lay-jury? Pretty well, I think. But stay tuned for the plaintiff's expert opine on the utility of an ECG.

### B. Is an ECG necessary?

**Continued cross-examination of defendant ED physician, Dr. Madison, by plaintiff's attorney, Mr. August:**

**Q.** So what about Mrs. Kamianka's presentation makes it OK not to do an ECG?
**A.** You're saying that with this presentation I'm obliged to rule out a cardiac origin. I'm saying that is not the case. There's no evidence that the patient had ischemic cardiac disease. The presentation was one of bronchitis and an infectious upper respiratory disease; and as such I'm not obliged to rule out a cardiac origin.

**Q.** What does a patient need to have as a minimum to get an ECG when they come to the ER with chest pain, if you're the one covering the ER?
**A.** Well, that patient certainly wouldn't present with a productive cough so [severe] she is throwing up with resulting chest pain.

**Author comments (Weinstock):** What does a guy have to do to get a drink around here?

### C. Diagnosis momentum: Can a patient have an URI and ACS at the same time?

**Q.** Can a patient who comes in with a productive cough that's coughing hard, coughing enough to vomit, can that patient still have a heart attack?
**A.** All things are possible.

**Q.** Can they still have a heart attack when their complaints include chest pain?
**A.** Yes, they can.

**Q.** And that's pretty important to rule out if you have a test that's easily accessible to you in the emergency room, isn't it?
**A.** To order that test, you need to have an indication.

**Q.** Truth is, doctor, you never even considered a cardiac cause of Mrs. Kamianka's chest pain complaints, did you?
**A.** It was in the differential but as I got further history and physical exam, it went further and further down the list.

**Author comments (Weinstock):** Do lawyers know about diagnosis momentum? You betcha!

**Q.** Doctor, isn't it true that once Mrs. Kamianka mentioned the fact that she had been to her family doctor and had a diagnosis of bronchitis some weeks before that you presumed the same diagnosis and operated accordingly?
**A.** No, absolutely not. I based my treatment upon my interview with the patient. Upon the history that I obtained, upon my physical exam and the treatment of the patient in the emergency department. I do not base my treatments and evaluations upon another physician.

**Author comments (Weinstock):** How about controversial observations such as the fact that women with cardiac symptoms present atypically? Is this even true? (Read commentary by chapter authors at the end of the chapter).

**D. Are the symptoms of ACS in women "atypical?"**

**Q.** A person can have an MI and still have pain between the shoulder blades?
**A.** Yes, they can.

**Q.** You talk about it as an atypical presentation of heart disease, is that what you said?
**A.** That's exactly what I said.

**Q.** You are aware of the fact that women more often present with atypical symptoms than men, right?
**A.** Yes, women can.

**Q.** Was it the cervical spine scoliosis that caused you to think this was not cardiac in origin?
**A.** No. It was part of the entire work-up. That, in and of itself, did not prevent me from getting an ECG. What you're doing is taking each finding specifically and singling it out, and I'm saying I took all those in context and as such did not order an ECG.

**Author comments (Weinstock):** Well done. In fact, the 2021 AHA/ACC/multi-society chest pain guidelines discourage the use of the word "atypical" as the symptoms present in women, diabetics, and the elderly might be "typical" for these demographics.[1] But we all understand what he means. How does the plaintiff's attorney wrap this up for the jury? The end of the questioning is always interesting; it is an attempt to leave a lasting impression. The following three questions have nothing to do with the medical decision-making or the quality of care rendered, and is clever on the plaintiff's part, as they can only be answered in one way and certainly don't make the physician look good. It is a clever approach since the attorney knows before he even starts how the doctor will answer—he knows the "glove will fit." See how he inserts the word "doctor" into the last question; my guess is that it wasn't said in the most respectful way.

**Q.** You don't have any reason to disagree with the coroner about the cause of death, do you?
**A.** No, I don't.

**Q.** [Was there any] evidence of bronchitis on autopsy?
**A.** No.

**Q.** As of November, Doctor, is it true and do you agree that cardiovascular disease was the number one killer of women in the United States?
**A.** Yes, I believe that it was.

**Mr. August.** Thank you very much.

**The Court:** Doctor, you may step down. Ladies and gentlemen, we're going to take our morning break. Break for about 25 minutes. You can go downstairs and have a cup of coffee. Please don't discuss this case among yourselves or with anyone else. Don't form or express any opinions until you have heard all the evidence. All rise for the jury.

**Author comments (Weinstock):** Remember that part about the ECG? The following is the plaintiff's expert's testimony. I will tell you this—I know this guy. He teaches nationally. And he doesn't come across as a medical "whore," he comes across as having a responsible thought process … if a bit judgmental … Mr. August cuts right to the chase:

**Direct examination of plaintiff's expert witness, Drew Florra, MD, FACEP (board certified emergency medicine physician) by plaintiff's attorney, Mr. August:**

**E. Standard of care:**

**Q.** Based on your training and experience as well as your review of the materials in this case, do you have an opinion as to whether Dr. Madison violated the standard of care in his treatment of Mrs. Kamianka on the morning of November 6th?
**A.** Yes.

**Q.** Are these opinions based upon reasonable medical probability?
**A.** They certainly are. All the opinions are more likely than not, at the very least. The opinion is that the standard of care—in other words, what a reasonably prudent physician would do under similar circumstances, was not upheld. That was not done.

**Q.** What is the basis of that opinion?
**A.** You can make it complicated or simple. I think simple is best. This was not an exceptional case in any way. This was a 39 year-old woman who came to the ED with chest pain about 5 in the morning and it's described many times in the chart. It's true it included some words like sharp, front and back, but also was described as pain between the shoulder blades, radiation down the arm, and also midsternal chest pressure. When a 39 year-old person comes in with those complaints, in our society, an ECG is mandatory. It's not a judgment. It's not a thought. It's mandatory. And that wasn't done. The tragic thing is 10 or 12 hours later the patient died of coronary disease. It is virtually certain that if a simple ECG, which costs almost nothing, they charge about $40 for it but the actual cost is nothing, and it's non-invasive … almost certainly would have been abnormal and would have saved her life.

**Q.** I want to back up a step here, Doctor. You said it's mandatory, it's required—it's not a matter of judgment. There has been testimony in this case that the physician has judgment when it comes to deciding what tests to order when a patient presents to the ER with various complaints. Why do you say in this instance there is no room for judgment?
**A.** I think that's a fair question because, you know, it's not like in emergency medicine most things are cut and dry. It's actually hard to think of things that are, but this is one. The fact is that this isn't a rare disease, this is coronary disease. Half the people in this room are going to die of it. Every single person has a relative or a friend that has died of a heart attack. We are in this business to find this disease. Amazingly enough, we have a pretty good test that's noninvasive, and it's pretty cheap: it's an ECG.

And it's just very clear that when people come in even without chest pain, [for example with] some of the other symptoms like nausea or vomiting, but certainly with midsternal pressure and radiation down the arm, in our society most lay people would know that—you have to do an ECG. Since it's such a common and lethal disease, that it is simply required. It doesn't matter if you think the person has bronchitis or is crazy, whatever you think, you still have to do the ECG.

**Q.** Does it matter what the potential risk is for the underlying condition when making the determination that an ECG has got to be done?
**A.** I think I see what you mean. Let's say, for example, a good careful physician honestly believed that the person was ten times as likely to have bronchitis as to have a heart attack. But you had a simple test that could rule out a heart attack with some good probability, or certainly could rule it in. Obviously, you would have to do it because if you miss the bronchitis, so what? It really doesn't matter. It's not even clear the treatment of bronchitis makes much difference. But when we're talking about ACS, that's one of about 5 conditions in emergency medicine that we are not allowed to miss. We only get one shot at it. So even when we have a very low suspicion, we have to go ahead and do the test to rule it out.

**Author comments (Weinstock):** Ok, ok, good arguments. Still, in the middle of cold and flu season? Did these arguments sway the jury?

## IV. The Verdict

**Judge's instructions to jury (shortened):** Good morning ladies and gentlemen. Welcome back. The evidence portion of the trial has now concluded. As I indicated, you're going to hear the instructions of law and the arguments of counsel this morning.

By agreement of the parties, instead of hearing closing arguments first, you're going to hear the instructions of law from me.

In determining whether an issue has been proven by a preponderance of the evidence, you should consider all of the evidence, regardless of who produced it. If the weight of the evidence is equally balanced, or if you are unable to determine which side of an issue has the preponderance, the party who has the burden of proof has not established such issue. Specifically, the plaintiff alleges that Dr. Madison as a treating emergency medicine specialist was negligent in failing to work Anna Kamianka up for a potential cardiac problem.

The issues for you to decide are the following. Number 1, has the plaintiff proven that the defendant was negligent in one or more of the respective claims against him? Number 2, if your answer to this first question is yes, was such negligence a proximate cause of the injuries and damages sustained, including death of the decedent?

**Author comments (Weinstock):** The judge goes on to define how the jury is to make their decision. Read closely, since this will be important later:

**Additional judge's instructions to the jury:** Although some other physician might have used a different method of diagnosis, treatment or procedure than that used by Dr. Madison, this will not by itself prove that Dr. Madison was negligent. The mere fact that Dr. Madison used an alternative method of diagnosis, treatment or procedure is not by itself proof of negligence. You are to decide whether the diagnosis, treatment, or procedure used by Dr. Madison was reasonable in accordance with the standard of care required of a physician in his field of practice.

**Plaintiff's attorney, Mr. August.** Objection! To preserve the record, your honor, I would like to renew the plaintiff 's objections to the charge or the absence of certain charges. First of all, the plaintiff objects to the inclusion of a charge on "different methods" because we believe the evidence in this case does not support the giving of that charge.
**The Court (Judge):** Okay, right, well, your objection is noted.

**Author comments (Weinstock):** Well, it all seems reasonable to me … but I'm no judge. The following is the jury verdict:

**The Court:** My bailiff has informed me you have reached a verdict
**Jury Foreman:** Yes.
**The Court:** Will the foreman please hand the verdict forms over? (Tendered)
**The Court:** All right. Has the plaintiff, Mike Kamianka, proven by a preponderance of the evidence that defendant, Timothy Madison, was negligent? (Reads.) The answer is "no." This is signed by seven jurors.

**Summary:** The jury found in favor of the defendant physician 7–1

## V. The Appeal—March 1st Approximately 1 1/2 years after the trial verdict

**Author comments (Weinstock):** But this was not the end of the story … The actual patient encounter occurred on November 6, and after an extensive legal process and a huge sigh of relief, the doctor is absolved. Now, almost five years after the initial patient visit, the doctor is informed the jury's decision has been appealed. Ugghh!

The following is the plaintiff's allegation for appeal and the defense argument against appeal.

**Plaintiff:** The trial court erred in instructing the jury, over plaintiff's objection, that there were different methods of diagnosing the plaintiff's decedent's medical condition when there was no evidence that more than one method is acceptable to diagnose coronary artery disease. Kamianka argues that the trial court should not have given the "different methods" jury instruction, because the expert testimony established that the only acceptable method of definitively diagnosing coronary artery disease is a cardiac work-up. Kamianka contends that this instruction misled the jury in a matter substantially affecting Kamianka's rights.

**Defense:** Dr. Madison argues that the instruction was proper because the trial testimony established that acceptable alternative methods of diagnosis existed for Mrs. Kamianka's condition, i.e., chest pain associated with a cough.

**Appeals court impression:** Although this instruction has been found appropriate under the facts of certain cases, it is concerning that different methods for diagnosis, treatment and procedure are all encompassed under this one instruction rather than parsed out. However, where the issue involved is whether the physician negligently failed to diagnose a particular disease from the observed symptoms, the instruction is misleading to the jury. In such a case, the instruction implies that even where multiple conditions may exist (bronchitis or coronary artery disease), as long as the physician followed a method for diagnosing one of the potential conditions, the doctor may be absolved of negligence. The question here is not whether the physician followed an accepted method for diagnosing bronchitis, but rather, whether the physician failed to recognize that the observed symptoms indicated the presence of heart disease.

Accordingly, we conclude that the trial court erred. The issue is not whether the doctors chose between two recognized methods of diagnosis, but whether they negligently failed to recognize that Mrs. Kamianka's symptoms required that they perform a cardiac work-up to rule out coronary artery disease. Chest pain and coughing were the symptoms, not the diagnosis. Kamianka's assignment of error is sustained.

**Judgment:** Reversed and remanded. It is ordered that appellant [plaintiff] recover from appellee [defendant] costs herein taxed. The court finds there were reasonable grounds for this appeal.

**Author comments (Weinstock):** Wow! How about going through years of depositions and a long trial which rules in your favor, only to have the defense verdict overruled two years later on what seems like a technicality?

## VI. The Twist

It is surprising what happens next: instead of proceeding to a new trial, the defense decides to settle. Settle? After winning? How much did they get? Below is an interview with the actual defense attorney, Mark Jones, who reveals their reasoning.

## VII. Guest Interview—The Legal Analysis

**Mark Jones, JD**
Roetzel & Andress, LPA
Cleveland, Ohio
(Actual defense attorney in this case)

**Authors.** We are doctors, trained to use our clinical judgment and not "cookbook" patients. How did you respond to the plaintiff's expert's allegations that an ECG always needs to be done?
**MJ.** Plaintiff focused on the complaint of chest pain and made the valid point that chest pain from coronary ischemia in women can deviate dramatically from the "classic presentation," placing the ED physician on notice that an ECG is always required. The defense focused on the primary presenting complaint being a severe cough, with associated chest pain. The defense argued that:

1. A presenting complaint of chest pain is so common in the ED and can arise from any number of causes that it would be unreasonable for the standard of care to demand ECGs for all chest pain presentations.
2. All chest pain is not the same, and medical judgment informed by experience and the particulars of the presentation establishes the standard of care.
3. It was reasonable for the ED physician to conclude from the totality of the presentation that the likelihood of coronary ischemia was very low and the likelihood of severe bronchitis was quite high.

**Authors.** Before the initial trial, did you consider settling? How confident were you that a defense verdict would prevail?
**MJ.** Yes, settlement was considered. Significant efforts to settle were undertaken prior to trial, but the demand remained too high. Plaintiff had a well-respected expert and much of the medical literature was supportive of his argument. Prior to the start of trial, it was felt that a defense verdict was a 50–50 proposition. As trial proceeded I became more confident of a defense verdict.

**Authors.** Were you surprised with the jury's verdict?
**MJ.** No. A jury is capable of coming to any result, and sometimes I am elated by the verdict, sometimes disappointed. Although I am often surprised by events during the trial of a case, I am never surprised by a jury verdict. In this case, it seemed the strident testimony of plaintiff's expert turned the jury off to his testimony; this was not his demeanor at his deposition some months earlier. I was pleasantly surprised by my client's testimony at trial; although he had never been a witness and was very anxious, he presented himself to the jury as confident, competent and thorough. It was this combination of plaintiff's expert's poor presentation and the defendant's very good presentation that carried the day.

**Authors.** Why did you lose the appeal?
**MJ.** Plaintiff appealed on an issue regarding the instructions of law given to the jury. Although it was unlikely that the one instruction faulted had any impact on deliberations, it was not an instruction supported by the evidence presented at trial. The appellate court found error in giving the instruction and sent the case back for trial on all issues.

**Authors.** If you won once, why did you think you couldn't win again?
**MJ.** The defense felt that in re-trying the case, plaintiff's counsel would adjust his presentation and avoid problems the defense took advantage of in the first trial, and therefore the likelihood of a defense verdict

would still be a 50–50 proposition. At trial I was able to take advantage of some inexperience on the part of plaintiff's expert witnesses, an advantage I would lose at a retrial. The doctor was also exhausted by the whole process and wanted to end it.

**Authors.** What was the settlement amount?
**MJ.** In settlement negotiations the demand became very reasonable (though I can't reveal the exact amount).

## VIII. Medical Discussion—Evaluation of Chest Pain

**Guest Authors:**
**Leen Alblaihed, MBBS, MHA**
Assistant Professor
Department of Emergency Medicine
University of Maryland School of Medicine

**Emilie C. Murray, MD, JD, MPH**
Medical Director of Quality & Safety
Attending Physician, Dept. of Emergency Medicine
MedStar Franklin Square Medical Center
Assistant Professor of Clinical Emergency Medicine, Georgetown University School of Medicine

**Amal Mattu, MD**
Professor and Vice Chair
Department of Emergency Medicine
University of Maryland School of Medicine

The American College of Emergency Physicians (ACEP) defines Emergency Medicine (EM) as "the medical specialty dedicated to the diagnosis and treatment of unforeseen illness or injury."[1] As such, we are trained to "rule out the worst" before considering the "most likely" cause for the patient's presenting symptoms.

In this case, Anna had chest pain, back pain, and shoulder pain. None of these were adequately assessed. Using mnemonics such as **"OLDCAAARS"** helps with cognitive unloading and to ensure that key aspects of the history of present illness (HPI) are obtained (a symptom-based approach). An alternative approach is to focus on the deadly causes of chest pain and tailor the history towards ruling those out (a diagnosis-based approach).

**O** – Onset
**L** – Location
**D** – Duration
**C** – Character
**A** – Alleviating/aggravating factors
**A** – Associated symptoms (ex. dyspnea, diaphoresis, nausea/vomiting)
**A** – Activity at onset

**R** – Radiation
**S** – Severity

When evaluating a patient with chest pain (or pain in any thoracic location), our primary focus is to risk stratify to a reasonably low level of suspicion the "killer causes of chest pain," such as acute coronary syndrome (ACS), pulmonary embolism (PE), aortic dissection, as well as pericardial tamponade/myocarditis, tension pneumothorax, and esophageal rupture Boerhaave syndrome. We can accomplish this by performing a thorough medical history and physical exam and, if necessary, obtaining appropriate lab work and imaging. Chest pain accounts for approximately 6% of all ED visits, with 10–20% suffering from an acute coronary syndrome (ACS).[2]

One approach to diagnosis is to think of the pain/concern area as a "box" filled with organs that might have "holes, plugs or inflammation." For example, the esophagus is an organ within the "chest box:" Is there a hole in the esophagus? (i.e., Boerhaave syndrome). Is there a plug (i.e., stricture, food impaction)? Is there inflammation or infection? (i.e., esophagitis). This approach can be applied to the other organs in the box including the heart and coronary arteries, the aorta and other blood vessels.

Missed or delayed diagnosis of acute myocardial infarction (AMI), just like in Anna's case, represents a very common reason for medical malpractice litigation in the United States.[3–6] In 2020, 2 in 10 deaths from CAD occurred in adults younger than 65 years-old.[7] AMI is not just a disease of the "elderly."

ACS is the umbrella term used for acute cardiac ischemia and/or infarction. Mortality has been increasing in women aged 35–54 with risk factors unique to women including autoimmune/inflammatory diseases, Polycystic Ovary Syndrome (PCOS), early menopause, preeclampsia, gestational diabetes and hypertension.[8] Traditional risk factors such as smoking and diabetes disproportionately increase the relative risk of ACS in women more than men. In one study, more than 7 times in women aged 35–44 when compared to men.[9,10] In addition, compared with age-matched men, women younger than 45 years of age with ACS are 6 times more likely to die.[11]

Chest pain is the most common presenting symptom in ACS but women are more likely than men to present without chest pain, especially in those younger than 45 years of age.[12] Interestingly, among women with ACS who presented without chest pain, "anginal equivalents" such as dyspnea, weakness, fatigue, and pain in the neck, jaw or upper back were reported instead.[13] Anna had many of these symptoms. Additionally, one wonders what was meant during the visit with her primary care doctor when she mentioned that she "doesn't feel well." Was this her anginal equivalent? In fact, the autopsy suggests that she recently had an MI, quite possibly 2 months previously when treated for "bronchitis" by her primary care physician. Autopsy diagnosis #3: *"Remote, organizing and acute myocardial infarcts."*

When we talk about "typical" chest pain we usually refer to pain that is severe and acute in onset, most often on the left side, exertional, associated with shortness of breath and a choking sensation. Further studies over the past years looked at chest pain features that best predicted AMI. Pain that was accompanied by diaphoresis or vomiting, radiation of the pain (especially to both arms), and pain that was worsened with exertion were among the greatest predictors of AMI. On the other hand, reproducible chest wall tenderness, pain that was pleuritic, sharp or positional were features that decreased the likelihood of ACS.[1,3] Dezman, et al. wrote a compelling article stating that in clinical practice it is not one factor that will make or break the diagnosis of ACS but the accumulation of many small factors that will tip the scale. In the case of chest pain and ACS, even if the patient has negative predictors of ACS noted above or the patient lacks any of the positive predictors, the remaining risk might still be too high for most clinicians to abandon the work-up. Therefore, the HPI and risk factors are often of limited value for "ruling in" or "ruling out" ACS unless there is a clear alternative reason for the chest pain.[3] Thus, almost always, patients with chest pain, especially chest pain with concerning features such as diaphoresis, vomiting, radiation, or exertional pain will require further evaluation with troponins, ECGs, and possibly provocative testing.

Over the past decade, many clinical decision support tools and accelerated diagnostic pathways (ADPs) have been developed, verified and are increasingly being used in the clinical setting to aid in the management and disposition of patients presenting to the ED with chest pain. The goal is to determine the level of risk for patients with possible ACS and support the appropriate testing and disposition.[2] Among the pathways used most frequently in the ED are the HEART Pathway and EDACS. EDACS had a sensitivity over 99% for major adverse cardiac event (MACE),[14] and the HEART pathway found that low risk patients had a 0.4% chance of experiencing death or MI at 30 days.[15]

Unfortunately, neither the HEART score/pathway or EDACS would be able to be calculated without an ECG or troponin, but even with an assessment of history, age and risk factors, Anna would have had a score of 4 on the HEART score, putting her at moderate risk.

In recent years, many emergency departments have begun utilizing highly sensitivity cardiac troponin (hs-cTn) assays when evaluating patients with chest pain. Approximately one-third of patients can have ACS ruled out with a single blood test, and up to two thirds could have an acute myocardial infarction ruled out with a second sample taken after as little as 1 hr.[16]

As we read through the case, a few things jump out:

1. The triage note has a scary description of chest pain "killers." "Chest pain plus back pain, vomiting, and pain radiating to the arm" elicit thoughts of thoracic aortic dissection and ACS. Pain that wakes anyone from sleep is concerning, as occurred here. Although her pain is not specified to be associated with exertion (it was unknown to the emergency physician that the patient had chest discomfort with exertion the night before), there are features concerning for ACS such as radiation to the right arm in addition to the vomiting. Furthermore, her pain was described as pressure on the triage note.
2. There are clear discrepancies between the physician's note and the triage note. In the physician's HPI, the chief complaint seems focused more on the cough rather than the pain itself, and the chest pain is described as "sharp" and worse with coughing. The vomiting is described as "post-tussive," related to severe bouts of coughing.
3. In the HPI, the documentation of chest pain is inadequate. There is little-to-no mention of the pain's onset, exact location, duration, alleviating or relieving factors, associated symptoms (this was mentioned partially), or radiation (not mentioned on HPI but mentioned in triage note). What about her back pain? What about any recent trauma? Are the symptoms she has now similar to when she was diagnosed with "bronchitis?"
4. It seems that the HPI is written to reflect what the physician wanted the diagnosis to be. Note that the HPI revolves around the cough. For example, the pain is when she coughs and the vomiting is described as post-tussive. All of this does not match what the triage note mentioned, which got our alarm bells ringing.
5. One point brought up by the plaintiff's attorney was that the ECG would have nailed the diagnosis. I am not sure that is an accurate statement. ECGs have a diagnostic sensitivity of approximately

40% for ACS.[17] However, the ECG is a relatively inexpensive medical test, and deferring its use in patients with chest pain is often difficult to defend.

6. The plaintiff's attorney pointed out that cardiac risk factors should have been elicited. What we have come to know of as the "classic" ACS risk factors (age, hypertension, hyperlipidemia, diabetes, obesity, smoking history, and early family history of CAD in a first degree relative) are effective for population use, but not necessarily for patients who come to the ED. Nearly 12% of patients will not report known classic risk factors with acute myocardial infarction.[18] On the other hand, recent literature states that early family history of CAD is an independent risk factor for MI, especially in first degree relatives in those younger than 55.[19] In the case we have, a young patient who presents with chest pain who has a brother who died at the age of 32 from an MI, and so, it should be difficult to dismiss concerns for ACS.

When all is said and done, who has the better argument?

- In favor of the plaintiff: Here's a 39 year-old woman with multiple cardiac risk factors, presenting with midsternal chest pressure radiating to the right arm and vomiting. The physician focused on her cough instead of doing what a good emergency physician is supposed to do—rule out the life threats! He did a lackluster history, didn't pay attention to the clues the nursing notes were giving him and didn't even do a cheap, simple test that would have saved her life. He took the easy way out by clinging to a benign diagnosis and now Anna Kamianka is dead!
- In favor of the defendant: This patient's presentation was entirely consistent with a non-cardiac presentation so much so that even an ECG was not indicated. As the chart shows, she had a cough productive of yellow sputum, post-tussive vomiting with back pain and sharp chest pain directly related to the cough. She improved after treatment. Show me the literature that indicates that ACS presents with a productive cough and wheezing that resolves with aerosols!
- We know that ECGs are usually non-diagnostic. So, if you are going to argue that this patient needed an ECG, you must also be arguing that this patient needed an admission and full work-up. That means that everyone showing up in the ED with a chest cold must be admitted!

This is a tough call. In fact, we the authors disagree on which side has the stronger argument, but we all agree that the case could go either way based on the likeability and believability of the expert witnesses and defendant. We also agree that extra time spent on the HPI and MDM would have likely prevented this lawsuit, and possibly the patient's bad outcome.

In conclusion, this case highlights important points and lessons to be learned:

- **Be thorough:** When it comes chest pain, it is tough to risk stratify for killer causes such as ACS without a thorough, detailed history, and physical exam.
- **Good documentation:** Many providers will habitually ask the patient all the right questions and obtain a detailed history and exam and exercise appropriate medical decision-making, but then fail to document it in the record. Remember the traditional lawyers' mantra: "If it was not documented, it didn't happen."
- **Address discrepancies:** The physician's documentation reflects a non-cardiac presentation of pleuritic chest pain and cough very consistent with bronchitis and relieved with aerosol medication. However, the triage note paints a different picture of a more sinister cause of chest pain, and these differences were not addressed or explained.

Without these approaches, the best a physician can do is cross their fingers when the summons and complaint are received.

## IX. Author Summary (Weinstock)

What can we learn from this case? Bronchitis is a dime a dozen—and who has bronchitis without any chest pain? We get that this was a tough diagnosis... but what if these points had been considered?

- When a patient has URI symptoms and chest pain, inquire about exertional pain or associated dyspnea or diaphoresis. If that had been done in this case, the doctor would have learned a fact we have not yet discussed: Though it may sound indelicate, it was brought up at trial that Anna and her husband had "relations" the night of her MI, and the exertion caused chest pain.
- Though multiple-complaint patients are time-consuming and often frustrating, each complaint still needs to be specifically addressed no matter how obvious the diagnosis, no matter how much static on the language line, no matter how long they have had fibromyalgia …
- Not to sound too much like a broken record, but "read the nurse's notes, read the nurse's notes, read the nurse's notes …"
- When the findings on evaluation do not mesh with the chief complaints, explain your thought process in a progress note. If the note is not convincing even to you, go back to the bedside, confirm the history and ensure life-threatening diagnoses are not occurring.
- Have a low threshold for performing an ECG in patients with chest pain.

It turns out the key to almost all of the cases in this book is low tech. Though this physician "won" the case (at least before the appeal), our goal is greater; to move from "standard of care" to "excellence in care"—our recommendations: Get a great history and document consideration of life-threatening illness!

## References


1. Gulati M, Levy PD, Mukherjee D, et al. 2021 AHA/ACC/ASE/CHEST/ SAEM/SCCT/SCMR Guideline for the evaluation and diagnosis of chest pain: A Report of the American College of Cardiology/American Heart Association Joint Committee on Clinical Practice Guidelines [published correction appears in Circulation 2021 Nov 30;144(22):e455]. Circulation 2021;144(22):e368-e454. doi:10.1161/CIR.0000000000001029.
2. Huis in 't Veld MA, Cullen L, Mahler SA, et al. The fast and the furious: Low-risk chest pain and the rapid rule-out protocol. West J Emerg Med 2017;18(3):474-78. doi:10.5811/westjem.2016.12.32676.
3. Dezman Z, Mattu A, Body R. Utility of the history and physical examination in the detection of acute coronary syndromes in emergency department patients. West J Emerg Med 2017;18(4):752-60. doi:10.5811/westjem.2017.3.32666.
4. Katz DA, Williams GC, Brown RL, et al. Emergency physicians' fear of malpractice in evaluating patients with possible acute cardiac ischemia. Ann Emerg Med 2005;46(6):525-33. doi:10.1016/j.annemergmed.2005.04.016.
5. Brown TW, McCarthy ML, Kelen GD, et al. An epidemiologic study of closed emergency department malpractice claims in a national database of physician malpractice insurers. Acad Emerg Med 2010;17(5):553-60. doi:10.1111/j.1553-2712.2010.00729.x.
6. Wong KE, Parikh PD, Miller KC, et al. Emergency department and urgent care medical malpractice claims 2001-15. West J Emerg Med 2021;22(2):333-338. Published 2021 Feb 15. doi:10.5811/

westjem.2020.9.48845.
7. Tsao CW, Aday AW, Almarzooq ZI, et al. Heart disease and stroke statistics—2022 update: A report from the American Heart Association. Circulation 2022;145(8):e153-e639. doi:10.1161/CIR.0000000000001052.
8. Young L, Cho L. Unique cardiovascular risk factors in women. Heart 2019;105(21):1656-60. doi:10.1136/heartjnl-2018-314268.
9. Yusuf S, Hawken S, Ôunpuu S, et al. Effect of potentially modifiable risk factors associated with myocardial infarction in 52 countries (the INTERHEART study):Case-control study. Lancet 2004;364(9438):937-952. doi:10.1016/S0140-6736(04)17018-9.
10. Njølstad I, Arnesen E, Lund-Larsen PG. Smoking, serum lipids, blood pressure, and sex differences in myocardial infarction. Circulation 1996;93(3):450-56. doi:10.1161/01.CIR.93.3.450.
11. Ricci B, Cenko E, Vasiljevic Z, et al. Acute coronary syndrome: The risk to young women. J Am Heart Assoc 2017;6(12):e007519. doi:10.1161/JAHA.117.007519.
12. Canto JG, Rogers WJ, Goldberg RJ, et al. Association of age and sex with myocardial infarction symptom presentation and in-hospital mortality. JAMA 2012;307(8):813-22. doi:10.1001/jama.2012.199.
13. Canto JG. Symptom presentation of women with acute coronary syndromes. Arch Intern Med 2007;167(22):2405-13. doi:10.1001/archinte.167.22.2405.14.
14. Than M, Flaws D, Sanders S, et al. Development and validation of the Emergency Department Assessment of Chest Pain Score and 2 h accelerated diagnostic protocol. Emerg Med Australas 2014;26(1):34-44. doi:10.1111/1742-6723.12164.
15. Mahler SA, Lenoir KM, Wells BJ, et al. Safely identifying emergency department patients with acute chest pain for early discharge. Circulation 2018;138(22):2456-68. doi:10.1161/CIRCULATIONAHA.118.036528.
16. Body R. Acute coronary syndromes diagnosis, version 2.0: Tomorrow's approach to diagnosing acute coronary syndromes? Turkish J Emerg Med 2018;18(3):94-9. doi:10.1016/j.tjem.2018.05.005.
17. Leisy PJ, Coeytaux RR, Wagner GS, et al. ECG-based signal analysis technologies for evaluating patients with acute coronary syndrome: A systematic review. J Electrocardiol 2013;46(2):92-7. doi:10.1016/j.jelectrocard.2012.11.010.
18. Body R, McDowell G, Carley S, et al. Do risk factors for chronic coronary heart disease help diagnose acute myocardial infarction in the emergency department? Resuscitation 2008;79(1):41-5. doi:10.1016/j.resuscitation.2008.06.009.
19. Ranthe MF, Petersen JA, Bundgaard H, et al. A detailed family history of myocardial infarction and risk of myocardial infarction–A nationwide cohort study. Aalto-Setala K, ed. PLoS One 2015;10(5):e0125896.

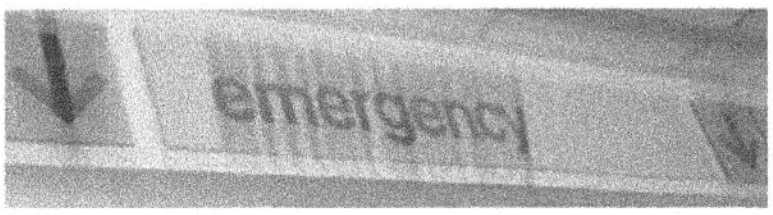


# Case 2

## A 42 Year-old Fireman with Shoulder Pain: When a Lifeline Becomes a Noose

**Primary case author:**
**David A. Talan**

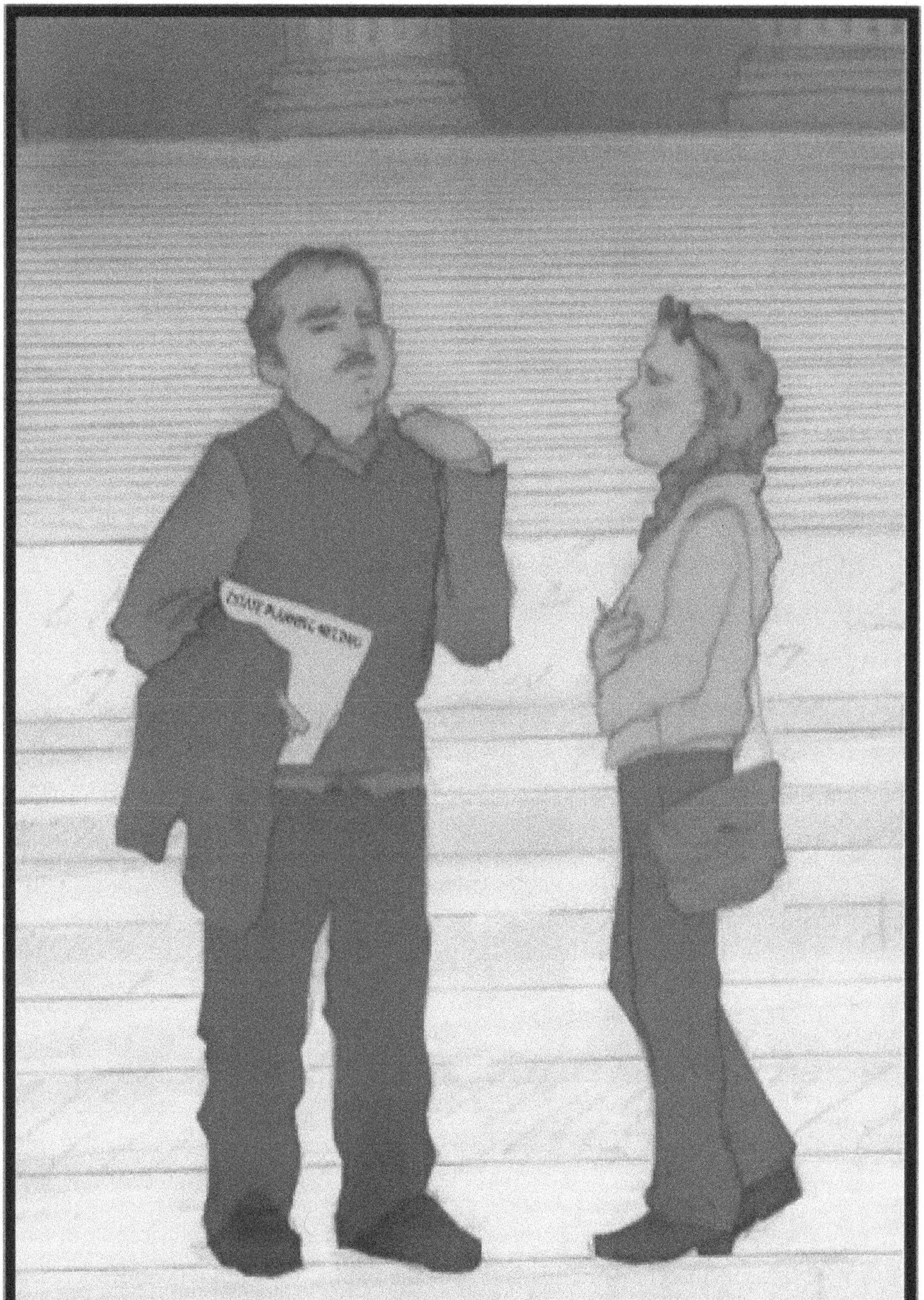

# Case 2

## A 42 Year-old Fireman with Shoulder Pain: When a Lifeline Becomes a Noose

This patient was initially seen by a PA who performed a history and physical, made a diagnosis, spoke with the primary care physician, and still asked the physician to see the patient and document a note. The physician re-examined the patient and documented a thorough note. This is curious; who goes to all this effort for a simple "shoulder strain?"

***Deep thoughts:***

1. *We are taught early in our careers that abdominal pain out of proportion to exam equals mesenteric ischemia. How about pain out of proportion to our diagnosis?*
2. *In addition to the HPI, what other historical information is important to obtain?*
3. *Does a referral from an urgent care or primary care physician obligate the ED doctor to perform certain tests?*
4. *How does a plaintiff's attorney use adverse outcomes to garner sympathy from a jury?*

**PART 1—MEDICAL**

## I. The Patient's Story

David Lykins is a loving father of three boys and devoted husband to Jill, currently 15 weeks pregnant with their 4th. His career started as a firefighter and paramedic, working his way up to Battalion Chief. David likes to spend as much time as possible with his family—Jill brings the boys to the firehouse every few days, and he spends several hours with them. His friend remembers, "To the kids, the firehouse was a big playground … he kept them running."

Co-worker John Bennett described David's approach as Battalion Chief: "He was very strict with us, but it was because he was concerned about our safety. You could tell he really cared. He was almost like a father, even though he was younger than [me]."

The following story of a squad run demonstrates David's dedication to his job. On February 24, a 911 call dispatched the team to the scene of a worker with his leg caught in an auger, "wrapped around like a piece of spaghetti." Though this was a new situation, David took charge and directed everyone, including officers of his own rank. During the 45 minutes that it took to extricate the worker, the worker said, "David talked to me, as I was laying there, waiting to get untrapped. [He] asked me how many kids I had and what my name was and, you know, tried to keep me conscious … After my accident I was in the hospital and Mr. Lykins came after a run and just checked on me to see how I was doing. I was lucky to be alive."

In the beginning of March, David begins to have problems of his own. He has severe left shoulder pain and presents to the Emergency Department at Shady Valley Hospital.

## II. The Doctor's Version (the following is the actual documentation of the provider)

**Chief Complaint per triage RN (March 2, at 10:30AM):** c/o left shoulder pain … (see below) Arrives via wheelchair (WC)

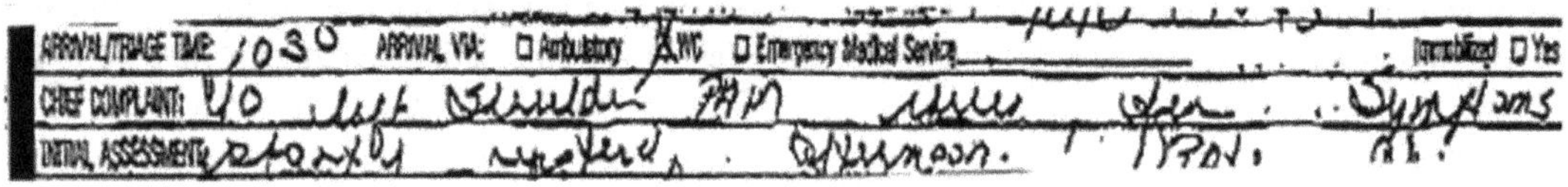


**Chief Complaint (physician assistant, Ed Heller) at 10:45:** This is a 42 year-old male who is a fire fighter for Fairtown. He says he was lifting patients yesterday. He complains of left shoulder pain. He says he is unable to move his left arm. He has had no trauma as far as a fall. He has done only lifting. He never had anything like this before. Review of systems is otherwise negative. There is no chest pain, shortness of breath, diarrhea or constipation. No dysuria. No numbness or tingling of the extremities. No peripheral edema.

**Past Medical History:**
**Allergies:** NKDA
**Meds:** None
**PMH:** He has a history of abdominal pain two weeks ago. CT scan was done. He does not know the results or what they were looking for. He is vomiting here possibly due to the pain.
**SH:** Unremarkable
**FH:** Unremarkable

**Date:** 3/2

Vital Signs

| Time | Temp(F) | Pulse | Resp | Syst | Diast |
|---|---|---|---|---|---|
| 10:30 | 97.8° F | 111 | 18 | 102 | 67 |

**Physical Examination:**
**Vital Signs:** As noted.
**General:** The patient is awake and alert.
**Extremity Exam:** He is somewhat inappropriate as far as pain and physical examination in relation to complaint and history. He refuses to move his arm. He is in an extreme amount of pain when I try to move his arm or touch him whether on his arm or on his clavicle. He has good grip. He is able to extend and flex his elbow and pronate and supinate. He has good distal light touch sensation, pulses and capillary refill.
**Abdomen:** Soft and nontender. He has good bowel sounds and no pain.
**Lungs:** Clear
**Heart:** Regular rate

**Testing (10:55):** Left shoulder and clavicle XR: No fracture of shoulder or clavicle

**Emergency Department Course:**
**11:05** – Dilaudid 1mg IM
**12:25** – Ondansetron 4 mg SL
**12:50** – Repeat vitals: Pulse 102, Resp 16, BP 102/65

**Medical Decision-Making Note (PA Ed Heller):** Left shoulder and clavicle X-rays show no acute fracture. We have given him 1 mg of Dilaudid and 4 mg of Ondansetron. We have put his arm in a left sling. We have told him to rest and no lifting. He is to return to the emergency department if worse. Soft diet. I talked with Dr. Oster [the primary care physician] who says the patient tends to sometimes overreact to his health care needs and it does not surprise him that the gentleman will not move his arm and that his physical examination is in proportion with his complaint and history. Dr. Oster will see him in the next two to three days. He is sent home with a prescription for Vicodin. He is to return to the emergency department if he is worse. The patient understands the instructions and agrees to comply. I have reviewed history, physical and clinical assessment of the patient with attending physician. Appropriate lab data, ECG and X-rays were discussed and agreed with final treatment plan and care. Patient was interviewed and examined by Dr. Vaughn.

**Diagnosis (12:57):** Left shoulder pain/strain

**Disposition:** Rx: Vicodin. Left arm in a sling with instructions to rest with no lifting. Apply ice and return to ED if worse. Soft diet. Dr. Oster will see him in the next two to three days.

**Attending Note:**
This is an attending note to accompany the dictation by the physician assistant.
HISTORY: The patient is a 42 year-old male who was seen with [Ed Heller] and disposition discussed. He is a healthy male firefighter. He apparently has had some left shoulder pain after doing some lifting of patients over the last couple of days. It is very painful with range of motion and any palpation. He has had no falls. He has no paresthesias or weakness to his arm. He has no abdominal pain, chest pain or shortness of breath. He has been vomiting. Apparently, these symptoms started roughly at the same time. He has had no fever. He has had no skin breaks to that shoulder. No other joints are involved.

**Physical Examination:**
**Vital Signs:** As noted.
**General:** The patient is awake and alert.
**Extremities:** He is very uncomfortable with any movement of his shoulder. On palpation, there is no erythema or swelling. No obvious injury to that area. Any movement of his shoulder causes pain. His left upper extremity neurovascular examination is intact.
**Abdomen:** Soft and nontender. He has good bowel sounds and no pain.
**Lungs:** Clear.
**Heart:**Regular rate.
**Medical Decision-Making Note (MDM):** I reviewed the X-ray of his shoulder and clavicle. The X-rays are normal. I do not see any evidence of a fracture or dislocation. The patient is vomiting and I do not have a good clue as to the cause of this, other than the pain from his shoulder. We have given him Ondansetron on two occasions with some improvement. We have put him home to bedrest with a sling for no greater than three days, Vicodin for pain, and Ondansetron as needed. He is in stable condition at this time. This looks to be more musculoskeletal and certainly I see no evidence of any referred pain.

This is very joint specific. There is nothing on his examination or in his history that makes me think this is a septic joint.

*Ed Heller, PA*
*Timothy Vaughn, DO*

## III. Risk Management/Patient Safety Opportunities (Weinstock)

**Author comments (Weinstock):** This seems like a straightforward shoulder strain, pain with motion and palpation. But is this the whole story?

**Risk Management/Patient Safety Opportunity #1:**

**Opportunity:** Not reading nursing notes.
**Discussion:** Can you decipher the hieroglyphics recorded by the nurse? Neither could the doctor. We get "complains of left shoulder pain" (barely). There was no effort to speak with the nurse to discover what was recorded. Her deposition testimony on November 8 (8 months after the patient presented), finally revealed the answer:

**Q. (plaintiff's lawyer):** Please read slowly so I can understand.
**A. (triage nurse):** "Complains of left shoulder pain, chills, fever."

If there is a discrepancy, hit this head on. For example: "The triage nurse documented that the child was 'lethargic.' I asked the patient to clarify and they stated that yesterday the child took a longer nap than usual, but currently is acting normally…or…I asked the patient about their complaint of fever and they said they checked their temperature, and it was 99.2 degrees." The triage nurse is part of the health care team, and the patient will sometimes provide information when they arrive that they do not relate to the clinician. Not reading the nurses'/triage notes is a common theme in medical malpractice cases.
✔ **Teaching point:** ALWAYS read the nurses' notes. If not able to be understood, speak with them personally.

**Risk Management/Patient Safety Opportunity #2:**

**Opportunity:** History inconsistent with the proposed mechanism.
**Discussion:** It is recorded that the patient had been lifting—but when? How soon after the lifting did the pain start? It brings to mind one of my favorite anecdotes in the vomiting patient, "I ate at McDonald's last night." OK. So did 30 million other people! If a patient lifts all day, every day and has shoulder pain one of those days, it is important to correlate if the pain started when lifting or at some point after.

This documentation does not build a case for a reliable mechanism. After all, most patients will offer a convenient history, convenient for you and for them. It isn't to intentionally mislead you, it's just what makes sense; patients don't want to be sick and will often offer an excuse to lead you toward the most benign diagnosis. You can choose to accept his "history" of overreaction without qualification or pursue further history to verify its relevance.
✔ **Teaching point:** Just because most patients with shoulder pain have a strain, doesn't mean they all do.

**Risk Management/Patient Safety Opportunity #3:**

**Opportunity:** Too narrow of a differential diagnosis.
**Discussion:** Could shoulder pain in a 42 year-old man be from a cardiac etiology? Absolutely! Questioning about exertional symptoms, associated symptoms of diaphoresis and dyspnea (which ***was*** recorded), and cardiac risk factors is advisable. An ECG is a simple and inexpensive screening test.
✔ **Teaching point:** Maintain a high index of suspicion for atypical presentations of life-threatening diagnoses. Everyone is sick until you prove they aren't.

**Risk Management/Patient Safety Opportunity #4:**

**Opportunity:** Including conjecture in the note.
**Discussion:** This point could be argued since it may be important to note that a "patient tends to sometimes overreact to his health care needs," but it does up the ante. We have a 42 year-old Battalion Chief with a new complaint of shoulder pain to the point that he needs to be brought back to his room in a wheelchair. That would be a serious overreaction. Additionally, how does this information factor into the medical decision-making process? Though not overtly stated, we can surmise from the note that for some reason, there was extra concern about this patient; who calls the PCP for a simple shoulder strain? If there was any doubt about the diagnosis before the call, it was laid to rest after learning about his "history" of overreaction.
✔ **Teaching point:** Be careful about including speculative comments in the chart. If you are right, it didn't matter anyway. If you are wrong, such comments will have a profound impact on your defense.

**Author comments (Weinstock):** As it turns out, our patient's pain actually started the day prior, on March 1. This is also part of the "ancient Egyptian writing" recorded by the triage nurse: "symptoms started yesterday afternoon."

**March 1:**
3:00 PM (one day before ED visit): David and his wife Jill have a meeting with a lawyer to discuss estate-planning matters. As they leave the office, David comments that his shoulder is bothering him.
11:00 PM: The pain is stronger and he has a low grade fever. Jill gives him two 800 mg ibuprofen.
**March 2:**
8:00 AM: Jill calls Dr. Oster, the PCP, and finds out David cannot be seen until 11 AM. He is unable to wait that long, so is referred to an urgent care.

**Back to the Future—The Urgent Care record per Dr. Benjamin Roth:**

**Triage (9:39AM)** - Complains of intense pain left shoulder which began yesterday
**History:** Pt. works for fire dept, was lifting patients, pain started hours after. Has headache, nausea, vomiting and feels dehydrated. Pt. feels it is not cardiac related but like it's in the muscle. Pt. iced and took ibuprofen. Unable to move shoulder, had fever all night, couldn't sleep secondary to the pain.
**PE:** Vitals: temp 97.5, pulse 116, resp 16, BP 120/78. Possibly swollen, extremely tender, no redness. ROM is zero. A&O x 3
**Urgent Care course:** Vomited in clinic x 1
**Diagnosis:** Severe left shoulder pain, needs septic arthritis ruled out
**Doctor Note:** Discussed with ER at Shady Valley. Will send him down there for evaluation.

*Benjamin Roth, MD*

**Author comments (Weinstock):** It is questionable if the ED doctor was aware that the patient was at the urgent care prior to the ED visit; he did note "This is very joint specific" but never specifically mentioned the referral. "There is nothing on his examination or in his history that makes me think this is a septic joint." Was this documented because of the concern of the urgent care doctor, because of a concern of David or Jill, or a concern of the ED doctor or PA? The same diagnosis that troubled the urgent care doctor is mentioned (septic joint), but no other reference is made to the urgent care visit.

When the records were eventually subpoenaed, the hospital was unable to find the urgent care "call-in sheet" or the urgent care record that was sent with the patient. However, the plaintiff's attorney was able to find them both, blowing them up into 4 × 5 foot posters displayed during the trial.

**Risk Management/Patient Safety Opportunity #5:**

**Opportunity:** Not speaking with the urgent care doctor.
**Discussion:** I have sent patients home without the testing recommended by the urgent care, but only after careful consideration and discussion with the patient and the family. For example, a child referred for brain scan after a fall has some radiation risk—with a parental expectation of imaging, they want to be involved in the decision-making process, but usually follow your recommendation to defer scanning. Was the urgent care doctor's concern reasonable? To summarize, we have a healthy 42 year-old man with severe shoulder pain, fever (possibly masked by the use of ibuprofen at home) and no definitive mechanism suggesting a muscle strain. Searching for another cause of fever would be helpful. Does he have rhinorrhea and cough (typical in March). Further defining what is meant by fever would also be helpful (felt warm or recorded temperature of 100.4° with thermometer). Discovering the timing of an antipyretic can be helpful.
✔ **Teaching point:** When there is a difference of opinion, speaking with the transferring/referring physician (urgent care or PCP doctor) may allow discovery of important information.

**Risk Management/Patient Safety Opportunity #6:**

**Opportunity:** Lost records.
**Discussion:** Thou shall not kill. Do unto others as you would do unto yourself. Medical records should not be lost. These statements are all so obvious that they don't really justify the ink and parchment that they are printed on, unless somehow, they are not obeyed.
✔ **Teaching point:** A mechanism needs to exist to ensure that the records provided by the referring doctor are available to the treating ED physician.

**Author comments (Weinstock):** As a closing thought, assuming he was aware of the urgent care visit, kudos to the ED physician who did an independent examination, assessment and documentation of the patient. This could have easily been omitted in a patient with a "simple shoulder strain."

## IV. The Bounceback

David is discharged from the ED at 12:57 PM, and his wife drives him to the pharmacy to pick up his prescription for Vicodin. On the way, they stop for gas. David vomits, then gets out of the car and urinates on the gas pump. When they arrive at home, David goes to bed. Jill can hear him moaning in pain.

- **Midnight** – His pain is increasing, and David asks Jill for pain medicine.
- **2:00 AM** – He asks for more pain medication.
- **3:30 AM** – Jill calls Dr. Oster (PCP). An "on call" doctor returns the call and tells her to go back to the ED if worse or wait until the morning and see Dr. Oster first thing. David says he does not want to return to the ED because they did not do anything for him when he was there earlier.
- **6:30 AM** – David is up and wants to take a bath before going to see Dr. Oster. Jill notices reddening and swelling of David's arm up to the shoulder. It looks like a bruise.
- **8:30 AM** – David presents to Dr. Oster's office with the complaint of shoulder pain and nausea. The pain is excruciating. "The patient is hyperventilating and is acutely ill appearing with edema over the left shoulder to the nipple and over the sternum, medially, but no discoloration, warmth or erythema. There is marked pain with motion of shoulder." He is sent immediately to ED.
- Per PCP, "Spoke with ED doctor who accepts the patient."

**ED visit #2—March 3**—Almost 22 hours after the initial ED discharge.

- **10:15 AM** – Temp 91.3, pulse 61, resp 20, BP 93/80. The ED team jumps into action.
- **10:25 AM** – David is seen by Dr. Timothy Vaughn (same doctor as yesterday): "Extremely ill-appearing and much worse than when I had seen him yesterday. Skin on chest is ecchymotic and some areas of necrosis and crepitation are noted underneath. We immediately initiated 2 large bore IV's."
- **10:40 AM** – Acute change in vitals: pulse increases to 145 and SBP drops to 70→IV fluids and dopamine.
- **10:50 AM** – Blood cultures taken. Started on Timentin and Clindamycin.
- CBC is normal. Creatinine is 2.5. Elevated LFT'S.
- **Assessment:** Extremely critical condition with probable multi-system failure, probably from sepsis secondary to some underlying myofascial infection. Dr. Anderson, general surgeon, is called to the ED to evaluate the patient and observes a discolored, darkened spot about the size of a fifty-cent piece which grows to the size of a softball in a short period of time.

**ED Diagnosis:**

1. Acute soft tissue infection left side of chest.
2. Septic shock.
3. Multiple organ failure with acute renal and hepatic failure.

- 11:30 AM – Taken from the ED to CT scan suite to define extent of the process. Results show necrotizing fasciitis of left anterior chest wall and possibly upper, anterior mediastinum.

**Hospital Course:**

- **12:15 PM** – From CT, the patient is immediately taken to surgery. Dr. Anderson performs extensive debridement of the left anterior chest wall. Following the surgery, Anderson was "a little encouraged" because the infection was not more extensive.
- David undergoes a second, "re-look" operation approximately 12 hours later. The infection has not extended beyond the margins of the first operation, no more necrotic tissue is discovered; it appears that the surgery has controlled the infection.
- David is found to have acute inflammation of the gall bladder and further surgery confirms this diagnosis, but also shows right colonic necrosis, which necessitates a right hemicolectomy. This is thought to be from the vasopressors.
- The renal failure worsens, requiring dialysis.
- He suffers extensive necrosis of the digits of both hands and feet.
- Diagnosis of ARDS—he remains on the ventilator.
- David continues a slow, but steady, downward spiral. After a multidisciplinary assessment, it is determined that he does not have a chance of recovering. This is discussed with the family, and comfort measures are taken.

- With his family in attendance, David expires on March 17, exactly 2 weeks after his bounceback visit.

**Final Diagnosis:** Necrotizing myositis, septic shock, ARF, ARDS, multisystem organ failure.

# PART 2—LEGAL

**Author comments (Weinstock):** It is sometimes tough when a patient arrives in the ED from the UC with an expectation of testing or care. "The doctor sent me here for an MRI of my knee. ..." Really? On a Sunday? The wrinkle in this case is we don't know if the ED doctor was aware of the Urgent Care visit or the history of fevers. Additionally, the nurse's triage note was illegible. Both these issues were pivotal to the plaintiff's case.

There are two ways to look at this patient. Imagine hearing it presented in one sentence at an M&M conference:

*1. This is a 42 year-old healthy fireman who was lifting patients and presents with shoulder pain, worse with movement. Impression: I see this patient every day. I see this patient ten times a day. I eat this patient for breakfast. ... ibuprofen, pain control, sling, bye bye. ...*
*2. This is a 42 year-old healthy fireman who has fever and shoulder pain so severe that the range of motion is zero. He was sent from an urgent care to r/o septic arthritis. Impression: Now I'm not so sure ...*

What happened at the gas station? ***La belle indifference:*** An apathetic demeanor observed in patients with necrotizing fasciitis/myositis. French term meaning "beautiful ignorance." This is a metabolic encephalopathy due to the underlying necrotic process.

Mr. Lykins was obviously in the throes of the disease at the initial ED visit, not even aware that urinating on a gas pump was out of the ordinary. Did the confusion start when he walked out the door of the ED or was it present, but unrecognized, during the initial ED encounter?

## I. The Accusation/Cause of Action

Soon after David's death, his wife Jill filed a lawsuit against the initial ED doctor, the physician assistant, Shady Valley Hospital and the primary care doctor. The main allegation was failure to diagnose necrotizing fasciitis/myositis with the subsequent fatal sequelae. The case was not settled, but proceeded to a trial lasting four weeks.

In the first chapter, we included the judge's instructions to the jury and the opening statements. In this chapter, we advance directly to the courtroom drama, an epic struggle between a hard driving plaintiff's attorney who had been friends with the deceased and two of the foremost experts in emergency medicine: Greg Henry and Dave Talan, both experts for the defense at trial. All three have contributed to this chapter. We complete the presentation with the attorneys' closing arguments.

## II. The Trial—The following is actual trial testimony, condensed from over 5,000 pages

Cast of characters (names changed, except where noted):
**The patient**: David Lykins (actual name) ED physician-defendant: Timothy Vaughn
**Physician assistant:** Ed Heller
**Primary care physician:** Dr. Jerry Oster
**Urgent care physician:** Benjamin Roth
**Plaintiff's attorney:** Dwight Brannon (actual attorney)
**Defense attorney:** Neil Freund (actual attorney)
**Defense expert witnesses:** Greg Henry and Dave Talan (both board certified emergency medicine, both actual expert witnesses in this case)

**Cross-examination of the defendant ED physician, Timothy Vaughn, by plaintiff's attorney, Mr. Brannon:**

**A. Triage note:**

**Q.** You never read the triage nurse's note about David Lykins before he was discharged, did you?
**A.** I—when a physician assistant presents a patient to us, it's my practice to look at the chart. I like to look at vital signs, medications, allergies, and I will glance at the triage note.

**Q.** You did not read the triage note on David Lykins on March the 2nd, did you?
**A.** I don't recall, sir.

**Q.** And when you attempted to read it, you said you weren't able to make out anything but complaint of left shoulder pain, correct?
**A.** If that is from my deposition, I would have to review that.

**Q.** Right. I'll let you look at page ten of your deposition. Excuse me just a second while I get it. May I approach the witness, Your Honor?
**The Court:** Sure.

**By Mr. Brannon:**
**Q.** First of all, Dr. Vaughn, is that a true and accurate copy, at least an enlargement, of what you looked at on the date of your deposition?
**A.** Yes, it is.

**Q.** When I asked you what the triage nurse had said in her report on March 2nd, you indicated you did not know unless you read the report. Am I correct?
**A.** I'm sorry. I don't follow your question.

**Q.** Well, when I said "what did the triage notes tell you about David Lykins on March the 2nd?" what did you tell me?
**A.** I'd have to look at my deposition, sir.

**Q.** Did you tell me that you had no independent recollection other than the medical records?
**A.** I don't understand your question.

**Q.** Alright. Tell me today, tell the ladies and gentlemen of the jury, what did Nurse Mayo's triage note say about David Lykins, without looking at the report.
**A.** He had left shoulder pain, fever, chills. He was pale.

**Q.** Did you know that on March the 2nd when you treated David Lykins?
**A.** Sir, I'm not sure what I recall about reading that chart.

**Q.** Would you read your answer [from the deposition] to the ladies and gentlemen?
**A.** (Reading his own deposition testimony): "The best I can tell is this, there is a complaint of— complaint of left shoulder pain. Then, the next thing I can pick up is symptoms started yesterday afternoon. That's all I can read."

**Q.** Well, you are not implying that at the time of your deposition in November, somehow there was some kind of trickery by showing up with copies you couldn't read but you could the original?
**A.** That's not what I'm implying, sir. You asked if I could read those. I could not read the copies.

**Author comments (Weinstock):** This plaintiff's attorney is sharp! The defendant physician tried to imply that he had read the triage note but was tricked during the trial into admitting that, during his deposition testimony months earlier, he had not been able to read the nursing documentation of fever, thereby revealing he was not aware of the complaint of this symptom during the ED evaluation. Ouch!

## B. Was the patient faking?

The plaintiff's attorney next moves to the patient's severe shoulder pain. He tries to establish that the providers did not take Mr. Lykins' pain seriously. Of course, a lot of patients overreact to their pain in the ED. I had a patient tell me once that he has had pain so long he now uses a logarithmic pain scale?! Is it possible to separate those patients who have organic disease from those seeking narcotics? In 1980, Waddell devised a set of physical signs to differentiate patients with the complaint of back pain.[1] Three or more physical signs on exam strongly suggest a non-organic component.

**Waddell's signs:**
Overreaction to the physical exam
Widespread superficial tenderness that does not correspond to an anatomical distribution
Pain on axial loading of the skull or simultaneous rotation of the shoulders and pelvis
Severe limitation on straight leg raise in patients able to sit forward with legs extended
Weakness or sensory loss that does not correspond to a nerve root distribution
Was the severity of the pain a factor which should have prompted the doctor to make the diagnosis? The plaintiff's attorney thinks so.

**Continuation of cross-examination of defendant ED physician, Dr. Vaughn, by plaintiff's attorney Mr. Brannon:**

**Q.** You saw excruciating pain, did you not?

**A.** I saw a gentleman with severe left shoulder pain, correct.

**Q.** Well, let's describe it. Let's describe it. I won't use my word. How did he seem to convey himself in regards to the amount of pain that he was in?
**A.** He seemed to be in severe pain when the shoulder was moved.

**Q.** Did he appear to be overreacting?
**A.** No, sir, I would never make that assessment.

**Q.** It's in your medical records, isn't it?
**A.** I did not dictate that. I would never make that assessment of a patient. I've been doing this for nineteen years, and I've never accused anyone of overreacting or faking.

**Q.** Didn't Dr … I'm sorry — Mr. Heller (the PA) come to you and say that he had talked to his family physician and that this patient "sometimes tends to overreact to his health care needs?"
**A.** At the end, sometime after Mr. Lykins had left and I saw Mr. Heller again, he did mention that the telephone conversation had occurred.

**Q.** Did that help you close the book on your diagnosis here?
**A.** No, sir.

**Q.** And, in fact, your diagnosis of shoulder sprain/strain was not correct, was it?
**A.** At the time, that was the diagnosis that I had arrived at, yes, sir.

**Q.** Was that the correct diagnosis that you had arrived at?
**A.** At that time, that was the correct diagnosis.

**Q.** So, it's your testimony here today that you can state within terms of a reasonable medical probability that David Lykins had no septic process such as necrotizing fasciitis ongoing on March the 2nd?
**A.** If that process was occurring, there were there were no external signs that would give us that indication.

**Q.** Well, is vomiting a sign?
**A.** Vomiting is a sign, yes, sir.

**Q.** And past fever is a symptom?
**A.** That would require some clarification. Many patients present to the emergency department complaining of fever.

**Q.** That's fair enough. Did you go to him and talk to him and say, now, I've heard that you have had this past fever; can you clarify it for me? Did you do that?
**A.** Yes, sir, I did.

**Q.** Did you ask either Jill or David if they had taken a temperature for fever?
**A.** Yes, I did.

**Q.** What did they tell you?
**A.** My–my response to that is twofold. When I ask a patient if they have had a fever, the first question is, "have you checked it?" If they haven't checked it, I would document no fever. If they have checked it and it is less than a hundred degrees, I would still document no fever. I don't feel that is a clinically significant temperature.

**Q.** Would you then ask if they have taken any medication for fever?
**A.** I had reviewed the chart, and there was no medications listed.

**Q.** Did you ask the patient? Did you ask David Lykins or Jill Lykins if he had taken any medication for the fever?
**A.** That is asked at triage. I don't specifically ask that question again.

**Q.** And at least at triage, they didn't report that he had Phenergan that day, did they?
**A.** That's correct.

**Q.** That would have been something for you to know?
**A.** Yes, sir.

**Q.** But you never asked the patient if he had had any medication, did you?
**A.** I don't recall if I had asked or not.

**Q.** Alright. Now, chills and sweats, would that be an important thing to know about?
**A.** In the face of a fever, yes.

**Author comments (Weinstock):** The patient had taken ibuprofen sometime before the visit, but the exact time is not documented. This is a tricky one, since many patients complain of fever, "My temperature was 98.7 but I normally run at 95 so that's a fever for me." Sometimes, they are wrong. Sometimes, they just want us to take them seriously, and sometimes, they have had a fever, which has been reduced by antipyretics.

Mr. Brannon prompted the defendant to admit that not only had he not read the nurse's notes, but that they contained essential information he should have been aware of. Additionally, the nurse's notes were not accurate, lacking any indication that the patient had received the medication Phenergan within the last several hours. The doctor admitted that the nurse's notes were inaccurate and that he did not independently ask about use of other medications, such as ibuprofen, which may have decreased the temperature.

During the trial, Mr. Brannon displayed a 4 × 5 foot poster defining the symptoms of necrotizing fasciitis for the jury. As we follow his questioning, he is going through all of the classic symptoms (fever, chills, severe pain, vomiting) to show the jury that these symptoms were present, but unrecognized, when the patient initially presented. The poster was actually a grease board with symptoms of necrotizing fasciitis and empty boxes next to each symptom. As he went through the testimony, he made a check mark next to each symptom present, but undocumented by the doctor.

On a side note, I thought the stories of 4 × 5 blow up posters were an urban legend meant to colorfully demonstrate a point to doctors in training. I will attest to the fact that this is no fable. For months, I had 20 of these stacked on my back porch.

### C. Symptoms of vomiting not accounted for:

**Q.** I'm not saying necessarily, but if you are considering throwing up, isn't it more likely that someone would throw up because they have an infection than because they have a shoulder sprain or strain?
**A.** Not at all, sir. We see many people with orthopedic injuries with nausea and vomiting.

**Q.** We? How many have you seen throw up from a shoulder sprain and strain?
**A.** Again, sir, I —I don't keep—I don't keep numbers. I evaluate everybody individually.

**Q.** Alright. Now, up here, is this a correct dictation of what you said?
**A.** I—yes, sir, it is.

**Q.** Would you read it to the ladies and gentlemen of the jury?
**A.** The patient is vomiting, and I do not have a good clue as to the cause of this other than the pain from his shoulder.

**Author comments (Weinstock):** The hospital was not able to find either the telephone triage note or the urgent care form. This was brought up repeatedly throughout the trial and was later the "hook" of the plaintiff's closing arguments.

**D. The urgent care note:**

**Q.** Did you see the Urgent Care form?
**A.** No, sir, I didn't.

**Q.** Did you see the phone form?
**A.** No, sir.

**Q.** Did you see any indication that Jill had brought David into the emergency room to rule out either septic arthritis or a septic joint? Did you see that?
**A.** At some point during our interaction, the Lykins' and I had discussed a septic joint. I'm not sure where that had come up. I have it dictated in my note. So, we talked about it.

**Q.** And they didn't mention that we're here because of the doctor sending us straight down from Urgent Care to rule out a septic joint or arthritis or some kind of infection?
**A.** Again, sir, I don't recall where that information came from.

**Q.** So, you don't deny here today in front of the jury that either one of the Lykins or both told you they had come in to have an infection ruled out?
**A.** That I don't recall.

**Q.** You've seen Urgent Care forms before, haven't you?
**A.** Yes, sir.

**Q.** And you have read them and used them, haven't you?
**A.** If the patients give them to us, we read them.

**Q.** And you are saying you never got this?
**A.** I never saw the Urgent Care form.

**Q.** Okay. Would you read from the bottom of Dr. Roth's [documentation]?
**A.** Severe left shoulder pain needs septic arthritis ruled out. Discussed with ER at [Shady Valley]. Will send him down there for evaluation.

**Q.** What about the phone form?
**A.** I did not see the phone form.

**Author comments (Weinstock):** The allegation that Mr. Lykins "Tends to sometimes overreact to his health care needs" was another frequent theme.

### E. Did the patient "overreact to his health care needs?"

**Direct examination of David Lykins' co-worker, John Bennett, by plaintiff's attorney, Mr. Brannon:**

**Q.** In the years that you worked with him, did you ever see him not do a job because of an injury, a sprain or a strain, or anything like that?
**A.** No.

**Q.** Did you ever hear him complain of an injury, sprain or strain?
**A.** No.

**Q.** Was David Lykins a complainer; "I'm hurt, I'm sore, I'm sick"?
**A.** Never.

**Q.** How about nausea, anything like that? Was he sick?
**A.** No.

**Q.** You knew people that worked with him. What was his reputation for truth and veracity?
**A.** Everybody trusted him. You knew he meant what he said. He would say what he meant. Mr. Brannon: Thank you. I have no further questions.
**The Court:** Thank you. Mr. Freund [defense attorney], cross-examine?

**Defense.** No questions, your honor.

**Author comments (Weinstock):** How did the defense rebut these arguments? The following are excerpts from two of the 12 defense expert witnesses (the plaintiff called 28 witnesses). Greg Henry is first and David Talan follows.

### F. The importance of history:

**Direct examination of Greg Henry, expert witness for the defense, by defense attorney, Mr. Freund:**

**Q.** For an emergency room physician, is history important?
**A.** Yes.

**Q.** And why?
**A.** History gives us at least some indication of the disease process which we're looking at.

**Q.** Okay. And in this particular case, was there any history other than the fact that this gentleman may have hurt his shoulder lifting a heavy object?
**A.** All we have is about a day and a half history of pain. The only thing we have related to it was lifting. And so at least on a temporal basis, on a time basis, they're related. We have no way of knowing whether those two are actually cause and effect.

**Q.** As far as the gentleman's physical appearance, his complaint was significant pain in the left shoulder. Is that correct?
**A.** Well, I don't want to use the term shoulder. It was up here. But it was somewhat broader than that. And that's why when they did his X-ray, they also X-rayed the clavicle, which is your collarbone, running from here to here. So, it was obviously not just a complaint of the shoulder, but of the upper chest area.

**Q.** OK. Now, as far as the particular patient is concerned, he had been to an urgent care. Is that correct?
**A.** Yes.

**Q.** And the urgent care physician believed that this individual may have what has been described as a septic joint or septic arthritis of the left shoulder. Is that correct?
**A.** Right. He didn't have that. He never had that in the course of this process. But that was a thought.

**Q.** Okay. Now, was that thought considered by Dr. Vaughn (the ED physician) and Mr. Heller (the ED PA) in the emergency room at Shady Valley Hospital on May 2?

**Mr. Brannon.** Object!

**The Court:** Overruled.

**A.** Yeah, by the nature of the write-up, the pertinent positives and negatives included, it was obviously considered because they commented on the temperature and skin coloration that you would see with an acute joint. And the purpose of taking an X-ray is for looking for fluid in the joint, which you would see with an acute septic joint.

**Q.** Okay. There's been some discussion, doctor, that Dr. Vaughn and Mr. Heller fell below the standard of care when they didn't stick a needle into the left shoulder joint and attempt to aspirate fluid. You're aware of that?
**A.** Yes.

**Q.** Okay. Would you tell the ladies and gentlemen whether or not Mr. Heller and Dr. Vaughn fell below the standard of care?
**A.** Absolutely not! You don't go sticking needles into joints. Joints are sterile areas. You don't go put a needle into areas until you have something palpable. You've got to know where you're going with the needle. So you've got to be able to feel fluid collection, and there was none palpable in this case, nor was there any seen on the X-ray. So, to stick a needle into a joint without a reasonable probability of coming back with fluid would be malpractice.

**Author comments (Weinstock):** What follows are the "even if" arguments. For example, even if the doctors knew the urgent care had sent the patient, he still would have been sent home. Even if the doctor had deciphered the nurse's note of fever, he still would have been sent home. These arguments speak to "causation," one of the two points a plaintiff needs to prove (together with standard of care). We know the patient was not correctly diagnosed, and these questions explore "would it have mattered?"

**G. The importance of an urgent care diagnosis and vital signs:**

**Continued direct examination of Dr. Henry, defense expert, by Mr. Freund, defense attorney:**

**Q.** Okay. Now, you are aware, of course, that Mr. and Mrs. Lykins were sent to Shady Valley Hospital [from an urgent care].
**A.** Yes.

**Q.** Alright. I want you to assume that Dr. Vaughn evaluated Mr. Lykins for what was described by Dr. Roth as a septic arthritis or septic joint.

**Mr. Brannon.** Object, your Honor.

**The Court:** I don't know the question yet.

**Mr. Brannon.** I apologize.

**The Court:** If I could hear the question.

**Q.** I want you to assume that Mr. Lykins was referred to Shady Valley Hospital to "rule out septic joint" or "septic arthritis." Just assume that as being true. When Dr. Vaughn and Mr. Heller evaluated this patient, is there an indication that they considered whether or not this individual had a septic joint?

**Mr. Brannon.** Object! Asked and answered.

**The Court:** Permit it. Overruled!

**A.** They checked those things which you would have with a septic joint. Again, this gentleman didn't have a septic joint.

**Q.** The fact that Dr. Roth, who in his work-up, thought [he] saw possibly a septic joint, does that mean that these physicians in doing their work-up, taking their histories and doing their assessments and their physical examinations should rely on somebody else and their provisional diagnosis?
**A.** They're obligated to do their own examination and come up with their own diagnosis.

**Q.** Okay. Now, you are aware, of course, that this individual did present, in addition to pain, with nausea and vomiting and a history of fever. Is that correct?
**A.** Yes.

**Q.** Now, when the patient presented at Shady Valley Hospital on March 2 with a history of fever, what would you think about that?
**A.** You take the temperature and see if they've actually got a fever.

**Q.** Did they take the temperature and see if he actually had a fever?
**A.** Yes.

**Q.** What was his temperature?
**A.** It was within the normal range.

**Q.** Alright. Now, are vitals important when you're trying to work a patient up and determine whether or not this patient is really sick?
**A.** Well, vital signs are an indicator. They're not a perfect indicator. But they are important in what we call the positive. They're not important in the negative.

**Q.** Okay. Why are they called vitals?
**A.** From the Latin vitae, meaning from the root is vitae, which we use for life.

**Q.** Vitals in the emergency room were basically what?
**A.** They were consistent with somebody in pain. Slight tachycardia. And otherwise they fell within the normal ranges.

**Author comments (Weinstock):** Would a CBC have been helpful, as alleged by the plaintiff?

**Q.** Alright. Let's assume for a moment that we accept the plaintiff's argument that a blood test should have been done on March 2, and there were clinical indications to do that test. What would a blood test have shown on the 2nd?
**A.** Well, we know that it [the CBC] was normal when the patient was sick on the 3rd. So, within the realm of reasonable medical probability, it would have been normal the day before as well.

**Author comments (Weinstock):** Did the PA and doctor meet the standard of care?

### H. Did the PA and doctor meet the standard of care?

**Q.** Okay. Now, doctor, in your examination, you have determined that there was no redness, no swelling, no portal of entry, no marks, no discoloration of the left shoulder. It has been shouted out in this courtroom many, many times that these physicians, Dr. Vaughn and Mr. Heller should have been thinking infection.
Now, what was to lead these physicians to think infection, infection, infection?

**Mr. Brannon.** Object! He's not stating the facts underlying.

**The Court:** Overruled!

**A.** Nothing at this point in time. He looks very similar to other patients who have shoulder pain. I would not be thinking infection at this moment in time.

**Q.** Do you send all patients out of the emergency room with a diagnosis?
**A.** I send them out with a clinical impression at that moment in time, because I understand that a diagnosis is sometimes not arrived at with one visit. Now, certain things are easily diagnosed. If you come in with a cut finger, we can pretty much make the diagnosis of laceration. If you come in with vague abdominal pain, in less than 50 percent of cases can we give you a [specific] diagnosis.

**Q.** As far as discharge, is it appropriate for a physician who has made a diagnosis to ask the patient to come back if the condition worsens? Is that usual or unusual?
**A.** Standard. The assumption is that we're open 24 hours a day, seven days a week. We'd expect if there's a change, that you come back. That's just the standard discharge line on the chart.

**Q.** Alright. Based upon your review of the record, from approximately 1:00 o'clock on, until presentation again the next morning, which would be March 3rd, maybe around 10:00 o'clock, did the patient get worse?
**A.** Oh, yes, dramatically worse. By the time they got in the next morning with the family practitioner, he was essentially in a pre-shock state.

**Q.** One final question, then, doctor. As you have reviewed the case and as you have reviewed the depositions of the physicians, do you have an opinion, based upon standards of care and reasonable medical probability and certainty, whether or not these physicians acted reasonably and met the standard of care?
**A.** Yes, my opinion is this is a very tragic and sad case, and my opinion is they met reasonable standards of care. I'm glad I wasn't the doctor who saw him because we will never know the outcome of the play until the [diagnosis] has actually presented itself.

**Mr. Freund.** No further questions.

**Cross-examination of defense expert witness, Dr. Henry, by plaintiff's attorney, Mr. Brannon:**

**Q.** Did you consider Dr. Roth's finding of possibly swelling and Mrs. Lykins' testimony that it looked swollen? [per the Urgent Care doctor's note and the testimony of Jill Lykins, David's wife, which is not reproduced here].
**A.** I read them both. I've got to depend on two healthcare professionals who saw him at that moment in time. They did not feel it was [swollen].

**Q.** Well, if they didn't do an adequate exam and Dr. Roth and Mrs. Lykins were correct, you would have a different opinion, wouldn't you?
**A.** Not from Dr. Roth, because he said "possible." So, I don't know what to do with that. That's not one way or the other. Again, his wife isn't medically trained. So, I would have less credibility in [her impression] than I would people who are medically trained.

**Q.** If I understand you correctly, March 2nd, when David Lykins came into the emergency room complaining of pain like he had never had before, giving a history of fever and chills, pale, screaming whenever he was touched, throwing up repeatedly, it was your opinion on examination or redirect by Mr. Freund that he wasn't sick. Is that correct?
**A.** Absolutely not. That's a mischaracterization of the testimony.

## I. Mortality from NSTI:

**Direct examination of Dr. Dave Talan, (ED physician triple boarded in EM, IM and ID) by defense attorney, Mr. Freund:**

**Q.** Would you describe for the ladies and gentlemen of the jury the mortality from necrotizing fasciitis and myositis?
**Mr. Brannon.** Object!

**The Court:** Overruled.

**A.** Both are obviously bad, but the fasciitis, which is the fibrous covering over the muscles, is 30–50%, so that's not very good. But if the muscle is involved, the mortality is in the range of 80%.

**Q.** Do you have an opinion upon reasonable medical certainty, as to whether the health care providers met the standard of care?
**A.** Yes. It's my strong opinion that reasonable physicians and physician's assistants would not have made the diagnosis of necrotizing fasciitis or myositis on that date. Their care was consistent with the community standard of care. This is a very, very rare condition that lacked many of the important features that would lead a reasonable physician to make the diagnosis
… and that's it in a nutshell.

**Closing statements:** The following are the shortened closing arguments from the plaintiff and defense attorneys. Plaintiff goes first, then defense:

**Mr. Dwight Brannon (plaintiff's attorney):**

What was the prize here? David Lykins wanted three things in his life. One, he wanted to do his very best for mankind. He wanted to be reasonable, responsible and accountable. He wanted security for his family. Worked hard at it. Triple jobs. And still had all that time for his family. Above all, he wanted to be there. He wanted to be there. Second, professionally, he wanted to give, he wanted to serve; it was obviously a token of his desire to serve mankind. Third, [serving] his community. This is about the community, accountability, responsibility: Those aren't hollow terms.

And I ask you in light of the testimony of Dr. Roth [the urgent care physician] who threw him a lifeline, "David, go to the emergency room." And at the emergency room, ladies and gentlemen, the triage nurse didn't meet the standard of care. Then, Mr. Heller didn't meet the standard of care. Then, Dr. Vaughn didn't meet the standard of care. That's the lifeline. And then they called Dr. Oster [the PCP] to close the loop. They closed the loop all right. (Taking a piece of rope from his pocket and tying a large knot.) Instead of giving him a lifeline, they gave him a noose.

This case really needs no convincing. I ask the question what is fair, what is just, what is the standard of care? Ladies and gentlemen, I await your verdict so I can tell the captain that his trip is truly over, his prize is truly won, and that you will post the conscience of this community so that these defendants stop, look, and listen to ordinary people. Because this courtroom is for the victims. This courtroom is for ordinary people. I ask you to realize how important it is and what an important thing [it is] that you do here. I believe that with all my heart. Thank you, ladies and gentlemen.

**Mr. Neil Freund (defense attorney):**

**The Court:** Mr. Freund, we're ready for the defense close.
**Mr. Freund.** Thanks Judge.

When we selected you folks as jurors, I played a portion of the tape to show you the beautiful family of David and Jill Lykins. I did that for a reason, and I'd like to share that reason with you.

I know from my life's experiences how I react to the death of loved ones. I know how you react to the death of loved ones. And yet, we expect you to come in here and judge us fairly and impartially. We ask that of you. And I know how difficult that is because I have experienced loss. And then we bring you in here and ask you to decide the case on the facts.

I was thinking, okay. Now, how are we going to go about this? And I thought that we would approach it like the doctors approached this case. In fact, what you are doing in this courtroom is making a diagnosis. And how are you going to make that diagnosis? You're going to look at the facts. You are going to render a verdict, which is your diagnosis. And you are going to go about this the very same way that the doctors did when they made their diagnosis in this case.

Common sense and reason. That's how doctors make their decision based upon their medical training. That's how I ask you to make your decision when you go back and talk to each other and deliberate with each other. Common sense and reason. Without hindsight or retrospect. Hindsight is 20/20. Put yourselves in the shoes of the caregivers. And what I mean by "put yourselves in the shoes of the caregivers" is simply, when you're judging my clients, judge them from the information they knew or should have known as the caregivers at that time. Independent of compassion or sympathy.

We have ranges on myositis from 80% fatality to as low as 20%. But you are being asked in this case to take the quantum leap that in this particular case with this particular individual that he would have survived this terrible deadly disease and not only that, but he would have survived it without disability. And you folks, when you are using your common sense, are going to reject that.

We didn't make the history up. Why is that important? Dr. Henry said in the emergency room, it's a snapshot at a particular moment in time. Everybody agrees; all the experts agreed that history was the most important part of the case. Alright. What history was given to Mr. Heller and Dr. Vaughn? He hurt himself lifting. That is the history that Dr. Roth got, and that's the history that we got at Shady Valley Hospital. None of the classic signs of redness, swelling, high temperature or vitals out of whack were present. I thought I would just highlight some of the testimony that was actually given in this case. When I was asked to represent Dr. Vaughn, Mr. Heller and Shady Valley Hospital, I wanted to find the best experts to review this case. So, I got the literature and found out who wrote more than anybody else. That was Dr. Johns, an infectious disease specialist (name changed, testimony not included here). He's written more, studied it more and seems to know more than anybody else.

Then I thought, but Mr. Heller and Dr. Vaughn are not infectious disease physicians. They specialize in emergency medicine. Then I thought, okay, I wonder if there's anybody out there who is an infectious disease person and an emergency medicine person. That was Dr. Talan, the fellow from UCLA. Did you notice he had sandals on? I couldn't believe it. He's from California; it figures. I was hoping he would stay in the box and not come out!

But anyway, he is one of only two doctors in the United States who is double boarded in emergency medicine and infectious diseases. One of two, and I got him to review the case. He said the case was defensible.

Then, I thought, I need somebody local. So, I went to Ohio State and I had Dr. Hankman (name changed) review the case. Professor, in emergency medicine … the works.

I'm going to do this some more. So, I sent the case to Dr. Henry. Now, Dr. Henry is from Ann Arbor. I wondered what the folks in Ohio will think about a guy from Michigan? I decided that he had the qualifications. Now, his qualifications were a little different, though, because he was boarded in emergency medicine. He also happened to be President of the whole United States of American College of Emergency Physicians, all 22,000 of them. He gave me a favorable review.

Did Mr. Lykins get worse between his discharge from the ER until he returned the next day? Yes. Actually, his condition changed very rapidly over several hours. Now, why does that make a difference? When they were discharged from the hospital at 1:00 o'clock in the early afternoon on the 2nd, they were given the specific instruction to return if the condition got worse. Well, it surely did get worse, and it got worse, according to Mrs. Lykins' own words, about midnight. Okay?

Now, what are we supposed to conclude from going from 1:00 o'clock at the time of the discharge to about 10:00 o'clock the next day until there was a change in condition? Mr. Brannon spent a lot of time talking about the fact that [David Lykins] was a paramedic. Think about that. Here's an individual who, from the testimony of the plaintiff, we're supposed to believe that his eyes were rolling up when he was in our institution on the 2nd. He had every ambulance in Fairtown available to him if he would have chosen to call. But, if we're supposed to believe that his condition was so bad, why didn't he want to go back to the emergency room on the 2nd. It is reasonable to conclude that surgery wasn't indicated on the 2nd?

I had a very good medical professor, a rheumatologist, [who] told me, and it's true, that there are diseases where at one point in time you cannot make the diagnosis and, therefore, you need to see the patient repetitively in order to establish a diagnosis. That's common, very common.

Whether or not you accept the idea that he suffered a strain and that's why the Strep A seeded in him or whether you believe that the Strep A seeded for some other reason, when you go back and discuss this among yourselves and consider the signs and symptoms, what was there for these doctors and Mr. Heller to diagnose? You will decide that the signs and symptoms were not sufficient to even suspect infection, much less this deadly disease.

Then, take Dr. Anderson [the general surgeon at Shady Valley who took him to surgery on March 3rd] and plug in his testimony that he would not have done surgery on the 2nd. That he would not have cut on what looked to be perfectly viable tissue. You would agree that the earliest time a diagnosis could be made was probably at about 6:30 in the morning [of March 3rd] when he actually had the discoloration, the swelling, and puffiness in his pectoral area.

Probably in hindsight and retrospect, if I had something to do over again in this case, with my client, you know what [that] would be? I would tell Mr. Heller, "Ed, don't use the word 'overreact.' "

When you go back there and you are deciding about whether the doctors and folks at Shady Valley met the standard of care, judge these folks as the facts existed and as the signs and symptoms existed at that time. And if you do, I am convinced that you'll make a decision that's favorable to them. This is not a "send a message to the world" case. I expect that you'll treat Jill Lykins and her family fairly, and we simply ask the same.

So, ladies and gentlemen, it's been a long four weeks. I thank you kindly for your attention. I hope I haven't bored you too much, and I look forward to your verdict. Thank you very much.

## III. The Verdict

As reported by The Dayton Daily news (combined articles, minimally edited and shortened). Note: Doctors' names have been changed to remain consistent within chapter. Written by Rob Modic:

DAYTON—An urgent-care doctor threw a "lifeline" to a Fairtown firefighter who had a deadly infection, but Shady Valley hospital and its staff turned it into a "noose" that killed the man, the lawyer for the firefighter's widow told a jury Thursday.

After 2½ hours of deliberations, a jury found for Shady Valley Hospital, an emergency room doctor, his assistant and a Fairtown doctor sued by the widow of a firefighter who died of a massive infection.

Mrs. Lykins later saw that a physician assistant, Ed Heller, had recorded that he had called Oster [the primary care physician] on March 2, who said Lykins "Tends to sometimes overreact to his health care needs." Oster denied he had said "overreact" and Heller said he mistakenly used the word. Plaintiff's attorney Dwight Brannon contended the remark caused the emergency room doctor and staff to doubt Lykins' claims of pain. But defense attorney Neil Freund countered that the conversation took place after doctors decided to discharge Lykins.

The eight-member Montgomery County Common Pleas jury, which needed at least six jurors to reach a verdict, gave six votes for the emergency room physician, Dr. Timothy A. Vaughn and his assistant, Heller. Four alternate jurors, who sat through the entire four-week trial, said they split 2–2.

Defense attorney Freund offered his condolences to Jill Lykins and claimed the victory that upheld the treatment David Lykins received as meeting the medical standards for care. "On behalf of Dr. Timothy Vaughn, Ed Heller and Shady Valley Hospital, we are grateful and thankful to the jury for their verdict," Freund said. "We believe the doctors associated with Shady Valley Hospital and all of the hospital staff give quality care within this community, and we are thankful that the jury agreed with us. This was a tragic case in which a fine family was devastated with a terrible disease, and we feel for the family and especially for Mrs. Jill Lykins and her children." Lykins' attorney, Brannon, said afterward that the case would be appealed.

**Why did the defense win?** The following are results of a jury perception study (conducted after the trial)

- Demographics:
  - 53% female
  - Age range: Young adult to sixties
  - Education: 20% with bachelor's or graduate degrees
- Facts supporting David Lykins (plaintiff):

- The ED staff didn't take the situation seriously.
- Vomiting should have indicated that David was suffering from more than a strained shoulder.
- ER staff did not communicate with each other in an efficient manner; they ignored the urgent care form, the telephone referral form and the triage nurse's notes.
- The fact that David was a paramedic should have factored into the diagnostic equation and led to a more proactive approach and recognition that he would not be exaggerating his condition.

- Facts supporting Shady Valley Hospital and defendants:
  - Mr. Lykins should have gone right back to hospital when he woke up instead of taking a bath (loss of valuable time).
  - Necrotizing fasciitis is an extremely rare condition with limited window of diagnostic opportunity, and it would not be fair to hold the staff responsible for failing to diagnose it.

**Thoughts of the actual attorneys:**

**Plaintiff's attorney, Mr. Dwight Brannon:**

- "Biggest case I ever lost—Was out-experted—I shouldn't have lost it."
- "I have tried six cases of necrotizing faciitis. This was my first [loss]. I have won all the others. I would like an opportunity to re-try this case."
- Note: Per Mr. Brannon, the unrecovered plaintiff expenses for the preparation and conduct of the trial were approximately $250,000.

**Defense attorney, Mr. Neil Freund:**

- "We got killed during the case, absolutely mauled by the newspapers."
- "According to Dr. Talan, expert witness for the defense: 9/10 or 10/10 ED physicians would have missed this diagnosis."

**Author comments (Weinstock):** When I initially contacted Mr. Brannon, he told me he wanted a chance to re-try this case, and he got his wish. At an Essentials of Emergency Medicine conference in San Francisco, CA, a mock trial was held with several participants from the original trial, including Dwight Brannon as the plaintiff's attorney and Dave Talan as the defense expert. With Mel Herbert as the judge, Billy Mallon as the plaintiff's expert, and Scott Weingart as the volunteer physician defendant, the four week trial unfolded over the course of an hour. A true jury of his peers, composed of six emergency medicine physicians, one physician assistant and a nurse practitioner ruled again for the defendant, 6–2. … but back to the original trial. This was not the end of the story.

## IV. The Appeal—The court's decision was appealed. The following is a brief summary of the 19-page appeals decision

From our review of the record, we conclude that any errors committed by the trial court were harmless. We further conclude that the record does not support the claim of improper conduct on the part of the defendants, defense counsel, or the defense witnesses.

There is competent, credible evidence to suggest that David's diagnosis of strain/sprain on March 2 was reasonable and that the proper diagnosis could not be made until the following day, when the signs of discoloration and swelling appeared.

We have found no evidence in the record to demonstrate any relationship between the failure to retain [the urgent care] records and the treatment of David Lykins. In other words, the timing of the diagnosis and David's death were not caused by the hospital's failure to keep those forms. It is clear from the record that Heller and Vaughn ruled out septic arthritis in David's shoulder, as requested by the urgent-care physician. It is further undisputed that David did not have septic arthritis of the shoulder.
All of Lykins' assignments of error having been overruled, we affirm the judgment of the trial court.
Judgment affirmed.

## V. The Legal Analysis—Guest Interview

**Jennifer L'Hommedieu Stankus, MD, JD**
Former medical malpractice defense attorney and military magistrate
Emergency Medicine physician
Former medical malpractice defense attorney

**Authors.** *You started out as a police officer then went to law school. Did it turn out to be what you expected?*
**JS.** When I started out as a medical malpractice defense attorney, straight out of law school, I believed the law was black and white; if there was no clear negligence, there could be no verdict for a plaintiff. As a hospital attorney, it was my job to determine the standard of care, and subsequently who should win and lose. If I found the standard of care was breached, with resultant harm, I felt obligated to reach a settlement that would adequately, but not excessively, compensate the patient for the harm suffered, and the patient would thank me for my efforts. I could not have been more wrong on every front.

These cases are about the money at stake, not about determining if negligence occurred or not. The cost to bring a case to trial can far exceed $100,000, usually paid out of pocket by the plaintiff's attorney. This is a huge risk. This impacts the award to the patient, as the attorney's contingency fees are subtracted from the settlement or judgment. Even with large awards, the patient is not compensated as much as one would expect. Standard of care is not always easy to determine; it is difficult for people to look only at a snapshot in time and remain objective. Even experts disagree, particularly in emotionally-charged cases such as this.

**Authors.** *Let's cut right to the chase, does the fact that the patient died increase the chance of a verdict for the plaintiff?*
**JS.** The worse the outcome, the better the plaintiff's chances. This case is horrific. The patient was a previously healthy, productive member of the community who was a loving father and husband. He went from a state of health to death in a matter of days. How can that be? How is it that a physician trained in emergency medicine could not see such an aggressive disease process? How could the patient be discharged with abnormal vital signs and told he had a mere shoulder strain, and within minutes of leaving become so encephalopathic that he urinated on a gas pump?

These are the questions that will go through the minds of the jurors. They are the questions that may go through the minds of other physicians. It is very difficult to get past the emotion of this vibrant firefighter's death and focus on the information available at the initial ED encounter. Even if necrotizing fasciitis was in the differential diagnosis, would it have changed the outcome? Dr. Talan argues no (below). Further, there was no physical sign of this disease, since it was likely deep in the muscle, not at the level of the skin. Labs may or may not have been useful. In hindsight, placing the patient in observation may have revealed the disease process, but with his symptoms at the time, this admission would not qualify at my hospital.

There have been many instances where juries render a verdict for the plaintiff, even where they believe that a physician was not negligent, merely because they wanted the patient or his or her family to have some compensation for their terrible loss … and this was a terrible, terrible loss.

**Authors.** *What were the biggest risk management mistakes at the initial visit?*
**JS.** Some have already been discussed, including knowledge of the referring physician's concerns, not inquiring when the triage note could not be read, inaccurate medication history from the nurse and discharge home with abnormal vital signs.

Two points deserve special mention. First, when things don't add up and the ED work-up is exhausted, strict instructions for return should be clearly communicated to the patient. The patient and family must feel comfortable about returning, and these discussions should be clearly and thoroughly documented in the medical record. I found it amazing that the patient's wife did not feel comfortable immediately returning to the ER, despite watching her husband urinate on a gas pump and vomit on the way home. That was a big change.

Second, never, ever, make a judgment about a patient or another provider in the medical record—ever. Not only is it unprofessional, but it is usually inaccurate. It makes the provider look uncaring, which fosters an assumption that the patient is not getting the best care. It is the "frequent flyers," chronic pain patients, drunks and "over-exaggerators" who are the most challenging because they need to be objectively examined every visit.

**Authors.** *Did the involvement of a PA increase the risk of a bad outcome?*
**JS.** I don't think so in this case. But, anytime there is communication between providers about patients, particularly with an unclear diagnosis, there is a strong risk of framing or anchoring bias. Here, the MLP presented the patient as having a shoulder strain. The patient himself related his symptoms to lifting on the previous day. He did not tie in the fevers and chills.

In cases such as this, biases are difficult to escape. But again, where things do not add up, take a step back and try to think of what else could be going on. Ask the history questions again. Physical exam was not useful here in terms of making this diagnosis, except to the extent that there was zero range of motion and extreme tenderness to palpation, but that wasn't until the following day. Still, pain out of proportion in a successful fireman is a bit unusual and probably deserves a second look (thus the second provider).

It is OK to tell a patient that you do not yet have a good explanation for what is going on and that is not unusual in many disease processes. Here, the patient's wife testified that the ED didn't do anything for her husband's condition, and she didn't feel that would change if she returned. Perhaps framing the aftercare instructions differently would have allowed her to feel more comfortable about returning.

**Authors.** *Who is legally more responsible, the doctor or MLP?*
**JS.** This depends upon state law. In some states, the MLP is acting under the physician's license, almost like a resident. In others, the MLP may practice independently. In this case it is a moot point, because the physician went and did his own exam and is therefore equally, if not more, responsible. The responsibility rests on the person with the highest level of training, who had direct involvement in the case.

**Authors.** *Are you surprised by the jury's decision in this case?*
**JS.** Absolutely. Even where the standard of care seems clear, one is not guaranteed a certain result. Anyone could have missed this case, and that at the time of presentation, proper care was given.

Yet, there were so many things that a jury could have latched onto. The first was the sympathy factor, since this was a shocking, sudden, horrific loss. The second was the judgment about the patient in the medical record. It gave the impression that the patient was not taken seriously and raises the question whether or not the outcome could have been better with a more thorough and thoughtful evaluation; would the physician have gotten more labs such as a CBC, sed rate, CK, or CRP? How about a chest CT? Juries love to latch onto anything that will allow them to help a sympathetic cause. The images of the patient urinating on a gas pump and vomiting right after leaving the hospital are powerful.

**Authors.** *How would you approach the plaintiff and defense strategies?*
**JS.** In terms of winning this case, the plaintiff should not have focused so heavily on the recommendation from the urgent care physician because that wasn't the diagnosis anyway. He should have focused on what else it could have been, given that things didn't add up. He could have emphasized what other diagnostic imaging could have been ordered to find the diagnosis. I would have hammered [the point] that this patient's significant signs of disease were discounted, as evidenced by the fact that within minutes of discharge he was not able to function normally. Was there really such a big change within minutes? I would argue that the patient and family must have been made to feel that their problem was insignificant because they chose not to go back to the emergency department, even despite these significant changes.

To win a case, there should be clear and convincing negligence. Here, that wasn't the case. Further, there has to be harm caused by a delay in diagnosis. One of two leading experts in infectious disease testified that this process was such that the patient would not have survived, regardless of the time of diagnosis. We are governed by a legal system in which physicians are afraid of being sued, even when they have met the standard of care or when the standard of care is not completely clear. Dr. Henry said, "This case represents what's wrong with the American system of justice." I agree.

## VI. Medical Discussion—Diagnosis and Management of Necrotizing Fasciitis and Myositis

**Guest Author:**
**David A. Talan, MD, FACEP, FIDSA**
Emeritus Professor of Emergency Medicine and Medicine/Infectious Diseases
The David Geffen School of Medicine at UCLA
Department of Emergency Medicine, Ronald Reagan UCLA Medical Center

Dr. Talan is board certified in emergency medicine, internal medicine, and infectious diseases. He has written and researched extensively on the intersection of infectious diseases and emergency department care. He serves on the editorial board of the Annals of Emergency Medicine and has numerous publications in high-impact journals, including The New England Journal of Medicine and the Journal of the American Medical Association.

I am primarily an emergency physician but have training and practice experience as an infectious diseases specialist. For over 30 years, through my research and teaching, I have focused on the diagnosis and treatment of infectious diseases in the ED. I am frequently asked to review medical-legal cases involving infectious disease issues during the course of ED care.

As you now know, I was a defense expert in this case. Additionally, a few years after the case concluded, my opinions and performance were tested in front of my peers at an EMRAP mock trial in San Francisco. I remember the case well, that is, all except wearing sandals, as the defense attorney joked. Apparently, his strategy to "connect" with the Ohioan jury members during his closing argument was to poke fun at his own expert who was from California. Anyway, they weren't sandals, they were flipflops. Delayed diagnosis and treatment of nec fasc is a poster child, along with spinal epidural abscess (SEA), for infectious disease ED malpractice cases. Both are rare and both present with pain, the most common symptom leading patients to come to the ED, typically related to injuries and musculoskeletal complaints. In the case of nec fasc, the pain is characterized as severe and out of proportion to exam findings. PA Heller wrote that Mr. Lykins was "inappropriate as far as pain and physical examination in relation to complaint and history." "Inappropriate" is quite a term to describe this responsible father and Battalion Chief, and appears both judgmental and dismissive. I cannot specifically recall the trial's discourse but can imagine Mr. Bannon saying, "What was inappropriate was David's negligent care." When we are confused by a presentation, we tend to look for more convenient explanations than our own ineptitude to figure things out. Perhaps PA Heller sold the idea that Mr. Lykins was "inappropriate" to his primary care doctor and then bought Dr. Oster's rationalized explanation that he overreacts. Be careful about dismissing a patient's extreme distress as drama and ascribing their severe pain to a simple musculoskeletal injury, which, in the absence of an accompanying fracture, is unusual. Having said that, I think that this would have been a difficult case to diagnose even if PA Heller had paged Dr. [Sir William] Osler, not our own Dr. Oster.

The problem is that pain is ubiquitous and subjective, and when the patient offers a possible explanation, as in this case, heavy lifting, one needs a hook to reasonably consider the diagnosis of nec fasc. Unfortunately, early on, these hooks are often absent. An NEJM review of these infections noted "pitfalls" in the diagnosis, many of which applied to this case: 1) attributing pain to injury, 2) absence of fever, and 3) absence of cutaneous findings.[2] Here, a possibly overlooked clue was the triage nurse's history of fever. Although providers should review nurses' notes, they also have an obligation to get their own history. It was very helpful to the defense that Dr. Vaughn documented that Mr. Lykins "has not had fever." He also clearly considered infection, a septic joint. Physical examination did not support that diagnosis. Point-of-care ultrasound (POCUS) could also have been used to exclude the presence of effusion.

Perhaps the use of over the counter (OTC) meds was overlooked and a fever in the ED was masked by prior ibuprofen use. Alternatively, a fever was unfairly absent as can sometimes occur in some of humankind's worst infections (present in only ~60% of nec fasc cases); we will never know. Keep in mind that the anti-pyretic effect of ibuprofen and acetaminophen wears off after about 4 hours.[3] Had a full set of vital signs, including temperature, been repeated prior to discharge, and a fever found, I suspect a different course would have been taken. If the ED has a policy requiring vitals to be repeated prior to discharge, and this is not done, this could be used as evidence of negligence when vitals are not repeated. A proxy for fever is that these patients just look plain sick. Additionally, in retrospect, vomiting was a clue, although a non-specific one.

The absence of the most common findings in nec fasc, redness and swelling (present in ~75% of cases), would lead us away from considering a skin and soft tissue infection, let alone a catastrophic one. A skin wound would be a clue, but in this case none was present. In the case of Group A Strep nec fasc, only about 50% have a portal of entry. Other cases are thought to arise from bacteremia complicating a preceding Strep infection. Perhaps Mr. Lykins had a mild case of pharyngitis that went unnoticed. Ecchymosis and bullae occur late, and crepitus is seen in infections caused by gas-forming organisms, (e.g., *Clostridium perfringens*), not Strep. It is also possible that Mr. Lykins had both muscle injury from lifting and early nec fasc. Experimental studies in animals have demonstrated that bacteria injected into the bloodstream tend to settle at the site of previously traumatized tissue. Check out this1904 reference![4] Also, since NSAID use is common in these cases, some have hypothesized their anti-inflammatory properties might predispose to this infection. However, since NSAID use is associated with pain severity, correlation does not prove causation.

A laboratory-based scoring system called the Laboratory Risk Indicator for Necrotizing Fasciitis (LRINEC) score[6,7] has been developed for the diagnosis of necrotizing fasciitis. It consists of the following components:

- elevated white blood cell count
- creatinine
- C-reactive protein
- glucose
- decreased hemoglobin
- decreased serum sodium

The problem with the LRINEC score is that its components were derived among patients with the final clinical diagnoses of nec fasc and cellulitis. Note that the percentages for the presence of fever, erythema, and swelling referred to above are at the time of diagnosis, not during the early stages of the disease. Since we first discussed this case, studies have found that the LRINEC score fails miserably when applied prospectively in practice for cases where uncertainty exists, which is when we most need the help. [5,6] Having said that, should you have a compatible presentation and get back some weird lab results, like a sodium of 124, it's something to keep in mind. And sometimes your surgeon consultant asks about it and it may be your job to point out the subsequently demonstrated poor sensitivity (~40–50% in the above referenced studies).

The white blood cell and hemoglobin counts are part of the LRINEC score and the plaintiff team suggested that labs should have been sent as an abnormal white blood cell count and differential would have led to an earlier diagnosis. Whereas this is possible, I think it's unlikely. Mr. Lykins' white blood cell count would have likely been elevated, consistent with infection but also with severe pain and inflammation related to a shoulder strain. In a case report, during panic attacks a patient's white blood cell count ranged from 15.5–20.5 compared to 5.4–10.0 during calm periods.[8] Similarly, the proportion of neutrophils could have been non-specifically elevated. The white blood cell count could also have been normal as it was normal the next day despite progression of the infection. Other tests that are sometimes helpful in confusing cases are creatinine kinase (CK) and CT or MRI imaging. However, these may fail to distinguish trauma-related muscle injury and infection unless due to a gas-forming organism. Of note, subcutaneous gas can also be seen at bedside on POCUS. The only diagnostic test that likely would have been of value in this case is inspection of the deep tissue in the operating room and, as supported by the surgeon's testimony, good luck getting one to take a patient without any local findings. This also gets to the issue of causation since even had Mr. Lykins been hospitalized, his surgery would likely have been deferred until some skin and soft tissue findings became evident.

The treatment of nec fasc is immediate surgical debridement or amputation of all non-viable tissue, antimicrobials, and hemodynamic support. In this case, the etiologic pathogen was Group A

*Streptococcus*, is an organism that is susceptible to many antibiotics, including penicillin. Both clinical and experimental data support the adjunctive use of antibiotics that inhibit protein translation at the ribosome, such as clindamycin and linezolid (with empiric broad-spectrum antibiotics, like vancomycin and piperacillin-tazobactam), in order to block toxin production and kill organisms that are metabolically active but at stationary growth. Controversy exists around the efficacy of intravenous immunoglobulin (IVIG), but it appears harmless and it's a Hail Mary that's typically thrown.

The reason that infectious diseases are among the most common diagnoses leading to malpractice suits is that they are potentially curable, provided that the diagnosis is suspected early enough. In this case, had a surgeon been willing to take Mr. Lykins to the operating room to explore his shoulder area for evidence of nec fasc on the evening of the first emergency department visit, it is likely that this diagnosis would have been confirmed about 24 hours earlier than it was. Logically, this would have increased Mr. Lykins' odds of surviving. However, his chance of survival would have to meet the legal standard of "more likely than not" (i.e., 51%), in order to be sufficient to support causation. No studies exist in which patients with suspected life-threatening infections were randomized to immediate or delayed therapy and then followed for their outcome. Therefore, causation is largely expert opinion based on known outcomes of the disease, the health of the host, the condition of the host and extent of the infection at the time of the possible earlier diagnosis, the virulence and susceptibility of the infecting organism(s), and the time difference between the possible earlier and actual treatment.

In this case, the overall mortality associated with nec fasc is about 30%.[9] Prognosis is worse in patients with advanced age and co-morbidities and if shock is present. In this sense, causation would be supported since Mr. Lykins was in good health and, at the time of the first emergency department visit, he was hemodynamically stable. However, the deeper the infection, the worse the prognosis, and when it substantially involves the muscle, (necrotizing myositis), mortality is much higher; one review suggesting it is uniformly fatal.[10] In addition, since debridement is the cornerstone of treatment, outcome also is greatly affected by the site of infection and the potential for tissue to be safely removed. In the case of truncal infections, as occurred here, options for full debridement may be limited, unlike extremity amputation. Since Mr. Lykins localized his symptoms to the shoulder and upper chest, even had he been diagnosed earlier, there was a very good chance he would not have survived.

## VII. Author Summary (Weinstock)

What can we take away from this tragic case?

- The medical decision-making note was well done; there was a lot of data from which to defend this case. Of course, it's better if it doesn't even go to trial in the first place ...
- Always read the nurse's notes. A history of fever without alternative explanation may have prompted consideration of an infectious process.
- Be careful about using conjecture in the chart. Even the defense attorney told the jury that use of the word "overreact" was unfortunate. Think of it this way: if the patient is overreacting, it doesn't help you. And if the patient actually has something bad, it definitely hurts you.
- Ensure protocols exist so records are not inappropriately discarded. Pen your initials, date and time on before scanning into the chart.
- At the completion of the evaluation, make sure the patient and family are aware if there is still diagnostic uncertainty. If this would have happened here, perhaps Mr. Lykin's wife would have brought him back when he urinated on the gas pump, instead of giving him pain pills through the night.

## References


1. Waddell G, McCulloch JA, Kummel E, et al. Non-organic physical signs in low back pain. Spine 1980;5:117–25.
2. Stevens DL, Bryant AE. Necrotizing soft-tissue infections. N Eng J Med 2017;377(23):2253-65.
3. Choi J, Chang S, Ahn JG. Comparison of fever-reducing effects in self-reported data from the mobile app: Antipyretic drugs in pediatric patients. Scientific Rep 2020;10(1):3879.
4. Miyaki H. Beitrage zur Kenntnis der sogenannten myositis infectiosa. Mitteilungen aus den Grenzgebieten Medizin und Chirugie 1904;Th 13:155-98.
5. Wong CN, Khin LW, Heng KS, et al. The LRINEC (Laboratory Risk Indicator for necrotizing fasciitis) score: A tool for distinguishing necrotizing fasciitis from other soft tissue infections. Crit Care Med 2004; 32(7):1535-41.
6. Fernando SM, Tran A, Cheng W, et al. Necrotizing soft tissue infection: Diagnostic accuracy of physical examination, imaging, and LRINEC score. Ann Surg 2019;269(1):58-65.
7. Cheng-Ting H, Chang C-P, Huang T-Y, et al. Prospective validation of the laboratory risk indicator for necrotizing fasciitis (LRINEC) score for necrotizing fasciitis of the extremities. PLos One 2020;15(1):e0227748.
8. Iskander JW, Griffeth B, Sampra M, et al. Panic-attack-indued leukocytosis in a healthy male: A case report. Gen Hosp Psych 2011;33(3):302:e11-302.e12.
9. Stevens DL. Invasive Group A streptococcus infections. Clin Infect Dis 1992;14(1):2-11.
10. Yoder EL, Mendez J, Khatib R. Spontaneous gangrenous myositis induced by Streptococcus pyogenes: case report and review of the literature. Rev Infect Dis 1987;9(2):382-5.

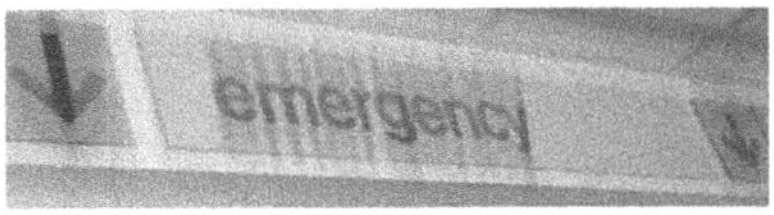


# Case 3

## A 15 Year-old Girl with Headache: A Grandmother's 9/11 Story

**Primary case author:**
**Jonathan Edlow**

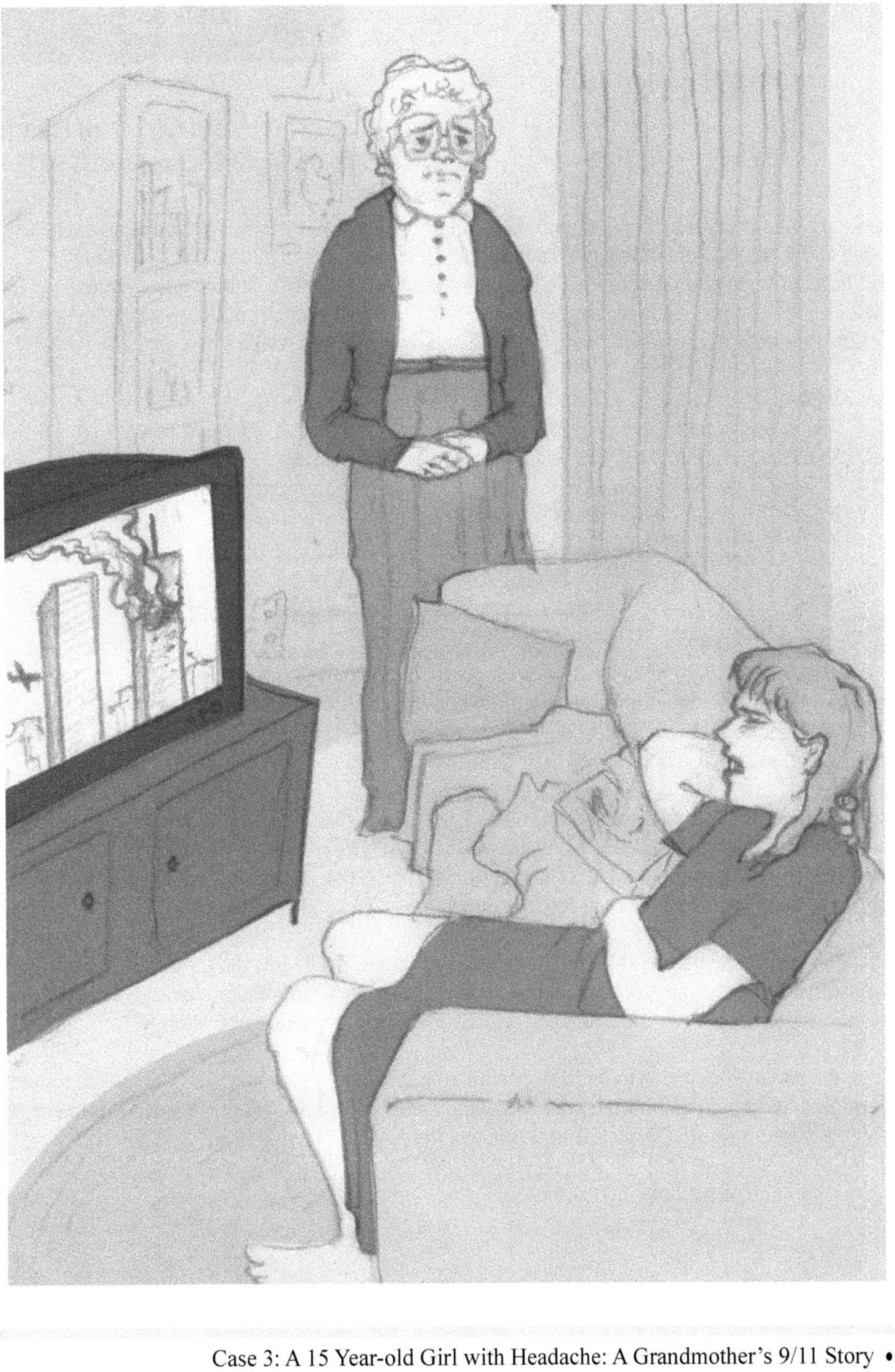

# Case 3

## A 15 Year-old Girl with Headache: A Grandmother's 9/11 Story

America has had many defining moments throughout the years. For many, we remember exactly where we were and what we were doing. On the morning of September 11th, 2001, I was working an 8 AM–4 PM shift in the Emergency Department. The day started slow. After I had seen a few patients, I checked the news on the computer; the report just before 9 AM was that a small commuter plane had crashed into one of the buildings of the World Trade Center. Soon, we knew the whole story.

***Deep thoughts:***

1. *Which historical factors are most important in the evaluation of headache?*
2. *Should we evaluate similar complaints differently when the patient presents per EMS?*
3. *How does the evaluation of headache differ in the pediatric population?*
4. *What role should "associated symptoms" play in the evaluation of a "chief complaint?"*

**PART 1—MEDICAL**

## I. The Patient's Story

Peggy is a 15 year-old high school student, usually to bed by 7:30 so she can be up at 5AM for school. She does not smoke or drink. She is one of three sisters, but is separated from her siblings and her parents; the other two sisters live with their father, and her mother lives in Phoenix, Arizona.

Peggy's home situation is unique; she lives with her grandmother, an engaged and caring person, founder of the Give the Children a Chance organization and host of Gospel Dimensions on WXYZ- FM. One of five grandchildren, Peggy has had some emotional issues, twice "cutting" herself, one time placing multiple parallel incisions on the left forearm and another time eight on the left shin.

On the afternoon of September 11, 2001, only hours after United 93 hits the ground in Stonycreek, Pennsylvania, Peggy begins to cough and develops a headache. Her grandmother tries to get her into the car to take her to the doctor, but is unable—at 2:15 PM Peggy's grandmother dials 911.

At 2:20, the paramedics arrive to find Peggy sitting on the couch. They record: "Patient had a sudden onset of neck and head pain this am after coughing. Denies dizziness, nausea, vomiting, numbness/tingling of extremities. ABC intact. Is able to move her neck."

They transport and arrive in the ED at 14:43.

## II. The Doctor's Version (the following is the actual documentation of the provider)

**Date:** September 11, 2001 at 14:53
**Chief Complaint:** Headache
**Nurse's Note:** Pt. c/o coughing and neck and head pains c/o stiff neck. Ears plugged – some nausea and vomiting of thin liquids. Pain scale 5/10

**History of Present Illness:** (Per physician assistant, Ms. Kelly McKinney): Patient complains of throbbing frontal headache(s) for a few hours prior to arrival. No n/v, blurred vision, photophobia, numbness, fever. Patient denies it is the worst headache ever. No trauma. Stated it started after a coughing spell. The condition has remained unchanged since onset. There has been no reported treatment prior to arrival.

**Review of Systems:** Unless otherwise stated in this report or unable to obtain because of the patient's clinical or mental status as evidenced by the medical record, the patient's positive and negative responses for constitutional, psych, eyes, ENT, cardiovascular, respiratory, gastro-intestinal, neurological, genitourinary, musculoskeletal, integument systems and systems related to the current problem—are either stated in the preceding or were not pertinent or were negative for the symptoms and/or complaints related to the presenting medical problem.

**Past Medical History:**
**Allergies:** NKDA
**Meds:** None
**PMH:** Asthma
**Soc Hx:** Nonsmoker

The History of Present Illness, Review of Systems, and Past and Social History are complete to the best the patient or the patient's representative was capable of reporting or could not be obtained because of the patient's clinical or mental status as evidenced by the medical record.

**Physical Examination:**

Vital Signs

| Time | Temp (F) | Rt. | Pulse | Resp | Syst | Diast |
|---|---|---|---|---|---|---|
| 15:00 | 97.8 | TM | 70 | 20 | 174 | 94 |

**Constitutional:** Alert and well developed
**Mental Health/Psychiatric:** Age-appropriately oriented to time, place, 3rd person. Affect appropriate for age.
**Head:** Without temporal or scalp tenderness, masses, or lesions.
**Eyes:** No discharge or conjunctival injection.
**Ears:** TMs without perforation, injection, or bulging. External canals clear without exudate.
**Nose:** Normal mucosa and septum.
**Throat:** Pharynx: without injection, exudate, or tonsillar hypertrophy. Airway patent.
**Face:** No tenderness or swelling.

**Neck:** Supple. No tenderness. No lymphadenopathy.
**Lungs:** Clear to auscultation and breath sounds equal.
**Heart:** RRR, nl heart sounds, without pathological murmurs, ectopy, gallops, or rubs.
**Neurological:** Cranial and cerebellar functions normal. Motor functions intact.
**Emergency Department Course:**
**16:00** – Ibuprofen 600mg PO. Soft collar neck. Ice pack

**Diagnosis:** Headache

**Disposition (16:39):** Patient was discharged home by the ED physician. Return in 2–3 days if no better. Condition upon discharge [undocumented]. Rx for ibuprofen 600mg TID. Return to ER if symptoms change.

*Kelly McKinney, PA-C*
*Bruce Hanninger, DO*

## III. Risk Management/Patient Safety Opportunities (Weinstock)

**Author comments (Weinstock):** There is a Bob Dylan line that comes to mind, "I can't help it if you might think I'm odd, if I say I'm not loving you for what you are, but what you're not." On the surface, the documentation seems good... but is there more to the story?

**Risk Management/Patient Safety Opportunity #1:**

**Opportunity:** Poorly defined onset of headache.
**Discussion:** When a patient presents with headache, fever, rash and confusion, my neighbor can make the diagnosis. The trick with headache is to find the life-threatening diagnosis lurking around the corner. Arguably the most important historical element in a headache patient is the onset.

Answers to the "onset question" can vary widely. Often, a patient will say the onset is sudden only to mean that it started over a period of a few hours. That may be "sudden" in relation to the time span of their life, but certainly not our definition of sudden; reaching maximum intensity in less than one minute. Consider asking a follow-up question, for example, "How long did it take from when the headache first started until it reached maximum intensity."
✔ **Teaching point:** Every headache patient needs to have a clearly defined documentation of onset.

**Risk Management/Patient Safety Opportunity #2:**

**Opportunity:** Inaccurate documentation.
**Discussion:** One of the most important aspects of the documentation is the general appearance of the patient. It is our Malcolm Gladwell's "Blink" moment. It is our gestalt as we walk into the room; "sick or not sick?" The appearance is documented here, but in a very general and nonspecific manner: "Alert and well developed. Age-appropriately oriented to time, place, 3rd person. Affect appropriate for age." To me, it sounds like it came from a computer pick-list or voice-activated "macro."

Consider this exchange during the deposition of the plaintiff's expert witness William Biggs by the plaintiff's attorney, Louis Latiff:

**Q.** When a patient presents in severe pain, do they always provide 100% accurate information?
**A.** Sometimes a patient in severe pain is unable to give a history until you've treated their pain and have them feeling better.

**Q.** Is it fair to say that Mrs. Rainey's (the grandmother) version of her interaction with Dr. Hanninger and Ms. McKinney (PA-C) is not entirely consistent with the [documentation provided]?
**A.** Yes.

**Q.** Is it fair to say that Mrs. Rainey's version describes Peggy as having severe pain and at some point screaming?
**A.** Yes, sobbing.

**Q.** That's not noted anywhere in the physician's report, is it?
**A.** That's correct.

Another interesting fact was unearthed during the trial; Peggy was examined while in the wheelchair. Her pain was so severe she was not able to even get on the cart.
✔ **Teaching point:** One of the most important parts of the documentation is describing if the patient appears sick or well.

<u>**Risk Management/Patient Safety Opportunity #3:**</u>

**Opportunity**: Contradiction between the triage note and the doctor's note.
**Discussion**: The triage note not only mentions vomiting, but describes the material Peggy vomited as "thin liquids." The specific nature of the description makes it believable, compared to the doctor's note which stated in the first ROS notation: "no nausea/vomiting." If there is a discrepancy between the triage note and the doctor's note, the more credible of the two wins, unless the physician addresses the discrepancy and declares the former inaccurate based on the findings.
✔ **Teaching point:** Just because your initials trump the nurse's initials doesn't mean your documentation automatically trumps theirs. Corny as it sounds, the providers should care for patients as a team.

<u>**Risk Management/Patient Safety Opportunity #4:**</u>

**Opportunity:** No exploration of associated symptoms of vomiting and neck pain.
**Discussion:** The primary complaint recorded by the nurse was headache, but there were other symptoms mentioned in the triage note, which were not explored further. Could the patient have had primary neck pain which then radiated up into the head, perhaps from a carotid or vertebral artery dissection? How about meningitis? She was coughing. Could pneumonia have been present? PE? Spontaneous pneumothorax?
✔ **Teaching point:** One complaint per customer doesn't fly in Emergency Medicine. When there is more than one complaint, they all need to be explored (remember Case 1?).

<u>**Risk Management/Patient Safety Opportunity #5:**</u>

**Opportunity:** No medical decision making (MDM) note.
**Discussion:** This is challenging, but no less necessary, in a busy community ED. Who has the time to write a progress note on every patient? Additionally, when ankle inversion is the mechanism and the X-ray is negative, it is easy to intuit from the chart why the physician arrived at the diagnosis of "sprain."

But there are some patients who leave the ED with diagnostic uncertainty; Peggy was one. The diagnosis recorded by the doctor was the same as the chief complaint, which is fine. But clearly, the exact cause of the headache was not defined. Writing a progress note will often force the physician to think through the decision-making process and differential diagnosis, often prompting them to re-check and re-examine the patient. If the progress note does not even convince you, it will definitely not convince a jury!

✔ **Teaching point:** Write a progress note on all high-risk patients.

**Risk Management/Patient Safety Opportunity #6:**

**Opportunity:** Reassurance because this is not the "worst headache of her life."
**Discussion:** I had a neurosurgeon see one of my patients in the ED, commenting to me later that the patient didn't have a headache with a "thunderclap" onset. Really? Get your head out of the textbook into the reality of ED headache presentations. What patient ever uses that terminology? If we sent home all chest pain patients not pointing to an elephant sitting on their chest, we would spend more time in court than at the bedside!

I personally never use the phrase "worst headache of life" and discourage the nurses from documenting it unless it is an unsolicited comment from the patient. After all, the first headache in your life is also the worst headache in your life (by definition). Besides, who would ever answer "no" to this question, particularly when the "questioner" is holding a syringe of Dilaudid and Phenergan?

What's most important is the onset and whether or not the patient's headache is unusual in any way. Reporting that the headache is the "worst of my life" is just one of many ways patients can relay to us that this headache is something unusual, unlike anything they have ever previously experienced. So, what makes a headache "unusual" enough to raise concern is the onset, intensity, new location, onset with exertion and certain associated signs or symptoms, such as syncope or neck pain, to name just a few. Another curious note in regard to our patient; here is a 15 year-old girl, who does not suffer from frequent headaches, being transported to the ED on 9/11 by squad because her grandmother couldn't even get her into the car. Here is a girl in such severe pain that she is examined in a wheelchair. Here is a girl screaming and sobbing in pain. And I ask this—how could this not be the worst headache of her life?

✔ **Teaching point:** Use caution when using catchphrases. Don't expect patients to conform to a textbook description of their symptoms.

**Risk Management/Patient Safety Opportunity #7:**

**Opportunity:** Gobbledygook! No. Not a medical term. But, nonetheless, I said "Gobbledygook!"
**Discussion:** Definition: unintelligible language, especially jargon or bureaucratese. We can trace its origins back to Maury Maverick, a man whose last name became synonymous with a politician who refuses to conform to the party line. (Though "mavericks" can change …) The term "gobbledygook" first appeared in print in the New York Times Magazine on May 21, 1944, being inspired by the turkey, "always gobbledy gobbling and strutting with ludicrous pomposity."

So, let me again reproduce the documentation from Peggy's chart: "Unless otherwise stated in this report or unable to obtain because of the patient's clinical or mental status as evidenced by the medical record, the patients positive and negative responses for constitutional, psych, eyes, ENT, cardiovascular, respiratory, gastrointestinal, neurological, genitourinary, musculoskeletal, integument systems and systems related to the current problem—are either stated in the preceding or were not pertinent or were negative for the symptoms and/or complaints related to the presenting medical problem." If anyone knows what this means, please write. If anyone thinks this protects you from a legal standpoint, please don't!

✔ **Teaching point:** Sometimes gobbledygook is just gobbledygook.

**Author comments (Weinstock):** A birds eye view of the case can boil down to a simple question; If there is an adverse outcome, does it help to document "Patient denies it is the worst headache ever?" (Especially if it is not true...)

## IV. The Bounceback

**September 15, 2001**—(PCP visit—four days after initial ED visit) Peggy goes to see her primary care physician. Her complaint is neck pain. He takes a history and examines the patient, prescribes flexeril for her neck pain and sends her home to return if worse. It is unclear whether the doctor knows she had recently been to the ED with a headache.

**October 7, 2001—The country wakes to the following headline: U.S. Strikes Afghanistan**

**October 8, 2001**—Peggy is not up for school. At 5:10 AM her grandmother goes to her room to see if she is awake and finds her unresponsive. The paramedics are called. There is no attempt at resuscitation. Peggy is pronounced dead.

**October 9, 2001**—As published in The Abdicator (compilation of two articles): Teen dies at home—Peggy Rainey, a 15 year-old South Kruesdale Avenue girl who had been hospitalized recently, died this morning at home and the County coroner's office removed her body, police said. They do not suspect foul play. The girl's grandmother found her unresponsive and not breathing at 5 AM. The coroner will determine the cause of death.

**Autopsy:**

Intracerebral hemorrhage due to ruptured berry aneurysm of proximal left posterior communicating cerebral artery

Acute "jet lesion" blood channel into left frontal lobe and left lateral ventricle with 30ml left lateral ventricle hemorrhage

No gross evidence of thrombosis or chronic hemorrhage of aneurysm. No hemosiderin staining around site of aneurysm

Acute pulmonary congestion and edema

No alcohol, drugs, carbon monoxide or growth from blood cultures

Mid and distal left forearm have multiple linear parallel incisional-type scars, some of which appear to be paired injuries. Inner mid left shin has 8 parallel linear incisional-type scars

**PART 2—LEGAL**

## I. The Accusation/Cause of Action

Plaintiff originally filed her complaint in September.

Plaintiff alleges that Peggy's pain and suffering and her death could have been prevented had the healthcare providers met their respective standards of care and detected or diagnosed Peggy's aneurysm. Had this aneurysm been detected, plaintiff claims that Peggy could have had life-saving surgery to clip the aneurysm.

Peggy's death was proximately caused by the defendants' negligence in failing to detect, diagnose, and treat her aneurysm.

## II. The Depositions/The Trial

Cast of characters (names changed, except where noted):
**The patient:** Peggy Rainey
**ED physician defendant:** Bruce Hanninger
**ED physician assistant:** Kelly McKinney
**Plaintiff's attorney:** Louis Latiff
**Plaintiff's Emergency Medicine expert witness #1:** William Biggs
**Plaintiff's neurology expert witness #2:** Leslie Neuman
**Defense attorney:** William Bonezzi (actual attorney)
**Defense Emergency Medicine expert witness:** Edward Eubank
**Forensic pathologist for defense:** Harry Manning

**Direct examination of plaintiff's expert witness Dr. William Biggs, board certified emergency physician, by plaintiff's attorney Louis Latiff.**

**Author comments (Weinstock):** The witness alleges that the history taken was incomplete and that if it had been adequate, the doctor would have been alerted of sentinel headache/bleed. His allegations are cleverly rebuffed later by the defense attorney.

**A. The importance of history:**

**Q.** Is the history taken adequate for an emergency room physician?
**A.** No.

**Q.** Why not?
**A.** First, the history of the present illness is totally inadequate. It does not meet the standards [for a patient] who presents with a headache. The review of systems is inadequate and inconsistent with other data. The physical exam records the blood pressure one time, and it's a crisis blood pressure. This is never addressed or repeated. One big deficiency is this record does not record a differential diagnosis, which is … which is a major feature of every encounter. And the discharge condition isn't given. There's no re-evaluation. There's nothing about response to treatment. It's an inadequate record.

**Q.** What is the nature of the history of present illness that you have cause for concern for?
**A.** The standard for history of present illness that every medical student is taught early in their training is that there are seven items that have to be addressed, and these items aren't addressed, and if they had been addressed, I think the outcome would be different. These items are the location of the pain. That is addressed. The character, throbbing. That is addressed. The onset and the time course. Is it sudden onset? That's a major thing that isn't addressed. The mitigating factors or precipitating factors, we know from the run sheet that this was precipitated by coughing, and that isn't addressed [by the doctor]. So, you know, by not addressing these important elements, the consideration of the cause of her headache was not there.

**Author comments (Weinstock):** Wow, this guy is tough! I'm glad he wasn't my attending when I was a med student … or maybe if he had been, I would be a better doctor. … He does have some good points, but would any of this have changed the outcome? Are the standards for a medical student the same as an ED attending? Does this equate to improved patient care? Whereas the onset is certainly important, would mitigating factors or location have made a difference in the evaluation? His answer about the HPI almost sounds like a rant, like he is responding to faculty in his institution or maybe a rogue student. Look what happens later. The defense's "cross" cleverly forces him to admit that many of these deficiencies actually were addressed.

**Cross-examination of plaintiff's expert witness Dr. Biggs by defense attorney William Bonezzi:**

**Q.** You indicated that the history and physical were deficient because not all of the items were obtained that should have been, those seven items that you talked about?
**A.** Yes.

**Q.** Well, he found out about the location of the pain, did he not?
**A.** Yes.

**Q.** He found out about the character of the pain?
**A.** That's true.

**Q.** He found out about the onset or the time course of the pain? "Patient complains of throbbing frontal headaches for a few hours prior to arrival."
**A.** Yes.

**Q.** Now, I note that on the history of present illness portion of the record, there is a statement there that says "Stated it started after a coughing spell."
**A.** Okay, I'm sorry. So that was addressed. I'm sorry.

**Q.** He also found out …
**A.** The time of onset, yes, but not the suddenness or its relationship to the cough.

**Q.** Well, was there suddenness?
**A.** He doesn't say. He does say it started after the coughing spell.

**Q.** Well, we just read what the grandmother said (not reproduced here), and her deposition said, "I don't think the neck and the head pain was brought on by the coughing." So, I guess what I'm looking at is, you know, there's nothing here or in the grandmother's testimony that would suggest that there was a sudden onset of headache, was there?
**A.** It's in the EMS note: "Patient had a sudden onset of neck and head pain this AM after coughing."

**Q.** Well, do you know whether or not the sudden onset of head and neck pain was brought on by the coughing? We don't know, do we?
**A.** Right. We don't know with an absolute degree of certainty, but putting the whole thing together, it all fits. And it's my opinion, and I hold this to a reasonable degree of certainty, that the sentinel bleed was brought on by the coughing and/or the hypertension.

**Q.** … are you aware that Dr. Harry Manning (the forensic pathologist) disagrees that there was a sentinel bleed?
**A.** No.

**Author comments (Weinstock):** What? What? Not a sentinel bleed? How is defense ever going to go there? Ever heard of hemosiderin? Yeah, I have too—many years ago in medical school.

**Continued cross-examination of EM expert witness Dr. Biggs by defense attorney William Bonezzi:**

**B. Was the final diagnosis of SAH even occurring at the initial visit?**

**Q.** You're aware of what hemosiderin is, right?
**A.** Yes.

**Q.** Okay. And are you aware of whether or not, if there is a subarachnoid bleed, that if the brain is examined in an autopsy, there'll be evidence of hemosiderin?
**A.** Actually, I never thought about it. I don't know. I don't know the answer to that.

**Q.** Fair enough. Did you review…
**A.** I practice in the emergency department.

**Q.** Did you review the deposition of Dr. Harry Manning, who is a forensic pathologist?
**A.** No.

**Author comments (Weinstock):** This guy is getting paid how much? Well, likely more for an hour on the stand than you made the last three shifts arguing with drunks at 3 AM and he didn't even read the path report? Really?

**Deposition (direct) of defense expert witness Dr. Harry Manning (forensic pathologist) by defense attorney William Bonezzi:**

**Q.** Did you reach any conclusions concerning Miss Rainey's cause of death?
**A.** Yes. The cause of death was a ruptured aneurysm.

**Q.** To what extent was the history important in determining the cause of death?
**A.** It had very, very, very little relevance.

**Q.** What factors did you take into account in coming to a decision on that?
**A.** The autopsy report and the microscopic slides. There was no evidence of thrombosis or clotting of the aneurysm. There was no evidence of chronic hemorrhage or evidence of a previous hemorrhage. There was no hemosiderin staining anywhere around the site of the aneurysm. There's no evidence that she suffered a previous bleed anytime more than four or five hours before she died.

**Q.** And you reached that conclusion based upon what factors?
**A.** The autopsy report findings call it an "acute jet lesion." There's no evidence of thrombosis and no evidence of hemosiderin.

**Q.** When you reached this conclusion, were you aware that Peggy Rainey had gone to the St. Steven's emergency room on September 11, 2001—and complained of a severe headache?
**A.** Yes.

**Q.** You are able to eliminate any consideration as to whether this history suggested that there may have been some earlier problem with this aneurysm that occurred prior to October 8th?
**A.** Although she may have had a headache and nausea and vomiting four weeks earlier, there is no evidence in the autopsy that she'd had a previous bleed. There is absolutely no evidence in the autopsy of anything being older than a couple of hours, and I concur with the pathologist who did the report and the coroner who signed it off.

**Author comments (Weinstock):** So there was no staining with hemosiderin, and therefore, she didn't experience a sentinel bleed. Maybe an enlarging aneurysm or other type of headache, but not a bleed. Even if a CT and LP had been done on September 11, 2001 he contended it would have been negative and not changed the outcome. The defense attorney further uses Dr. Manning's testimony to focus on the extremely rare occurrence of this diagnosis:

**C. This is a rare diagnosis in a 15 year-old:**

**Q.** How common is it for a 15 year-old to have an aneurysm of the nature that Peggy Rainey did?
**A.** Rare.

**Q.** How rare?
**A.** Very rare.

**Q.** How many cases?
**A.** Out of about 6,000 autopsies, I think I remember personally seeing two.

**Author comments (Weinstock):** The whole crux of the plaintiff's allegation is that if a CT and LP had been done, the sentinel bleed would be confirmed and the aneurysm would have been diagnosed and clipped. The following is this allegation played out by Dr. Biggs (plaintiff's ED expert witness) and then by Dr. Leslie Neuman, a neurologist also hired by the plaintiff as an expert witness:

**Direct examination of plaintiff 's EM expert witness Dr. Biggs by plaintiff's attorney Louis Latiff:**

**D. Should a CT scan have been done?**

**Q.** Should Dr. Hanninger have ordered a CT scan?
**A.** Yes.

**Q.** What would the CT scan have shown?
**A.** The CT scan has a 95 percent sensitivity to see a subarachnoid hemorrhage.

**Q.** What if the CT scan hadn't shown it?
**A.** If the CT scan does not show a subarachnoid hemorrhage and it's a high-suspicion case, then the standard of care is to perform a lumbar puncture, which is sensitive to detect virtually 100% of subarachnoid hemorrhages.

**Q.** Is it your opinion, Doctor, that Dr. Hanninger's failure to order a CT scan for Peggy Rainey was beneath the standard of care?
**A.** Yes.

**Q.** Is it also your opinion, Doctor, that Dr. Hanninger's failure to order a lumbar puncture was beneath the standard of care?
**A.** Yes. I know that the risk for someone who has a sentinel bleed, the risk of a re-bleed within three weeks is 50 percent, and the risk of death from a re-bleed is about another 50 percent. For the first month after a sentinel bleed, the risk of a re-bleed is about 1 to 2 percent each day, and neurosurgical interventions greatly reduce this risk. And I would say to a reasonable degree of medical certainty, looking at the whole time course and all the data … That's my opinion. Is it absolute? No, nothing in medicine is ever absolute. But it's more likely than not, in my opinion.

**Author comments (Weinstock):** Another of the plaintiff's expert witnesses was Leslie Neuman, a neurologist. He gives testimony, but it seems that his standards are of a neurologist, not of an ED physician.

**Direct examination of plaintiff's expert witness Dr. Leslie Neuman (neurologist) by plaintiff's attorney Louis Latiff:**

**Q.** You have many patients who come into your office with neck pain and a headache, do you CT scan [all of] them?
**A.** Do you want the real answer?

**Q.** I do.
**A.** Yes. Every patient that I see that has a headache gets a CAT scan.

**Q.** Is there any difference in the standard of care and treatment between neurologists and emergency room physicians?
**A.** I don't think so. I do not—I don't believe so. I mean, there are certain things that transcend certain specialties, where there is a lot of crossover. In this case, I think an emergency room physician [and] a neurologist, those front-line specialties could evaluate this type of situation.

**Q.** Was the standard of care met in the emergency room on September 11, 2001?
**A.** I believe it was not met.

**Q.** What is the basis of your opinion?
**A.** … the many issues we talked about, unusual headache, first time severe headache unusual enough to warrant transport to an emergency room, headache onset with coughing, some nausea and vomiting, complaints of neck stiffness, high blood pressure, all of those factors together …

**Author comments (Weinstock):** Well, how about the high blood pressure? It was checked once and was 174/94, certainly high for a 15 year-old girl (who probably usually runs 90/60), but not unexpected for someone in severe pain. A recheck might have been nice since the elevated BP was brought up more than once by the plaintiff as a risk of SAH. Her blood pressure was elevated on 9/11, but did she have a diagnosis of hypertension?

Additional considerations are whether or not the hypertension was a physiologic response to an acute CNS event? It is a well-known phenomenon that acute stroke results in a hypertensive responsive to preserve cerebral perfusion pressure. If the claim is made that the hypertension is due to severity of pain (you see where I'm headed with this), how can we claim this wasn't an unusual headache, based on the intensity alone?

**Continued cross-examination of plaintiff's expert Dr. Biggs by deense attorney William Bonezzi:**

**E. Is the elevated blood pressure a "red flag?"**

**Q.** You have a concern with the blood pressure?
**A.** This was another big "red flag." She had a blood pressure of 174/95. This is a 16 year-old girl with no record of hypertension who comes in with this high blood pressure. Hypertension is a major risk factor for severe headaches. Those readings are equivalent to a middle-aged man coming in with a blood pressure of 250/150. We see strokes in adolescents with blood pressures of 150, 160, 174. That's a serious red flag flapping in the breeze that something's wrong here.

**Q.** (By Mr. Bonezzi): [tries to interrupt]: Dr. Biggs …
**A.** Hypertension is a risk factor for subarachnoid hemorrhage, and acute headache in a 16 year-old with that blood pressure in itself is a neurological emergency. The blood pressure was never addressed.

**Author comments (Weinstock):** Ever see the movie "A Few Good Men?" When Tom Cruise has Jack Nicholson (Col. Jessup) up on the stand and decides to go for broke and provoke him into revealing what actually happened with a new recruit who died, with the Nicholson's subsequent, famous line, "You can't handle the truth!" Though the plaintiff's attorney's comparison to an adult BP of 250/150 sounds outlandish to me, I couldn't say for sure if he actually did have data to support that statement. The defense attorney must have been less sure, but decides to go for broke.

**Continued cross-examination of plaintiff's expert William Biggs by defense attorney William Bonezzi:**

**Q.** Get me the article or give me the study that you're referring to that compares her blood pressure with a male's blood pressure that would be 250/150.
**A.** I don't have an article that compares that. I'm just telling you that in medical practice, I've been taught this by my professors and so forth, that an adolescent with a blood pressure in that range is serious, particularly an adolescent girl.

**Q.** You don't have anything to support what you're saying, is that right?
**A.** Yes, I do. I have 25 years of experience as an emergency physician.

**Q.** Doctor …
**A.** I have some fine professors who have taught me that over the years.

**Q.** Doctor, that doesn't count in a courtroom.

**Author comments (Weinstock):** Embarrassing. Ever thought of being an expert witness? Maybe think again...

Did she have hypertension or transiently-elevated blood pressure? Is the contention that her elevated BP was a cause of the stroke acutely, that she had chronic hypertension setting her up for the aneurysm or more likely that cerebral autoregulation was responding to some CNS insult? She did have a recheck, but not in the ED. It was at the PCP office four days later.

**Cross-examination of plaintiff's expert witness Dr. Leslie Neuman (neurologist) by defense attorney William Bonezzi:**

**Q.** And, oh, by the way, you are aware that when she went to see her PCP a couple days later, her blood pressure was normal?
**A.** Right.

**Author comments (Weinstock):** We've heard a lot from the plaintiff's folks. How does the defendant rebut this witness? Enter Edward Eubank, Professor of Emergency Medicine. Board certified in emergency medicine, internal medicine, and critical care medicine. He has over 100 original publications, over 50 textbook chapters or invited review articles, and over 100 research abstracts. One of his main contentions is that the primary consideration in a 15 year-old girl with headache, neck pain and vomiting is meningitis.

**F. Is the very act of her presenting to the ED enough confirm that a "serious illness" is occurring?**

**Cross-examination of defense ED expert Dr. Edward Eubank by plaintiff's attorney Louis Latiff:**

**Q.** [Would it] be unusual for a 15 year-old girl to come into an ER complaining of a severe headache?
**A.** That isn't the most common age group that comes in with primary headache complaints.

**Q.** And you're aware that she went to the ER on 9/11, the day that the Twin Towers were struck by the terrorists?
**A.** I am.

**Q.** Wouldn't you find it even more unusual that a teenager would present herself to the ER complaining of a severe headache if it was simply a common headache where she never presented to the ER with headache?

**Defense, Mr. Bonezzi.** Objection!

**A.** No, not necessarily. In fact if anything it could almost be the other way around, that could have induced a stress reaction.

**Q.** I'd like to give you a hypothetical: A patient's headache was bad enough to present herself to the ER on September 11, 2001. The patient arrives in an ambulance. She was not able to walk as she normally would and was only able to be transported via wheelchair. The patient complains of a headache described as one that is killing her, a stiff neck, nausea and vomiting, the inability to walk and talk. Would your treatment differ in any regard to the treatment given by the ER physician in the file that you reviewed?
**A.** Well, you're outlining a hypothetical case that has some differences from the documented record in this case. If I picked up that chart [my] number one concern would be meningitis. The number two would be possible meningitis. It would not be subarachnoid hemorrhage. It's very uncommon in 15 year-olds.

**Q.** And I gather that you would not have ordered a CT scan for this patient?
**A.** I do not have sufficient information to be able to answer whether a CT scan would be indicated. There are a whole number of additional questions including [questions related to infection, history of headaches, severity of headache] and dependent to the answers to those questions, [I would decide].

**Q.** Isn't the arrival of someone in an ambulance an indicator that the condition is serious?
**A.** Yes and no. We have patients that come in by ambulance who are taken off the gurney and sent to the waiting room. Some people use ambulances like taxis. We do a very careful evaluation of a patient that comes in by ambulance, but that doesn't always mean they get put at the top of our priority list.

**Author comments (Weinstock):** Can we causally relate her headache on September 11, 2001 to the ruptured aneurysm on October 8?

**Q.** In your view, you're not convinced that the patient had a sentinel bleed on 9/11?
**A.** I don't believe we know whether she had a sentinel bleed on September 11th. I'm not a pathologist. I addressed the standard of care in getting a CT scan for working up a possible hemorrhage. Given her symptoms complex, given the course of her subsequent symptoms and how long they went on, I would say there's a very good chance that she did not have a sentinel bleed.

## III. Guest Interview—The Legal Analysis

**William Bonezzi, JD**
Bonezzi, Switzer, Murphy & Polito
Cleveland, Ohio
(Actual defense attorney in this case)

**Authors.** *The doctor was obviously concerned about the patient by asking her if this was the worst headache of her life, but failing to define onset. There were also some discrepancies between the documentation and testimony of the grandmother. How was this rebutted in court?*
**WB.** The grandmother was cross-examined regarding her recollection of the ED encounter. Her testimony did not comport with the statements she gave to the EMS upon their arrival. The complaints the granddaughter gave to EMS were also contrary to what the grandmother said. The documentation by EMS was important to set the stage regarding what was said to the first responders. I did not argue with the grandmother; instead, I brought out each discrepancy of her testimony vis-à-vis the documents. I knew that was going to be important to the jury, and arguing with someone who was grieving for the loss of her grandchild was inappropriate. The testimony of the PA was very important in supporting what the documents indicated. I ended my questioning with the significance of "the worst headache in your life." I asked what would have been done had the answer been affirmative as opposed to being negative.

**Authors.** *What were your main arguments to the jury?*
**WB.** I felt that I had a good standard of care witness, and an even better proximate cause witness. I explained, both in my opening and closing, what a sentinel bleed was, its signs and symptoms and what one would expect to see on autopsy. I also discussed a "jet lesion," the lack of hemosiderin and the fact that it was greater than 21 days from the time the plaintiffs claimed there was a sentinel bleed until the SAH. I indicated that the further out one goes from the original symptoms [of headache] the less likely the original problem was a sentinel bleed. My forensic pathologist was very good at explaining the dynamics of a sentinel bleed, the sequelae of same, and the medical reasoning why the 9/11/01 event was not a sentinel bleed. Plaintiffs did not engage a forensic pathologist and were left only with crossing my expert.

**Authors.** *Peggy was a "cutter," as described in the autopsy. Were you able to use this as an argument at trial that she was somehow overreacting or not giving accurate story?*
**WB.** I did not go into the "cutting" because I chose not to retain a psychiatrist to explain its significance. I did not feel that it aided in the defense of the case, which in my estimation needed to be focused on the medicine. Of interest was the fact that the decedent's sisters lived with their father and only Peggy lived with their grandmother. They all lived within the same city. The mother lived in Arizona and rarely came back to visit. Neither the mother nor the father were witnesses in the case.

**Authors.** *If there is a choice, a standards defense is always preferable, but in this case, causation (hemosiderin) was extremely important. What was your "hang your hat" argument at the trial?*
**WB.** I will always try to defend a case on both standard of care (SOC) as well as causation. If I do not have a standards defense, I will at times even admit that the SOC was breached. In those circumstances, I literally have to show that the breach of the standard did not cause the injury or death, and concentrate on cause. The more I focus on that, the more the plaintiff's attorney has to follow suit. It is then a trial of medical experts. To proceed with a true cause defense requires a good expert who has the talent to educate and explain to the jury the significance of cause, why the injury or death was not avoidable, and that under the best of circumstances, the outcome would have been the same.

**Authors.** *When the jury was out, what did you think were your chances of winning?*
**WB.** I felt very good about the case, but with every case that involves a lot of technical details, I questioned whether I did an adequate job of explaining the medicine and its significance. My physician was very well-prepared, as were my experts. I believed that if my explanations were appropriate, we would win on SOC, but I always felt that the best argument was causation, which this jury never had a chance to decide!

## IV. The Verdict

On September 13, Judgment Entry concluded in part that as a neurologist, Dr. Neuman was not qualified to testify as to the standard of care in the emergency department. One week into the trial, the family physician, Dr. Hernandez, was dismissed with prejudice. The trial continued on into the second week with the defense of Dr. Hanninger (defendant ED physician). At the conclusion of the trial, a verdict of 7–1 returned for the defense on Standard of Care. The jury never deliberated on causation.

**Summary of verdict:** For the defendant-physician.

## V. Guest Interview

**Dr. Leslie Neuman** (named changed)
Neurologist for the plaintiff

**Authors.** *What were your main contentions about the evaluation at the ED visit?*
**LN.** This was not an ER frequent flier. If her headache was bad enough to come to the ER, she should have had a CT scan.

**Authors.** Were you surprised with the verdict?
**LN.** I thought money would be paid.

## VI. The Appeal (September 5)

***Continuation of guest interview:*** **William Bonezzi, JD**
Bonezzi, Switzer, Murphy & Polito
Cleveland, Ohio.
(Actual defense attorney in this case)

**Authors.** *The case was appealed due to the trial judge's determination that the neurologist, Dr. Neuman, was not qualified to testify concerning standard of care in the ED. How did this occur?*
**WB.** The jury never decided the cause issue because they found 7–1 that the physician met the standard of care (SOC). The appeal was a formality, and the defense verdict was upheld. Originally plaintiffs retained Dr. Neuman as both a SOC expert as well as a cause expert. I was able to demonstrate that Dr. Neuman did not work in an ER, did not know protocols and procedures of an ER, and was not a neurosurgeon. He could not provide testimony relative to what would be done on behalf of Peggy Rainey had a CT scan been ordered and demonstrated a leak. He could not answer whether this "leak" if found would have been "coiled" or removed surgically. As a result, the original Judge was going to rule that his intended testimony would be limited. As a result, plaintiff's counsel dismissed the case with the right to re-file within one year. The case was re-filed, but counsel never retained a neurosurgeon and did not retain a forensic pathologist. As the case progressed, it was apparent that plaintiffs did not have an ER expert. I moved once again to have the case dismissed.

**Authors.** *Any other thoughts or interesting observations from the trial/ordeal?*
**WB.** As with any case, preparation was key. I felt that the case was analyzed correctly and the proper experts were retained. The issues were crystallized and testimony was obtained to support the arguments. The most important aspect, however, was the defendant physician's testimony. He had gone over the records thoroughly, he had reviewed his deposition so that he was extremely familiar with it, he was available for many preparation meetings, and he worked with me through the case. I also felt that plaintiff's counsel did not appreciate the nuances of the issue involving hemosiderin, and as a result was not prepared to counter it at trial.

## VII. Medical Discussion—Evaluation of Headache, Diagnosis of Subarachnoid Hemorrhage (SAH)

**Jonathan Edlow, MD, FACEP**
Professor of Medicine and Emergency Medicine, Harvard Medical School
Attending Physician, Department of Emergency Medicine
Beth Israel Deaconess Medical Center

Dr. Edlow was Chair of the June 2008 American College of Emergency Physicians (ACEP) Headache Clinical Policy Task Force.

In addition to clinical duties, Dr. Edlow has authored two books for the general public: *Bull's Eye: Unraveling the Medical Mystery of Lyme Disease*, which was featured on Terri Gross' NPR show *Fresh Air*, and his newest book: *The Deadly Dinner Party and Other Medical Detective Stories.*

### A. Intro:

I will start out by disclosing that although I was not involved in this case, I do act as an expert witness on medical malpractice cases, both for plaintiff and defense. Also, the diagnosis of subarachnoid hemorrhage (SAH) is a strong academic interest of mine. With those caveats, let's dissect the case that has just been presented. First, for at least two decades, SAH has been identified as one that emergency physicians have been taught to "never miss." Of course, "never" is not only a lofty goal given the variations with which patients can present, but an unattainable one that would require doing every test on every headache patient every time, at huge financial cost including working up all the incidental findings. That said, the most common reason for misdiagnosis is not getting a CT scan.[1,2] The notion, as the neurologist testifies, that "every patient with a headache" gets a CT scan is ridiculous. I doubt that it is true for a neurologist, but it is certainly not true (nor should it be) for emergency physicians.

### B. So which patients with headache SHOULD have a CT?

There were no well-derived and validated decision rules to answer this question when the first edition of this book was published. Since then, the Ottawa SAH rule has been published and validated.[3,4] Patients without any of the 6 criteria do not need an evaluation for SAH. It is important to remember that the patients who were studied had a new onset of a severe non-traumatic headache that reached maximal intensity within an hour, so they already had a "high'ish" pre-test probability.[4] Because thunderclap headache is one of the six criteria, ALL patients with thunderclap headache need to be evaluated beyond history and physical examination! If one were to decide to not work-up a patient with one of these six Ottawa criteria, you should have a very good reason and document that reason in the chart. Remember that the rule applies to patients with a modestly high pre-test probability to start with.

| Clinical decision rules to rule out subarachnoid hemorrhage for acute headache (high risk findings) |
|---|
| Symptoms of neck pain or stiffness |
| Age $\geq$ 40 years |
| Witnessed loss of consciousness |
| Onset during exertion |
| Thunderclap headache (peak intensity immediately) |
| Limited neck flexion on exam (meningismus) |

This "rule" is only meant for SAH and not for other serious causes of headache. Also, in this particular case, I would equate onset with coughing as "onset with exertion" since they both share the common physiology of a Valsalva maneuver that would transiently increase intracranial pressure (ICP). We don't know from the testimony about a "thunderclap" onset because it was not recorded. I would not over-think "immediately" versus "over seconds" versus "over a several of minutes," because patients are often unable to make this distinction reliably.[3] I consider this as a "tie goes to the runner" event. When it's a "rapid onset," it gets my attention. I always ask patients, "What were you doing when headache started?" Sometimes this jogs their memory about rapidity of onset. The important thing with headache history-taking is to ask a few questions to sort out the onset; it takes less than a minute (and if the patient cannot answer because she's in too much pain, I default to a worst-case scenario and work them up.)

This patient is a 15 year-old girl with a severe headache, no clear-cut history of a prior headache syndrome, that started with a coughing fit and associated with vomiting. There is considerable discussion in the depositions and in the chart (remember the paramedics wrote "sudden onset") regarding if it was sudden-onset or not. Although the lawyers can parse out different statements from different individuals, the reality is that the defendant could have and should have obtained this simple piece of history. However, let's give him the benefit of the doubt on this point. The absence of prior headaches is another issue. It's one thing if the patient has a history of multiple prior similar headaches and a migraine diagnosis and quite another if this is a first unusual headache. Add in the vomiting that the nurse documented, and in my book, this buys a CT scan.

She is neurologically intact with a supple neck. Does a normal neuro exclude SAH? Unfortunately, no. There are many serious, treatable neurological diagnoses that can present with a normal exam, including SAH. Meningismus from SAH may not develop for 12–24 hours and might not be present at all. So, like many physical findings, they are helpful when present, but useless when not.[5]

There is one other important clue, however, from the viral signs. A blood pressure (BP) of 174/94 is important. Whether this number is equivalent to 250/150 (as was alleged) in a male adult is irrelevant. What is relevant is that 174/94, in a 15 year-old girl (whose normal pressure is likely closer to 90/60) is an extraordinarily high value. For me, this BP is a big red flag — but not for the reason that the plaintiff's expert opines. He suggests the patient was hypertensive and therefore at risk for SAH. To me, the significance is that such a high pressure suggests (and only suggests) that a central nervous system process may be occurring and that the elevated BP represents autoregulation to improve cerebral perfusion pressure to an injured area the brain. Yes, it could be due to pain, or anxiety. However, 174/94? That's off the chart for me. At this level of blood pressure in a 15 year-old, the burden is on the physician to prove that this reading is not significant.

At an absolute minimum, treat the pain and anxiety and re-check the blood pressure. Failure to do this is an error. She had a normal BP four days later in the pediatrician's office, demonstrating that she is not chronically hypertensive, but the later pressure does not mean that the pressure was benign, since it could have signified a serious intracranial problem four days prior in the ED and which has subsequently stabilized. Another thought here is that if a CT had been done and was normal, a lumbar puncture (LP) would have allowed one to directly measure the ICP to test that hypothesis, or if one is skilled in ocular ultrasound, the optic nerve sheath diameter could be measured to approximate the ICP.

## C. SAH in children:

Aneurysms are rare in children; only a few percent of patients with symptomatic aneurysms are children.[6] In one single-institution review, there were only 77 aneurysms found over 27 years.[7] So, I can easily imagine not thinking about an SAH in a 15 year-old with a headache but SAH is not the only potential cause of this girl's headache. One should have a checklist of "serious" or "cannot miss" diagnoses (things that cause big problems and that are treatable) for every headache patient, at least to consider by history and physical examination. This patient could have hypertensive encephalopathy, meningitis, a non-SAH intracranial bleed (AVM, tumor, vasculopathy), cerebral venous sinus thrombosis, pituitary apoplexy, arterial dissections and other possible diagnoses. All are uncommon, but the bottom line is that the presentation of a severe, unusual headache in the presence of severely elevated blood pressure (which may have developed abruptly) demands an evaluation. Therefore, I would have done a CT followed by an LP if the CT was non-diagnostic. I believe that it was a violation of the standard of care not to perform these tests. The date of occurrence (9/11/01) is noteworthy. The first plane hit the North tower at 8:46 AM, and the second plane hit the South tower at 9:03. The ambulance arrives at the ED at 2:43 PM. So, the headache is already approximately about 5 ½ hours in duration, meaning that unless she had a CT immediately upon triage, she would not have been scanned within 6 hours of onset.

All that said, would the results have changed the outcome? I don't think so. The forensic pathologist's testimony is key. If her aneurysm had bled at the time of the first visit, there should have been gross or microscopic signs of the bleeding. Our old friend, hemosiderin, should have been present, and it wasn't. The fact that the plaintiff's expert had not read the pathologist's deposition is astonishing; for an expert not to know the facts of the case is sloppy and irresponsible. The absence of hemosiderin is the key to the case. The aneurysm had not bled at the time of the first visit; the glove does not fit!

Sentinel headache and sentinel bleed are two different terms that are often used interchangeably, but they actually describe two very different things. A sentinel headache is a severe, unusual headache that precedes a subsequent SAH. A sentinel bleed is an actual bleed that precedes a subsequent SAH. Sentinel bleeds are a subset of sentinel headaches. The vast majority of sentinel headaches are actually bleeds that, in retrospect, were not diagnosed as bleeds at the time (either because the patient never sought medical care or the clinician did not do a work-up). If all sentinel headaches were worked up, the vast majority would be found to actually be bleeds (in other words, a first, clinically mild SAH).

## D. What about CT without LP?

Are "reports of the death of LP greatly exaggerated" or should it "rest in peace?" There is variation of practice amongst emergency physicians about following a negative or non-diagnostic CT with an LP for a SAH evaluation. One argument is that modern CT is so sensitive that there is little value in an LP, which takes us time and is uncomfortable for patients. Another is, let's just do a CTA and if there is no aneurysm, then there's no need to look for bloody spinal fluid (CSF).

Maybe I am just old-fashioned, but I continue to perform an LP for cases in which the CT scan was done beyond 6-hours after headache onset. Negative CTs done within 6 hours essentially rule out SAH.[8] Although increasing data show that the number of SAHs that are diagnosed by LP is very low, in some studies zero at up to 24 hours after headache onset,[9] the longer out from onset, the more likely a false negative CT. CT hardware and software may have changed over the last 20 years, but biology hasn't. There is a brisk flow of CSF, which turns over three times per day. Thus, any blood in the CSF is being continuously diluted. The flow of CSF is why a simple trick can be helpful to distinguish a traumatic tap from a true SAH: waste 10–15 mLs of CSF between tubes 2 and 3, trying to get tube 4 as close to zero as possible.[10] Since the body makes 20 mLs of CSF per hour, those 15 mLs will be replaced by the time you even get the lab result back.

And by the way, it's not just my own opinion that LP should follow a negative CT done beyond 6 hours. The latest (2023) AHA guidelines on SAH still recommend LP "In patients with acute onset of severe headache who present >6 hours from symptom onset or who have a new neurological deficit, a non-contrast head CT and, if negative for an SAH, lumbar puncture (LP) should be performed to diagnose/exclude an SAH."[11] Another consideration about the LP issue is "who's reading the CT?" I don't think you need a neuroradiologist. I am OK if it's an experienced general radiologist who has been told that the clinical consideration is SAH, but I am not OK with a radiology trainee or most emergency physicians' reads (myself included).

What are the data that a normal CT and CSF analysis are sufficient? In a pooled analysis of 813 patients with thunderclap headache, normal CT and CSF, 0/813 patients had SAH or sudden death on long-term follow-up. This fact is in part the basis for the ACEP clinical policy on headache that states that patients with thunderclap headache can be safely discharged after a negative CT and LP.[12] However, occasional patients with acute, severe headache will have a cerebral aneurysm that is symptomatic (dissected, thrombosed or acutely expanded) but not ruptured.[13–16] Despite the number of references, these are the stuff of case reports and should not guide routine care. Some have suggested that CTA should be done to rule out SAH,[17] but I am against this strategy for many reasons too numerous to outline here.[18] I am not aware of any head-to-head studies comparing LP to CTA as a second line test and the new AHA guideline also does not recommend CTA as a primary diagnostic investigation.

One last caution about the CTA. There is a misconception that small aneurysms don't rupture and so can be disregarded. Although it is true that larger aneurysms are more likely to rupture than those ≤ 5mm, smaller aneurysms are far more common, so although a smaller proportion of them rupture, multiple series of aneurysmal SAH report that half of ruptured aneurysms were < 5mm is size.[19] Even aneurysms of 3mm can rupture,[20] so when you are doing a CTA for acute headache, consult a neurosurgeon or neurovascular specialist for any aneurysm found, no matter the size.

**E. The bottom line:**

My bottom line with this case: Take a good history. Don't over-think (or under-think, as was done here) a case. In patients with unusual, severe headache with vomiting (and extremely high blood pressure that is not otherwise explained), do the CT and LP including opening pressure. If these are negative, you have done a standard work-up, and although you can still be sued if an SAH is missed, it is far more easily defended.

Should she have had an MRI/A or CTA? This is a matter of judgment.[21,22] I would not testify against a physician who made a thoughtful decision not to pursue work-up beyond CT and LP. In this particular case, an MRA or CTA would have likely diagnosed the aneurysm, which presumably had acutely expanded, thrombosed or dissected. The outcome would likely have been far better, but vascular imaging is not standard of care for all patients with thunderclap headache.

In summary, I think that the standard of care was violated, but the negligence in this case was not the direct and proximate cause of the injury. The pathological evidence shows that she did not bleed at the time of the first ED visit. Therefore, had the standard work-up been done, the CT and the CSF most likely would have been normal, and the outcome would have been the same.

## VIII. Author Summary (Weinstock)

The initial ED record seemingly reads well, but during deposition and trial testimony, was revealed to be inaccurate. How could her headache have been 5/10 when she was at one point screaming and sobbing in pain?

There was a discrepancy between the triage note and the physician's note (triage: "vomiting thin liquids" vs. clinician "no vomiting"), indicating that the triage note was likely not read.

There was at least some diagnostic uncertainty; the presenting symptom was headache and the final diagnosis was headache, indicating that a definitive diagnosis had not been found. This is fine, but in these situations:

- Discuss this uncertainty with the patient and family so they can become "health care partners" and return if symptoms change, worsen, or persist.
- Repeat and record your evaluation after some time has passed.
- Document a progress note to explain why you do not think the most serious causes of the presenting symptom are occurring.
- One technique is to apply what we, the authors, call the "front door-back door" approach:
- Front door: A symptom-based approach to diagnosis (see Chapter 1 and OLD CAAARS mnemonic).
- Back door: A diagnosis-based approach, to gather data (H&P) with consideration of the differential.
- This chapter in no way recommends obtaining CT scans on all HA patients. It does argue for an appropriate history, specifically concerning the onset of HA, and an accurate description of the clinical picture.

## References


1. Edlow JA, Malek AM, Ogilvy CS. Aneurysmal subarachnoid hemorrhage: Update for emergency physicians. J Emerg Med 2008;34(3):237-51.
2. Kowalski RG, Claassen J, Kreiter KT, et al. Initial misdiagnosis and outcome after subarachnoid hemorrhage. JAMA 2004;291(7):866-9.
3. Perry JJ, Stiell IG, Sivilotti ML, et al. Clinical decision rules to rule out subarachnoid hemorrhage for acute headache. JAMA 2013;310(12):1248-55. doi:10.1001/jama.2013.278018.
4. Perry JJ, Sivilotti MLA, Émond M, et al. Prospective Implementation of the Ottawa Subarachnoid Hemorrhage Rule and 6-Hour Computed Tomography Rule. Stroke 2020;51(2):424-30. doi:10.1161/

STROKEAHA.119.026969.
5. Edlow JA, Caplan LR. Avoiding pitfalls in the diagnosis of subarachnoid hemorrhage. N Engl J Med 2000; 342(1):29-36.
6. de Rooij NK, Linn FH, van der Plas JA, et al. Incidence of subarachnoid haemorrhage: A systematic review with emphasis on region, age, gender and time trends. J Neurol Neurosurg Psychiatry 2007;78(12):1365-72.
7. Hetts SW, Narvid J, Sanai N, et al. Intracranial aneurysms in childhood: 27-year single-institution\ experience. AJNR Am J Neuroradiol 2009; 30(7):1315-24.
8. Dubosh NM, Bellolio MF, Rabinstein AA, Edlow JA. Sensitivity of early brain computed tomography to exclude aneurysmal subarachnoid hemorrhage: A systematic review and meta-analysis. Stroke 2016;47(3):750-55. doi:10.1161/STROKEAHA.115.011386.
9. Vincent A, Pearson S, Pickering JW, et al. Sensitivity of modern multislice CT for subarachnoid haemorrhage at incremental timepoints after headache onset: A 10-year analysis. Emerg Med J 2022;39(11):810-17. doi:10.1136/emermed-2020-211068.
10. Edlow JA. Managing Patients with nontraumatic, severe, rapid-onset headache. Ann Emerg Med 2018;71:400-08.
11. Hoh BL, Ko NU, Amin-Hanjani S, et al. 2023 Guideline for the management of patients with aneurysmal subarachnoid hemorrhage: A guideline from the American Heart Association/American Stroke Association. Stroke 2023;54(7):e314-e370. doi:10.1161/STR.0000000000000436.
12. Edlow JA, Panagos PD, Godwin SA, et al. Clinical policy: Critical issues in the evaluation and management of adult patients presenting to the emergency department with acute headache. Ann Emerg Med 2008;52(4):407-36.
13. Neuman JA, Piepgras DG, Pichelmann MA, et al. Small cerebral aneurysms presenting with symptoms other than rupture. Neurology 2001;57(7):1212-6.
14. McCarron MO, Choudhari KA. Aneurysmal subarachnoid leak with normal CT and CSF spectrophotometry. Neurology 2005; 64(5):923.
15. Raps EC, Rogers JD, Galetta SL, et al. The clinical spectrum of unruptured intracranial aneurysms. Arch Neurol 1993;50(3):265-8.
16. Witham TF, Kaufmann AM. Unruptured cerebral aneurysm producing a thunderclap headache. Am J Emerg Med 2000;18(1):88-90.
17. McCormack RF, Hutson A. Can computed tomography angiography of the brain replace lumbar puncture in the evaluation of acute-onset headache after a negative noncontrast cranial computed tomography scan? Acad Emerg Med 2010;17(4):444-51.
18. Edlow JA. What are the unintended consequences of changing the diagnostic paradigm for subarachnoid hemorrhage after brain computed tomography to computed tomographic angiography in place of lumbar puncture? Acad Emerg Med 2010;17(9):991-5; discussion 6-7.
19. Edlow JA. Managing patients with nontraumatic, severe, rapid-onset headache. Ann Emerg Med 2018;71:400-08.
20. Park GT, Kim JH, Jung YJ, et al. Characteristics of patients with ruptured very small intracranial aneurysm sized less than 3 mm. J Cerebrovasc Endovasc Neurosurg 2021;23(1):1-5. doi:10.7461/jcen.2020.E2020.07.001.
21. Moussouttas M, Mayer SA. Thunderclap headache with normal CT and lumbar puncture: Further investigations are unnecessary: Against. Stroke 2008;39(4)1394-5.
22. Savitz SI, Edlow J. Thunderclap headache with normal CT and lumbar puncture: Further investigations are unnecessary: For. Stroke 2008;39(4):1392-3.

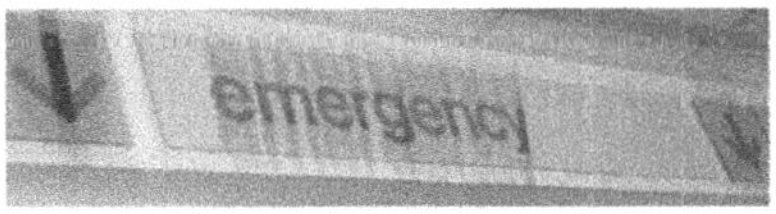


# Case 4

## A 36 Year-old Man with Chest Pain: The Double Bounceback

**Primary case author: George Willis**

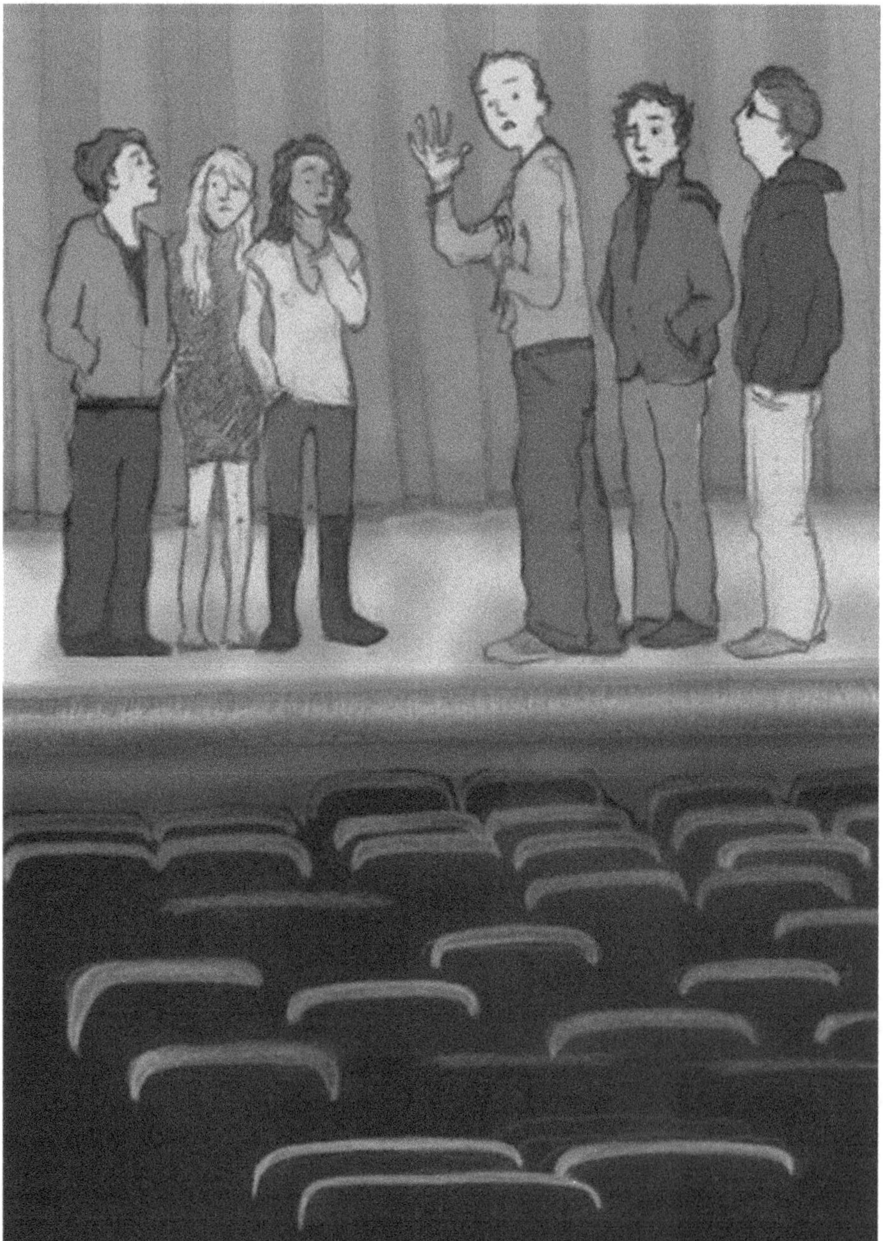

# Case 4

## A 36 Year-old Man with Chest Pain: The Double Bounceback

How much credence do we place in normal tests when the history screams otherwise? This case explores one of the most common and most devastating risk management hazards: failure to read the nurses' notes. Because of this case these emergency departments have changed their procedures.

***Deep thoughts:***

1. *Since we have more training than paramedics and nurses, can we ignore their documentation?*
2. *Is the "double bounceback" more legally troublesome than a single erroneous ED discharge?*
3. *Does a bizarre therapy in the face of a misdiagnosis hurt the physician legally?*
4. *How do we reconcile a patient with anxiety and potentially life-threatening complaints?*

**PART 1—MEDICAL**

## I. The Patient's Story

At the age of 22 Jonathan moves to New York City to pursue his dream of writing a musical. Like most struggling artists, life isn't easy. He spends weekends waiting tables at the Moondance Diner in Soho. He spends weekdays at his keyboard writing songs. His tattered four-story walk up is so tiny, there is a bathtub in the kitchen. Through the years, he has some success writing for Sesame Street and cabarets, but not the big break he has been hoping for.

In the late 80's, he begins work on a new project; he has a vision to create a modern version of "La Boheme." He doesn't merely want to update the opera, but to transform the American musical tradition, appealing to a younger audience raised on MTV, modern film, and changing social values. After two years of hard work, the project is suspended, but he returns to it with a passion after three young friends die of AIDS.

Finally, in 1994, he receives a grant to develop his musical at The New York Theater Workshop. He sends his dad a note: "Dear Dad, I quit work. Love, Jon."

In December 1995, dress rehearsals begin. One month later, on Sunday January 21st, he is in the theater for the final week of rehearsals, visualizing his last seven years of hard work. After dinner, at 6:30 to be exact, he is suddenly struck by intense chest pains. He is short of breath and dizzy. He tells a friend, "You'd better call 911, I think I'm having a heart attack," then falls to the floor between the theater's last two rows.

An ambulance rushes him to Cabrini Medical Center. On the way, the paramedics record their diagnosis: "Pleuritic chest pain."

## II. The Doctor's Version

**Date:** Sunday January 21, 1996 at 18:45
**Place:** Cabrini Medical Center, New York City

**Chief Complaint (per nurse at 18:45):** Inspiratory chest pain. Rates pain as 7/10
**Chief Complaint (per physician at 19:00):** Epigastric abd. pain

**History of Present Illness (19:00):** Pt. states he ate a turkey sandwich, which didn't taste right. Had dinner and smoked marijuana prior to developing Sx. Hx of ulcers but no hx cardiac disease, no smoking or cardiac risk factors—just finished producing a play—increased stress. Review of systems negative for nausea, vomiting, or diarrhea.

**Past Medical History:**
**Allergies:** NKDA
**Meds:** None
**PMH:** Ulcers, stress
**PSH:** Negative, non-smoker
**FH:** No family history of heart disease

**Physical Examination:**
**Vital Signs:** Normal
**Constitution:** A&O x 3, in no apparent respiratory distress
**Resp:** Breath sounds clear and equal bilaterally; no wheezes, rhonchi, or rales
**Card:** Regular rate and rhythm, no murmurs, rubs or gallops
**ABD:** Soft with minimal epigastric tenderness to palpation, no rigidity/rebound/guarding
**Skin:** Normal for age and race; warm and dry; no apparent lesions

**Testing:** ECG, CXR, blood work are performed but results are not recorded on the chart

**Emergency Department Course (additional info from interview later is included below):**
Dizzy spell while in the radiology department. Nursing documentation records breathing problems and dizziness while in the ED including the patient saying, "I can't take a breath." It is unclear from records whether the doctor was informed of this episode.
"He was pale and clammy," says best friend Jonathan Burkhart, who met him at the hospital. "You've never seen a person breathe as hard as he was breathing."
Jonathan's friend asks the doctor for an update and is told, "I can't find anything wrong."
You'll be out of here in one hour since I want to pump his stomach."

**Treatment:**
Gastric lavage with NG tube
50g activated charcoal per NG
Toradol 30mg IVP

**Diagnosis:** Food poisoning

**Disposition (22:15):** Instructed to eat a bland diet for 24 hours and return to the ED if necessary

**Note:** The next morning, the radiologist over-reads the CXR as normal *Michael Meirs, MD*

## III. Risk Management/Patient Safety Opportunities (Weinstock)

**Author comments (Weinstock):** We see this identical patient on every shift... or do we? This patient provided us with the diagnosis (food poisoning), which is nice, since we can just put it in the bottom box and move on. But wait—which medical school did he attend? No one wants to be sick, and in many cases, patients explain away their symptoms as a benign cause. In this case, there are few historical factors which support the patient's self-diagnosis.

**Risk Management/Patient Safety Opportunity #1:**

**Opportunity:** Not reading or acknowledging the nurse's notes.
**Discussion:** We have all had the medical school experience of presenting a patient's history only to find the attending gets a different history, usually with you feeling nine inches tall. Just because a nurse records a history does not mean the patient needs thousands of dollars of tests: "the worst headache of his life," "child turned blue," "pleuritic chest pain." But it does mean the documentation needs to be acknowledged and either confirmed or refuted by the physician. The options include:

1. Record that you have read the nurse's note and have discussed it with the patient (and/or family), and they deny saying the documented phrase. I usually note that I have confirmed this twice. Two doctors beat one nurse, even if it's just the same doctor asking twice.
2. Seek other ways to confirm which party is getting the most accurate information, such as family members or a squad report. (Note: realize patients may change their story, such as an adolescent who told the triage nurse he was suicidal, but denies it to you since he now realizes he will be "pink slipped").
3. Speak with the nurse to confirm that the history documented is actually the history received

Just as speaking with the nurse is important, valuable information can be discovered from the paramedics.Their observations are particularly valuable in seizure patients, motor vehicle accidents ("When we got there he was completely alert") and with altered-consciousness elderly patients ("Doc, we run on this guy every week, and he is always non-verbal.") In this case, the paramedics found a patient complaining of inspiratory chest pain who had just had a syncopal episode—not a story easily swallowed as food poisoning.

✔ **Teaching point:** Ignore the nurse's documentation at both your patient's and your own peril.

**Risk Management/Patient Safety Opportunity #2:**

**Opportunity:** Not digging deeper.
**Discussion:** A patient with food poisoning would be expected to have more symptoms than mere epigastric abdominal pain (i.e., vomiting or diarrhea). These associated symptoms are not essential for the diagnosis, but without them an alternative explanation should be considered. Was anyone else who had the turkey sandwiches sick? Is there any dizziness or sweating, or at least some nausea? Are there other symptoms (chest pain) which would lead the physician to an alternate diagnosis?

✔ **Teaching point:** When the story is not consistent, return to the bedside and:

1. Confirm the history.
2. Inquire about other important symptoms based on Ddx of "can't miss" diagnoses.

3. Re-examine the patient.
4. Ensure disease process is not progressing.
5. Record a progress note.

**Risk Management/Patient Safety Opportunity #3:**

**Opportunity:** Performing bizarre therapy.
**Discussion:** We barely pump stomachs for drug overdose anymore; it is hard to see how it would be helpful to remove a "food-poisoning" toxin already far enough downstream to be causing symptoms. Singer, et al. evaluated 1,171 procedures and reported that NG tube insertion was the most painful.[1] Was the doctor trying to be vengeful or thorough? The old adage, "Doctor, don't just stand there, do something," sometimes needs to be replaced with "Doctor, don't just do something; stand there," particularly when the therapy is unpleasant and ineffective.
✔ **Teaching point:** First, do no harm.

**Risk Management/Patient Safety Opportunity #4:**

**Opportunity:** Not addressing documented complaints, i.e., syncope and chest pain.
**Discussion:** Question: "Doctor, have you ever seen a case of_______?"
Answer: "No, I have never seen a one."
Question: "Never seen, or never diagnosed?"
The physician started with a chief complaint of epigastric pain, but after he heard about the bad turkey sandwich, it was all over. The complaints of syncope as documented by the paramedics and chest pain documented by the nurse should throw this differential wide open. Even if the chief complaint was accurately noted to be epigastric pain, there are non-abdominal etiologies that can be responsible for this constellation of symptoms, cardiac ischemia being one of the most serious. An ECG was performed, meaning this diagnosis was considered, but a progress note was not present to explain why the life-threatening diagnosis was not occurring. Additionally, a good history could have easily explored this potentially serious diagnosis with questions about an exertional component, radiation to the shoulder(s) or jaw, associated symptoms of dyspnea or diaphoresis, and of course, risk factors.
✔ **Teaching point:** If it's not in the differential, it won't be in the diagnosis.

**Risk Management/Patient Safety Opportunity #5:**

**Opportunity:** Poor communication between staff and physician.
**Discussion:** The patient had a dizzy spell while in radiology. (Why was a patient with food poisoning in ***radiology?***) There is no evidence this was communicated to the doctor. With the additional history of dizziness and dyspnea, the diagnosis of food poisoning would need to be reconsidered. One of the great advantages of diagnostic testing in the ED is that it prolongs a patient's course, allowing for the disease process to evolve. This seems to have occurred in this case. The doctor was either uninformed about, ignored or chose to not address the change in condition.
✔ **Teaching point:** Empowering staff to communicate with the physician will improve patient care and decrease legal risk.

**Risk Management/Patient Safety Opportunity #6:**

**Opportunity:** No repeat abdominal exam.

**Discussion:** Incorporating a repeat abdominal exam before discharge on all patients with abdominal pain will go a long way in finding the serious/surgical causes. Of all the stomach flus and food poisonings, a few will turn out to be something more serious, perhaps appendicitis or a bowel obstruction. If we see 150,000–200,000 patients in our careers, how many times can we afford to be wrong?

✔ **Teaching point:** Perform a repeat abdominal exam on all patients before discharge.

## IV. The Bounceback

**Monday, January 22, 1996—Jonathan returns home**

Jonathan is discharged from the hospital at 22:15 Sunday night, and upon wakening Monday morning, he calls the hospital to see if the tests had shown evidence of food poisoning.

"They couldn't find the results," says Jonathan's friend Eddie, who spent the day nursing him. "But he was told they were sure if there was something wrong he would have been notified."

The same Monday evening, his roommate Brian returns to their apartment to find Jonathan in bed, short of breath and speaking in a quiet mumble. Brian describes Jonathan's color as "pale and off-greenish." He is only able to eat Jell-O and tapioca pudding. Jonathan asks him to stay and sleep on the living room floor. Brian sets an alarm and wakes up every couple of hours.

**Tuesday, January 23, 1996**

When Jonathan wakes up, his symptoms have improved, but come evening, his chest pains have again become intense. His roommate Brian calls Cabrini and a hospital attendant says the hospital is unable to get access to the records from Larson's previous visit, so he takes Jonathan by cab to St. Vincent's Hospital and Medical Center, which is closer than Cabrini.

**Ed Visit #2: St.Vincent's Hospital And Medical Center**

**Date:** Tuesday, January 23, 1996 at 23:00
**Place:** St. Vincent's Hospital and Medical Center, New York City

**Chief Complaint:** Chest pain

**Triage (23:00)** – The nurse triages patient as "urgent" and records chief complaint of right-sided "inspiratory chest pain" for 4 hours. "The patient thinks his pain may be from heartburn."

**History of Present Illness (00:40):** Pt. complains of fever and right sided, inspiratory chest pain which is a tightness, which he rates as 7/10. Pt. complains of "not feeling right." Pt. denies malaise, cough, diaphoresis, myalgia, N/V/D

**Physical Examination:**
**Vital Signs:** Temperature 100.4 degrees, elevated heart rate of 100, respiratory rate elevated to 22, wide difference between systolic and diastolic blood pressure
**Constitutional:** Alert and oriented LUNGS: Clear to auscultation bilaterally
**Card:** Regular rate and rhythm without m/r/g ABD: Soft and nontender without r/r/g
**Testing:** CXR and ECG—Both read as normal by ED physician
**Emergency Department Course:** Vital signs not repeated.
**Diagnosis:** Viral syndrome with instructions to follow with his own physician. Condition: Improved.

*Paul Votapek, MD*

**Author comments (Weinstock):** A friend later describes Jonathan's appearance in the ED. "He was slumped over in a chair with his head in his hands, just completely out of it, white as a ghost, sweating and pissed off." He remembers Jonathan saying, "I just don't know what it is. I feel like shit, but they can't find anything, and I just don't feel right."

## V. Risk Management/Patient Safety Opportunities—ED Visit #2 (Weinstock)

**Author comments (Weinstock):** You can call a bounceback annoying, or be thankful for a second chance to "get it right." Often, the ED return patient is irritating to the staff; "That headache lady with the sunglasses is back ***again.***" In this case, it is hard to know if the physician was even aware that the patient had been seen several days earlier.

**Risk Management/Patient Safety Opportunity #7:**

**Opportunity:** Diagnosis momentum.
**Discussion:** In 2002, Croskerry described "bias" in medicine, later popularized in ***How Doctors Think***, a best-selling book by Jerome Groopman. Croskerry termed "diagnosis momentum" to describe a physician who gets locked into a diagnosis too early in the evaluation and is unable to escape[2]—sort of like the Eagles' song "Hotel California" where " … you can check out anytime you want, but you can never leave."
✔ **Teaching point:** The biggest impediment to a correct diagnosis is often a previous diagnosis.

**Risk Management/Patient Safety Opportunity #8:**

**Opportunity:** Not repeating vital signs.
**Discussion:** This is becoming a recurring theme. Elevated heart rate not rechecked in a patient who is "white as a ghost," diaphoretic and has his "head in his hands" is never a good sign. A re-evaluation and progress note are in order.
✔ **Teaching point:** Address abnormal vital signs and test results.

**Risk Management/Patient Safety Opportunity #9:**

**Opportunity:** Not recognizing a bounceback patient as high risk.
**Discussion:** A bounceback patient is high risk and has a higher chance of misdiagnosis, and a higher likelihood of needing admission.[3] Here is a suggested approach to the bounceback patient:

1. Thank the patient for returning
2. Sit down when taking history
3. Perform a complete evaluation with each visit—do not be misled by ***diagnosis momentum***
4. Specifically ask the ***main reason*** for the return visit
5. After history is taken, summarize to the patient what was just told to you
6. Ensure all documented complaints are evaluated
7. Review the documentation from the ***previous visit*** looking for:
    - Symptoms that were not evaluated
    - Abnormal findings not addressed
    - Accuracy of initial diagnosis
    - Appropriateness of treatment

8. Document a progress note explaining the medical decision-making process
9. Address concerns with family members
10. Provide after-care instructions which are action and time-specific.

✔ **Teaching point:** Though often seemingly annoying, treat the bounceback patient gently.

## VI. The Revelation and Outcome

The writer we have been discussing is Jonathan Larson, author of the musical Rent, one of the longest-running shows on Broadway.

**Wednesday, January 24, 1996—ED Discharge to Home**

- In the early hours of Wednesday morning, during a cab ride home from St. Vincent's, Jonathan complains of continued pain and tightness in his chest saying, "Nothing has changed."
- In the morning, the radiologist over-reads the CXR: "Heart size upper limit of normal."
- Later, a cardiologist reads the ECG, writing "question lateral MI." There is no follow-up with the patient.
- Larson calls his father and tells him he has chest and lower back pain and a low-grade fever.
- Around 7:30 PM Wednesday night Jonathan arrives at the theatre for a preview with 200 invited guests. His musical receives a standing ovation, but Jonathan is noticeably different. "He was moving slowly and didn't speak loudly," the director noted. "Jonathan was usually an exuberant guy, and he was behaving gently."
- He meets with a New York Times reporter around midnight who says the music is tremendous and would change the direction of musical theater. Jonathan says he needed to respond in some way to celebrate the lives of his friends who have died young. "It's not how many years you live, but how you fill the time you spend here," Jonathan said, prophetically in hindsight, about the meaning of his play. He leaves the theater in a cab, planning to meet with the director in the morning. He arrives home at 12:30 AM.

**Thursday, January 25, 1996**

- At 3:40 AM, Jonathan's roommate Brian returns home to find a gas flame burning under a scorched tea kettle and Jonathan lying on the floor. Brian opens his shirt and begins chest compressions, yelling, "Wake up! Wake up, Jon!" The police arrived shortly after and pronounce him dead. It is the day before opening night.

**Friday, January 26, 1996**
**Autopsy:**

- Cystic medial degeneration of the aorta, likely from undiagnosed Marfan's syndrome
- Twelve-inch aortic dissection from base of aorta 1½ cm superior to the aortic valve to the bifurcation of the common iliac arteries
- Hemopericardium and cardiac tamponade with 700cc blood in pericardial sac

***RENT* Preview**—Later that night, the curtain rises on the first preview. The rock opera's opening night ended with no applause. The audience, cast, and crew sat completely silent until an unidentified voice said, "Thank you, Jonathan Larson." Within a few months RENT moves to Broadway, where it wins the Pulitzer Prize, four Tony Awards, six Drama Desk awards and three Obie awards.

## PART 2—LEGAL

## I. The Accusation/Cause of Action

Family sues with an initial demand of $250 million, estimating revenues from RENT, in a negligence lawsuit against both hospitals. A report on PrimeTime Live raises serious questions and results in an investigation by the New York State Health Commissioner, Dr. Barbara DeBuono. The investigative process includes extensive review of the ED visits, 29 interviews, plus the advice of eight physicians, including three with expertise in emergency medicine and five board-certified radiologists.

[As quoted]: "Mr. Larson's condition was misdiagnosed at both hospitals," said State Health Commissioner Dr. Barbara DeBuono. "We do have concerns about the appropriateness and medical soundness of the treatment Mr. Larson received in their emergency rooms." (Note: one of the emergency physicians and the medical director of ED #1, Cabrini, shed light on the process later in this chapter.)

## II. What Would Greg Do (WWGD)?

**Greg Henry, MD**
Past President of The American College of Emergency Physicians (ACEP)
Past Professor of Emergency Medicine at the University of Michigan

Greg discusses care of the double bounceback patient, defense of the case and how a State Board review differs from a standard negligence lawsuit.

**"[In the ED] we have oceans of mediocrity surrounded by moments of terror and regret"**

I have to confess having knowledge of the case. Not only have I known of this case, everybody in the country knows of this case—we also know of the similarly tragic deaths of John Ritter and Richard Holbrooke.

Most of the things that we see in the emergency department are nothing. In truth, we have oceans of mediocrity surrounded by moments of terror and regret. In my 140,000 patient experiences, I don't ever remember seeing a young man of this age with Marfan's syndrome and an aortic dissection. It is easy to forget the rarity of this disease. There are only 3,000 to 4,000 thoracic aortic dissections in the United States each year, which means the average emergency physician might see one, even in a busy institution, every seven or eight years. Do the math.

Goethe said, "We see only what we know." When "what we know" is a diagnosis, we try and make the history and physical fit that diagnosis. The presenting complaints of this patient are syncope and chest pain, but we dress it up with everything else: "I ate a bad turkey sandwich." To ascribe causation to the turkey sandwich is to spell disaster. If the standard of care is what actually happens, in this disease it is to have missed it on the first one or two presentations. The diagnosis is always eventually made—unfortunately when it occurs post-mortem, it doesn't count for much.

Paramedics' and nurses' comments are equivalent to the physicians' in a courtroom: these are healthcare professionals that have both training and experience and a right to put their opinions on paper. The expectation of the public is that the physician will have accounted for the pre-hospital and triage notes when formulating a diagnosis. Ignore Allied Professional notes at your peril!

The concept of the "double bounceback" always needs to be sung as an emergency medicine anthem. If they are in for the second time, take a really good look; if they are in for the third time, admit. It doesn't really matter why they returned—if they have been back three times and the diagnosis is confusing, the problem is not resolved. In this particular case, the initial evaluation and bizarre therapy probably didn't do much to establish the physician's credibility, but they also didn't do much to harm him intellectually or legally.

Patient safety opportunities begin and end with diagnosis momentum. We get channeled as we see patients. When you see the patient for the second visit, listen to that little voice that says, "Something here isn't right." An even greater attribute is to look at a previously-assigned diagnosis and question its basis. There is no substitute for actually putting fresh eyes on a case. I'm aware of at least two insurance companies who request that return visits are seen by different eyes and unbiased neurons.

The defense in this case will be obvious:

- We are talking about rare disease
- The patient believes he has a cause for his symptoms that seems plausible to the emergency physician
- The vast majority of patients who present with such vague symptoms have no easily discernable medical problem

That doesn't mean we have a right to miss everything, but on the same basis we can't work up everyone for everything.

A decision to settle or try this case is more based on sensationalism than science. A famous person has died; the reasons for such a death may be secondary to the emotional appeal to a jury. There is definitely harm to the defense from the sensationalism and this would force me, as the representative of the insurance company, to seriously consider a reasonable settlement.

It is important to point out that families often don't just want money but may need some form of recognition or plan for quality improvement. I have settled cases in which part of the settlement was attaching a plaque in a room in the ED dedicated to the family member who they lost. I have seen cases where a family wants the physician to listen to their story of grief as a part of their settlement agreement. It is the wise attorney who takes all of these things into consideration when deciding on the resolution.

As was noted, this case was turned over to a State Board for review. State Board reviews are much different than standard negligence lawsuits. It depends on the state, but I have seen Boards with unbelievable power. It is clearly the uninformed and uninitiated who would go to such a meeting without proper counsel.

(Note: This case was presented initially as an EM RAP bounceback presentation in January 2009.)

## III. Review by the State Medical Board

Cast of characters:<br>**The hospitals: Cabrini and St. Vincent's**<br>**The family**<br>**The State Medical Board of New York**<br>**37 physicians and witnesses interviewed under the watchful eye of the press**

## IV. Guest Author

**Diane Sixsmith, MD, MPH, FACEP**
Emergency Medicine, New York Hospital Queens
Assistant Professor of Emergency Medicine, Weill Medical College of Cornell University
Expert witness for the NY Office of Professional Misconduct (OPMC) in the case of Jonathan Larson

The death of Jonathan Larson was a front-page item in all the local newspapers. The analogy to his own musical was too great to ignore. A later feature article in the New York Times was even titled "A Composer's Death Echoes in His Musical." The tabloids emphasized the fact that Jonathan had visited not one, but two New York City EDs in the days before his death; every ED director's worst nightmare.

Faced with the media attention, the Office of Professional Medical Conduct (OPMC) of New York State felt compelled to investigate whether the care met accepted standards. The Office is the working arm of the New York State Board of Professional Medical Conduct, one of 70 state medical and osteopathic boards in the U.S. and its territories. In New York, the Board is composed of hundreds of physicians in all the recognized specialties who are appointed to a voluntary three-year term by the governor. Another hundred or so members are laypeople.

While the OPMC investigates complaints about physicians, physician assistants and specialist assistants and monitors practitioners who have been placed on probation, it refers its findings for final decision to the State Board. Such decisions usually involve the medical license, but also may deal with substance abuse treatment, medical or psychiatric evaluation and practice monitoring.

In New York, physicians come to the attention of the OPMC through a variety of channels besides high-profile media cases. Malpractice claims, individual patient or family complaints, and referrals by other physicians or hospitals are all funneled through the OPMC and then reviewed for significance. If a particular incident or complaint appears to have merit, a medical investigator and a physician employed by the OPMC assemble the relevant medical records and interview the relevant parties, including the physician under investigation. They may also ask to see individual physician peer review or credentialing files, looking for other evidence of problematic conduct or care. The findings are then sent to an outside reviewer of the physician's own specialty.

I was the outside reviewer in Jonathan Larson's case. My job as a reviewer was to determine whether there were deviations from the accepted standard of care and whether these constituted negligence or gross negligence, incompetence or gross incompetence. My opinions were summarized in a written report, which was then used by the Office to determine whether the physicians should be charged and brought to a hearing before the Board. The main purpose of the hearing would be to determine whether the physicians should be allowed to continue to practice medicine, since the overarching mission of the State Board is to ensure public safety.

I reviewed the medical records from both EDs and the transcripts of interviews that had been taken with all the providers involved. A segment of PrimeTime Live had an interview with a cardiologist who opined that Jonathan's X-ray clearly showed aortic abnormalities, so I had his case blindly and anonymously reviewed by cardiologists, radiologists and ED physicians at my own hospital in an attempt to bring some objectivity to my review. To each of my colleagues, I presented the information in the ED record regarding history, vital signs and physical findings and then asked them to review the X-rays and ECGs and come to a tentative diagnosis and disposition. They were all surprised at the final diagnosis. None of them considered the chest X-ray significantly abnormal, and none of them considered the diagnosis of aortic dissection.

I was considerably bothered about the fact that in the first ED, Jonathan had an NG tube placed and was given activated charcoal, and I expressed this in my report. While I felt that this was not something that the majority of physicians would have done, we give other physicians considerable latitude in administering therapies that they believe may have efficacy.

I suspected that a better history could have been elicited at both ED's. The one essential aspect of the history that may have changed the outcome, the "bounceback," appeared not to have been known by the second ED providers. Was the failure to impart knowledge of the previous visit Jonathan's or the ED staff's failure to record it? I also was concerned that the dizzy spell while in the radiology suite at visit #1 was not more fully evaluated. But in the end, I felt that "there but for the grace of God go I" or any of my colleagues. In adhering to the information as it appeared in the records, without giving in to my own unproved suspicions about cursory histories or incomplete examinations, I concluded that on neither visit did Jonathan appear to have any red flags that warranted further work-up or criteria that justified further observation or admission.

Per the guidelines of the OPMC, incompetence is defined as acting without sufficient knowledge or skill; negligence is failing to provide the care that a reasonably competent ED physician or the majority of ED physicians faced with similar circumstances would provide. Since I felt that most physicians would have ended up doing a similar work-up and then discharging Jonathan, I concluded that there was no negligence or incompetence. Moreover, I felt that aortic dissection was a diagnosis that almost no one would have included on his or her differential diagnosis list.

**Author comments (Weinstock):** If you had to choose, which is preferable, a State Board review or a standard, run of the mill grilling in the courtroom? Neither? We agree!

## V. Guest Interview

**Tim Whiteside, MD**
One of the physicians interviewed, as well as named in the lawsuit, was Tim Whiteside, a very capable physician, double boarded in EM/IM.
Dr. Whiteside was the ED director at Cabrini Medical Center (ED visit #1)

**Authors:** *Did you see the patient at the initial visit?*
**TW:** No. I first learned about the patient from the Nurse Manager the next day. The nurses were concerned that a patient diagnosed with food poisoning was treated with lavage and charcoal since they had never seen that before. I reviewed the case and discussed this with the physician and was still a little unclear about the reasoning.

**Authors:** *What did the ED doctor say about the case?*
**TW:** His impression was that the patient would be better in 24 hours. He did not specifically address the chest pain with the patient. He was really focused on this being GI-based.

**Authors:** *The CXR was over-read the next day. Was there a discrepancy?*
**TW:** There was no discrepancy in the CXR report from radiology.

## VI. The Verdict/Settlement—Per the State Medical Board (Obtained under the Freedom of Information Act)

June 9, 1997: Whereas the New York State Department of Health has conducted surveys and inspections of [Cabrini Medical Center and] St. Vincent's Hospital and Medical Center and has found alleged violations of Article 28 of the Public Health Law and Title 10 (Health) of the Official Compilation of Codes, Rules and Regulations of the State of New York and Whereas the parties wish to resolve this matter by means of settlement instead of an adversarial administrative hearing;

### A. Cabrini Medical Center (ED #1):

ED doctor did not fully evaluate the chief complaint of chest pain. No information was presented that considered or eliminated the possible causes of chest pain.
There is no evidence the physician interpreted the CXR or CBC prior to ED discharge, contrary to established emergency room procedures.
The diagnosis of food poisoning was not supported by patient symptoms or complaints except for possible epigastric tenderness and description of turkey sandwich with a bad taste. Use of NG tube was inappropriate and unnecessary.
No repeat vital signs despite nursing documentation of breathing problems and dizziness.
**Summary:** Not correctly diagnosed and incorrectly treated.
**Penalty:**
Issued statement of deficiency and fine of $10,000.
Required plan of correction which would relate to the care of all patients. The plan must be generic in nature, aimed at preventing such deficiencies in the future. It must include intended completion dates and mechanisms established to assure ongoing compliance.

### B. St. Vincent's Hospital (ED #2):

Vital signs including pulse were abnormal and were not repeated, as required by hospital's own protocol.
Patient was triaged as "urgent" but not evaluated by a physician for 1 hour and 40 minutes after triage, not consistent with written triage procedures mandating evaluation within one hour.
With exception of fever, diagnosis of viral syndrome was not supported by Mr. Larson's condition or presenting symptoms. There was no malaise, cough, diaphoresis, myalgia, nausea, vomiting, nor diarrhea.
**Summary:** Not correctly diagnosed and incorrectly treated.
**Penalty:**
Issued statement of deficiency and fine of $6,000.
The respondent shall develop, submit and implement an acceptable plan of correction within time frames acceptable to and subject to the department's monitoring.
The respondent shall submit quarterly progress reports to the Department on each of the components of this Stipulation and Order for a one-year period commencing with the effective date of this Stipulation and Order with assessment of effectiveness.

## VII. The Press

**State Faults Hospitals for "Rent" Tragedy**—NY Daily News
by Joe Nicholson and Anne E. Kornblut—December 13, 1996 (shortened)

The author of the hit musical "Rent" was twice misdiagnosed and sent home from hospitals to die, just days before he was about to unveil the work that brought him international acclaim, state health officials said yesterday. As the main artery from his heart was about to burst, Jonathan Larson went to two of the city's most prestigious hospitals with excruciating chest pains, dizziness and shortness of breath. But doctors told him he had food poisoning or a viral syndrome and sent Larson, 35, home, where he died of an aortic aneurysm on his kitchen floor.

Larson's health problems were "not correctly diagnosed and inappropriately treated" at Cabrini Medical Center and St. Vincent's Medical Center, investigators said. The hospitals were hit with unusual fines totaling $16,000 after the state's four-month probe, and doctors at both hospitals were referred for investigation by the state's Office of Professional Medical Conduct.

"A number of deficiencies exist between the department's report and the medical facts in this case," said a statement from St. Vincent's Medical Center. "Our exhaustive review indicates that Mr. Larson's evaluation at St. Vincent's was medically thorough and appropriate."[State health commissioner] Dr. DeBuono conceded that diagnosing the aortic aneurysm "would pose a challenge to the best clinician," particularly because of Larson's young age and lack of history.

The musical, a modern version of "La Boheme" depicting life on the lower East Side, played to sellout performances at the New York Theater Workshop before it moved to Broadway's Nederlander Theater, where it won prestigious Tony and New York Drama Critics' Circle awards. Three months after Larson's death, "Rent" won the 1996 Pulitzer Prize.

**On Anniversary of a Son's Death, Contracts and Awards Are Small Comfort**
The New York Times—by Rachel L. Swarns—January 26, 1997 (shortened)

Allan Larson buries his grief in the stacks of paper towering precariously on his desk, in the pages of the book about and in the cards and letters from fans overwhelmed by his son's creation, the hit musical "Rent" And sometimes at night, in the hazy place between wakefulness and sleep, he finds himself believing that his son is still alive, that the telephone will ring and that Jonathan Larson, the curly-haired, ebullient playwright and composer, will be on the line, humming the riff of a newly penned song.
"I have my moments, when I still can't believe, because it shouldn't be," said Mr. Larson in an interview yesterday, on the one-year anniversary of his son's death. "But you wake up and it's the same nightmare," said Mr. Larson, who flew to New York from New Mexico with his wife, Nanette, to spend the day with the cast of the musical. "This year has been a roller-coaster ride from hell, and it continues to this day."

Last night, about 100 friends and relatives commemorated his death. Gathered on the stage of the Nederlander Theater, where the show is performed, they sang the anthem, "Seasons of Love." The actors in "Rent," a contemporary American version of the Puccini opera "La Boheme," have had to get used to working without him. But some say they still feel his presence. "Every time there's an empty seat in the theater, we like to think that Jonathan's there," said Anthony Rapp, the actor who plays the character Mark.

Yesterday, before the stage gathering, the actors shared their memories of the young playwright, who grew up in White Plains pounding on the family piano. "His big eyes, his smile, his laugh, his big ears, his curly hair, the way he always looked like he was up to some mischief, that's what I remember," said Daphne Rubin-Vega, who plays the role of Mimi in the musical. "A year ago today, we just sat there on the stage, huddled together," she said. "We spoke. We cried. And today we want to be together."

Mr. Larson's father, who scattered some of his son's ashes on Broadway, said he could think of no better place to spend the day than with the actors. "You want to be with family," he said. "They're family now."

## VIII. The Legal Outcome

The suit was settled for an undisclosed amount. Part of the money is currently used to fund educational efforts by the National Marfan Foundation.

## IX. Guest Interview—The Legal Analysis

**Greg Rankin, JD**
At the time of this interview, Mr. Rankin was the managing partner at Lane, Alton & Horst in Columbus, Ohio
Over 30 years of medical practice defense
Recognized as one of The Best Lawyers in America in the specialty of medical malpractice

**Authors.** *What is the difference between defending a case against an allegation from a patient and from a State Medical Board?*
**GR.** There are many differences between *civil litigation*, in which a patient is suing a physician for negligence, and an *administrative proceeding*, in which a state medical board is taking action against a physician's license. One of the main differences is the stakes involved:

- In a civil malpractice action, the consequence to the physician is an award to the plaintiff of money damages, which are typically covered by professional liability insurance. There are, of course, exceptions to this when the amount sought and/or recovered by the patient against the physician exceeds the physician's policy limits, in which the physician's personal assets are subject to garnishment. In a malpractice action, the rules of evidence govern. They typically preclude a plaintiff from introducing evidence of prior acts and/or findings of negligence on the part of the physician.
- In an action filed by a state medical board, the potential is for the physician to lose his license to practice medicine, either temporarily or permanently. Typically, there is no monetary sanction against the physician. In a state medical board proceeding, prior claims against the physician can be introduced.

**Authors.** *Is the first or second ED physician at greatest legal risk?*
**GR.** With respect to the conduct of the first ED doctor, there are a number of factors which could have made his case more defensible. First, had he reviewed (and noted in the chart), the EMT/nursing note, this likely would have sent him down a path different from food poisoning. The physician should have noted that he had reviewed these records, as well as the diagnostics studies and blood work. The physician should have set forth his thought processes and/or a differential diagnosis to reflect that he had

considered other etiologies besides food poisoning. Finally, there is no mention of the patient's condition at the time of discharge.

The second ED doctor did err by failing to note that this was a "bounceback." This information should have been elicited in the history, either by the nurse or the physician. Bounceback patients should be assessed at higher risk for this reason and should trigger an even more detailed and thorough assessment than usual.

Because Mr. Larson died from an undiagnosed condition does not mean that the physicians are automatically liable for the death. Aortic dissection is an extremely rare condition, which places it further down the differential. Though the first physician also missed the diagnosis, that physician may have less exposure at trial since the second physician should have been able to build upon the initial failed diagnosis and continued symptomatology of the patient. The second ED physician had the "last clear chance" to arrive at the correct diagnosis and commence treatment at a time that likely would have saved the patient's life.

**Authors.** *What factors play into the decision to settle or go to trial?*
**GR.** A settlement is arrived at by looking at the following considerations:
What are the chances of a defense verdict?
Is this case defensible on the standard of care or proximate cause?
If there is a plaintiff's verdict, what is the likely and maximum monetary exposure?
What medical expenses were incurred by the plaintiff?
What are the lost wages or lost earning capacity of the patient?
What are the non-economic damages to the plaintiff, i.e., pain and suffering, emotional distress, mental anguish?

Other less predictable factors include:

The venue where the case will be tried
Whether the jurors are generally considered to be conservative or liberal
Are there aggravating circumstances in the underlying case, such as gross negligence on the part of the defendant or an attempt to modify or dispose of records?
Will there likely be adverse publicity surrounding this case?
Are there significant sympathy factors favoring the plaintiff, such as the death of children?

**Authors.** *Would you have settled this case or gone to trial?*
**GR.** I would have attempted to settle this case for a reasonable sum. However, the plaintiff's demand of $250 million is far beyond the scope of potential jury verdict range. It appears that the plaintiffs were more focused on extracting a "pound of flesh," rather than a reasonable settlement figure. Sometimes we are forced to try cases that are going to lose because the plaintiffs are unwilling to accept a reasonable sum as a settlement.

**Authors.** *When a case is settled, is the doctor still entered in the National Practitioner Data Bank?*
**GR.** All cases which are settled on behalf of the physician are reported to the National Practitioner Databank regardless of the amount. The physician does have the opportunity to submit his own statement explaining the circumstances under which the case was resolved. Cases are typically subject to a confidentiality clause so as to prohibit either side from discussing the terms of the settlement publicly. This is done to encourage settlement and to prevent situations where a settlement will be used to cause embarrassment or harassment to a physician.

**Author comments (Weinstock):** This settlement was also subject to a confidentiality clause; we spoke with the Larson family attorney who was helpful and supportive, but would not reveal specifics of the settlement.

## X. Medical Discussion—Aortic Dissection Presentations, Diagnosis, and Case Commentary

**George C. Willis, MD, FACEP, FAAEM**
Associate Professor
Department of Emergency Medicine
University of Texas Health Science Center at San Antonio

**Chest Pain and Aortic Dissection and Legal Statistics:**
Chest pain is the third most common complaint for emergency department (ED) visits in the United States. Emergency clinicians must consider 5 deadly diagnoses for patients who present to the emergency department with chest pain including:

- Acute coronary syndrome
- Pulmonary embolism
- Pneumothorax
- Cardiac tamponade
- Acute aortic dissection

Most of these diagnoses are ruled out with a good history and physical examination or a rapid diagnostic test such as an ECG, blood testing, or chest radiograph. However, this is not the case for acute aortic dissection and the mortality is higher than the others.

In the medical malpractice world, this diagnosis is a frequent cause of medical litigation.[4]

- 41% of the time, the emergency physician is the main defendant.
- 72% of the time, it is for failure to diagnose and treat.
- 41% of the time, the verdict rules in favor of the plaintiff or is settled in court with the average payout being 1.3 million dollars.

That's not including the mental anguish the defendant clinician has to endure in defending their care of the patient.

It is well-established that aortic dissection's variable presentations make it difficult to diagnose. Some pundits even postulate that it is not in the scope of practice for the emergency clinician to make this diagnosis, suggesting that it is more luck than skill. In my opinion, the difficulty in making the diagnosis hinges upon three very related facts: 1) the incidence of aortic dissection is rare; 2) most emergency clinicians may not consider the diagnosis; 3) the lack of a rapid diagnostic modality to make the diagnosis.

The incidence of acute aortic dissection is around 3–4 per 100,000 person-years, but[5] it is difficult to calculate the true incidence as about 20% die before making it to the hospital. Additionally, most of these population-based studies are based on collections of large referral centers or single centers. Regardless, it is well-established that the incidence of aortic dissection is relatively low leading to lack of consideration when evaluating patients presenting with chest pain.

**Clinical Presentation of Aortic Dissection (including IRAD data):**
Most emergency clinicians use the history and physical exam as a tool to rule out diagnoses. The history and physical exam are primary tools in ruling out diagnoses. The classic triad for patients who present with aortic dissection is:

- chest/back pain
- hypertension
- pulse deficit

Clinicians are taught that the pain will be described as "tearing" or "ripping" and going into the back, often between the shoulder blades. Additionally, the pain is described as "severe" and usually abrupt in onset. The International Registry of Aortic Dissection or IRAD reports that 79% of patients present with chest/back pain, which means that about 21% do not.[6-7] There is a small study from China of 141 patients presenting to the ED who were subsequently diagnosed with aortic dissection of which 61 presented without chest pain; those patients were more likely to present with abdominal or back pain alone and were more likely to have shock.[8] In patients who present with abdominal pain alone, one study showed a delay in diagnosis which led to higher mortality.[9] Syncope is described in 13% of cases and is more likely to present with painless aortic dissection but is also more likely to present with some complication such as tamponade or stroke from cerebral malperfusion.[6]

I personally think aortic dissection should be considered with any acute torso pain. Whether it be pain in the back, abdomen, or chest. If the pain abruptly occurs and reaches maximum severity within minutes, an evaluation should be considered. In my charting, I make a habit to use a mnemonic for pain complaints. OLDCAAR or OPQRST are a couple to consider. I do make a point to note the Onset, describing the acuity of the onset, the Character or Quality, describing it as sharp or dull or tearing in nature and any associated symptoms (which I'll cover in the next section). Also, any patient with migrating chest pain or pain that is moving from one area of the chest or back into another should have an evaluation of their aorta. Lastly, unexplained syncope should have aortic dissection considered in the differential diagnosis.

**Chest Pain "Plus:"**
The aorta has multiple arterial branches that supply blood to the brain, heart, gastrointestinal organs, kidneys, spine, and extremities. Some pundits recommend that if there is pain above and below the diaphragm, an aortic work-up should be considered. I would take it one step further: by thinking about "chest pain plus." If a patient presents with chest pain plus another pain-related complaint or neurologic deficit, consider evaluation for aortic dissection. This is especially true of neurologic symptoms, as the presence of both is almost pathognomonic for aortic dissection. Any patient I evaluate for stroke, I inquire about chest pain preceding or coinciding with the neurologic deficit. Too often, clinicians focus on the chest pain and disregard the other complaint, subsequently missing this critical diagnosis.

Hypertension is thought to commonly occur in patients with aortic dissection and, indeed, hypertension is the leading risk factor for patients to develop an aortic dissection. However, IRAD paints a different picture; 49% of patients who presented with aortic dissection were found to have systolic blood pressure greater than 150 mmHg, which means that 51% of patients were found to be normotensive or hypotensive on presentation.[7] This could be due to tamponade, aortic insufficiency, or simply taking the blood pressure in an arm that has a malperfused brachial artery from the intimal flap. Regardless, emergency clinicians should not rely on the absence of elevated blood pressure to rule out aortic dissection.

Other risk factors exist for aortic disease; most patients are older than 50 years old, but younger patients can develop the disease as well, commonly as a result of connective tissue disorders such as Marfan Syndrome or Ehlers-Danlos Syndrome. Unfortunately, some of these patients are unaware of the diagnosis at presentation. Cocaine use causes a catecholamine surge and vascular changes that can cause an intimal tear and subsequent dissection. Pregnancy can also cause aortic dissection although it is rare, only occurring in about 1% of women in the IRAD database.[10] However, about 19% of women less than 35 years old presented during pregnancy or within 12 weeks postpartum,[10] most having an underlying undiagnosed connective tissue disorder.

Lastly, pulse deficits are thought to commonly occur. If a pulse differential exists, consider aortic dissection, but according to IRAD, this was only present in 15% of patients diagnosed with an aortic dissection.[7] The problem with relying on this finding is that the deficit can be located in the upper or lower extremities and often emergency clinicians compare the upper extremities to each other and neglect the lower extremities.

**Diagnosing Aortic Dissection:**

There have been many attempts to create clinical decision rules and to find a blood test which would rapidly rule out aortic dissection. Chest radiographs are only about 62% sensitive for diagnosing aortic dissection, according to IRAD.[7] Therefore, a chest radiograph is inadequate as a rule out diagnostic tool. If the chest radiograph shows any concerning findings, CT imaging is warranted. D-dimer is claimed to have very good sensitivity while poor specificity for diagnosing aortic dissection in several studies and has been presented as a potential rule out diagnostic modality.[11-13] However, the large majority of the studies evaluating D-dimer had low numbers, were retrospective, had very high incidences of aortic dissection in their populations, or were metanalyses. Until there is a good prospective trial, D-dimer should not be utilized for ruling out of aortic dissection, and this is supported in The American College of Emergency Physicians (ACEP) clinical policy statement.[14]

Lastly, there are two clinical decision rules: Aortic Dissection Detection Risk Score (ADD-RS) and the AORTAs score. The ADD-RS combines high-risk historical features, high-risk predisposing conditions, and high-risk physical exam findings to estimate pretest probability. It was, however, found to be an inferior scoring system when used alone. However, Nazerian, et al. retrospectively and, in a separate study, prospectively combined the ADD-RS with D-dimer to propose a diagnostic algorithm with promising results, claiming a near 100% sensitivity for patients with an ADD-RS score of 0 with a negative D-dimer and 98.8% sensitivity for patients with an ADD-RS score of 1 with a negative D-dimer.[15-16] The problem with these studies is that the prevalence in the patient population studied was 13%, which is very high. Nazerian is part of the study team also for the AORTAs score which combines 6 of the clinical features of the ADD-RS and again combines with the D-dimer. As seen in the ADD-RS trial, near 100% sensitivity, but the specificity plummeted to 48% and, again, the prevalence was elevated at 11%.[17]

The gold standard diagnostic modality is CT angiogram (CTA). In addition to confirming the diagnosis, the CTA confers additional benefits including diagnosing any malperfusion of organs from the intimal flap occluding the arterial branches of the aorta. Some clinicians think that CTA chest PE protocol is sufficient to help rule out PE and aortic dissection. However, the timing of the contrast bolus is different for PE vs. aortic dissection studies and is insufficient to rule out aortic dissection. Therefore, it is recommended to order the appropriate study for the diagnosis that is the most likely based on the clinical presentation. In unstable patients who clinicians are hesitant to transport to CT, transesophageal echocardiogram is also very sensitive and specific for aortic dissection. Transthoracic echocardiogram is not very sensitive but has a specificity of greater than 90%. Both latter modalities are operator-dependent.

There is certainly a risk of radiation and contrast with over-testing, but a risk of missing disease with under-testing, so how do we decide? With the presence of the aforementioned findings on history or physical exam and certainly in conjunction with risk factors, this should warrant consideration of aortic imaging. Documentation of the absence of these findings and decision-making to forgo testing will lower the medicolegal risk if aortic dissection is missed.

**Jonathan Larson's Case:**
Describing Jonathan's case as difficult is an understatement! We have the benefit of hindsight, but, clearly, the first emergency physician had a few things going against them. First, Jonathan was young. Second, he had a previous diagnosis of "ulcers." His symptoms began after eating a sandwich that he said, "didn't taste right." The consideration of a gastrointestinal malady would be a logical conclusion. However, it doesn't really explain the necessity of pumping the stomach and then giving a medication (ketorolac) that is known to increase gastrointestinal upset and increase the likelihood of peptic ulcer disease. I do question some of the decision-making here.

A few things in this initial presentation stick out like a sore thumb. First, the physician's final diagnosis of food poisoning and Jonathan's clinical presentation don't make sense. Food poisoning is almost always accompanied by some gastrointestinal symptoms such as nausea, vomiting, or diarrhea, which the emergency physician notes are absent. Second, he has a dizzy spell with reported breathing problems in radiology. Now, it is entirely possible that the physician was not made aware of this episode, but it's hard to imagine a nurse noting it in documentation but not telling the doctor about it. A patient who is volume-depleted from vomiting and diarrhea may have dizziness, but recall, he didn't have either of those symptoms. Lastly, what about the chest pain and syncope? There is no documentation of the syncope in anyone's notes from EMS, nursing, or the physician. However, the chest pain was reported by EMS and by nursing. It is not even addressed by the physician that there is acknowledgement of the EMS report or the nursing documentation. Not addressing the history obtained by an initial provider has come back to bite many a clinician!

The second visit is a little more worrisome. Any bounceback should be considered an opportunity for broadening the diagnostic work-up. It is not evident that the clinicians at this second visit, which is at a different hospital, even knew about the first visit. However, the triage nurse and the physician both note a complaint of "inspiratory chest pain" in their notes. Additionally, abnormal vital signs with fever, tachycardia, and tachypnea (at 22 breaths per minute) were noted, which means someone actually counted. Most notably "a wide difference between systolic and diastolic blood pressure" was documented. Pulmonary embolism should have certainly been in the differential with his tachycardia, tachypnea, and pleuritic chest pain, and it is entirely possible that, had a CT scan been performed, an aortic dissection may have been diagnosed by pure chance. Again, the final diagnosis doesn't coincide with the presentation. Yes, viral syndrome can present with fever, but I've never heard of nor seen a viral syndrome cause chest pain at 7/10 in severity and have absence of any other viral symptoms, notably cough, myalgias, malaise, nausea, vomiting, or diarrhea. What virus causes isolated inspiratory chest pain?

**Bottom Line:**
Aortic dissection is one of the 5 most deadly causes of chest pain. Although its incidence is rare, it is incumbent upon emergency clinicians to gather appropriate data to avoid missing this deadly diagnosis. Be thorough in your evaluation, and make certain your documentation reflects a logical conclusion about the final diagnosis; this will most importantly improve patient safety, but also lower your risk of malpractice.

**Pearls:**

- Aortic dissection is a difficult diagnosis to make. Consider in patients with elevated risk and remember that young people can get sick also.
- Consider aortic dissection in all patients with acute torso pain or pain plus another complaint, especially if it is neurologic.
- There are no shortcuts, such as D-dimer, to making this diagnosis. CT angiogram is the modality of choice.
- If the final diagnosis has atypical symptoms or absence of typical symptoms, consider starting over and asking further questions or broadening the work-up. The medical decision note should reflect why it is not in the differential.

## XI. Author Summary (Weinstock)

Mr. Larson had pain described by friends as severe, with associated shortness of breath and two near-syncopal episodes. In retrospect, in a patient with probable Marfan's syndrome, these symptoms fit neatly into a picture of aortic dissection. But it is easy to see how this unusual diagnosis could have been missed, especially if it wasn't in the physician's differential.

Like many of our patients, Jonathan Larson did not want to have a serious diagnosis, telling the first physician about a bad turkey sandwich and the second that he thought he had heartburn. Both physicians were led astray. But both missed opportunities to make the diagnosis, including reading the nurses' and paramedics' notes, getting additional history from his friends in the ED, reassessing Jonathan after he deteriorated during his initial ED visit with a near syncopal episode, and having time and action-specific follow-up in a patient who is discharged with diagnostic uncertainty.

The second visit was more troubling because he was now a bounceback patient, putting him at higher risk of having a serious underlying problem. Jonathan also had another serious risk for misdiagnosis: a previous diagnosis. His tachycardia was not recognized or reassessed. His CXR was possibly misread, and over-reliance was certainly placed on testing above clinical findings. The ECG was abnormal with an unrecorded impression.

Jonathan's father, Allan Larson, summed up the feelings of any parent who survives his child: "Parents should never have to cry for their lost children."

Thanks to:

1. Allan Larson, Jonathan's father, who supported this work and clarified details of Jonathan's life during the course of several telephone calls
2. Jonathan Martin, Director of Education at the National Marfan Foundation
3. Sora Newman, from National Public Radio, for focusing the commentary
4. The State of New York Department of Health

## References


1. Singer AJ, Richman PB, Kowalska A, et al. Comparison of patient and practitioner assessments of pain from commonly performed emergency department procedures. Annals Emerg Med 1999;33:652-8.
2. Croskerry P. Achieving quality in clinical decision making: Cognitive strategies and detection of bias. Acad Emerg Med 2002; 9:1184-204.
3. Martin-Gill C, Reiser RC. Risk factors for 72-hour admission to the ED. Am J Emerg Med 2004;22:448-53.
4. Choinski K, Sanon O, Tadros R, et al. Review of malpractice lawsuits in the diagnosis and management of aortic aneurysms and aortic dissections. Vasc Endovascular Surg 2022;56(1):33-9. doi:10.1177/15385744211026455.
5. DeMartino RR, Sen I, Huang Y, et al. Population-based assessment of the incidence of aortic dissection, intramural hematoma, and penetrating ulcer, and its associated mortality from 1995 to 2015. Circ Cardiovasc Qual Outcomes 2018;11(8):e004689. doi:10.1161/CIRCOUTCOMES.118.004689.
6. Evangelista A, Isselbacher EM, Bossone E, et al. Insights from the international registry of acute aortic dissection: a 20-year experience of collaborative clinical research. Circulation 24 2018;137(17):1846-60. doi:10.1161/CIRCULATIONAHA.117.031264.
7. Hagan PG, Nienaber CA, Isselbacher EM, et al. The International Registry of Acute Aortic Dissection (IRAD):New insights into an old disease. JAMA 2000;283(7):897-903. doi:10.1001/jama.283.7.897.
8. Fan KL, Leung LP. Clinical profile of patients of acute aortic dissection presenting to the ED without chest pain. Am J Emerg Med 2017;35(4):599-01. doi:10.1016/j.ajem.2016.12.037.
9. Upchurch GR, Jr., Nienaber C, Fattori R, et al. Acute aortic dissection presenting with primarily abdominal pain: a rare manifestation of a deadly disease. Ann Vasc Surg 2005;19(3):367-73. doi:10.1007/ s10016-004-0171-x.
10. Braverman AC, Mittauer E, Harris KM, et al. Clinical features and outcomes of pregnancy-related acute aortic dissection. JAMA Cardiol 2021;6(1):58-66. doi:10.1001/jamacardio.2020.4876
11. Suzuki T, Distante A, Zizza A, et al. Diagnosis of acute aortic dissection by D-dimer: The International Registry of Acute Aortic Dissection Substudy on Biomarkers (IRAD-Bio) experience. Circulation 2009;119(20):2702-7. doi:10.1161/CIRCULATIONAHA.108.833004.
12. Fan QK, Wang WW, Zhang ZL, et al. Evaluation of D-dimer in the diagnosis of suspected aortic dissection. Clin Chem Lab Med 2010;48(12):1733-7. doi:10.1515/CCLM.2010.337.
13. Asha SE, Miers JW. A systematic review and meta-analysis of D-dimer as a rule-out test for suspected acute aortic dissection. Ann Emerg Med 2015;66(4):368-78. doi:10.1016/j.annemergmed.2015.02.013.
14. Diercks DB, Promes SB, Schuur JD, et al. Clinical policy:Critical issues in the evaluation and management of adult patients with suspected acute nontraumatic thoracic aortic dissection. Ann Emerg Med 2015;65(1):32-42.e12. doi:10.1016/j.annemergmed.2014.11.002.
15. Nazerian P, Morello F, Vanni S, et al. Combined use of aortic dissection detection risk score and D-dimer in the diagnostic workup of suspected acute aortic dissection. Int J Cardiol 2014;175(1):78-82. doi:10.1016/j.ijcard.2014.04.257
16. Nazerian P, Mueller C, Soeiro AM, et al. Diagnostic accuracy of the aortic dissection detection risk score plus d-dimer for acute aortic syndromes: The ADvISED Prospective Multicenter Study. Circulation Jan 16 2018;137(3):250-258. doi:10.1161/CIRCULATIONAHA.117.029457
17. Morello F, Bima P, Pivetta E, et al. Development and validation of a simplified probability

assessment score integrated with age-adjusted D-dimer for diagnosis of acute aortic syndromes. J Am Heart Assoc 2021;10(3):e018425. doi:10.1161/JAHA.120.018425

## Additional reading:

Elefteriades JA, Barrett PW, Kopf GS, et al. Litigation in nontraumatic aortic diseases: a tempest in the malpractice maelstrom. Cardiology 2008;109(4):263-72.

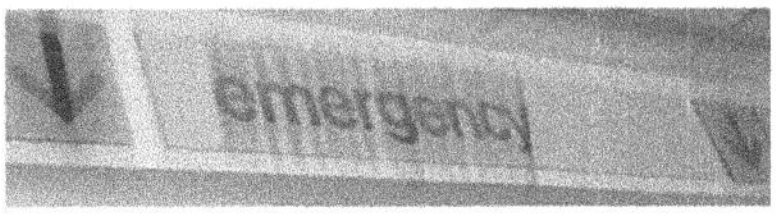


# Case 5

## A 42 Year-old Man with Dizziness: Common and Trivial, or a Brainstem Bomb?

**Primary case author:**
**Jonathan Edlow**

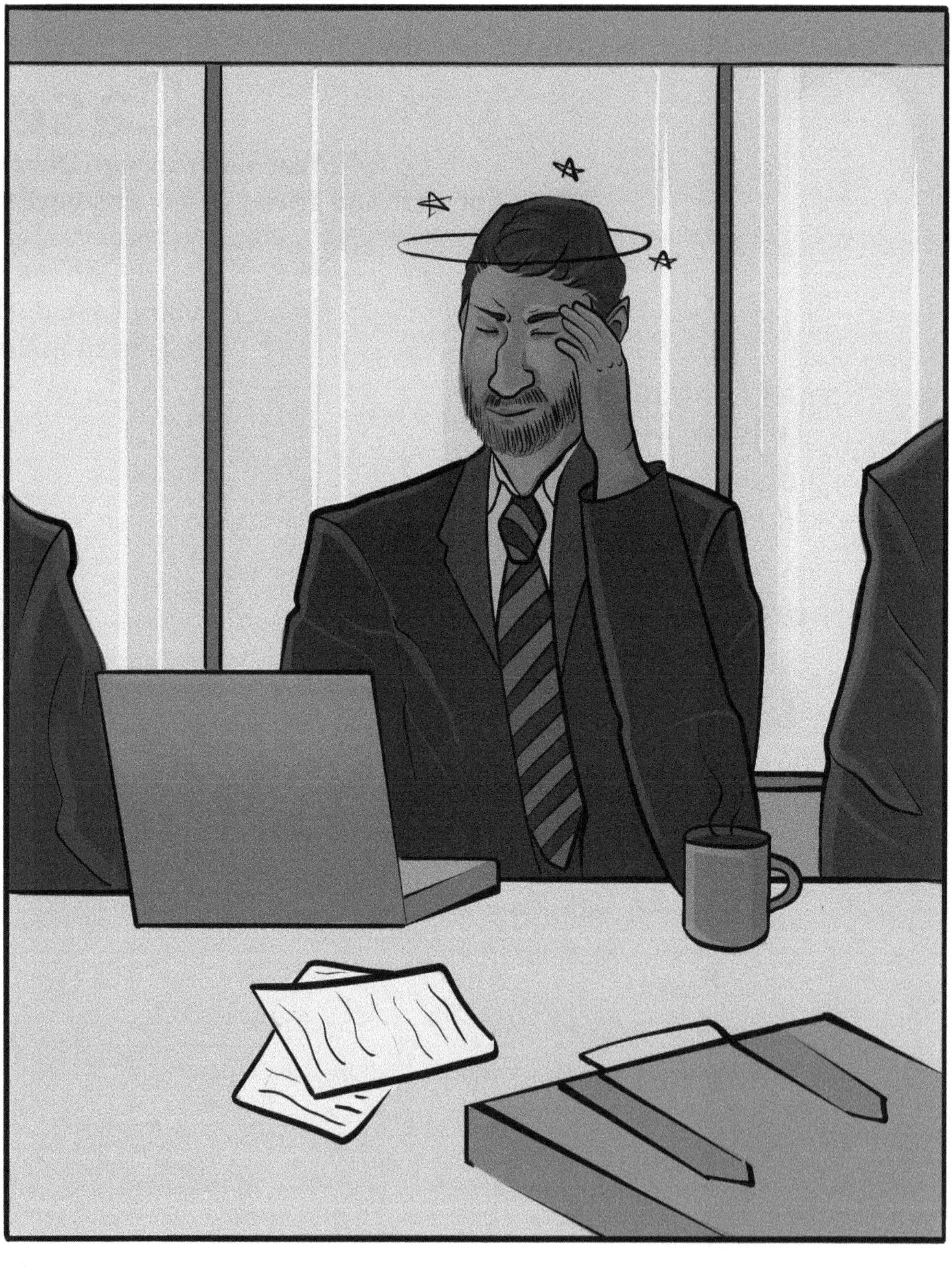

# Case 5

## A 42 Year-old Man with Dizziness: Common and Trivial, or a Brainstem Bomb?

***Deep thoughts:***

1. *Which features of dizziness should increase our suspicion of a serious cause?*
2. *Is it legally risky to list a broad differential in the chart, but then to not explore those possibilities in the H&P or with testing?*
3. *Should a patient who can't ambulate at discharge trigger a reassessment?*
4. *In a previously non-hypertensive patient who presents with new neurological symptoms, is a severely elevated blood pressure a significant finding?*

**PART I—MEDICAL**

## I. The Patient's Story

Joe Spinoza is a 42 year-old man who is married and lives in a small to medium sized community in the western United States. He earned a law degree from a prestigious university. His career started initially as a self-employed attorney, but after a few years working in a solo practice, he joined a larger group, which grew over time. He has an income of about $150,000 dollars a year. On Wednesday morning at 9 AM, he is in a meeting and becomes dizzy. It becomes so severe to the point that he seeks medical care, arriving at the ED by car around 9:30 AM.

## II. The Doctor's Version (the following is the actual documentation of the provider)

**Chief Complaint per RN at 09:32:** Dizziness (in a meeting and became dizzy and nauseated)

**History of Present Illness (Physician):** Joe Spinoza is a 42 year-old male who presents to the ED today for evaluation of dizziness onset this morning at 0900. The patient reports initially feeling as if he was going to pass out while in a meeting and then felt dizzy as if his "head was spinning." He reports associated nausea and balance issues. He also reports having a headache intermittently for the past two weeks that is different from his normal tension headaches but states he does not have one today. The patient vomited during the exam. Currently, the patient rates his discomfort as a 0/10 in severity, exacerbated with changing positions and improved with lying down with his eyes closed. No at-home therapies reported. He denies smoking tobacco or drinking alcohol. The patient otherwise denies fever, congestion, visual/hearing changes, chest pain, shortness of breath, abdominal pain, urinary symptoms, diarrhea, numbness, weakness, or any other acute concerns.

**Review of Systems:** The following systems were reviewed individually and are negative except as noted in the HPI: Constitutional, neurologic, cardiovascular, respiratory, GI, genitourinary, integument, musculoskeletal, hematologic/lymphatic, endocrine, and allergy/immunology.

**Past Medical History/Past Social History:** Negative
**Social History:** Married, never smoked

Vital Signs

| Time | Temp(F) | Pulse | Resp | Syst | Diast | Sat (room air) |
|---|---|---|---|---|---|---|
| 09:33 | 98.3 | 90 | 16 | 177 | 111 | 96% |
| 09:42 | | 67 | 18 | 167 | 108 | 96% |
| 10:42 | | 61 | | 142 | 104 | 94% |

**General:** Nontoxic appearance
**Head:** normocephalic; atraumatic
**Eyes:** sclerae are clear; extra-ocular muscle movement intact; conjunctivae are moist; no exudates
**Ears:** The tympanic membranes are clear bilaterally
**Oropharynx:** oral mucosa moist and pink
**Neck:** supple
**Pulmonary:** lungs [are clear], no retractions; no wheezes; no rales; no rhonchi; No respiratory distress
**Cardiovascular:** heart with regular rate; no murmur; no gallops; no pedal edema
**Gastrointestinal:** abdomen soft; no tenderness to palpation; no guarding; no rebound tenderness
**Genitourinary:** no suprapubic tenderness; no costovertebral angle tenderness to percussion
**Back:** normal range of motion
**Neuro:** alert and awake; Cranial nerves normal as tested; normal mental status; no focal motor or sensory deficits; Dix-Hallpike maneuver was positive on the right; the patient had fatigable vertiginous dizziness which was consistently reproducible with head movements
**Skin:** warm, dry; normal turgor; no rash; no petechia or purpura
**Musc/Skel:** no apparent deformity; no tenderness

**Differential Diagnoses:**
A partial list of diagnoses considered of the evaluation of this patient included benign positional vertigo, vestibular neuritis, basilar artery migraine, Meniere's disease, sensorineural hearing loss, CVA, Ml, ear infection, intracranial bleed.

10:40: Diazepam (VALIUM) 5mg, NS 1,000 mL
12:23: Ondansetron 8mg PO

**Medical Decision-Making:** I performed Epley maneuver on the patient. This provided modest relief of his symptoms. Based on the combination of history and exam and work-up, the dangerous diagnoses considered in this case were determined to be unlikely. I specifically felt that intracranial pathology was particularly unlikely because of the fatigability and reproducibility as well as the absence of neurologic deficits. I did not feel that further work-up would be likely enough to benefit the patient to justify. Explained the patient's diagnosis and gave the signs that would indicate a need to return. I answered all questions to best of my ability. We also discussed the importance of following up as instructed.

**Diagnosis:** Peripheral vertigo, unspecified laterality (primary)

**Follow-up:** Follow up with Dr. PCP, your primary care physician, in 1 week and with [a] hearing and balance center [contact info given to the patient] in 5 days

## III. Risk Management/Patient Safety Opportunities (Weinstock)

**Author comments (Weinstock):** Is standard of care (SOC) enough? Whereas this is the minimum standard during a legal proceeding, the purpose of this book is to strive for "excellence in care" (i.e., the care we would want for our family and friends and patients). This case is challenging as we know dizziness is incredibly common and mostly benign, but we need to "balance" the risk of testing including radiation exposure, expense, time, and false positives with the risk of missing clinically relevant disease. Though this physician did a good job in the evaluation reflected in the documentation… were there opportunities to improve patient safety at the initial visit?

**Risk Management/Patient Safety Opportunity #1:**

**Opportunity:** Data gathering/history – Was the dizziness constant or intermittent? Was the onset sudden?
**Discussion:** When we think of benign paroxysmal positional vertigo (BPPV), one of the hallmarks is the intermittent nature… after all… it's in the name! (paroxysmal). That said, some patients with BPPV will not give this classic history of intermittent episodes, especially after a first attack, probably due to nausea which lasts longer than the dizziness, or anxiety about head movement. With a positive Dix-Hallpike test, it is clear the physician thought the diagnosis was BPPV, but it might have been more likely if the vertigo was documented as resolving between episodes. Additionally, the classic "sudden" onset of BPPV occurring while rolling over in bed did not occur in this case. Of course, we should never rely on a "classic" history for just about anything; BPPV is no different. Though less common, BPPV can certainly occur in a meeting. It is also not 100% clear from the history if the onset is truly sudden or not and if symptoms are intermittent or constant. Does "improved with lying down with eyes closed" mean that the dizziness completely resolved or just improves? All that said, given the fact that the dizziness (and we are using the terms "dizzy" and "vertigo" synonymously because use of one word versus another has little diagnostic utility)[1, 2] started in a meeting suggests a sudden onset. The truly sudden onset of any symptom should suggest a blocked vascular supply (think MI) or an obstructed tubular structure (think ureteral colic), but it is not uncommon for BPPV to start abruptly but vestibular neuritis and vestibular migraine can also start suddenly. In fact, when persistent dizziness begins abruptly, neuritis is about three times more likely than stroke.[3]
✔ **Teaching point:** Sudden onset of persistent dizziness should at least suggest the possibility of a vascular cause; however, it is by no means specific.

**Risk Management/Patient Safety Opportunity #2:**

**Opportunity:** Data gathering/history – What is the significance of dizziness that gets worse with head movement?
**Discussion:** While position changes exacerbate the dizziness in BPPV, (again, it's in the name—positional); however, changes in head position will also exacerbate most central causes of dizziness. It is a common misconception that dizziness that worsens with head movement confirms that it is peripheral in nature. Furthermore, the positional exacerbation of BPPV is very specific, depending on which of the semi-circular canals and which side is involved. In this case, the fact that Dr. Garcia documents that the Dix-Hallpike test is only positive on one side is an important detail to recognize and document.
✔ **Teaching point:** Dizziness that is exacerbated by head movement does not equate with a peripheral cause.

**Risk Management/Patient Safety Opportunity #3:**

**Opportunity:** The symptoms of headache were only minimally explored.
**Discussion:** The patient gave a history of tension headaches, but lately is having a "different" headache (though not present at the time of the visit). Were these headaches sudden in onset (concern for subarachnoid hemorrhage or cerebral venous thrombosis) or associated with visual changes (giant cell arteritis or pseudotumor cerebri) or associated with weight loss (malignancy)? Additionally, headache is not a symptom of BPPV. The history of headaches here is a little bit of a teaser; I want to know more! If it is important enough to mention in the documentation, further exploration might be useful. In all fairness, the physician did explore this issue to a certain extent, but we don't know if further details would have been diagnostically useful. In addition, the documented details clearly show that he was not simply using a "macro" or checking off boxes. Clearly, he was taking a detailed history on this individual patient.

✔ **Teaching point:** When there are 2 complaints, both should be explored and explained.

**Risk Management/Patient Safety Opportunity #4:**

**Opportunity:** Data gathering/vital signs: Severe hypertension in a patient without a history of hypertension and with new neurological signs or symptoms should be considered in the diagnostic evaluation.
**Discussion:** With the obvious caveat that many ED patients will have a high measured blood pressure due to pain or anxiety, or chronic hypertension that is poorly controlled, when a patient has new severe hypertension in the presence of a neurological presentation, we should at least consider that the hypertension is the body's neuro-protective response to autoregulate blood pressure in an ischemic or injured area of the brain. This patient's initial blood pressure was 177/111, which is fairly high and it never normalized. Although there is no hard and fast way to definitively answer this question, one should at a minimum factor in new severe hypertension into one's decision-making.

✔ **Teaching point:** Elevated blood pressure may be present due to a neuro-protective response.

**Risk Management/Patient Safety Opportunity #5:**

**Opportunity:** Understanding limitations of testing.
**Discussion:** The Dix-Hallpike test is diagnostic for posterior canal BPPV, but the details are super important[4,5] and we know that in routine practice, emergency physicians do not always use the Dix-Hallpike test correctly.[6] The physician is later questioned to the predictive nature of the Dix-Hallpike test but states he does not know how accurate it actually is. First, the Dix-Hallpike test is mostly useful for posterior canal BPPV, not for horizontal canal (the second most common type), so a Dix-Hallpike test might be negative in a patient with BPPV of the horizontal canal. But for the posterior canal (the most common type) a truly positive Dix-Hallpike test is diagnostic. Secondly, a truly positive Dix-Hallpike test is positive on one side and negative on the other; Dr. Garcia documents ("positive on the right"). This detail was quite important to the jury. Finally, and most importantly is that a positive Dix-Hallpike test shows torsional-upbeating nystagmus that develops with the positional maneuver, then resolves over a minute or so with holding the head in that position. This is because the otoliths fall in the canal with gravity and when they have settled at the bottom of the canal, the symptoms and the nystagmus stop.[4] Imaging is not recommended in patients with a positive Dix-Hallpike when BPPV is the target diagnosis.

✔ **Teaching point:** The Dix-Hallpike test, when performed correctly and when the typical upbeating torsional nystagmus is present unilaterally has excellent predictive value for posterior canal BPPV. Know what nystagmus pattern to look for.

**Risk Management/Patient Safety Opportunity #6:**

**Opportunity:** Understanding limitations of the therapeutic interventions.
**Discussion:** In a patient whose Dix-Hallpike test is unilaterally positive (as defined above), the Epley maneuver is extremely useful with a Number-Needed-to-Treat of ~3; making it one of the most effective treatments in all of medicine. Of course, this maneuver needs to be done properly (watch a YouTube video before you go into the room). Often, more than a single Epley is needed.[4,5] A good practice is after the Epley, go off and do something else then re-do the Dix-Hallpike again and if it is still positive, repeat the Epley. When it succeeds in reducing or eliminating the patient's symptoms and converting a positive Dix-Hallpike test to a negative one, not only is it therapeutic but it helps to confirm the diagnosis. Although this physician documented better than many may have, ideal documentation would include, "After an Epley maneuver, the patient's symptoms were X% better and there was less nystagmus on repeat Dix-Hallpike testing." Even better would be to document, "After a second Epley, repeat Dix-Hallpike was negative, and the patient's symptoms were nearly totally resolved." Details (and documenting those details) matter.
✔ **Teaching point:** A therapeutic Epley maneuver is useful but often needs to be repeated a few times.

**Risk Management/Patient Safety Opportunity #7:**

**Opportunity:** We should list our differential diagnosis, and if you don't think that a given serious condition is occurring, this should be explained in the MDM.
**Discussion:** We should certainly consider a wide range of causes for patient's symptoms, and it is fine to list these items in the MDM as a Ddx, but we don't get partial credit! If an item is listed and we think it is unlikely, we should then explain why (after our data gathering) we don't think it is occurring. It doesn't help our cause to list an item in the Ddx, but then to not further explore it or document its exclusion on clinical grounds... Take 3 of the items in the Ddx cited above:

- CVA – This seems less likely with a lack of numbness or weakness and (likely per the thought process of the physician) of a positive Dix-Hallpike test (alternative diagnosis), but we know that a posterior circulation stroke can occur with isolated vertigo and without focal neurological signs or symptoms. Kudos that this was mentioned in the MDM, but it would have been useful to further explain why it was unlikely to be occurring. A major argument of the defense expert was that not only is basilar stroke a very rare entity in a young patient with isolated dizziness and the patient had no vascular risk factors. Further, BPPV is literally orders of magnitude more common, and a truly positive unilateral Dix-Hallpike test does not occur in basilar stroke.
- MI – This is another diagnosis which can present atypically. The question is: How do we enhance patient care (or billing) by mentioning something which has such a low likelihood of occurring? With no chest pain or shortness of breath in a healthy 45 year-old man, how is anything benefited by including this in the Ddx? If it is mentioned, then one is compelled to explain why they don't think it is occurring?
- Intracranial bleed – Could this have been spontaneously occurring? Of course. The history of several weeks of headaches could have been important to explore further. How was it excluded from the Ddx based on the patient's history of present illness? It might have been nice to mention that there was no trauma, specifically that he had no use of anticoagulant medications, and headache wasn't currently present, making this Dx very unlikely.

✔ **Teaching point:** The MDM should explain why any serious condition listed in the Ddx is sufficiently unlikely to be the actual diagnosis and that no further testing is needed.

**Risk Management/Patient Safety Opportunity #8:**

**Opportunity:** Sharing with the patient any "diagnostic uncertainty."
**Discussion:** When patients (who have an adverse outcome after their ED visit) are asked why they didn't return, sometimes they (or family) will say something to the effect of, "I was already in the ED, and they did all the indicated tests and told me everything was fine." Allowing for some diagnostic uncertainty and informing the patient accordingly might allow for a return if symptoms change, progress, or don't resolve. Dr. Garcia considered stroke as a cause of Mr. Spinoza's presentation in the differential which might have been included due to the severity of the vertigo, the loss of balance and even possibly because of the different type of headache (though headache is not usually a symptom of an ischemic stroke), but it did not seem that the patient was aware of this consideration upon leaving the ED.
✔ **Teaching point:** When the diagnosis is not definitive, informing the patient of items on the Ddx not completely excluded at discharge, informs them of when and why to return. This may lead to a productive conversation about the patient's values and is probably a good risk management tool.

## IV. Bounceback Visit (24 hours later)

**History of Present Illness:**
This is a 42 year-old male who presents today with his wife via EMS for evaluation of altered mental status. The patient's wife states that the patient was evaluated yesterday in the ED for dizziness and was diagnosed with vertigo and given Antivert. The wife states that she woke him up at 0530 and helped him to go to the bathroom. The wife notes that his child found him at 1100 unresponsive on his bed. EMS states that the patient has some neurological response and had high blood pressure reading. The wife notes that the patient has been complaining of a headache over the past 3 days that has been around the right temple consistent with his prior tension headaches. The wife also notes that the patient has been seeing "stars" intermittently. Currently, the patient's symptoms are severe. At-home therapies were not pursued. The patient's review of systems was not obtained due to the patient's condition. The patient denies any aggravating or alleviating factors associated with his symptoms.

**Physical Examination (shortened):**
**General:** unresponsive with sonorous respirations
**Head:** normocephalic; atraumatic
**Eyes:** sclera clear; the right pupil measures approximately 1 cm and is not appreciably reactive to light while the left pupil measuring approximately 3–4 mm
**Pharynx:** gag reflex is present
**Neck:** supple; no cervical adenopathy; no tenderness to palpation
**Pulmonary:** Sonorous respirations are present; equal bilateral breath sounds are clear
**Cardiovascular:** Heart with regular rate; sinus rhythm
**Gastrointestinal:** abdomen soft; no tenderness to palpation; no guarding; no rebound tenderness
**Neuro:** Patient has his eyes closed and does not appear to be able to open them; his pupils are unequal; there is purposeful movements of his bilateral upper and lower extremities; no posturing; he is obeying commands by holding his thumbs up when asked; he moves his feet on command; sensory exam is grossly intact

**Author comments (Weinstock):** OK folks, get ready for the best and most complete MDM note you have ever read:

**Medical Decision-Making:** I was called to the bedside to assist in the evaluation and management of this patient who was found unresponsive and in bed at home. I awaited this patient's arrival in the ambulance bay and began my evaluation when the ambulance arrived. The last known well according to his wife was 5:30 this morning. He was found at 11 AM in bed unable to follow commands or be aroused. It was reported that he was seen yesterday in the emergency department for vertigo symptoms. He has been taking Antivert for his symptoms.

Differential diagnoses I have considered include CVA versus intracranial hemorrhage versus medication reaction versus brain herniation versus intracranial mass versus electrolyte derangement versus sepsis versus acute cardiac event versus dysrhythmia versus pulmonary embolus versus transient ischemic attack versus seizure disorder versus syncope versus overdose among other things.

I accompanied the patient to the resuscitation bay and I had a high suspicion that this patient required emergent intubation given his sonorous respirations. As we were preparing for intubation, it was found that he had a gag reflex and is able to obey commands with moving his extremities. He is unable to open his eyes or speak. His pupils are unequal with mydriasis on the right.

It was my decision at that time to postpone intubation and obtain an emergent CT scan and we took him directly to the CT suite. I initiated a stroke protocol CT in order laboratory studies including CBC, metabolic panel, troponin, urinalysis, lactic acid level as well as a chest X-ray and urinalysis. I had several conversations with the patient's wife and briefly reviewed his records from his last visit to the emergency department. Given this presentation, I was highly suspicious of an acute neurologic event.

My interpretation of the noncontrast portion of the CT of his head is that there were no findings of intracranial hemorrhage. This was confirmed when I was called by the radiologist with the wet read of the CT. We proceeded with the contrast portion of his CT angiogram of the head and neck. A short time later, I received another call from the radiologist who was interpreting the CT angiogram of the head and neck. He reported to me that there was a basilar artery occlusion as well as occlusion of his posterior cerebral artery and left vertebral artery. It was felt that this represented a vertebral artery dissection potentially causing emboli in the vessels mentioned. Given that the patient was greater than 6 hours his last known well, I did not feel that the patient was a candidate for systemic TPA. His NIH stroke scale was considerably high as well.

**Testing: CT angiogram head and neck w/wo contrast:** Intermittent occlusion of left vertebral artery. Occlusive basilar tip thrombus. Occluded right P2 segment. Question underlying dissection. No brain ischemia seen by noncontrast CT.

**EM Physician Medical Decision-Making (continued):**
I rapidly contacted Dr. [Neurologist] who is on-call for neurology. We discussed this patient's presentation, work-up thus far and my findings on physical examination. Dr. Neurologist agreed that the patient was not a candidate for systemic TPA but felt that the patient may benefit from interventional radiology consultation. Efforts had been made to contact the interventional radiologist on-call after the radiologist spoke to me. Instead of waiting for the interventional radiologist to get in touch with me, I called him directly and he was reviewing the images of the CT angiogram. He had concerns about the patient's findings and his ability to intervene on this patient's behalf. In his opinion, this would be a risky procedure. As he was reviewing the remaining images, I had a discussion with the patient's spouse about the further findings we obtained an CT angiogram and indicated to her the serious nature of these findings. I answered her questions to the best of my ability and called the interventional radiologist back

so that he could have a direct discussion with the patient's wife about intervention. During the time that she was on the phone, I decided to perform endotracheal intubation for airway protection since the patient was less consistently following commands. He continued to have a gag reflex as we tried to put a nasal trumpet in place. The patient was intubated using a GlideScope without incident. He was preoxygenated and had no desaturation after he was given etomidate and succinylcholine as his induction and paralytic agents. No immediate complications were noted and a chest X-ray confirmed placement of the ET tube.

After this, I spoke directly with the pulmonologist on-call at the downtown ICU. He has kindly agreed to take care of this patient after he gets out of interventional radiology. The CBC shows a mildly elevated white cell count, but the patient does not have anemia or thrombocytopenia. The metabolic panel shows a glucose that is slightly elevated. His coag studies are not significantly abnormal. Lactic acid level is normal. The chest X-ray does not show any concerning opacity. The orotracheal tube is in good position.

Emergent transport was arranged and soon after the chest X-ray was performed, the patient was taken directly to the interventional radiology suite at the downtown hospital. Transfer paperwork was filled out. Then I had my last discussion with the patient's wife, I indicated the critical nature of his illness at this time, and we discussed the risk of interventional radiology. We both felt it was reasonable to pursue any aggressive intervention since it remained unknown how much injury was already sustained by the brain secondary to the occluded vessels. The patient was then transferred.

**X-ray Chest:**
I. Endotracheal tube terminates 4 cm above the carina.
2. Low lung volumes with left greater than right perihilar opacities, likely atelectasis and/or aspiration.

**Receiving Hospital Procedures:**
**Pre-Procedure Diagnosis:** Basilar Artery Stroke and Left vertebral dissection.
**Post-Procedure Diagnosis:**
1. Embolus in the distal basilar artery occluding both posterior cerebral arteries with collateral flow to the posterior cerebral arteries through the posterior communicating arteries as well as collateral flow from the right middle cerebral artery to the right posterior cerebral artery.
2. Occluded left vertebral artery due to an atherosclerotic occlusion. No vertebral artery dissection identified. Extensive clot identified in the left vertebral artery following crossing the occlusion but complete removal of the clot following aspiration embolectomy.
3. Recanalization of the basilar artery as well as left posterior cerebral artery following embolectomy. Partial recanalization of the right posterior cerebral artery with persistent occlusion at the P3 segment.
4. Successful stent assisted angioplasty of the proximal left vertebral artery occlusion.
**Procedure:** Basilar artery thrombectomy, cerebral angiogram, and stent-assisted angioplasty of the left vertebral artery origin.

**Pulm/Crit Care Admit Note:**

**Impression:**
1. Cerebrovascular accident secondary to left vertebral artery atherosclerotic occlusion, with embolic occlusion of basilar artery, and bilateral posterior cerebral arteries. Neurologic status at this time is unknown as he is just returned from procedure and remains on propofol. Exact ischemic time is also unknown, though it is concerning that he may have had a relatively prolonged ischemic time. He is now status post stents to the left vertebral artery and embolectomy.

2. Hypotension, transient. Likely related to propofol. Was transiently on phenylephrine, which has since been discontinued.
3. Acute respiratory failure, secondary to #1.

**Plan:**
1. Patient is admitted to the intensive care unit.
2. Continue mechanical ventilatory support.
3. We will gradually lighten propofol for neurologic assessment.
4. Check lipid panel, and start statin therapy. Continue clopidogrel and low-dose aspirin, with next dose in the morning. Clearly antiplatelet therapy in the setting of possible prolonged ischemia raises the risk for hemorrhagic conversion; however, at this point in time this risk is definitely outweighed by the risk of stent reocclusion.
6. Strict BP control, to keep systolic blood pressure less than 140. We will utilize nicardipine if needed.

**Long Term Follow-up Status:**
Mr. Spinoza's subjective complaints include inability to ambulate, visual impairments and difficulty speaking. He is able to use a walker, although his wife does not allow him to be alone in the event he falls backwards. He uses a wheelchair but is not able to push himself. His home is no longer accessible to him due to his condition.

# PART 2—LEGAL

**Author comments (Weinstock):** Before a legal action occurs, the plaintiff's attorney retains expert(s) to decide if there even is a case. If the case does not settle and the jury decides for the defense, the plaintiff does not recover any of the money they spent, which can certainly be in the hundreds of thousands of dollars. If the expert agrees there is a case, they are then asked to write an opinion (below).

Eventually, the plaintiff will need to decide how much money to ask for in their initial demand. Below is an estimate of the medical costs which the defendant (patient) will incur, as well as loss of past and future earnings. Mr. Spinoza was an attorney and had a high income, with "expectations to earn $129,000 per year and maintained a work-life expectancy similar to that of non-disabled males with a master's degree. Post-injury, Mr. Spinoza's projected earnings are zero. This analysis considers a projected 1.73% increase per year."

## I. Monetary Demands of Plaintiff

| Category | Reference | Amount |
|---|---|---|
| Present Value of Future Medical Costs | Schedule 5 | 8,504,429 |
| Present Value of Future Household Services Costs | Schedule 9 | 441,002 |
| Past Lost Earnings | Schedule 3 | 576,493 |
| Present Value of Future Lost Earnings | Schedule 3 | 2,413,637 |
| Total | | $11,935,561 |

**Author comments (Weinstock):** Following is the [shortened] opinion of the emergency medicine plaintiff's expert witness. Suffice it to say, that this was not a "hired gun," but a true, respected academician, with a CV reflecting an impressive number of positions and publications; they are critical of so many aspects of this patient's care. Do any of the points strike home... or is this opinion overly critical? Following the formal opinion of the plaintiff's expert is the defendant physician's response to these allegations.

## II. Opinion of Plaintiff's Expert (shortened)

Dr. [Plaintiff's expert witness] will testify that Dr. Garcia breached the standard of care applicable to board certified emergency medicine physicians practicing in [this geographic area]. His opinions, detailed below, are based upon the foundation set forth in his disclosure as well as the documents and items [he]reviewed as documented in Section __ of this disclosure. Dr. [Plaintiff's expert witness] will testify that he holds these opinions to a reasonable degree of medical certainty and on a more likely than not basis.

**A. There is a national standard of care that applies to board-certified emergency medicine physicians regardless of geographic location:**

Dr. [plaintiff's expert witness] will testify regarding the process of becoming board-certified with the American Board of Emergency Medicine ("ABEM"). Additionally, he has acted as an oral board examiner for the ABEM. In his roles with both the ABEM and the American Heart Association, Dr. [plaintiff's expert witness] has helped develop and institute stroke protocols that reflect evidence-based standards in the treatment of strokes. Such protocols have been widely accepted and used throughout the country and help establish the national standard of care for timely treatment of strokes. The stated mission of the ABEM is "To ensure the highest standards in the specialty of Emergency Medicine." The purpose of initial certification is to objectively and independently confirm that physicians who complete an emergency medicine residency demonstrate core knowledge, skills, and abilities needed to practice emergency medicine at the highest standards. It is expected that Dr. [Plaintiff's expert witness] will testify that for board-certified emergency physicians, the standard of care for evaluating and diagnosing patients with stroke symptoms was a national standard of care, with no significant deviations [depending on geographic location]. Due to his specialized training and board certification during his treatment and care of Mr. Spinoza, Dr. Garcia was subject to this national standard of care.

**Author comments (Calvert):** In a civil legal case against a doctor, the standard of care can be defined as that of "ordinary care," or that degree of care that an ordinary and reasonable physician in the same or similar circumstances would exert in like or similar circumstances. Of note, guidelines should provide guidance rather than a required template of care. Once there is talk about "the highest standards," it is arguably leaving the realm of ordinary care.

Next, it is well documented that when reviewers know the outcome, this impacts their opinions. I think this syndrome is even more likely with those experts who we lovingly refer to in our business as "Ivory Tower" critics; they cannot imagine missing this diagnosis! So, it is important to mention the hindsight nature of the criticism and the somewhat haughty position that this could not happen to a reasonable doctor. Having supportive expert witnesses discuss these points at trial is very helpful.

**B. Board certified emergency medicine physicians are taught to utilize a differential diagnosis and to perform a complete history and physical:**

Board certified emergency medicine physicians are taught to utilize a differential diagnosis to differentiate between two or more conditions that may be causing a patient's symptoms. This is an important tool as it guides the physician in their decision making. Adequate steps should be taken to eliminate or "rule out" dangerous potentials, such as stroke. When symptoms suggestive of a stroke are present, the standard of care requires stroke as a cause of the symptoms to be considered. These are basic and fundamental standard skills and competencies familiar to all board-certified emergency medicine physicians which do not vary by geographic location.

Board certified emergency medicine physicians are taught that a complete history and physical of the patient is required. The standard of care requires the provider to gather a complete history of a patient's complaints and symptoms in order to fully assess potential causes of the patient's complaints. This can be done in a variety of ways including asking the patient and/or their family if accompanied to the emergency department. Information provided should be considered when determining potential causes of the patient's complaints and deficits.

**C. A board certified emergency medicine physician are trained to recognize symptoms of stroke and to perform tests for stroke:**

Board certified emergency medicine physicians are taught to recognize symptoms of stroke, based on their presentation and examination. Face drooping/asymmetry, extremity weakness, speech deficits, balance problems, difficulty/inability to walk, dizziness, nausea/vomiting, neck pain and severe headache can be symptoms of stroke. Recognizing these symptoms and signs does not require any specialized equipment or specialized facilities. Board certified emergency medicine physicians, regardless of geographic location, are trained to recognize these symptoms and to understand that they are suggestive of a potential stroke.

When stroke or other neurological injury is on the differential, board certified emergency medicine physicians are taught that a complete neurological work-up is required in order to determine whether the patient is suffering from any deficits to their nervous system. Such findings can help differentiate between potential causes of the patient's symptoms (i.e., stroke versus vertigo). The standard of care requires a complete assessment of motor and sensory skills, balance, coordination, reflexes, strength, and mental status. This evaluation can be done through a variety of tests, depending on the clinical presentation of the patient. Such information is critically important in determining whether the patient is potentially suffering from a stroke. This is a basic and fundamental standard which does not vary by geographic location.

**D. A board certified emergency medicine physician is required to test for stroke if it is on the differential:**

The standard of care requires the emergency medicine physician to order and implement appropriate stroke testing, such as a non-contrast CT, CT angiogram, CT perfusion or MRI to evaluate the potential stroke. If the facility does not have such testing available, transfer may be required. If stroke is on the differential, the standard of care does not allow the physician to simply ignore the potential of stroke without imaging or testing. More must be done to either confirm the diagnosis or eliminate that possibility as a cause of the patient's symptoms.

**E. Most patients will be admitted, but if discharged the standard of care requires an assessment of their needs at discharge:**

Most patients with a concern for stroke will be admitted to the hospital for further evaluation, treatment and secondary prevention. If the physician is considering discharging a patient with symptoms suggestive of a stroke, the standard of care would require that the patient be assessed for their needs at discharge, that a plan of care be developed and implemented, and that the discharge plan and follow-up instructions be appropriately documented. This would include close consultation and a timely follow-up appointment with a neurologist or primary care physician who is comfortable managing stroke as an outpatient. In addition, stroke risk factor modification strategies would be initiated which may include initiation of an anti-platelet medication, a statin, and tight blood pressure and glucose management. It is widely accepted and known that the highest risk for a recurrent stroke is within the first days to week after the initial presentation of stroke symptoms. These are basic and universal standards of care for a patient being discharged from an emergency room. When there is a concern for a possible stroke, the patient and/or the patient's family must be informed and educated about ongoing medical concerns, signs, and symptoms of a recurrent stroke and exactly when to return to the emergency department.

**F. Dr. Garcia's care was beyond negligent:**

Removing stroke from the differential diagnosis and informing the patient that he was not suffering from a stroke was a breach of the standard of care because such statements were made without medical justification. Without an adequate documented neurologic work-up, Stroke/CVA could not reasonably be eliminated from the differential diagnosis. In fact, a finding of such neurologic symptoms makes the diagnosis of benign positional vertigo highly unlikely and the possibility of a stroke or other CVA more likely.

Benign Positional Vertigo is best understood as a cluster of symptoms, rather than a diagnosis. Benign Positional Vertigo (BPV) is not typically associated with sudden, persistent, and severe symptoms. BPV symptoms normally come and go and commonly last less than a few minutes. Ultimately, making a final diagnosis of benign positional vertigo in these circumstances was a breach of the standard of care.

It was a breach of the standard of care to rely on either the Dix-Hallpike Maneuver or the Epley Maneuver to rule out a stroke. Dr. Garcia failed to document Mr. Spinoza's visual field and to assess any nystagmus. Dr. Garcia recognized and testified in his deposition that he understood that such tests, in the presence of other neurologic signs or symptoms, are inadequate to rule out a stroke. In such an instance, such tests neither have the necessary sensitivity or specificity to rule out a stroke.

Dr. Garcia chose not to have Mr. Spinoza walk and not to document any neurologic testing that would confirm or exclude neurologic symptoms including weakness. Despite this, he chose to eliminate stroke from the differential. Any board-certified emergency medicine physician should know that such actions create a high probability of a misdiagnosis of stroke. Dr. Garcia's care was beyond negligent.

**G. Causation:**

More likely than not, had Dr. Spinoza properly initiated the stroke code, appropriate imaging, including non-contrast CT and CT angiogram, would have been performed. Had the stroke procedures been properly followed, appropriate interventions could have been initiated. Had the stroke procedures been properly followed, neurology would have been consulted, an NIHSS would have been completed, and appropriate IV tPA or mechanical thrombectomy would have been considered. The breaches of the standard of care outlined above were substantial factors in the misdiagnosis of the stroke Mr. Spinoza was suffering from.

**Author comments (Weinstock):** So, what just happened??!! Let's bring it all home. The plaintiff's expert alleged not only that the data gathering (H&P) was poorly done, but also that the medical decision-making was "beyond negligent, it was reckless."

But just because we consider the diagnosis or stroke... or pulmonary embolism... or acute coronary syndrome... are we required to do objective testing? Certainly not. In fact, a patient with slurred speech might be concerning for stroke on initial presentation, but when the patient's family member reveals that they just finished a fifth of vodka, we now move it way lower on the Ddx! But yet, some of these allegations have a ring of truth.

When the EM defendant was deposed, they were asked to respond to many of these allegations. Here is how the deposition unfolded:

## III. Deposition of Defendant-Physician

**A. Dr. Garcia testified as to the standard of care as it relates to evaluating neurologic symptoms including questions as to the Dix-Hallpike test:**

**Q.** (Plaintiff's attorney). So, one of the standards of care that you're taught, that you understand based on all your education and training, is that you would want to rule out neurological signs and symptoms as a way of differentiating between vertigo and a stroke?
**A.** (Dr Garcia). That's correct.

**Q.** And that's the standard of care that you would apply in [your geographic location at the time of the patient encounter]?
**A.** Yes.

**Q.** Okay. What are the elements of a neurologic examination regarding the cerebellum?
**A.** Cerebellum would generally be more coordination-type activities.

**Q.** Like?
**A.** Finger-to-nose testing, the hand flipping, heel-to-shin testing, those sorts of coordination activities.

**Q.** Did you ever offer or suggest to the Spinoza's that they could be admitted for observation and a neurologic work-up?

**Defense Attorney.** Asked and answered.

**The Witness:** I don't believe so.

**Q.** That's one thing you could do if you're concerned about a stroke or a stroke developing; isn't that true?
**A.** I don't think I've ever heard of anyone doing that. I mean, I've heard of people admitting because

the symptoms, that they didn't feel that the patient would be able to care for themselves at home. But typically, if you're still worried about that possibility, you would do an MRI.

**Q.** I guess if I'm understanding your answer, there are tests that you can run to help rule out the possibility of a stroke?
**A.** Correct.

**Q.** And name some of those. I think you said MRI. What else?
**A.** MRI would help you identify whether there was an actual stroke in the brain. Not a perfect study but it's good. A CT angiogram would identify problems with the blood vessels but would not be an effective way—consistently effective way of identifying a stroke early in the process.

**Q.** Okay. And with respect to a Dix-Hallpike, do you know what the sensitivity and specificity are with respect to whether you can rule out a central stroke?
**A.** By itself, no, I do not know.

**Q.** Do you know whether that's—that's been studied or considered by people who look at these things?
**A.** I don't know of a specific study on that.

**Q.** Are you aware that with respect to a Dix-Hallpike, you—it is not specific or sensitive enough to rule out a central stroke if there are other neurologic signs?

**Defense Attorney.** Object to the form.

**The Witness:** I have not heard that. I have heard the contrary; that if there are no other neurologic signs, then that they have an exam suggestive of peripheral stroke, that that is adequate to exclude it.

**Q.** But if there are other neurologic signs, a Dix-Hallpike is not sensitive or specific enough to rule out a stroke. Is that your understanding?
**A.** If there are other neurologic signs that are indicative of a stroke, correct.

**B. For documenting the medical chart regarding testing for the presence or absence of neurologic findings, Dr. Garcia testified:**

**Q.** You don't recall, at least, having him do leg lifts or stand or walk; is that true?
**A.** I don't remember the specifics of my neurologic exam.

**Q.** Okay. And that would be something you'd want to document; isn't that true?
**Defense Attorney.** Object to the form.

**Q.** The specifics of a neurologic exam bears on stroke symptoms, that's something you would document, isn't that true?
**Defense Attorney.** Object to the form.
**A.** In varying degrees of detail, yes.

**C. As it relates to discharging the patient and providing instructions for monitoring and follow-up, Dr. Garcia testified:**

**Q.** Did you give any instructions to the patient with respect to monitoring him for ongoing signs or symptoms of a stroke once they left?
**A.** I don't remember specifically the instructions that I gave them. All I can speak to is my usual practice.

**Q.** Which is?
**A.** Usually speak with them about sorts of things that would be worrisome that would indicate that there was a problem that would need to be brought back and have further assessment.

**Q.** Well, with respect to what you understand about Mr. Spinoza's evaluation in the ER and your discharge of him, what would that have been specifically in this case?
**A.** Oh, things such as decreased function, decreased strength or sensation of a part of his body, symptoms that did not resolve with remaining still, changes in level of consciousness.

**Q.** Was it important to you for him to be monitored once he left the hospital for any developing symptoms of a stroke?
**A.** Oh, certainly.

**Q.** Is it the standard of care to inform the patient about ongoing medical concerns that they need to watch out for?
**A.** Oh, yes.

**D. Finally, Dr. Garcia agreed that there were no deviations in the way board-certified emergency medicine doctors practiced in [this geographic location]?**

**Q.** Is training for learning how to assess and diagnose a stroke something they teach you in medical school?
**A.** Yes.

**Q.** And is that something that's also trained as part of your residency?
**A.** Yes.

**Q.** And that's something that I think you told me is tested as part of your board certification in emergency medicine?
**A.** Yes.

**Q.** And as far as you're aware, that's a pretty uniform training and approach that's done at medical schools all over the country?

**Defense Attorney.** Objection; foundation, calls for speculation.

**Q.** As far as you're aware?
**A.** I would assume that the signs of stroke are taught broadly.

**Q.** And the same thing with respect to the board certification. I think we've already discussed that this a board that you take if you want to be board certified, regardless of where you went to medical school and where you're going to practice.
**A.** Correct.

**Q.** As far as you're aware, you know of no deviation in that training with respect to the board certification as it relates to [your geographic location]?
**Defense Attorney.** Objection; foundation, speculation.
**A.** Correct, that is my knowledge.

## IV. The Verdict

This case did proceed to trial.
**Verdict:** Defense.

## V. The Legal Analysis

**T. Marc Calvert, JD**
Medical malpractice defense attorney with over 35 years of experience
Calvert, Leever & Ostler
Cypress, Texas

**Approach to this discussion:**
Because we know there is an adverse outcome, I have tried to remove the outcome bias by writing almost all of this before reading about the bounceback visit.

**The case...and the documentation:**
Our patient is a relatively young patient, a lawyer, and someone who may not go to the doctor at the drop of a hat; should the physician have been more concerned about a serious condition?

The MDM has some language which may pose some risk, especially with good cross-examination: "(T)he dangerous diagnoses considered in this case were determined to be unlikely." The wording could be bothersome for a jury of lay people. "Unlikely" could technically be 49%, for goodness sake! That is pretty high. And if it was truly felt that it was the toss of a coin, then I think non-medical people (the jury) will be bewildered that more effort was not deployed to rule out a dangerous condition. On the other hand, if it was felt that brewing disasters were basically and reasonably ruled out, and the "unlikely" is really meant to convey that it is so remote that the chances are nil, then it needs to be stated in that manner with the reasons included. I would recommend a modifier to underscore the remoteness; highly or very unlikely, come to mind.

The next phrase in the MDM has similar language; "I did not feel that further work-up would be likely enough to benefit the patient to justify." Again, the opposing attorney may try to exploit this word choice. Open to interpretation is the word "justify." Justify it in terms of time? Justify in terms of money? Because the downside could be so catastrophic, the imagery of the risk benefit analysis being a close call "but it is just not worth it" is potentially concerning to an average juror. Most patients, and keep in mind that jurors are patients, simply are not comfortable with a doctor playing Russian roulette when a gun is pointed at the patient's head. It is easy to be risky with another's life or money. These are the type of feelings that a skilled plaintiff's attorney will try to evoke. It will be alleged that this approach shows a lack of respect and concern for the risk of this patient having a significant untoward health event that is possibly treatable and the outcome avoidable.

**What is a better way to document?**
List why the more serious diagnoses are not occurring. If you cannot exclude the concerning diagnoses to an acceptable level of reliability, then do the tests. A specific example of phrasing could read, "Based on the patient's presentation and results of the testing in the ED, the risk of a posterior circulation stroke or mass or bleed are highly unlikely, therefore additional testing was not indicated/performed."

Additionally, the follow-up language should be more precise and strict. An example would be "Contact PCP ASAP to follow up within the next 2–3 days and return to ER immediately if symptoms persist." I agree with Dr. Weinstock's comments in the risk management section; depending on how the doctor comes across in testifying, there is some bona fide risk that the jury wants more for the standard of care.

**Was reasonable care provided?**
The overarching issue is whether reasonable care was provided. Dr. Edlow mentions the difference between a thoughtful error and a negligent error; this is helpful, and a good way to build a defense. The key is whether the doctor acted reasonably (not necessarily correctly) at the time based on what was known, because the end game was not known at that first visit. Again and again, it will return to the question of "was it reasonable to not suspect a serious condition such that more detailed testing was indicated?" It will be pivotal that, on the witness stand, the doctor comes across as caring, competent, and to have a reasonable explanation for not digging deeper with this patient. I would not have been surprised if the jury had gone against the doctor; this is a tough case to defend.

## VI. Medical Discussion—Dizziness and Posterior Circulation Stroke: Thoughtful Error vs. Negligent Error

**Jonathan Edlow, MD, FACEP**
Professor of Medicine and Emergency Medicine, Harvard Medical School
Attending Physician, Department of Emergency Medicine
Beth Israel Deaconess Medical Center

Dr. Edlow was Chair of the June 2008 American College of Emergency Physicians (ACEP) Headache Clinical Policy Task Force.

In addition to clinical duties, Dr. Edlow has authored two books for the general public: *Bull's Eye: Unraveling the Medical Mystery of Lyme Disease*, which was featured on Terri Gross' NPR show *Fresh Air*, and his newest book: *The Deadly Dinner Party and Other Medical Detective Stories.*

This case illustrates many of the important aspects of care in general and management of patients with acute dizziness in particular.

As for the care in general, there are elements of this case that Dr. Garcia did quite well and a couple things that he could have done better. Having reviewed many malpractice cases over the last 20 years, both for the defense and for the plaintiff, I thought that the documentation in this case was far better than the vast majority of those that I have reviewed. I have practiced emergency medicine for nearly 40 years, and I have made my share of mistakes. In my practice, my teaching and in my review of malpractice cases, I differentiate what I call "thoughtful error" and a "negligent error."

For the last 25 years, our department has conducted an M&M conference, with 2–3 cases being presented each week. Many of these cases involve patients whose diagnoses, in retrospect, prove to be missed or delayed. Although the members of the audience know that something bad has happened (after all, it's being run at M&M), the case is presented as it unfolded in real life, literally minute by minute and the audience is blinded both to the outcome and to subsequent facts that the actual treater was not yet in possession of. Occasionally, the member of the group spot errors that might have resulted in the misdiagnosis. However, it is not at all uncommon that nobody in the audience makes the correct diagnosis before it was made in real life. What is the difference between a "thoughtful error" and a "negligent" one? It has to do with gathering the right information in the history and physical examination, understanding the accuracy and limitations of our tests (including history and physical examination), and most importantly, thoughtfully documenting one's medical decision-making.

**What did Dr. Garcia get right?**

He considered stroke, even though this was a young patient had no vascular risk factors. It was interesting that most of the vascular imaging referred to atherosclerosis in the left vertebral artery although even at trial, it was never clear if the arterial pathology was atherosclerotic or dissection. Although the notion that dizziness that worsens with head motion confirms a peripheral cause is wrong, Dr. Garcia did the diagnostic test for posterior canal BPPV and although he may or may not have correctly interpreted the nystagmus, he did document that it was positive only on one side. This finding should not be seen in stroke. Although it is unlikely that Mr. Spinoza had simultaneous BPPV and stroke, the logic (given his age and absence of vascular risk factors and no other neurological physical findings), for me that he had an extremely common condition (BPPV) rather than stroke makes this a "thoughtful error." That said, this case represents a missed diagnosis of a posterior circulation stroke.

Perhaps the most important thing that Dr. Garcia did right, and a lesson we've all heard before, was his excellent documentation. Sure, one can almost always find things that could have been documented better, but Dr. Garcia's documentation, especially of his MDM, allowed for a vigorous defense. It is very clear that Dr. Garcia is not simply checking a box or inserting a macro. He has specific, detailed language in his MDM that clearly shows what he was doing and why he was doing it. Thoughtful, specific documentation helps!

It is also worth noting that BPPV is very common. If you work twelve 8-hour shifts per month and you see 2.5 patients per hour (pretty standard), you should be seeing at least 6–8 BPPV patients per year. If you're not, you're probably missing them. But basilar stroke is rare and usually presents with symptoms beyond isolated dizziness,[7] like when this patient represented. I have only knowingly seen it a handful of times in my 40 years and delayed diagnosis is common.[8] Posterior circulation strokes are simply more difficult to diagnose than anterior circulation strokes, but they ***are*** diagnosable.[9–11] With BPPV (and vestibular migraine) being so common and basilar stroke being so rare, it is no wonder that we are far more often right than wrong when we diagnose a benign cause of dizziness.[12,13] And because we don't get "burnt" very often, we tend to downplay the stroke risk in these patients.

One other issue that played a role in the trial is the plaintiff's expert and plaintiff's lawyer use of language of "differentiating vertigo from stroke" and that "BPPV is best understood as a cluster of symptoms rather than a diagnosis." At trial, this was exposed as a lack of understanding by the plaintiff side. "Vertigo" is not a diagnosis but a symptom. "BPPV" is ***not*** a cluster of symptoms but a very specific, well defined and very common condition. Thus, some of the plaintiff side's argument fell flat, which helped the defense expert to educate the jury on these issues and may have allowed the members of the jury to question the plaintiff's arguments.

**What did Dr. Garcia get wrong?**

In the information gathering phase, he describes the "different than usual tension" headaches that the patient had been having for the two weeks prior to the first ED visit. He did document that the patient was not having a headache at the time of his ED visit, and this was important. But the co-presence of recent atypical headaches and possible stroke symptoms should at least raise the suspicion of an arterial dissection. Because the headache was not present in the ED, this factor did not play out as being super important at trial. As well, the vascular pathology (atherosclerosis versus dissection) was never clear, even at trial.

Another issue is the blood pressure of 177/111. In a patient without a prior history, this is higher than one typically sees with anxiety from being in the ED and we know there was no pain. This did not play out as important at the trial, but in retrospect, one has to wonder if this was the body's autoregulatory attempt to optimize perfusion to an ischemic brainstem or cerebellum. The second thing that Dr. Garcia could have better documented was the absence of other neurological findings. He does a pretty good job and again, it's clear he's not simply inserting a macro, but he might have been more emphatic about brainstem signs that were not present in his MDM. Finally, he did not document cerebellar function, visual fields and gait, nor, from his deposition testimony, did he remember testing them. These are common things that non-neurologists do not test and visual fields and gait cover a lot of neuro-anatomic territory.

The terminal branch of the basilar artery is the posterior cerebral artery, which nourishes the occipital lobes and the neurological deficit of occipital lobe is a visual field cut. In a cooperative patient, this takes less than a minute to test and if positive, completely changes how you would think about this patient, since having any hard neurological deficit would not be consistent with BPPV. This finding also did not seem to play an important role at trial.

**Gait testing:**

The issue that did play a major role at trial was ***gait testing***. Dr. Garcia did not recall testing the gait and did not document gait testing. There was no nursing documentation of his gait and Mr. Spinoza was discharged from the ED in a wheelchair. I am critical of him for not testing and documenting the gait; however, in this case, there was trial evidence based on text messages from Mrs. Garcia to a friend that he needed assistance with walking, but that he ***was able*** to walk. This text message was enough for the jury to belief that although his gait may not have been normal, he was able to walk with some assistance. If a patient cannot walk (and it's a new issue), I would never diagnose BPPV without other testing and/or consultation. Patients with BPPV should be able to walk unassisted. I believe that ***the gait should be tested and documented in every dizzy patient***. The ability to walk independently is also a useful finding that helps distinguish neuritis from stroke.[14] Gait testing does not require any special training or learning curve to master. In addition to having diagnostic utility, if a patient cannot walk safely, then one needs to consider if it's a safe disposition to discharge the patient. I cannot overemphasize the importance of gait testing. Were it not for those text messages and the clear documentation of a positive Dix-Hallpike test, it is quite possible that this case might have been decided in favor of the plaintiff.

**General thoughts:**

There are gaps in how emergency physicians manage patients with acute dizziness. Using the history, I try to place the patient into a timing and triggers category, the same as we would do with a chest pain or an abdominal pain or headache patient.[1,15–18] Then, depending on what category they fall into, I apply various bedside techniques to sort through the differential diagnosis of each timing and triggers category. In patients with persistent ongoing dizziness and nystagmus, I apply the HINTS exam. Some emergency physicians may prefer to use the STANDING algorithm, which does not require defining the timing and triggers category. However, these bedside physical examination elements, which are extremely useful when applied correctly, have not yet permeated general emergency medical practice.

Over the past 10 years, I have gradually modified my approach to these patients.[16] Like most emergency physicians, dizziness used to be my least favorite chief complaint. There are many reasons for this. First, the old "what do you mean, dizzy?" paradigm, that was universally taught to my generation of physicians (and unfortunately, still is) rarely seemed to work for me. Basing the differential diagnosis purely on the descriptor that a patient used should not inform the differential diagnosis. Rather, the timing and triggers of the dizziness are more important. Secondly, my training in vestibular problems was either non-existent or taught in a way such that I did not remember any of it. Finally, my understanding of nystagmus (discussed below) has dramatically improved. For the first two decades of my practice, I had no clue what I was supposed to look for, how to describe it or what it meant.

**Nystagmus:**

By now, it should be clear that knowing a thing or two about nystagmus goes a long way towards improving our care of patients with acute dizziness. After graduating from medical school and finishing my residency training, I confess that I knew next to nothing about nystagmus. And yet, this one finding is incredibly important to me now, not the mere presence or absence of nystagmus but its characteristics – is it persistent or does it only develop with positional testing? What is the direction of the fast-beating component? These characteristics of the nystagmus will often allow a very specific and confident diagnosis to be made.[4, 18, 28]

**Standard of care:**

The issue of "standard of care" was important in this trial. As someone who has been intensely interested in the ED management of patients with acute dizziness, our collective standard of care (what the average emergency physician would have done in similar circumstances) is not great and is far from what "excellent care" should be. As a specialty, we need to improve our care of patients with acute dizziness. The specific ways of doing this are the following (each of which should also be documented):

- Use the history to characterize the timing and triggers of the dizziness
- BPPV is very common – master it!
- Learn nystagmus – it is your friend!
- Always test the gait
- Learn to perform and correctly interpret the HINTS exam, the Dix-Hallpike test and the Epley maneuver (or learn the STANDING algorithm)
- Physical examination is often more helpful than brain (or vascular) imaging (and getting imaging is not protective against malpractice suits)[29]

**Figure 1: Overarching diagnostic algorithm for patients with acute dizziness Developed by Jonathan Edlow, MD**

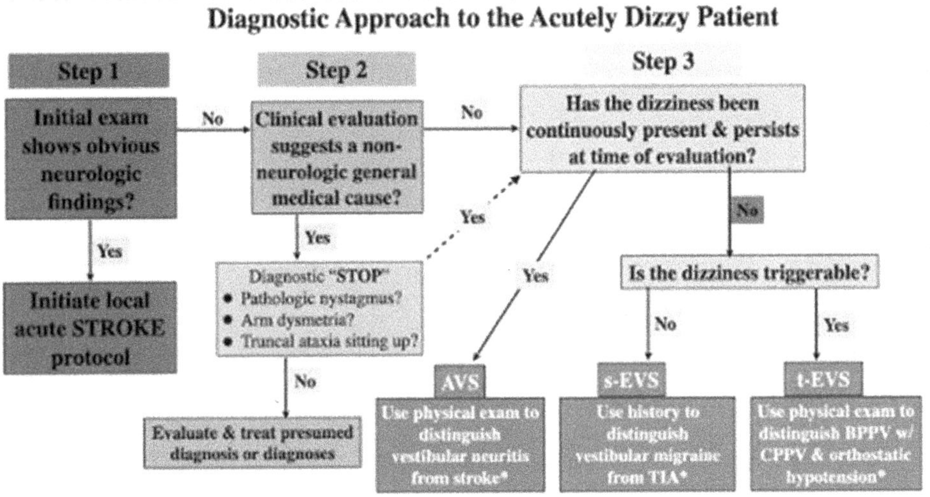


AVS: acute vestibular syndrome, s-EVS: spontaneous episodic vestibular syndrome, t-EVS triggered episodic vestibular syndrome. TIA transient ischemic attack, BPPV benign paroxsmal positional vertigo, CPPV central paroxysmal positional vertigo; only the most common diagnoses listed

This algorithm developed by Dr. Edlow starts by trying to eliminate obvious strokes with clear exam findings beyond isolated dizziness. The second step moves on to looking for general medical causes of acute dizziness, which, in an emergency medicine practice, accounts for half of all dizzy patients.[19] These causes are usually suggested by elements of the history of present illness, co-complaints, or abnormal vital signs (e.g., dizziness plus fever and urinary symptoms or dizziness plus starting a new antihypertensive medication). It then breaks down the differential diagnosis and diagnostic testing by category (Table 1).

**Table 1 – Timing and triggers approach to patients with acute dizziness**

| Timing & triggers category | Definition | Common or important causes | Bedside testing | Notes |
|---|---|---|---|---|
| Acute vestibular syndrome (AVS) | Sudden or rapid onset of persistent dizziness, often with nystagmus | Vestibular neuritis<br>Posterior circulation stroke | HINTS or HINTS plus testing | HINTS is only useful in patients with spontaneous nystagmus.<br>Physicians must acquire some proficiency with the HINTS exam. |
| Triggered episodic vestibular syndrome (t-EVS) | Brief episodes of dizziness triggered by some obligate | BPPV<br>Orthostatic hypotension<br>CPPV | Positional maneuvers for BPPV<br>Orthostatic vital sign measurement | Dix-Hallpike test for posterior canal BPPV<br>Supine head roll test for horizontal canal BPPV<br>A successful therapeutic maneuver helps to confirm the diagnosis |
| Spontaneous episodic vestibular syndrome (s-EVS) | Variable duration episodes of dizziness that are not triggered by anything | Vestibular migraine<br>Posterior circulation TIA<br>Meniere's disease | none | Migraine is by far the most common diagnosis in this category |

The 3-component HINTS or HINTS plus (HINTS plus bedside test of hearing by finger rub) have been used to differentiate peripheral causes of AVS (neuritis) from central ones (stroke).[20, 21] In the hands of experts, it is more sensitive than MRI with diffusion-weighted imaging in the first 48 hours after symptom onset.[20] However, it is critical that the person doing the exam is proficient in the techniques since data clearly show that in current routine emergency medicine practice, we are not.[22, 23] The traditional teaching was always that if hearing and balance were both involved simultaneously, it argued for a peripheral localization because the cochlea (hearing) and the semicircular canals (balance) are co-located peripheral structures – "labyrinthitis." However, it has become apparent that the peripheral structures and the area of the exit for cranial nerve eight (a combination of both the cochlear and the vestibular nerve) can be simultaneously affected by strokes in the AICA territory (anterior inferior cerebellar artery). It is important that to call a HINTS or HINTS plus "peripheral," ALL 3 or 4 components must suggest a peripheral cause; if ANY ONE component suggests a central cause, it should be managed as central.

**Table 2: HINTS test HINTS plus**

| Component | Result in peripheral cause | Result in central cause |
|---|---|---|
| Head impulse test | Presence of a corrective saccade | Absence of a central saccade |
| Nystagmus testing | Unilateral direction-fixed horizontal nystagmus | Torsional, vertical or direction-changing nystagmus |
| Test of skew (alternate cover test) | Absent (no vertical refixation) | Presence of a vertical refixation |
| Bedside hearing test by finger rub* | Normal (symmetric) hearing | New unilateral hearing loss |

*this test is the fourth component that makes the HINTS "plus" test

**Table 3: The STANDING algorithm**
**Developed and modified by Jonathan Edlow, MD[24]**

Another way to approach dizzy patients is with the STANDING protocol (Table 3).[24, 25] This 4-step algorithmic approach is centered on the presence or absence and quality of nystagmus. Another distinguishing feature is that it is "agnostic" to the timing and triggers category. However, it is important to know that the STANDING examination still involves knowing the elements of HINTS testing (except for test of skew) and also involves knowing how to perform the positional tests for both posterior canal (Dix-Hallpike) and horizontal canal (supine head roll) BPPV. Gait testing is also a part of the STANDING protocol. This protocol was validated not only by the original investigators[25], but also in two other studies, one involving trained senior emergency physicians[26] and the other involving family practice and emergency medicine interns.[27] One of these studies also validated HINTS testing by emergency physicians.[26] Collectively, these three studies provide proof-of-concept that emergency physicians can learn to effectively use both HINTS testing and the STANDING protocol. My own personal experience corroborates this.[16]

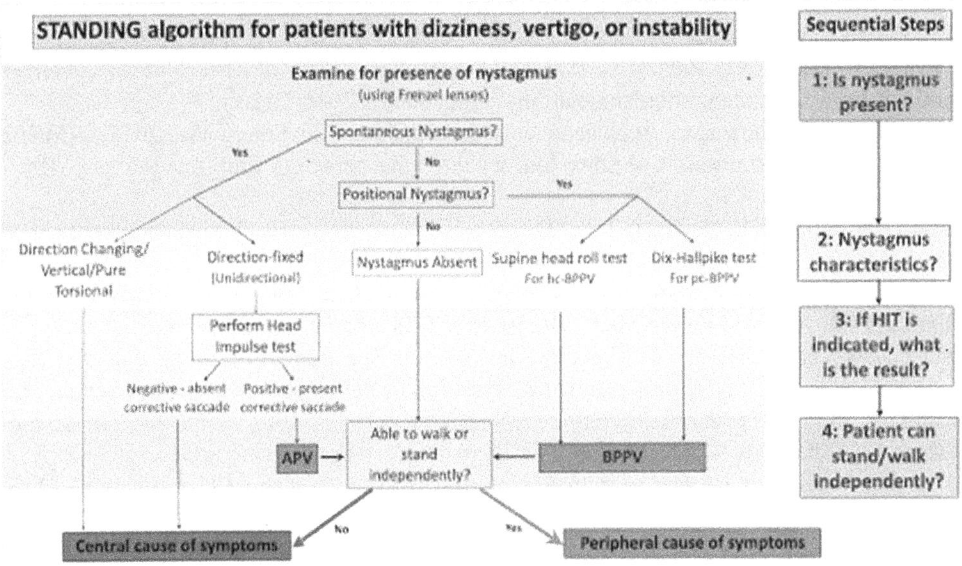


## References


1. Edlow A. Diagnosing dizziness: We are teaching the wrong paradigm! Acad Emerg Med 2013; 20(10):1064-6.
2. Newman-Toker, DE, Cannon LM, Stofferahn ME, et al. Imprecision in patient reports of dizziness symptom quality: A cross-sectional study conducted in an acute care setting. Mayo Clin Proc 2007;82(11).1329-40.
3. Tarnutzer AA, Berkowitz AL, Robinson KL, et al. Does my dizzy patient have a stroke? A systematic review of bedside diagnosis in acute vestibular syndrome. CMAJ 2011;183(9):E571-92.
4. Edlow, JA, Kerber K, Benign paroxysmal positional vertigo: A practical approach for emergency physicians. Acad Emerg Med 2023;30(5):579-88.
5. Kim JS, Zee DS. Clinical practice. Benign paroxysmal positional vertigo. N Engl J Med 2014;

370(12):1138-47.
6. Dmitriew C, Bodunde O, Regis A, et al. The use and misuse of the Dix-Hallpike test in the emergency department. CJEM 2021;23(5):613-16.
7. Mattle HP, Arnold M, Lindsberg PJ, et al. Basilar artery occlusion. Lancet Neurol 2011;10(11):1002-14.
8. Burns JD, Rindler RS, Carr C, et al. Delay in diagnosis of basilar artery stroke. Neurocrit Care 2016; 24(2):172-9.
9. Gurley KL, Edlow JA. Avoiding misdiagnosis in patients with posterior circulation ischemia: A narrative review. Acad Emerg Med 2019;26(11):1273-84.
10. Salerno A, Strambo D, Nannoni S, et al. Patterns of ischemic posterior circulation strokes: A clinical, anatomical, and radiological review. Int J Stroke 2022;17(7):714-22.
11. Saro-Buendia M, Torres-Garcia L, Angel NJ, et al. Dizziness evaluation and characterisation of patients with posterior circulation stroke in the emergency department; A case series study. Arch Acad Emerg Med 2023;11(1):e12.
12. Kerber KA, Zahuranec DB, Brown DL, et al. Short-term risk of stroke after dizziness presentation. Reply. Ann Neurol 2014;76(5):767-8.
13. Yang L, Bai HX, Zhao X, et al. Short-term risk of stroke after dizziness presentation. Ann Neurol 2014;76(5):766-7.
14. Carmona S, Martinez C, Zalazar G, et al. The diagnostic accuracy of truncal ataxia and HINTS as cardinal signs for acute vestibular syndrome. Front Neurol 2016;7:125.
15. Edlow JA, Managing patients with acute episodic dizziness. Ann Emerg Med 2018;72(5):602-10.
16. Edlow JA, Acute dizziness: A personal journey through a paradigm shift. Acad Emerg Med 2023;30(5):598-02.
17. Edlow JA, Gurley KL, Newman-Toker DE. A new diagnostic approach to the adult patient with acute dizziness. J Emerg Med 2017;54(4):469-83.
18. Edlow JA, Newman-Toker D, Using the physical examination to diagnose patients with acute dizziness and vertigo. J Emerg Med 2016;50(4):617-28.
19. Newman-Toker DE, Hsieh Y-H, Camargo, Jr. CA, et al. Spectrum of dizziness visits to US emergency departments: Cross-sectional analysis from a nationally representative sample. Mayo Clin Proc 2008;83(7):765-75.
20. Kattah JC, Talkad AV, Wang DZ, et al. HINTS to diagnose stroke in the acute vestibular syndrome: three-step bedside oculomotor examination more sensitive than early MRI diffusion-weighted imaging. Stroke 2009;40(11):3504-10.
21. Newman-Toker DE, Kerber KA, Hsieh Y-H, et al. HINTS outperforms ABCD2 to screen for stroke in acute continuous vertigo and dizziness. Acad Emerg Med;2013:20(10):986-96.
22. Dmitriew C, Regis A, Bodunde O, et al. Diagnostic accuracy of the HINTS exam in an emergency department: A retrospective chart review. Acad Emerg Med 2021;28(4):387-93.
23. Ohle R, Montpellier R-A, Marchadier, et al. Can Emergency physicians accurately rule out a central cause of vertigo using the HINTS examination? A systematic review and meta-analysis. Acad Emerg Med 2020;27(9):887-96.
24. Vanni S, Pecci R, Casati C, et al. STANDING, a four-step bedside algorithm for differential diagnosis of acute vertigo in the emergency department. Acta Otorhinolaryngol Ital 2014;34(6):419-26.
25. Vanni S, Pecci R, Edlow JA, et al. Differential diagnosis of vertigo in the emergency department: A prospective validation study of the STANDING algorithm. Front Neurol 2017;8:590.
26. Gerlier C, Hoarau M, Fels A, et al. Differentiating central from peripheral causes of acute vertigo in an emergency setting with the HINTS, STANDING, and ABCD2 tests: A diagnostic cohort study. Acad Emerg Med 2021;28(12)1368-78.

27. Gerlier C, Fels A, Vitaux H, et al. Effectiveness and reliability of the 4-step STANDING algorithm performed by emergency interns and seniors for predicting central causes of vertigo. Acad Emerg Med 2023;30(5):487-500.
28. Gurley KL, Edlow JA. Diagnosis of patients with acute dizziness. Emerg Med Clin North Am 2021; 39(1):181-201.
29. Ghaith S, Voleti SS, Bellolio F, et al. Dizziness as a missed symptom of central nervous system pathology: A review of malpractice cases. Acad Emerg Med 2023;30(5):589-91.

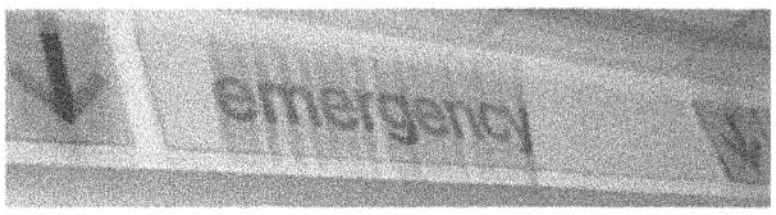


# Case 6

## A 32 Year-old Woman with Headache: We Own This Diagnosis

**Primary case author:**
**Vishnu Mudrakola**

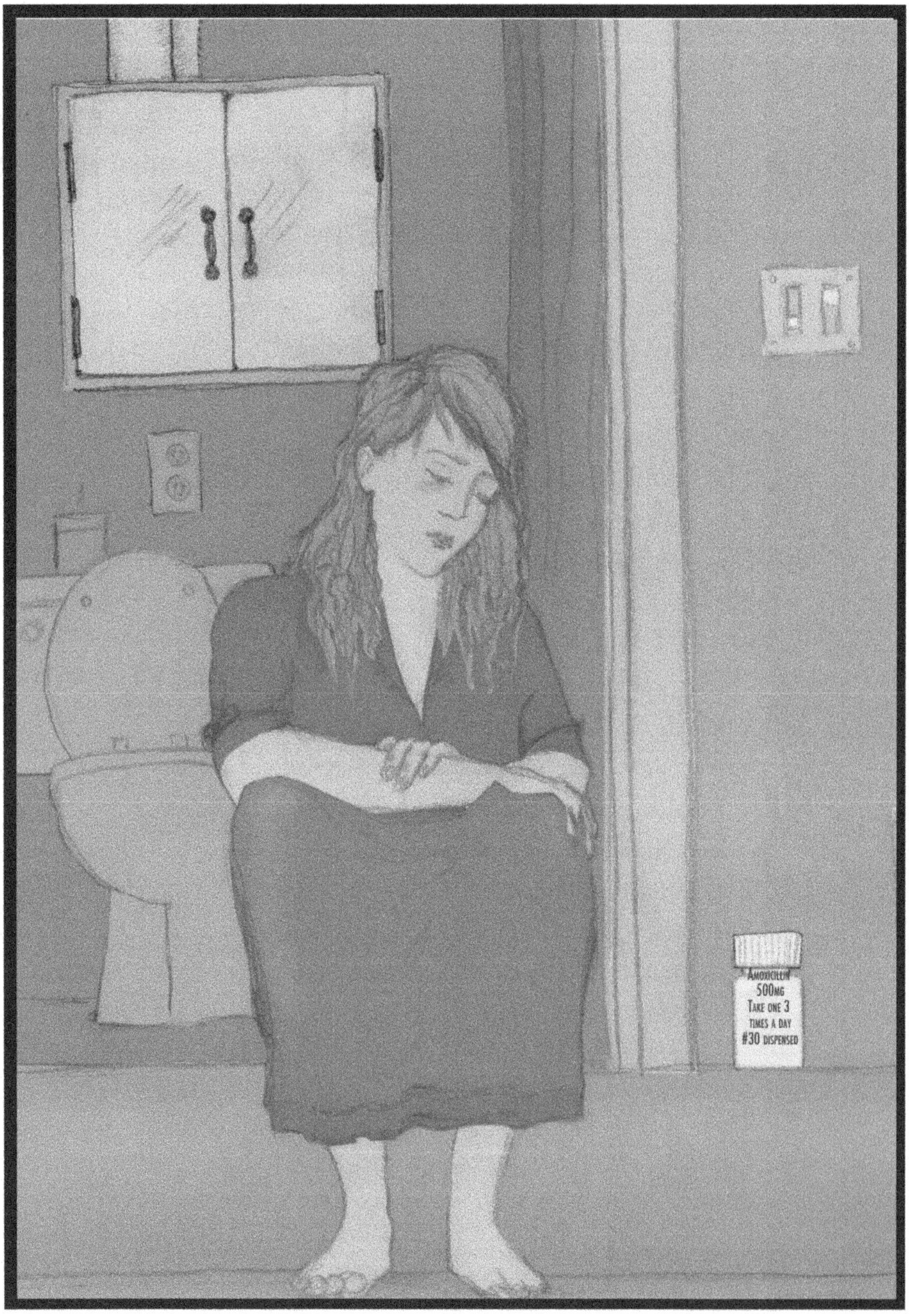
AMOXICILLIN
500MG
TAKE ONE 3
TIMES A DAY
#30 DISPENSED

# Case 6

## A 32 Year-old Woman with Headache: We Own This Diagnosis

Some days I am so good I can diagnose patients from my workstation; sudden onset flank pain is a stone; positional low back pain is a lumbosacral strain … but sometimes I need to see the patient. Headache is a complaint which causes us to put our guard down, particularly if the patient has a history of chronic pain … or sinusitis. The "big two" in evaluating nontraumatic headaches are subarachnoid hemorrhage and meningitis, but there are a few other causes which need to be included in the differential.

***Deep thoughts:***

1. *Is the "worst headache of your life" pathognomonic for ANYTHING?*
2. *How do we reconcile positive test results with a conflicting clinical story?*
3. *Have you ever been a victim of "diagnosis momentum?"*
4. *What is the role of advanced line antibiotics in the treatment of sinusitis?*

**PART 1—MEDICAL**

## I. The Patient's Story

Kelli Flood has a good job selling advertising. She is smart, has a sharp wit and a good work ethic. She and her second husband, Shane, are active parents. They recently married, on October 28, 1998, and took a honeymoon at a Sandals resort.

Several days after the birth of, Jacob, on July 30, Kelli presents to her primary care physician with a headache and is diagnosed with sinusitis; she is placed on amoxicillin. The headaches continue to the point that on August 8th she says her head pain is "indescribable, like my head was going to come off, or split in two."

She presents to an emergency department in rural Ohio.

## II. The Doctor's Version (the following is the actual documentation of the provider)

**Date:** August 8, at 18:32
**Chief complaint:** Throbbing head [pain], migraine comes on suddenly
Nurse's note: Headache has happened 3 times in past 7 days, c/o pain in the forehead and back of head. This headache was of sudden onset a ½ hour ago. Had an epidural. Ice to forehead, crying, headache 10/10.
**History of Present Illness (18:55):** This patient is a 32 year-old female, who is 8 days postpartum. She describes this [headache] as the worst one of her life. She has no known history of direct or indirect trauma to the head. Apparently, 5 or 6 days ago, she was identified as having sinusitis and placed on Amoxicillin 500 mg t.i.d. Since that time, the patient has had 2 other headaches, which were not quite as severe as this one. The patient describes frontal as well as bi-temporal discomfort with photophobia and nausea, but no vomiting. There is no phonophobia, numbness or tingling. The patient had been asleep and woke up with the discomfort.

**Past Medical History:**
**Allergies:** Sulfa (swelling)
**Meds:** Amoxicillin, Tylenol extra strength, prenatal vitamins
**PMH/PSH:** Negative
**Surgery:** c-section, broke arm 16 years ago, laparoscopic surgery
**FH:** Father - diabetes

**Physical Examination:**

Vital Signs

| Time | Temp(F) | Rt | Pulse | Resp | Syst | Diast | O2 sat RA |
|---|---|---|---|---|---|---|---|
| 18:42 | 97.0 | 0 | 68 | 18 | 156 | 95 | 97% |

**Constitutional:** She is a well developed and well nourished female, alert and oriented X3. She does appear to be moderately uncomfortable.
**Skin:** In general has normal texture and turgor. No lesions are identified.
**Eyes:** EOMI. PERRL. The external lids and conjunctivae are clear. Fundi are normal.
**Nose, Mouth, and Throat:** There is minimal nasal mucosal erythema. The pharynx is normal. The uvula is in midline. There is bifrontal region tenderness to palpation and pressure.
**Neck:** Supple without masses, no lymphadenopathy.
**Lungs:** CTAB. No respiratory distress.
**Heart:** RRR without rubs, clicks or murmurs. Carotid pulsations are 2+ and symmetric.
**Neurologic:** Evaluation including sensory, motor, cerebellar, and cranial nerve II-XII examination is intact. No meningeal signs present.
**Emergency Department Course:**

**19:20 – Brain CT:** (reading per ED doctor): No evidence of intracranial bleeding or mass lesion. The bone windows do show evidence for mucoid material within both frontal sinuses with possible ethmoid involvement.

**19:50** – After discussing the situation and the possible effect of narcotics on the baby, who is breast fed, mother did agree to an injection of pain medication and nausea medication.

**20:15** – Repeat vitals: Pulse 64, respirations 18, BP 176/50.

**Doctor progress note:** The patient had moderate relief of her discomfort. The patient has cephalgia, which I believe is related to sinusitis and I will switch her to a different antibiotic, pain medicine and decongestant. I recommend liquids and rest. Recheck in 3 to 4 days if there is no improvement in the overall symptoms, sooner if there is significant worsening.

**Diagnosis:**
1. Acute sinusitis.
2. Acute cephalgia.

**Plan:** Released ambulatory at 20:35

*Seth Hockenberry, MD*

**Note:** A later overread by the radiologist finds the brain CT normal.

**Author comments (Weinstock):** It is obvious from the note that he cared about his patient. He not only spent a lot of time with her, but also informed her when and why to return. The following are some considerations about the initial evaluation.

## III. Risk Management/Patient Safety Opportunities (Weinstock)

**Risk Management/Patient Safety Opportunity #1:**

**Opportunity:** Differential diagnosis too narrow.
**Discussion:** Whereas two immediately concerning ED diagnoses in patients with nontraumatic headache remain SAH and meningitis, there are other "can't miss" secondary headaches, including:

1. Meningitis/Encephalitis
2. Temporal arteritis
3. Pseudotumor cerebri (idiopathic intracranial hypertension)
4. Carbon monoxide toxicity
5. Acute angle closure glaucoma
6. Carotid artery dissection
7. Brain mass (sometimes seen and sometimes not)
8. Preeclampsia/eclampsia
9. Post-LP headache–our patient did have an epidural…
10. Cavernous sinus thrombosis (able to be visualized on noncontrast brain about half the time)
11. Subarachnoid hemorrhage (SAH). According to Perry, et al. within 6 hours we should see 100% of SAH, but at 1 week we are only around 50%...
12. Posterior reversible encephalopathy syndrome (PRES)
13. Reversible cerebral vasoconstriction syndrome (RCVS). Risk factors include:
    i. Pregnancy and postpartum state
    ii. Prescribed medications (triptans, decongestants, SSRIs)
    iii. Illicit drug abuse (typically sympathomimetics such as cocaine)
    iv. Hypertension
14. Pituitary apoplexy: May present with thunderclap headache

Preeclampsia is concerning in our patient since she not only had increased blood pressure when she arrived, but it was actually higher just prior to discharge. Preeclampsia/eclampsia can occur up to 6 weeks postpartum.[1] The problem is that a headache (pain) can also cause the blood pressure to go up. Additional findings with preeclampsia may include hyperreflexia/clonus, abdominal pain, proteinuria and lack of a previous history of hypertension.

Another consideration is post-dural puncture headache. These are worse when sitting up and better when lying flat. If this diagnosis was firmly established, the elevated blood pressure could be explained as a response to the often severe pain.

Primary headaches include the following; however, none of these were consistent with our patient's presentation:

1. Migraine
2. Tension
3. Cluster
4. Narcotic withdrawal
5. Stress HAs

In addition to pregnancy and the perinatal period, other high risk factors for headache patients include:

1. Immunosuppression
2. Age over 50
3. Systemic anticoagulation
4. Hypercoagulability (Cancer, Behcet's disease, OCP use, pregnancy, lupus, factor 5 Leiden deficiency, etc.)

✔ **Teaching point:** Maintain a high index of suspicion for high-risk headache patients.

**Risk Management/Patient Safety Opportunity #2:**

**Opportunity:** Overreliance on test results.
**Discussion:** The phrase "worst headache of life" means a lot to patients and lawyers, but it is really questionable how much it should mean to emergency physicians. If you are going to document this and do a brain CT, it is important to realize the limitations for diagnosis of subarachnoid hemorrhage (SAH).[2-4] At seven days it drops to only 58%. Our patient had already had a week of pain when she presented to the ED.
✔ **Teaching point:** Understand the potential benefits as well as limitations of testing.

**Risk Management/Patient Safety Opportunity #3:**

**Opportunity:** Anchoring bias and diagnosis momentum.
**Discussion:** It is difficult to determine exactly which diagnosis was to be excluded with a head CT, but once the physician saw sinus thickening, he anchored on sinusitis. This was likely coupled with ***diagnosis momentum***, since the patient was actually taking amoxicillin for a sinusitis diagnosis from the primary care doctor. Curiously, there was no documentation of clinical sinus symptoms such as rhinorrhea, postnasal drip, facial/tooth pain or fever, but the patient did have sinus pain with palpation.
✔ **Teaching point:** When a test shows an unexpected result, historical confirmation should support it as the source of the patient's symptoms or it should be discounted.

**Risk Management/patient safety opportunity #4:**

**Opportunity:** Overreliance on antibiotics for sinusitis.
**Discussion:** Sinusitis is usually viral, with a "number needed to treat" (NNT) with antibiotics between 8 and 12. When the decision is made to use a second-line antibiotic (macrolide, quinolone) instead of a first-line antibiotic (amoxicillin, TMP/SMZ, doxycycline), the NNT skyrockets to 100.[5] If 100 patients with a diagnosis of sinusitis are treated with advanced line ATB, one patient will get better sooner. Whereas it is OK to "bump up" the antibiotic from amoxicillin to Biaxin with our patient, the fact that she failed an antibiotic in the first place should cause pause in the diagnosis of sinusitis.
✔ **Teaching point:** Sinusitis is overdiagnosed and therapy overrated.

**Risk Management/patient safety opportunity #5:**

**Opportunity:** Misreading CT.
**Discussion:** The ED physician did document a thorough discussion of the CT reading. Unfortunately, his reading was in contradiction to the radiologist's final reading. When there is a question, teleradiology should be employed to confirm the correct interpretation. A mechanism must be in place to identify all ED radiology discrepancies after the patient leaves the ED. Regarding CT scans, the standard of care is for radiology to provide the contemporaneous reading. Providing an interpretation of a CT without

the assistance of the radiologist may increase risk for the patient and the emergency physician. Sinus findings on CT are very sensitive, but not specific.

✔ **Teaching point:** Avoid interpreting brain CTs without the input of Radiology.

## IV. The Bounceback

August 9th, the day after ED discharge, Kelli, Shane and Jacob are running some errands, but upon return to the house, her headache starts to worsen. She fixes dinner, but doesn't eat anything because "I just can't." She asks, "Shane, [will] you please run me a bath?"

Per Kelli: "I went into the bedroom because that's where Jake was, and I couldn't see him. I yelled for Shane and I said, 'Shane, I can't see the baby.' He came. I said, 'For that matter, I can't see you.' I rubbed my fingers together clear up by my face and I couldn't see them. So, I sat down on the steps of the bathroom and I just don't remember anything else. That's as far as I go." Shane noticed that Kelli "seemed to be in somewhat of a daze and was rubbing her hands together." She begins to shake all over, her eyes roll back in her head and she is foaming at the mouth. Shane dials 911.

August 9 (21:05): Quincy County EMS receives a call for a patient having a seizure. At 21:08 they are enroute, arriving on location at 21:10 to find their patient sitting on the steps leading into the bathroom. She does not respond to verbal commands and is disoriented to time and place. She experiences short episodes of body tremors, lasting less than 10 seconds each. Finger stick glucose is 92, monitor shows NSR. Here is the actual report (redacted):

At 21:28 they arrive at the ED.

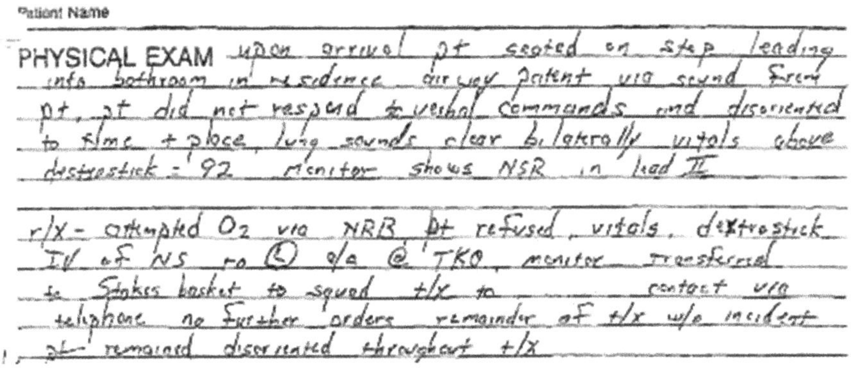
Patient Name

PHYSICAL EXAM upon arrival pt seated on step leading into bathroom in residence airway patent via sound from pt, pt did not respond to verbal commands and disoriented to time + place, lung sounds clear bilaterally vitals above dextrostick = 92 monitor shows NSR in lead II

r/x - attempted $O_2$ via NRB pt refused, vitals, dextrostick IV of NS to (L) f/a @ TKO, monitor transferred to Stokes basket to squad t/x to contact via telephone no further orders remainder of t/x w/o incident pt remained disoriented throughout t/x

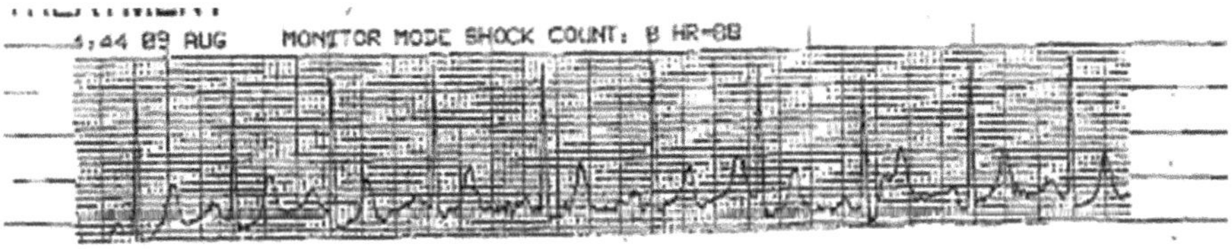


**ED record:** August 9 at 21:32:
**Chief complaint:** Possible seizures
**HPI:** A 32 year old white female accompanied by her husband and transported to the Emergency Department by ambulance from her residence after a possible seizure. The patient's illness began

yesterday, with the patient presenting to the Emergency Department with a headache that she has had since the birth of her latest child on 07/30. Headache had been mostly of her forehead, and her occipital area. A more severe headache then began about a half an hour before the patient arrived at the Emergency Department yesterday at 1832 hours. The Emergency Room physician on duty at the time ordered a CT, that was read as normal, both by the Emergency Room physician and later by the Radiologist. It was felt that the patient had an acute sinusitis causing the acute cephalgia. The patient was started on [antibiotics, decongestants, pain medication]. According to the husband, the patient did go home and rest and slept through the night well. The following day, her headache did persist, but seemed not severe until about 6:00 p.m. The patient had been somewhat more fatigued before that and had fallen asleep apparently at the dining room table. Later this evening the husband was running the patient's bath and noticed the patient seemed to be in somewhat of a daze and rubbing her fingers together, and then began to have shaking allover, and with her eyes rolling back, and husband describes what he thought was generalized seizure. There is no history of seizures. This lasted for about a minute or more. Thereafter, the patient appeared confused and did not respond appropriately but was screaming about her severe headache. The patient also has a history of migraine headaches but this was much more severe. Ambulance was called and the patient was transported to the Emergency Department, remaining alert through the transfer.

According to the paramedics transporting the patient, upon their arrival, the patient was seated on a step leading into the bathroom. The patient did not respond to verbal commands and seemed to be disoriented to time and place. Cardiac monitor revealed a normal sinus rhythm. O2 was given by mask, but the patient refused, during transport, the patient remained disoriented and was crying out about her headache. The patient has no history of neurological problems, except the migraine headaches. She did have an epidural for delivery of her child, but apparently had no complications with a normal vaginal delivery. This was her second child. There is no history of herpes simplex infections, including no cold sores in the past. There is apparently no one in the family with herpes simplex infections.

**Physical exam:**
**Vital signs: Temp 97.4, pulse 78, resp 16, BP 172/99, sat 97% (RA)**
**PE (shortened):**
A well developed, well nourished white female, moaning with pain and shaking her head at times from side to side and crying. Known answers to questions at times, and at times appeared to ignore the questions. Did answer positively when I asked about her headache. Answers questions mostly with moans and very infrequent words. Appears at times to answer appropriately as when asked if she could see my fingers clearly when up before her. She answered also positively with her husband when he held up his fingers and asked how many fingers he held up, then she would begin moaning and crying again, and shaking her head. She was having periods when she would shake her head and shake her extremities, but apparently this was different than what husband witnessed as a possible seizure. Slight pallor. No gross neurological deficits were noted,

**Progress note:** Although [a brain CT] was done yesterday, there was question of whether she may have had a herald subarachnoid bleed yesterday [so CT was repeated]. Rule out encephalitis, possibly herpes simplex.

**CT brain (radiologist):** Normal computed tomography of the brain.

**Labs:** WBC 12.8, Hb 14.3, plt 434. Chemistry and coags nl. Calcium and magnesium normal. CXR – no infiltrates. UA normal.

**ED course:** Patient's blood pressure did go up to 190/115 and the patient's headache seemed to increase with increased shaking of her head and crying. Lasix 20 mg was given IV and Nipride was started at 0.25 micrograms per kilogram per minute or at 16 micrograms per minute. Blood pressure was to be decreased to 160/90. Over a short period of time, the patient's blood pressure then did decrease to 140/90. O2 saturation remained at 95%. Patients headache did appear to decrease somewhat though it was still very severe. She was given [pain medication] with further apparent lessening of her headache and the patient seemed to be resting more comfortably; however, she continued with periods of shaking her head and crying and indicating she had a severe headache, and her mental status remained unchanged, with varying stages of alertness as when she first came in. Cardiac monitor revealed no dysrhythmia throughout. I spoke with the husband several times, giving possible differential diagnoses and after the CT appeared to be normal, except for possible some cerebral edema, I stated to the husband that she may be having an encephalitis, and an LP was indicated. Further, Zovirax would be started intravenously depending upon the results of the LP. I then spoke with the physician covering for Dr. [private physician]. I then spoke with Dr. [Neurologist] on call. The above was summarized, and the decision was made not to do the LP here since our lab is limited and would be able to only do the cell count. The patient was thus admitted directly to the Intensive Care unit where the appropriate further testing and medications will be undertaken.

**Final Diagnosis:**

1. Severe cephalgia, with acute mental status change, and possible first time seizures.
2. Consider encephalitis, herpes simplex.
3. Cannot entirely rule out a herald bleed, with undetectable subarachnoid hemorrhage at this time.
4. Rule out other inflammatory Central Nervous System problems.

*Robert Carozza, MD*

**Author comments (Weinstock):** Hmmm … who has ever called a neurologist and been talked *out* of an LP? There were still several diagnostic possibilities on the table which the second ED physician had not ruled out, including subarachnoid hemorrhage, herpes encephalitis, meningitis and eclampsia. A young, healthy woman with a first-time seizure, and consideration of any of these entities would call for an LP. Of course, we all know she has eclampsia—or does she?

**Hospital Course:**

- MRI showed ischemic changes in the right cerebellar cortex. EEG was unremarkable. LP: WBC 1, RBC 84, protein 77, glucose 46. Bacterial cultures and India ink stain were negative. Urinalysis with trace proteinuria. Sed rates ranged from 16–32.
- Repeat MRIs showed cerebral infarcts in the frontal, parietal and occipital lobes. She was placed on Dilantin and Ativan and high-dose Solu-Medrol. SBPs ranged from 110–190. She had visual loss and speech delay after the occipital event, but was able to communicate with her husband.
- On 8/19/99, ten days after admission, Kelli is sitting in her hospital bed, playing cards with her husband, when she has another seizure. An emergent CT shows attenuation in right occipital lobe and question of vertebral vasospasm.

**Transfer to The University Hospital Medical Center:**

- Initial note: Since arrival has been unresponsive and stuporous with decerebrate posturing.
- MRA showed diffuse arterial "beading" of the small and medium vessels in both the carotid and vertebral vascular distributions.

- At that time the differential diagnosis included postpartum cerebral angiopathy, cerebral vasculitis and eclampsia. She was treated presumptively with high dose IV steroids and magnesium.
- Nicardipine drip was continued to keep her BP 160–170 mm Hg.
- Mental status remained unchanged for the next two weeks.
- On 9/4/99 she developed a temperature of 106°. Indwelling lines were removed, and she was pan-cultured.
- Attempts to reestablish central venous access were unsuccessful, and shortly after those attempts, she developed neck edema and became stridorous, which did not respond to racemic epinephrine.
- Anesthesiology is consulted for difficult airway management, and ENT placed an emergent tracheostomy. The stridor was thought to be secondary to an allergic reaction and the neck manipulation during central line attempts.
- Blood cultures returned positive for *Klebsiella* so the patient was started on Zosyn and tobramycin.
- Throughout the rest of the hospital course, she had slow improvement in neurological status and at discharge was mildly responsive and occasionally interactive.

**Final Outcome:** Kelli is triplegic. Her condition has stabilized but not improved. She lives at home and is cared for by her husband.

## PART 2—LEGAL

Why sue? This patient had a horrible outcome; a young mother now triplegic, requiring life-long medical care and assistance. Before her turn for the worse, she was sitting in the hospital room playing cards with her husband, waiting to go home to be with her family and newborn child. Suddenly, she experienced a seizure from which she would never recover. It is not difficult to see why this family would file suit.

**Plaintiff's attorney:**
**Q.** [Kelli,] would you generally describe your family and how it's functioning, in broad terms? What about you and Shane, and Sarah, Lindsey, and Jacob?
**A.** We're a close family.

**Q.** As to Jacob, would you describe Jacob for us?
**A.** He's a wonderful little boy. He's three and a half. He is extremely active. He's just … I can't say enough about him. I'm a very proud mother.

**Q.** What are some of the things that you like to do with Jacob?
**A.** I like to play Leap Frog with him. If you have children you'll understand. It's a computer game. I like to help him count and teach him his alphabet. I like to play "This Little Piggy" with him. He climbs up and sits on my lap. I let him brush my hair. He likes to read to me. He can't read, but he likes to tell me stories that he makes up. He pretends. He likes to help me with anything that I ask him to do. If I ask him to get mommy a drink of water, "would you, Jacob," he'll run and get it. If I need a Kleenex, he runs and gets it.

**Q.** Does Jacob love you?
**A.** Yes, he does.

**Q.** How do you know that?
**A.** Because he tells me so. He throws his arms around my neck and says, "Mommy, I love you."

## I. The Accusation/Cause of Action

Barton County, OH Court of Common Pleas four years later: Plaintiff requires the use of a wheel chair and has only the use of her left hand. Prior to this event, plaintiff was the active mother of three children. She sought past medicals of **$561,266**, future medicals of **$10,393,754** and future wage loss of **$1,300,000**.

At trial, plaintiff argued that doctors Hockenberry and Carozza failed to differentially diagnose her with postpartum preeclampsia and/or eclampsia (together PE/E) and failed to presumptively treat her with magnesium sulfate, which led to her ultimate brain injury and related paralysis. Specifically, plaintiff argued that any life-threatening illness which appears on the differential diagnosis should be treated presumptively and/or the patient should be admitted if the diagnosis of a life-threatening illness cannot be ruled out.

There was also a lawsuit against the neurologist, Dr. Quinn, which was dropped several days into the proceedings.

## II. The Trial (January four years later)

**Judge's instructions to jury:** Good morning ladies and gentlemen. Today is the 15th of January. We convene in Flood vs. Hockenberry.

Opening statements will give you a preview of what the respective attorneys believe this case will show. Opening statements are not evidence. These are given by the attorneys to assist you and to set the framework, the table of contents, or the coming attractions. Ultimately, the decision of what the evidence [shows] is yours.

Now, in any lawsuit, the plaintiffs go first because they have the burden of proof. They get to go first in presenting evidence. The plaintiffs [also] will get to go first in closing arguments.

This is not a criminal case and the burden of proof that you may have heard of about "beyond a reasonable doubt" does not apply. In a civil lawsuit the plaintiffs have the burden of proving their suit by a preponderance of the evidence, which is the greater weight of the evidence. That is evidence that you believe because it outweighs in your mind the evidence opposed to it. Are counsel ready to proceed with opening statements?

Cast of characters (names changed, except where noted):
**The patient:** Kelli Flood
**ED physician defendant #1:** Seth Hockenberry
**ED physician defendant #2:** Robert Carozza
**Plaintiff's attorneys:** Mr. Lutz and Mr. O'Neil (actual attorney)
**Plaintiff's expert witness (ED physician):** Dr. Geller
**Defense attorney:** Lawrence Huffman (actual attorney)
**Defense expert witness (Neurology):** Dr. Baja Sabdur
**Defense expert witness:** Dr. Stan Kapplan

**Opening Statement—Mr. Lutz (plaintiff's attorney):**
Good morning ladies and gentlemen. I want to first start out by talking a little bit about some rules that doctors follow, rules they learn in medical school and apply every day. Doctors have a duty to use ordinary care; what a reasonably cautious doctor would do in the same situation. Those are rules you'll follow, too, when you decide this case. There's going to be a word mentioned by every doctor that testifies in this case. That word is eclampsia. It has been known for many, many years.

A couple of things about eclampsia. Number one, fifty thousand people a year die from eclampsia. Number two, that's in the world; okay? In the United States, ninety thousand to a hundred thousand are diagnosed with a condition called preeclampsia. It is the second leading cause of maternal death in the United States. Every textbook talks about it. Every doctor knows, or should know, what it is.

What is eclampsia? Eclampsia is a disease. These are not disputable things. Any woman that is pregnant or has recently delivered a baby can get it. Some people used to think that it was a toxin, a poison that would go through your body. That's why it was called toxemia. I look at it like a snake bite. If you get a snake bite you've got to do something quick. If the poison goes through, well, what do you do? You go get the serum, right, to stop the poison. Well, there's a serum [for] eclampsia. It's a drug called magnesium sulfate. Doctors say "drug of choice." It's the drug. It's been known for a hundred of years. It's the drug of choice.

Now, I mentioned preeclampsia; you have preeclampsia before you have eclampsia. The body gives out warning signs. There's not much dispute here. Number one, you've got to be pregnant or postpartum. Number two is high blood pressure. There's often a severe headache, visual disturbances like [sensitivity to light], protein in the urine, nausea and upper quadrant [abdominal] pain.

How does a doctor go about finding these signs? Easy. He takes a history. What happened? Are you pregnant? Recently been pregnant? Have you had headaches? Visual disturbances? Nausea? What's the second way they do it? Lab tests, for example proteinuria. What's the third? An exam. So, history, exam and testing.

Some other things about eclampsia that will be interesting to you. I call them truisms. Number one, it gets worse if untreated. It can move from preeclampsia to eclampsia in a short amount of time. That's why it's a medical emergency. How do you treat it? Mag. Sulfate.

Okay. July 30th, we've got a couple proud parents. Kelli Flood delivered a baby. It was a pretty happy time. July 31st, Kelly and Jacob leave the hospital. On August 8th, eight days postpartum, it's the first opportunity to help Kelli. Kelli is seen by the first emergency room doctor, Dr. Hockenberry. Kelli was in bad shape on August 8th. It was Sunday night at 6 PM. She was crying. She had the worst headache of her life. She had visual changes, photophobia, nausea. He takes a blood pressure. It's 156/95. Dr. Hockenberry thought that a cold was causing the most severe headache of her life and that the high blood pressure was caused by the pain. So, he gave her a shot of Demerol. The headache got better, but the blood pressure went up. The pain was less, and the blood pressure was more. It went from 156 to 176.

Do you know what he didn't do? Order a urinalysis. This is no big complicated test; you pee into a bottle and check it with a dipstick. He didn't do that. He didn't check her reflexes. He didn't refer her to her OB.

When Kelli returned to the ED, the second ED doctor did two things that the first ER doctor didn't do, he ordered a urinalysis for protein which was abnormal. He also checked her reflexes, which were hyperactive. He didn't call her doctor of the last nine months, her OB. He thought that it was herpes. So, that's the first opportunity and the second opportunity.

On the 14th, they finally got around to calling Doctor Garcia [the obstetrician]. He was there within minutes. He looked at Kelli and diagnosed eclampsia. At this point, it was too little, too late. She left the hospital on the 21st near death. Her family was told to hope for the best and prepare for the worst. She was life-flighted on August 21st to University Hospital. She was 20 days in a coma.

They're going to have doctors come in and in hindsight say it [was not eclampsia]. The discharge summary from St. Margaret's says postpartum eclampsia. Doctor Garcia, the obstetrician [diagnosed] eclampsia. The discharge summary at University Hospital and the Specialty [rehab] Hospital admission [was for] eclampsia. They're going to say in hindsight, it wasn't eclampsia.

They're going to say it was something else; Call-Fleming. Hypertension isn't part of the diagnosis. Proteinuria isn't part of the diagnosis. Seizure is not part of the diagnosis. It comes on all at once. Kelli earned $45,000 a year. She hasn't worked since and will never work again. This is a picture of her family, her kids (shows picture to jury). She can do a few things. She can read to them if the print is big or if she has a magnifying glass. She can count numbers a little bit. But, she can't throw a ball. She can't drive to soccer. Kelli is frozen in her own body and it was preventable.

**Author comments (Weinstock):** If I ever get eclampsia (which is highly unlikely), I want this guy working for me! Though it seems clear the diagnosis was preeclampsia, the defense is about to throw a wrench into the mix; they argue the patient did not even have preeclampsia, but a syndrome called Call-Fleming, a progressive disease resulting in large cerebral infarcts. Ever heard of it? Neither have I.

**Opening Statement—Mr. Huffman (defense attorney):**

Well, good morning ladies and gentlemen of the jury. As we promised you yesterday when we opened this trial, there are, of course, two sides to every story. Mr. Lutz has presented the side of the story represented by the plaintiffs. I'd like to talk to you a bit about the side of the story that has to do with my clients Drs. Hockenberry and Carozza.

First, I'd like to have you meet my clients. Dr. Hockenberry is the gentleman in the center who has just nodded to you. He did a combined internal medicine and pediatrics residency. He's been doing emergency room medicine since then. He's a highly qualified and a highly skilled emergency room physician.

My other client is Dr. Carozza [the second ED physician], who is seated there on the left, in the gray jacket. He practiced family medicine for a number of years and then became board-certified in emergency medicine.

Mr. Lutz stated the occurrence of eclampsia is 50,000 world-wide. The facts are that eclampsia is a disease solely limited to pregnant women. The treatment of choice for preeclampsia is delivery of the baby. Almost every time, when the baby is delivered, preeclampsia is over. That's it. You're finished.

Postpartum preeclampsia is very, very rare, and all the witnesses are going to [confirm this]. Furthermore, it is even rarer for her to have postpartum preeclampsia or eclampsia if she had no symptoms during the pregnancy, and Mrs. Flood had no symptoms whatever of preeclampsia during her pregnancy.

As each day goes by after the delivery, the prospects of her having preeclampsia get even more distant.

The only witness who will say that Dr. Carozza or Dr. Hockenberry did anything wrong is Dr. Geller. He's going to say, yes, they should have recognized this disease in the emergency room. I asked Dr. Geller when we took his deposition, I said, "Dr. Geller, how many cases have you ever seen in your professional life of a woman who had eclampsia after the birth of the child?"

Do you know what he said? "One." That was back in the early nineties. He saw one case. My expert witness, Dr. Wendel Johnson, who is the head of the emergency room service at [his] hospital testified in the depositions, "I have never seen a case of eclampsia postpartum. I haven't seen it." Dr. Kevin LaHue, who is a second emergency room expert witness says, "I think I may have seen one or two cases years ago when I was training in [a big hospital] in New York City." That's how rare this disease is. So, keep in mind when people are talking about eclampsia; are they talking about before birth or after birth?

Plaintiffs contend that there's kind of a magic bullet here of magnesium sulfate. But it can be a very dangerous drug, causing respiratory distress and death. Mr. Lutz mentioned a study in which 1,049 people who were given mag sulfate and none of them proceeded to have seizures. In the same study, there were a similar of number of patients who had the same symptoms and who were not given magnesium sulfate and 12 of them may have proceeded on to a seizure. So, whether mag sulfate is a magic bullet that heals everything will be open to serious question. There are some countries, for instance England and Canada, that never use magnesium sulfate; it's unheard of.

All of this talk about eclampsia makes good theatre, but in fact, doesn't really mean anything if, in fact, Mrs. Flood did not have postpartum eclampsia. It's going to be part of our evidence that she did not have postpartum eclampsia. She had a condition which is known as postpartum cerebral angiopathy; a disease lumped together called Call-Fleming syndrome.

We will bring in a physician who is the Chairman of the Department of Obstetrics and Gynecology at the University Medical School and when you hear him state his qualifications, you will recognize why he is considered the world's leading expert on eclampsia. He's written 40–50 articles which are "the Bible" of eclampsia.

We will also present to you the testimony of Dr. Louis Kapplan, Chairman of the Department of Neurology at the [very prestigious] Medical School. He is considered to be the leading expert in America on Call-Fleming syndrome.

Dr. Kapplan [will explain] that the reasons she had Call-Fleming syndrome is that the arteries were found to have "beading," similar to an old-fashioned handful of frankfurters. You do not have that in postpartum eclampsia.

Dr. Kapplan indicates that in Call-Fleming syndrome you have large infarcts of the brain, but in postpartum eclampsia you have some brain swelling and maybe some small infarcts. In Call-Fleming syndrome the brain damage is extensive and is in the cortex part of the brain. In postpartum eclampsia, it's mostly in the white part of the brain. Magnesium sulfate may prevent seizures, but it does not prevent the brain damage in Call-Fleming syndrome. There are clear distinctions between the two diseases. One other distinction in the two disease processes, which will be pointed out by Dr. Sabdur, is that eclampsia is not a progressive disease. This is the crucial issue in this case. You do not get it on October 8th and then get worse and worse and worse and worse and worse and worse and worse, as Mrs. Flood did. That's not the way eclampsia acts. In the Call-Fleming syndrome, you get progressively worse, as she did.

In the end, she didn't have postpartum eclampsia. She was suffering from Call-Fleming syndrome, a rare condition with some of the same symptoms as postpartum eclampsia, for which there is no known treatment. The unfortunate physical situation in which she is now is not the result of any medical malpractice on the part of my clients, Dr. Hockenberry and Dr. Carozza.

**Author comments (Weinstock):** So, it is a bit curious. What seems so obvious on initial read of the ED chart (preeclampsia) has now been drawn into question by the alleged world's leading experts on eclampsia and Call-Fleming. His argument is not so farfetched. Has anyone seen someone become quadriplegic after a simple seizure? How about the "beading" in the carotid and vertebral vessels? Is there even consensus on how to treat postpartum eclampsia? Does a patient need to be admitted and placed on a magnesium drip until they reach the "magic number" of 30 days postpartum?

In the end, a "standard of care defense" is always preferable to arguing "proximate cause" (we missed the diagnosis, but that miss was not the sole cause of her quadriplegia); i.e., "we screwed up but it wouldn't have mattered."

The deposition is a way for each side to see how its witnesses will respond to questions and to discover each other's strategy. The deposition is how the plaintiff's attorneys in this case knew the defense was going to argue Call-Fleming and their subsequent attempt to preempt it in their opening statement.

Let's travel back in time to the deposition of the main plaintiff's witness, Dr. Geller. He seems sure of himself during the plaintiff's "direct," alleging the first three items on the differential were eclampsia, but is then blindsided by the clever defense attorney, who grills him on the progressive nature of the disease process. Dr. Geller seems taken by surprise about the importance of this distinction. In fact, it seems as if he doesn't even understand the question.

## III. The Depositions

### A. Should this diagnosis have been on the differential?

**Deposition (direct) of plaintiff's expert witness Dr. Geller by plaintiff's attorney Mr. O'Neil:**

**A.** No, I wouldn't agree to that actually.

**Q.** You would agree that Mrs. Flood had a condition difficult to diagnose?

**Q.** I take it that you have criticisms of the emergency physicians?

**A.** That's correct.

**Q.** In your review, were you able to formulate a diagnosis as to Mrs. Flood's condition?

**A.** Yes.

**Q.** And would you please tell me what your diagnosis was in that regard?
**A.** I believe at both times she had eclampsia. It is a continuum of the disease, and she presented in two different stages.

**Q.** Did you make a differential diagnosis?
**A.** Yes. First was eclampsia, second would be eclampsia, third would be eclampsia, fourth would be other causes of an intracranial process. And I'm going to lump them together for you; various forms of stroke, vasculitis or infection, but that would fall far beneath that. Given the symptom complex and its findings, [eclampsia] is far and away the most likely diagnosis.

## B. Were the CT and MRI scans consistent with the diagnosis?

**Cross-examination of plaintiff's expert witness Dr. Geller by defense attorney Mr. Huffman:**
**Q.** Is it your understanding that her brain films became progressively worse?
**A.** I'm not sure what you mean by brain films.

**Q.** Is it your understanding that the strokes which appear on the serial brain films became progressively worse as time went on?
**A.** It is my interpretation from the record that both her clinical course and her radiographic studies showed increasing injury to the brain. How we characterize them, whether it's strokes or other events isn't really fundamentally the issue. She did become worse both subjectively and objectively over time.

**Q.** Are you aware of whether or not a progressively worsening condition is consistent with postpartum eclampsia?
**A.** I didn't review the records to seek to draw an opinion about that in either direction so I can't offer you an opinion.

**Author comments (Weinstock):** Oops! Defense goes on to ask about the "beading" of blood seen in the vasculature. He is continuing to build the case for Call-Fleming, to the seemingly unaware plaintiff's expert.

**Q.** Are you aware that "beading" of blood was manifested on the MRAs?
**A.** I'm not sure what you are asking me exactly.

**Q.** Are you aware of whether "beading" of blood on MRAs is consistent with postpartum eclampsia?
**A.** I did not review the records seeking to draw conclusions or opinions about that so I can't offer you anything.

**Author comments (Weinstock):** The defense is using the witness' own description of symptoms of preeclampsia against him. Earlier, the witness had discussed abdominal pain as a component of preeclampsia/eclampsia. He is now forced to admit the patient did not have this symptom.

## C. Should systemic findings have been explored?

**Q.** Another sign of postpartum eclampsia is abdominal pain; would you agree with that?
**A.** That's one sign along with nausea or vomiting.

**Q.** She had no abdominal pain?
**A.** She had no abdominal pain but again that is not an invariant finding in patients with eclampsia even at severe forms.

**Author comments (Weinstock):** How about edema?

**Q.** Alright, when Dr. Hockenberry saw her on the 8th, she did not have any edema. Did she?
**A.** He did not document any excessive amount of edema. I don't know whether or not there was the absence of edema in its totality. That would be a very rare event in someone who had just delivered a baby recently.

**Q.** When she was admitted to St. Margaret's on the 9th, Doctor Quinn (the neurologist) specifically noted at that time that there was no edema. Didn't he?
**A.** I believe that's correct.

**Q.** Okay. So, if it was specifically noted on the 9th on her admission history and physical that there was no edema, you don't contend that there was probably or might have been edema on the 8th, do you?
**A.** Yes. I believe that there might have been. I can't possibly … all I know is that it wasn't directly assessed. It's not possible for me to offer an opinion about something that's not clearly sought after and documented.

**Q.** You can form an opinion based upon the circumstantial fact that we know there was no edema on the 9th. Why would there be edema on the 8th?
**A.** All I know is that one physician believed there was not edema to meet his individual criteria for abnormal. That doesn't mean that it was absent in its totality on either day, and I wouldn't be able to offer you an opinion about it. There's not enough information to even offer conjecture about it.

**Author comments (Weinstock):** We have heard from the attorneys and some of the experts. How does the physician defend himself?

**D. Differential diagnosis of headache:**

**Cross-examination of physician defendant Dr. Hockenberry by plaintiff's attorney Mr. O'Neil:**
**Q.** Now, with headaches, especially severe headaches, there are some conditions that can become very serious and others that are just transient.
**A.** That's correct.

**Q.** And as part of the triage of emergency room medicine the doctor is to find out if any of the short list of items on the very bad list are present, isn't that correct?
**A.** That's certainly part of the job, sir.

**Q.** Okay. And what items are on the short bad list for severe headache?
**A.** Thc bad list includcs such things as mcningitis, cnccphalitis, brain absccss. It would includc various forms of intracranial bleeding whether it be from aneurysm or intravenous malformation—trauma, but that's usually pretty obvious when the patient presents.

**Q.** Okay. What about with a woman who is just recently postpartum, is there a list of serious conditions with a severe headache that you have kind of a check-off sheet in your mind?

**A.** With a headache, you always have to think about any of those things that are listed. Could the headache be associated with something like eclampsia or pre-eclampsia? What to remember is that pre-eclampsia and eclampsia are generally diagnoses of pregnancy and the treatment is delivery. I also recall there have been some reported cases 24 or 48 hours after delivery.

**Q.** And based on that memory, did you not then consider the issue of pregnancy-induced hypertension, pre-eclampsia and eclampsia?
**A.** It was something that I considered, but based on historic elements and the physical examination, I felt it was much lower on the list of items in the differential diagnosis.

**Author comments (Weinstock):** This is tricky terrain. The physician doesn't want to appear stupid or give the impression that he wasn't thorough, so he says he considered preeclampsia. The problem is that, in a legal setting, consideration of a diagnosis can imply that that diagnosis, especially if potentially life-threatening, should be further explored. See comments below by Bob Bitterman, MD, JD, on the "believability" and advisability of this line of testimony.

I was taught in medical school that if you consider a diagnosis (the classic example was pulmonary embolism) you needed to test for it. I categorically disagree with this line of reasoning. Putting this case aside, I contend that every patient with chest pain needs to have the emergency evaluation start with a consideration of the differential diagnosis of the five life-threatening causes of chest pain, which can be rapidly whittled down based on the history and physical exam. Does the 45 year-old with onset of chest pain while lifting a refrigerator have angina from the exertion or a muscular strain from the lifting? Both need to be considered, but all patients with chest pain do not need to be admitted—we are doctors after all, not robots.

## IV. Judge's Instructions to Jury (January 29)

The Court has given you the instructions on the law applicable to this case. In a civil case, at least six members of the jury [out of a total of eight] must agree upon a verdict. When you have reached a verdict you will select and complete the verdict forms according to your decision. In fulfilling your duty as jurors, your efforts must be to arrive at a fair and just verdict. Each of you must decide this case for yourself, but, you should do so only after a discussion of the case with your fellow jurors.

## V. The Twist

As the jurors leave the courtroom to deliberate, there is a flurry of activity on both sides. A defense offer of $500,000 to settle had already been declined, but an emergency call from the insurance company reaches the defense attorney, cell phone in hand; their new offer is increased to $750,000. This is conveyed to the plaintiff 's attorney who, after deliberating with the client in a hotel room across the street, declines the offer. Panic ensues as the insurance company is told of the rejection and the ante is upped to $1,000,000. Additional telephone calls are placed, but the offer is again rejected by the plaintiff.

**Per the defense attorney, Mr. Huffman:** "I felt from a scientific standpoint we had a winner, but I kept looking at a lady in a wheelchair. I was not confident [the jury] would walk away from her. They were asking for almost $15 million, which I did not think they would get, but I would not have been surprised with $4–5 million. Our defendant was very good."

## VI. The Verdict

**THE COURT:** It's January 29th. The record should reflect that the parties are all present, with counsel. The jury has indicated that they have reached verdicts. Mr. Spino, I understand you were selected as the foreperson.
**JURY FOREMAN:** Yes, your Honor.

**THE COURT:** Congratulations. Have you reached verdicts?
**JURY FOREMAN:** Yes, we have, sir.
"We, the jury, being duly impaneled, sworn and affirmed, find for the defendants with respect to the claim against the defendant:

**Number One—Seth Hockenberry [ED doctor first visit]:** "Do you find that defendant Dr. Seth A. Hockenberry was negligent?" It's circled "no." The same seven jurors signed that verdict form.

**Number two—Robert Carozza [ED doctor second visit]:** The second verdict is signed by seven jurors. "Do you find that defendant Dr. Robert Carozza was negligent?' The answer circled is 'no.' "

**THE COURT:** Ladies and gentlemen of the jury, this obviously was a long case and a very difficult case. Throughout the trial, as I would look over and watch you folks, I know you didn't take your job lightly. I appreciate your willingness to sacrifice the time that you put into this. The parties had a dispute they couldn't resolve. Our system says that we call upon eight citizens to help resolve the issues. You did everything you were called upon to do—you should be proud of your service.

You are now free of any obligations. You can discuss this case now with anyone you want. That's entirely up to you. You are free from any of the other restrictions that I have been saying throughout about discussing the case or talking it over with anyone. Anything else from any counsel before I excuse the jury from the case? Plaintiffs?
**MR. O'NEIL:** Nothing, your Honor.
**MR. HUFFMAN:** No, sir.

**Author comments (Weinstock):** The jury split 7–1, voting for the physicians-defendants. After the trial, the lead defense attorney was standing in the hall and saw the plaintiff being wheeled out of the courthouse. The wheelchair was being pushed by two people, one was the lone juror who voted for the plaintiff. When they exited the courthouse, she helped load the defendant into the van.

## VII. Legal Insight per Attorneys in this Case

**Thoughts from defense attorney:**

- The jury didn't buy whether two ED doctors ought to have been able to diagnose postpartum eclampsia when an OB who has testified at 450 trials had only seen it once.

**Thoughts from plaintiff's attorney:**

- I think about this case at least once a week.

- The ED docs won the case as they [the jury] thought "if neurologist couldn't diagnose it, how could we expect an ED doc to [make the diagnosis]."
- Once the case was settled with the neurologist, the case against the ED docs was lost.

**Author comments (Weinstock):** The "Empty chair" defense is an excellent tool when available. Although it is inadmissible, it is glaringly obvious to the jury when a critical defendant is missing, such as the neurologist in this case. The jury is free to draw their own conclusion, which is often that liability was alleged and a settlement reached, thus pointing the finger of liability at the empty defendant's chair (that was vacated by the neurologist).

## VIII. The Legal Analysis—Guest Author

**Robert Bitterman MD, JD, FACEP**
Dr. Bitterman is a physician-attorney consultant who has specialized in compliance issues related to the Emergency Medical Treatment and Labor Act (EMTALA) and emergency department (ED) risk management.

My perspective stems from 30 years practice in busy inner city emergency departments, as well as being the attorney, director of risk management, and faculty member of a large academic emergency medicine teaching program. Additionally, I have been an owner, board member, chair of claims committees and chairman/CEO of malpractice insurance companies which insure only emergency physicians.
**I'll comment on five aspects of this case:**

A. How does knowledge bias influence retrospective review of cases?
B. What were the four main diagnostic failures in this case?
C. Should EPs interpret CT scans?
D. Is the EP's liability resolved when the patient is admitted?
E. Which factors determine the outcome of medical malpractice lawsuits?

### A. How does knowledge bias influence retrospective review of cases?

Everything is easier in retrospect, especially when you are biased by knowing the ultimate outcome of the case. Unscrupulous plaintiff's attorneys are particularly adapt at intentionally inducing knowledge bias in their experts; they hurriedly tell you the negligence, adverse consequences and poor medical outcome before you can inform them you really only want to know what the emergency physician knew at the initial encounter. If the care at an initial ED visit is what's in question, as it is in this case, I think it's much more valuable and fair to all parties to provide an expert opinion without knowing the eventual outcome. The government is frequently guilty of inducing the same bias when obtaining peer review for physician quality improvement hearings.

That said, I hope, but can't guarantee, that my comments on the two emergency department visits described herein would be the same even if I hadn't been provided the second visit data, the ultimate medical facts, expert opinions, trial evidence and author comments.

### B. What were the four main diagnostic failures in this case?

I don't know if either emergency physician should have made the correct diagnosis, but a few things are certain. First, the diagnosis of sinusitis should not have been made; it was clear error. Second, the physicians should have done an LP. Third, the patient's obstetrician should have been involved. And fourth, better medical decision-making would have led either physician down a different pathway, and may have led to an earlier diagnosis.

1. Sinusitis?

Three distinct episodes of head pain described as sudden, spontaneous and "worst of her life," woke her from her sleep, and "indescribable, like my head was going to come off, or split in two" just isn't sinusitis. No way. To even entertain that diagnosis may be an error, and non-improvement after treatment should cause the provider to question the diagnosis. The sinuses on the CT scan were completely normal; the described findings are routinely seen and provide no evidence of sinus infection, let alone a sinus infection sufficiently rip-roaring to cause severe headaches.

2. No lumbar puncture (LP)

The first physician clearly entertained the diagnosis of subarachnoid hemorrhage (SAH), and even wrote in his progress note that "at this time, I can find no evidence of intracranial bleeding." Well, it's hard to find evidence if you don't look properly.

The second physician considered the diagnosis even more and still didn't do the LP. He notes in the chart that there was a question of a herald SAH bleed yesterday, so he repeated the CT, and then as a final diagnosis writes, "Cannot entirely rule out a herald bleed, with undetectable subarachnoid hemorrhage at this time." This alone mandated an LP.

Furthermore, on the second visit the patient is postseizure, with no clear diagnosis, and the physician entertained encephalitis as a possibility, going so far as to even put on the chart, "I stated to the husband that she may have encephalitis, and an LP was indicated." Ouch.

To skip the LP because he was dissuaded by a consultant or "since our lab is limited" is also clear error and faulty reasoning, particularly in a confusing case where more data may be helpful. The CSF may reveal SAH blood, cells or protein and can be sent for cultures and saved/frozen for later testing with a lab less "limited."

3. Failure to involve the patient's obstetrician

In an otherwise healthy woman with no significant past history, new onset severe headaches, hypertension and no clear etiology, the obvious question is what's different in her life that is temporally related that could be causing her symptoms? Pregnancy, delivery, epidural anesthesia and recent hospitalization jump out as obvious considerations! The obstetrician's knowledge of those events may be invaluable.

If the first physician truly considered postpartum preeclampsia as stated in his deposition (I'll comment more on this assertion below), he had even more reason to talk with the patient's obstetrician. The second physician, though, was faced with a still more confusing picture in a much sicker patient; there's no excuse for not utilizing the obstetrician's expertise. There is every reason to believe the obstetrician would have suspected a vascular event and advised the emergency physician to obtain an MRI, which likely would have revealed the culpable pathology.

4. Failure to consider less common disorders

Emergency physicians should continually ask themselves the question, "What if I'm wrong— what serious diagnoses can be causing the patient's symptoms?" This is especially true when considering whether to accept the diagnosis of "sinusitis" in a patient with symptoms that could be from a lethal disease, such as SAH, preeclampsia or other intracranial vascular pathology.

The emergency physician doesn't need to know all the odd or rare diseases, but should know enough to consider that this patient is in the sphere of the unusual and needs to be evaluated for an uncommon disease or an uncommon presentation of a more commonly-seen problem (such as SAH). To make a diagnosis, you must first think of it. Pain from ischemia with hypertension as a reflex autoregulatory response to maintain tissue blood flow should be considered, particularly postpartum. Whether it's an odd vascular event or some rare cause of ischemia, such as "Call-Fleming syndrome" isn't the point. What matters is that the emergency physician recognizes that the clinical picture isn't in the ordinary category and that it needs further investigation to determine the etiology, including specialty consultation.

## C. Should EPs interpret CT scans?

Should emergency physicians read head CT scans themselves? Absolutely not! First, it is not standard practice for EPs to read CT scans. So if you do read your own head CTs, no matter how good you think you are, you had better be formally credentialed by the hospital, and you had better be right—every single time. In this case, the physician's misinterpretation of the CT led to an incorrect diagnosis.

Second, certain deadly conditions, such as subarachnoid hemorrhage (SAH), can be quite subtle, particularly early on; precisely when you need to catch it. It can also be subtle later in its course, when blood becomes difficult to detect. Patients rightly expect someone with the training, expertise, experience and appropriate hospital privileges to read studies that can make the difference between life and death.

Where was the ED Medical Director, the hospital's risk manager or the insurance carriers which insured the hospital or the physician group? How could they allow the emergency physician to interpret head CT scans and discharge the patient without first obtaining a reading by a qualified radiologist? The plaintiff's attorney should have sued the hospital, the ED administrator, and the ED Medical Director right along with the emergency physicians; these individuals were equally to blame for the CT error, and it would have made the care provided look "sloppy" (just another word for "negligent").

Skilled radiologists make enough errors, and their interpretations or communication of their interpretations creates a great deal of liability for emergency physicians. It might surprise emergency physicians to learn that about 20–25% of hospitals don't even keep a copy of the preliminary reading in the patient's permanent medical record. Instead, they discard the preliminary interpretation and replace it with the final interpretation, which is contrary to recommendations of the American College of Radiology.[22]

This practice is medically and legally untenable. It doesn't honestly or accurately reflect the true course of events related to the patient's care, and it unnecessarily creates additional risk for the emergency physicians and the hospital. We frequently make very consequential medical decisions based on these preliminary interpretations.

With today's digital technology, all special studies (CT, MRI, etc.) should be read by a radiologist in real time while the patient is still in the ED—not the next morning—and any acute significant findings communicated immediately by the radiologist directly to the physician. The preliminary interpretations must be ***in writing***, must be ***signed*** by the radiologist interpreting the images and must be ***maintained in the patient's permanent medical record***, exactly like the final reading of that same study is kept in the patient's records.

## D. Is the EP's liability resolved when the patient is admitted?

Admitting the patient, even to an ICU as in this case, does not necessarily relieve the emergency physician of malpractice liability. There are a whole host of reasons that emergency physicians are successfully sued related to admissions, such as:

- Failure to admit to the appropriate level of care
- Failure to timely order the clinically indicated diagnostic studies
- Delay in consulting the appropriate specialist
- Delay in starting treatment in the ED
- Failure to communicate the seriousness of the patient's condition to the admitting physician

In this instance, failure to do the LP, failure to consult with the patient's obstetrician and perhaps even failure to order an MRI prior to sending the patient to the ICU, all fall squarely into this category. Failure to administer parenteral antibiotics in the ED to admitted patients with serious infections is perhaps one of the more common theories of litigation against emergency physicians related to admitted patients.

Whenever you know what a patient needs, "just do it"—don't assume it will get done in a timely fashion, or get done at all, by the admitting physician.

## E. Which factors determine the outcome of medical malpractice lawsuits?

Physicians routinely underestimate the influence of non-medical issues on the outcome of malpractice suits. Good medicine is not good enough to prevent lawsuits, or to win lawsuits. Only 20% of lawsuits filed contain negligence; the vast majority of cases are focused on the care provided. Were you nice to the patient and family, did you answer all their questions, did the hospital systems break down?

The degree of damages incurred by the patient has a much greater correlation with the amount of settlement payment or jury award than the presence of negligence. The universal mantra of medical malpractice reinsurers is "how bad are the damages," prodding claims managers to set aside reserves.

In most cases, however, the prime factor in the outcome is the credibility and believability of the defendant. In this case, the emergency physician was not very credible. The comment made at deposition (which, by the way, is where defendants-physicians win or lose most malpractice cases) that "I thought of [preeclampsia]" is not logically consistent with his actions.

Any physician who actually considered preeclampsia would have checked for peripheral edema and hyperreflexia, obtained a urinalysis for proteinuria, documented their presence or absence and likely discussed the issue with the patient's obstetrician. It sounds too self-serving to say that and likely wouldn't sit well with the jury.

<u>Why didn't the case settle during jury deliberations when the defendants made a million-dollar offer?</u>
Many factors impact settlement decisions, including the amount of money sought and the unpredictability of juries. But a major factor is sympathy for the plaintiff, especially when coupled with terrible damages. The woman in this case was smart, had kids and a husband, and a good job, but now is triplegic, requiring life-long care. As the defense attorney noted, "I kept looking at a lady in a wheelchair." The lone juror who favored the plaintiff and helped push her wheelchair out of the courthouse evidences the sympathy that the plaintiff's attorney hoped to engender, which would lead to

a multimillion-dollar award. The attorney had reasonably good expert witnesses, some medical issues to chew on and physician credibility issues to bolster his case. He chose to seek the $15M megascore, and ended up leaving a million bucks on the table.

The defense attorney was clearly concerned with the sympathy factor, but the settlement offers were forced by the insurance carrier or the defendants-physicians themselves. The physicians may have been concerned that they would be personally liable for any amount over their policy limits, typically $1M each, and demanded that the insurance company attempt to settle the case within policy limits. The plaintiff's rejection and failure to offer an amount within policy limits forced the verdict, and also saved the insurance company a potential "bad faith" claim from the doctors if it didn't accept a counteroffer within policy limits. (For additional discussion of a "bad faith" claim, see "Help! I am being sued.")

Why did the physicians "win" at trial?

First, whatever this patient had was extremely rare, regardless of whether it was postpartum preeclampsia/eclampsia or a progressive postpartum cerebral angiopathy. Second, as the two attorneys involved opined, the jury didn't expect two small-town emergency physicians to be able to diagnose something so rare that the plaintiff's obstetrician expert had only seen once a zillion years ago, or that the neurology "specialist" wasn't able to diagnose either. Lastly, the jury may have believed the causation defense, that even if the physicians and hospital were negligent, their actions didn't materially affect the patient's preordained clinical outcome.

This case, in essence, presents poor physician care, lousy medical decision-making and incompetent, or at least inattentive, ED administrative leadership but a lucky legal result. It didn't have to end up that way.

## IX. Medical Discussion—Headaches and Postpartum Preeclampsia

**Vishnu Mudrakola, DO**
Emergency Medicine
Summa Health
Research Director, Assistant Program Director, Peer Review Committee Member

From the outset, the main issue with the doctors' medical decisions is not considering the patient's postpartum state. The postpartum state is a very fragile time both emotionally and physically with an increased risk of hemorrhage, clotting (pulmonary embolism/cerebral venous thrombosis), vasculitis, cardiomyopathy, and postpartum preeclampsia.[2-4] The physician on the first did not consider diagnoses that are specific to the postpartum state. Even though sinusitis is a common cause of headaches, the history and exam were not consistent with sinusitis. Sinus headaches are typically constant not episodic, throbbing, and worse with positional change.[1] Due to significant ambiguity over the term sinus headache, the International Forum of Allergy and Rhinology released diagnostic criteria to classify primary headache secondary to sinus disease.[5]

Headaches from sinus disease should have developed in temporal relation to the onset of chronic rhinosinusitis and usually wax and wane in parallel with the degree of sinus congestion. The headache is also exacerbated by pressure applied over the paranasal sinuses.[6] This does not match the documented exam at all. Further, there is no reason to believe that the patient would have such high pain levels especially with no prior history of chronic pain issues and no air fluid levels or severe inflammation of the sinuses on CT. In general, CT imaging has poor specificity (40-60%) for diagnosing sinusitis, as up to 40% of adults without acute sinusitis will still have abnormalities on CT.[7] The clinical practice guideline by the American Academy of Otolaryngology – Head and Neck surgery in 2015 recommends that radiologic imaging not be obtained in patients who meet diagnostic criteria for diagnosis of acute rhinosinusitis unless a complication or alternative diagnosis is suspected.[8]

While the physician clearly empathized and did his best to treat Kelli's pain, there is no evidence in the documentation that she had sinusitis; here we have a patient that is not even two weeks postpartum presenting with acute onset severe headache with no recent URI, no significant nasal congestion, no facial swelling or focal sinus tenderness, and no real CT findings to explain her symptoms. Most crucially, the abnormal vitals both at presentation and at time of reassessment are never addressed. Per the American College of Obstetrics and Gynecology (ACOG) recommendations, features of headache that warrant prompt attention include "thunderclap" headache, rapid onset, elevated blood pressure (BP), visual changes, altered level of consciousness, and fever.[9] A non-contrast head CT this far out from the onset of the first headache essentially rules out nothing aside from, perhaps, a large brain tumor!

The blood pressure (BP) reading should stand out as a big red flag in the context of the postpartum setting with no prior history of hypertension. Blaming pain for abnormal vitals is a very slippery slope. Yes. Pain and anxiety can cause BP elevation. However, based on previous experiments, usually the increase in BP is 30mmg Hg or less.[10] A recent study noted that patients with increased BPs in the ED without prior diagnosis of hypertension had persistently increased BPs at home.[11] Persistent BP elevation even after pain improves should raise suspicion for a different cause of headache including postpartum preeclampsia, which can occur up to six weeks after delivery. Of note, even without postpartum preeclampsia, ACOG recommends treatment of severe hypertension (SBP>160) if persistently (greater than 15 minutes) elevated.[12]

At this point in the work-up, elevated BP from autoregulation due to ischemia, vasospasm, bleeding, clotting, or another vascular phenomenon need to be considered. For a successful defense to say, "The doctor considered the elevated BP but did not think it needed further work-up," there should be some explanation in the medical decision-making (MDM) note. In Dr. Hockenberry's note, there is no explanation for the elevated BP, no explanation for why the BP increased when rechecked (despite the patient receiving pain medication), why an LP was not necessary, and why a urinalysis, liver function tests, fibrinogen, and D-dimer levels were not obtained. Further, if preeclampsia/eclampsia were truly considered, reflexes and muscle tone should have been assessed and documented.

The neurological exam is crucial here but is documented poorly with vague terminology. It is hard to elucidate what specific tests were done to conclude "sensory, motor, and cerebellar system … is intact" Did the doctor simply see the patient from across the room, sitting upright in a chair and talking and call it a day? In addition to not fully considering additional causes of her symptoms, the first ED doctor falls into the trap of trying a different therapy for sinusitis; which seems like a classic case of diagnosis momentum (when a previous diagnosis becomes established and prevents consideration of an adequate differential on subsequent visits). [13]

On the second visit, there are now additional symptoms that are not consistent with primary headaches. Vision change and witnessed seizure-like activity are significant symptoms but it is clear from the second ED doctor's documentation that the differential has been widened to mostly infectious and possibly auto-immune etiologies. Meningitis and encephalitis can certainly cause vision changes and seizures but are less likely in the absence of a fever, rash, and other risk factors. Herpes simplex is specifically discussed as well. This is a reasonable thought in undifferentiated headache and altered mental status but again, Kelli is an otherwise healthy, immunocompetent postpartum female. In addition, part of routine prenatal and antepartum testing is to check for herpes, HIV, GBS, and rubella status. Barring any abnormal results, the patient may have neglected to mention, these already seem like low probability diagnoses.

ACOG defines preeclampsia as new onset hypertension (SBP ≥ 140mm Hg, or diastolic ≥ 90 Hg) with any other manifestation of organ dysfunction.[12] It is important to note that preeclampsia is a spectrum. In its mildest form, preeclampsia demonstrates elevated BP with proteinuria. As the disease process progresses, organ dysfunction evolves.

| Severe Features of Preeclampsia[12] |
|---|
| Thrombocytopenia: Platelets < 100 x109/L |
| Renal insufficiency: serum creatinine > 1.1 |
| Abnormal liver function tests |
| Pulmonary edema |
| Significantly elevated BP (SBP ≥ 160mm Hg, or diastolic ≥ 110 Hg) |
| Neurologic symptoms: unexplained new headache or visual symptoms |

Kelli clearly meets the BP criteria, with a repeat reading of 176/50, putting her in the "severe features" category. When her condition worsens, she is essentially in eclampsia as evidenced by her seizures. There is likely some dogmatic thinking occurring; since Kelli already delivered and did not have preeclampsia prior to delivery, eclampsia is less likely or not even possible. This is not uncommon, as a study by Yancy, et al. showed that over half of patients with postpartum preeclampsia did not have antepartum or peripartum precampsia.[14] Most patients with postpartum preeclampsia/eclampsia do not have a history of preeclampsia during pregnancy and present between day 3–10 of postpartum, which is similar to Kelli. [15,16] Even if there was some diagnostic uncertainty, at least the initial magnesium loading dose should have been given while waiting for the dust to settle with additional tests and consults. This is a cheap, safe, effective, and easy treatment that was entirely omitted in Kelli's care until she arrived at the tertiary care center.

Another glaring omission from both doctors' care is not involving the obstetrician. Based on the vitals alone, any obstetrician would have significant concern for preeclampsia and recommended BP management and a magnesium load. ACOG is appropriately aggressive in their recommendations for patients with headache and elevated blood pressure. They specifically note that it is important to consult the obstetrician and consider RCVS (reversible cerebral vasoconstriction syndrome) and PRES (posterior reversible encephalopathy syndrome), especially if the patient is altered or vomiting.[9] RCVS is a group of disorders that cause severe headache due to vasoconstriction or other acute vascular processes in the brain. While the exact pathophysiology of the process has not been established, 50-60% of cases have postpartum state as the most significant contributor.[17] PRES commonly presents with headache, altered mental status, vision changes, and seizures (similar to Kelli's presentation). In a retrospective study, PRES was found in more than 90% of eclamptic patients and 20% of preeclamptic patients with neurological symptoms.[18] So, even if the ED physician did not, the obstetrician, if consulted, would have a high index of suspicion for these conditions.

The defense throws a curveball with the argument for Call-Fleming syndrome. It is a rare disease that matches some of Kelli's findings but most notably has beading of the arteries noted on angiography. The difficulty here lies in the classification and cause of this syndrome. The exact cause and pathophysiology are still poorly understood. However, it has been associated with postpartum patients.[19,20] Call-Fleming is part of the spectrum of the larger group of conditions within RCVS.[21] This is a difficult condition to diagnose and usually has normal CSF results and initial imaging. The diagnosis is best made on angiography which shows focal areas of vascular constriction and associated infarcts.[22] Similar to Kelli, patients diagnosed with Call-Fleming syndrome do present with headache, visual changes, vomiting, and seizures. Based on the limited case reports, Call-Fleming syndrome does appear to be reversible, and the vasospasms usually respond well to nimodipine.[22] It has an excellent prognosis if discovered early. The key takeaway is that this condition is part of RCVS, which in turn is a complication of preeclampsia/eclampsia and should be considered per ACOG guidelines.

Even if these physicians did not think of the rarer complications like RCVS and PRES, treating the patient appropriately and aggressively with magnesium, BP control, and consulting the obstetrician is simple. Having a high index of suspicion for specific postpartum related complications is invaluable. Even at the tertiary care center, after all the advanced imaging and consultations, the main treatment was magnesium along with BP control and steroids. This is in line with ACOG recommendations for treatment of secondary headaches with preeclampsia/eclampsia symptoms and severe features.[12] Evaluation of secondary causes of headache and treating preeclampsia early would likely have affected Kelli's severe morbidity.

The take home points in this unfortunate case are to not ignore abnormal vitals, create a broad differential diagnosis, and understand what diagnoses are more likely in the postpartum state.

## X. Author Summary (Weinstock)

Is there harm in getting unwarranted tests? Does this "therapeutic radiation" increase patient satisfaction? (I had a great doctor—he was really concerned—ordered tons of tests!)
Our patient's CT may have harmed her in another way; forget the radiation, the brain CT wasn't falsely negative, it was falsely reassuring.
Let's try and follow the thought process of the initial EP who ordered the scan. He has a patient with a severe headache and CT seems a logical choice—it's a headache, let's image the head—but what was he looking for?

1. Brain cancer—This would be a bizarre coincidence in a postpartum woman with less than a week of headaches and no neurological symptoms. Has it happened in the history of the world? Yes. Was it happening here? No.
2. Subarachnoid hemorrhage—With around a week of symptoms, sensitivity of CT is just over 50%; if this life threatening diagnosis was a legitimate concern, an LP should have followed.
3. Meningitis—Well … would need some awfully good resolution.
4. Carbon monoxide toxicity, acute angle closure glaucoma, pseudotumor cerebri, temporal arteritis, carotid artery dissection, cerebral venous thrombosis—if these serious entities are seriously considered—a brain CT is not the test.

Was this radiation therapeutic or misleading? Did it help the patient—did it help the doctor? You be the judge …

This case strikes to the heart of the EM encounter; how do we find bad disease in the routine complaint? As our contributing authors point out, there were more than several elements of this ED visit which were not routine, including the severity of the headache, the increased blood pressure and the "special-population" patient, a woman eight days postpartum. Headaches are usually nothing. But as EM physicians, we will see 150–200,000 patients over the course of our careers ... playing the odds is not good enough.

## References


1. Cashman EC, Smyth D. Primary headache syndromes and sinus headache: An approach to diagnosis and management. Auris Nasus Larynx 2012;39(3):257-60. doi:10.1016/j.anl.2011.05.003
2. Bukhari S, Fatima S, Barakat AF, et al. Venous thromboembolism during pregnancy and postpartum period. Eur J Intern Med 2022;97:8-17. doi:10.1016/j.ejim.2021.12.013
3. Honigberg MC, Givertz MM. Peripartum cardiomyopathy. BMJ 2019;364:k5287. doi:10.1136/bmj.k5287
4. Wheaton N, Al-Abdullah A, Haertlein T. Late pregnancy and postpartum emergencies. Emerg Med Clin North Am 2019;37(2):277-286. doi:10.1016/j.emc.2019.01.013
5. Orlandi RR, Kingdom TT, Smith TL, et al. International consensus statement on allergy and rhinology: Rhinosinusitis 2021. Int Forum Allergy Rhinol 2021;11(3):213-739. doi:10.1002/alr.22741
6. Kim R, Patel ZM. Sinus headache: Differential diagnosis and an evidence-based approach. Otolaryngol Clin North Am 2020;53(5):897-904. doi:10.1016/j.otc.2020.05.019
7. Quality ID #333: Adult sinusitis: Computerized tomography (CT) for acute sinusitis (Overuse). Updated Nov 2019. Accessed 7/5/2023, 2023. https://qpp.cms.gov/docs/QPP_quality_measure_specifications/CQM-Measures/2020_Measure_333_MIPSCQM.pdf
8. Rosenfeld RM, Piccirillo JF, Chandrasekhar SS, et al. Clinical practice guideline (Update): Adult sinusitis. Otolaryngol Head Neck Surg2015;152(S2):S1-S39. doi:10.1177/0194599815572097
9. Guidelines-Obstetrics ACoCP. Headaches in pregnancy and postpartum: ACOG clinical practice guideline No. 3. Obstet Gynecol 2022;139(5):944-72. doi:10.1097/AOG.0000000000004766
10. Saccò M, Meschi M, Regolisti G, et al. The relationship between blood pressure and pain. J Clin Hypertens 2013;15(8):600-05. doi:10.1111/jch.12145
11. Tanabe P, Persell SD, Adams JG, et al. Increased blood pressure in the emergency department: Pain, anxiety, or undiagnosed hypertension? Ann Emerg Med 2008;51(3):221-9. doi:10.1016/j.annemergmed.2007.10.017
12. Gestational hypertension and preeclampsia: ACOG practice bulletin summary, number 222. Obstet Gynecol 2020;135(6):1492-95. doi:10.1097/AOG.0000000000003892
13. Croskerry, P. Achieving quality in clinical decision making: Cognitive strategies and detection of bias. Acad Emerg Med 2002;9(11):1184-204.
14. Yancey LM, Withers E, Bakes K, et al. Postpartum preeclampsia: Emergency department presentation and management. J Emerg Med 2011;40(4):380-4. doi:10.1016/j.jemermed.2008.02.056
15. Chames MC, Livingston JC, Ivester TS, et al. Late postpartum eclampsia: A preventable disease? Am J Obstet Gynecol 2002;186(6):1174-7. doi:10.1067/mob.2002.123824
16. Lubarsky SL, Barton JR, Friedman SA, et al. Late postpartum eclampsia revisited. Obstet Gynecol 1994;83(4):502-5. doi:10.1097/00006250-199404000-00003
17. Sattar A, Manousakis G, Jensen MB. Systematic review of reversible cerebral vasoconstriction syndrome. Expert Rev Cardiovasc Ther 2010;8(10):1417-21. doi:10.1586/erc.10.124
18. Mayama M, Uno K, Tano S, et al. Incidence of posterior reversible encephalopathy syndrome

in eclamptic and patients with preeclampsia with neurologic symptoms. Am J Obstet Gynecol 2016;215(2):239.e1-5. doi:10.1016/j.ajog.2016.02.039
19. Hadhiah KM, Alshagawi ZA, Alzahrani SK, et al. Reversible cerebral vasoconstriction syndrome in a background of eclampsia responding to milrinone infusion. Am J Case Rep 2021;22:e934528. doi:10.12659/AJCR.934528
20. Neudecker S, Stock K, Krasnianski M. Call-Fleming postpartum angiopathy in the puerperium: A reversible cerebral vasoconstriction syndrome. Obstet Gynecol 2006;107(2 Pt 2):446-9. doi:10.1097/01.AOG.0000187945.61146.e6
21. Calabrese LH, Dodick DW, Schwedt TJ, et al. Narrative review: Reversible cerebral vasoconstriction syndromes. Ann Intern Med 2007;146(1):34-44. doi:10.7326/0003-4819-146-1-200701020-00007
22. Pop A, Carbonnel M, Wang A, et al. Posterior reversible encephalopathy syndrome associated with reversible cerebral vasoconstriction syndrome in a patient presenting with postpartum eclampsia: A case report. J Gynecol Obstet Hum Reprod 2019;48(6):431-34. doi:10.1016/j.jogoh.2019.03.019

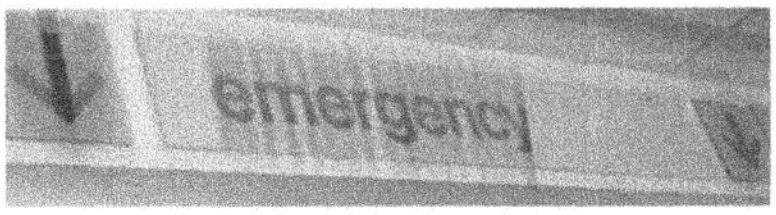


# Case 7

## A 42 Year-old Woman with Shortness of Breath: How Wide Should We Cast the Differential?

**Primary case author:**
**Matthew DeLaney**

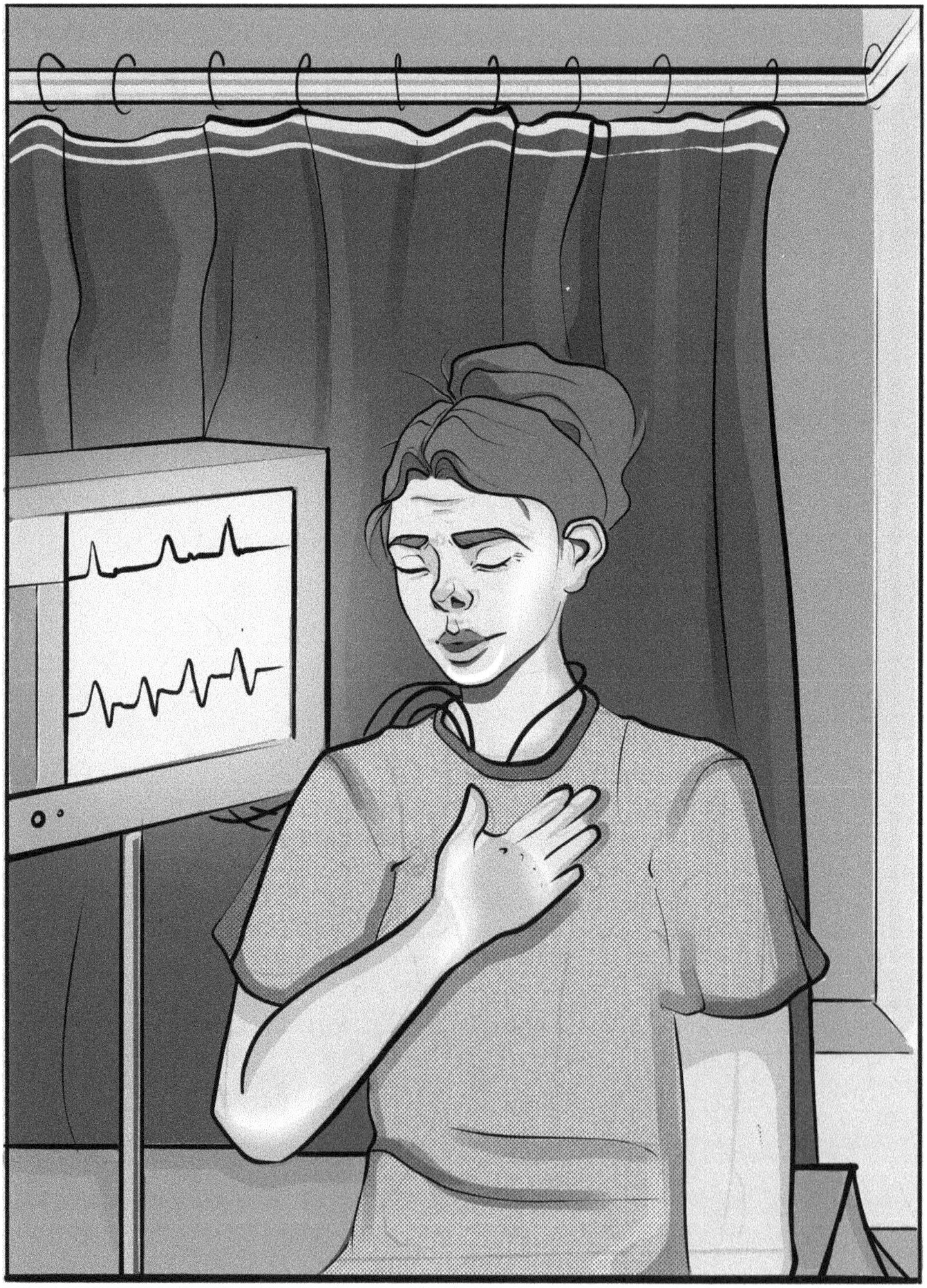

# Case 7

## A 42 Year-old Woman with Shortness of Breath: How Wide Should We Cast the Differential?

Shortness of breath (SOB) is a common complaint but unlike chest pain where we have a defined number of diagnoses to rule out in the ED. Many group this into the "Big 3" of acute coronary syndrome (ACS), pulmonary embolism (PE), and thoracic aortic dissection (TAD) and the "Second 3" of cardiac tamponade, tension pneumothorax and esophageal rupture. The differential of SOB is broad ranging from causes from airway, pulmonary, cardiac, systemic, or neuro/psychiatric. How do we distinguish between a respiratory process such as a URI or pneumonia compared to more serious pathology?

***Deep thoughts:***

1. *How do we balance the risk of misdiagnosis with the risk of over testing and false positive results?*
2. *Could myocardial ischemia or pulmonary embolism have been excluded at the bedside?*
3. *What is the legal exposure of the emergency physician when an outcome occurs more than a week after the ED visit?*

**PART 1—MEDICAL**

## I. The Patient's Story

On April 26th, Barbara Noon presented to an outpatient Medical Office with complaints of pelvic pain and pain in the bilateral legs. She weighed 170 pounds and was 5 foot and 3 inches tall. It was noted that her pulse rate was 104 beats per minute. She was evaluated by the primary care physician, Dr Roger Shiland, with a negative examination of the lower legs, no signs of trauma or cellulitis, and prescribed a NSAID and asked her to return in one month.

Instead, she returned just 3 days later on April 29th with complaints of shortness of breath, cough and dizziness for two days. At this time her pulse was 100 beats per minute. She was evaluated by Dr. Wolff, who noted that she had a heavy period with a history of fibroids and anemia, including a hemoglobin of 10 G/DL from the previous visit. He noted no complaints of chest pains, headaches or palpitations. Her physical examination was reported to be within normal limits. He diagnosed anemia secondary to uterine fibroids as a cause of the dyspnea and dizziness. Her prescription for iron was increased and she was referred to the emergency department (ED) for further evaluation of her dyspnea.

The next day she presented to the emergency department (ED) [a different hospital than below] for what is described in the chart as "exertional shortness of breath for four days." A chest X-ray and electrocardiogram were done and read as negative. Blood tests were unrevealing. She was discharged home with a diagnosis of anxiety and bronchitis. She was still taking Naprosyn for pain.

On May 4th, she returned to the outpatient medical office and again saw Dr. Wolff (the second primary care doctor she had seen). She continued to complain of mild shortness of breath and wheezing. Her pulse rate at this time was 114 beats per minute. The physical examination was reportedly within normal limits. Another electrocardiogram was done which showed sinus tachycardia. Dr. Wolff's note indicates his impression that her dyspnea was most likely secondary to recent bronchitis/pneumonia. He advised to continue antibiotics. A nebulizer treatment was given, reportedly with good results. She was given prescriptions for pulmonary function testing and an echocardiogram. His note indicates his impression that decedent's tachycardia was due to multiple factors, including pneumonia and anxiety. She was reportedly referred to a cardiologist and prescribed a low dose beta blocker for her tachycardia.

Two days later she was back in the ED.

## II. The Doctor's Version (the following is the actual documentation of the provider)

**Chief Compliant: May 6th (13:02):** "Difficulty breathing"
**Triage (nurse):** Patient arrived from home. Patient arrived ambulatory via private auto accompanied by immediate family member to the ED's external triage
**Chief Complaint quote (nurse):** sob x 1 week, with coughing. The patient complains of a mild cough that began gradually I week(s) ago. The symptoms have worsened in the last 1 day(s). The cough is non-productive. It has been associated with fever and difficulty breathing. patient was seen by private doctor on [May 3rd] for sob, told to come to er

**History of Present Illness (physician): (15:20)** 42 Fem denies any past medical history p/w [presents with] worsening SOB for the last 1 week. As per patient for the first few days she saw a PMD ordered a PFT and prn albuterol. After a few days patient had worsening SOB even at rest, no cough, subjective fevers, generalized malaise, and body pains. No sick contact, no travel history
ROS: +fever/chills. No arthralgias/myalgias, vomiting, chest pain, diaphoresis, hemoptysis, syncope, ankle edema, unexplained weight change. Patient has uterine fibroma
NKDA
PMH: Neg
PSH: Neg
Meds: Proventil puffs PRN

Vital Signs

| Time | Temp(F) | Rt. | Pulse | Resp | Syst | Diast | Pos | $O_2$ Sat |
|---|---|---|---|---|---|---|---|---|
| 13:06 | 98.4 | 0 | 108 | 24 | 117 | 80 | S | 94 |
| 14:27 | | | 100 | 22 | | | | 97 |
| 15:33 | 100.5 | 0 | 86 | 20 | 121 | 81 | L | 95% NC2L |
| 20:00 | 97.8 | 0 | 108 | 20 | 134 | 58 | L | 95 |

**Physical Examination (15:30):**
**Constitutional:** mild distress, speaks in phrases, oriented, can lie flat, tachypneic
**Eye:** Pupils are equal and reactive to light. Extraocular muscles are intact
**Hent/Neck:** Normal pharynx; mucous membranes pink/moist; no erythema; neck supple
**Cardiac:** Regular rate and rhythm; normal S 1, S2: no murmurs, rubs, or gallops

**Resp/Chest:** good airway, clear lungs, use abdominal muscles to breath
**GI/Abdominal:** + BS, soft, non-tender, slightly enlarged abdomen

**Orders:**
**13:26:**
Albuterol Inhalation 2.5 mg
Atrovent HFA Inhalation 0.5 mg
Biaxin Oral 500 MG
**17:50:**
Ceftriaxone 1 gm
Normal Saline (0.9%) Intravenous 1 liter

**Attending Assessment and Plan (15:52):** 42 female complaining of shortness of breath for the past three days; worse today. Fluids, CXR, labs, observe. May need admit if she does not look better

**Results:**

| Test | Flag | Value | Units | Ref. Range |
|---|---|---|---|---|
| WBC: | H | 11.2 | K/mcL | 4.5 – 11.0 |
| Hgb: | L | 10.9 | (g/dl ) | 12.0 – 16.0 |
| Plt: | | 265 | (K/mcL) | 130 – 400 |
| | | | | |
| Sodium: | | 140 | (mEq/L) | 136 – 152 |
| Potassium: | | 3.7 | (mEq/L) | 3.5 – 5.3 |
| Chloride: | | 104 | (mEq/L) | 98 – 112 |
| BUN: | | 10 | (mg/dl) | 8 – 22 |
| Creatinine: | | 0.8 | (mg/dl) | 0.4 – 1.6 |
| $CO_2$ Content: | | 24 | (mmol/L) | 23 – 32 |
| Glucose: | | 114 | (mg/dl) | 70 – 110 |
| | | | | |
| Alk Phos: | | 65 | U/L | 30 – 115 |
| ALT (SGPT): | | 21 | U/L | 2 – 50 |
| AST (SGOT): | | 23 | (U/L) | 2 – 40 |
| Calcium: | | 9.1 | (mg/dl) | 8.5 – 10.5 |
| T Protein: | | 6.5 | (g/dl) | 6.5 – 8.5 |
| Albumin: | | 3.3 | (g/dl) | |
| T Bili: | | 0.6 | (mg/dl) | 0.0 – 1.5 |

**CXR Radiology Report:** Faint infiltrate, probably pneumonia, is seen in the left upper lobe. There is no pneumothorax. The costophrenic angles are clear and the contour of the heart is normal
**IMP:** 1. PNEUMONIA, LEFT UPPER LOBE

**Progress Notes:**
**17:58:** pneumonia—antibiotics given at triage. Will not draw blood cultures until patient on inpatient service
**21:40:** Patient has improvement of her symptom and VS after IV hydration and antibiotic treatment. Will discharge with Biaxin and follow up with OPD. Patient is ready to go home

**Diagnosis:**
Shortness of breath (SOB)
Pneumonia

**Disposition (21:48):**
Disposition is discharged. Follow-up: pt will f/u w/ pmd
General Discharge Instructions – Spanish
Rx Biaxin

## III. Risk Management/Patient Safety Opportunities (Weinstock)

**Author comments (Weinstock):** Try and remove your perspective of this case being presented in a Bouncebacks! book (yeah, something bad happened…) and consider that this is a patient you are seeing in the middle of a busy shift. She has SOB, fever, myalgias, perhaps a cough (nurse says yes and doctor says no), and an XR "confirming" an infiltrate (an "infiltrate" or pneumonia); sounds like an infectious process. The care was pretty well done. Later the legal system will figure out if it met standard of care. However, was there an opportunity to widen the differential or to gather data which would have helped us to suspect the actual diagnosis? You be the judge…

**Risk Management/Patient Safety Opportunity #1:**

**Opportunity:** Correlation between nurse chief complaint and physician chief complaint/HPI.
**Discussion:** This is a constant theme in med mal cases. Though, in this case, probably not the sine qua non which would have helped make the diagnosis, it is curious that the nurse gives a pretty detailed description of a cough, but the physician simply says there is no cough.

Nurse: Documentation of the severity (mild), the onset (gradually), the duration (1 week), that is worsened the last 1 day, and that it is associated with fever and difficulty breathing.

Physician: No cough

As physicians/PAs/NPs, how do we reconcile a statement in the nursing note that we don't find to be the case in our data gathering (H&P)? The answer is by simply acknowledging that it was present in the nursing notes and that we addressed it in our own patient encounter. An example could be:

Made-up example: *"I read the nurse notes and asked the patient about presence of cough and she confirmed that she had a cough a few days ago, but it is no longer present and has not coughed in 48 hours."*

Though the lack of cough in this patient is unlikely (the nurse's description of cough is so detailed that it is probably what was occurring), the "made-up" example above is one way that a discrepancy could be addressed in our documentation.

✔ **Teaching point:** Make sure all nurse/triage chief complaints and discrepancies are addressed.

**Risk Management/Patient Safety Opportunity #2:**

**Opportunity:** Expanded HPI and Ddx.
**Discussion:** Though this history was fairly well done, diving deeper, there are some other aspects which might have been helpful to expand upon. What do we know about the SOB? We know the duration (1 week), previous therapy (albuterol), that it is worse, and it is present at rest. We also know that the primary care doctor ordered pulmonary function testing (PFT). In the context of the second part of the HPI which confirms subjective fevers, malaise and body pains, this certainly seems infectious. But would

an expanded history as to the onset (sudden vs. gradual), response to therapy (did the albuterol make it better?), orthopnea, or paroxysmal nocturnal dyspnea, helped to expand or contract the Ddx? As a thought exercise, let's consider some items on the Ddx for SOB:

- *Heart failure?* Seems unlikely as there is no history of heart disease and no ankle edema or weight changes. It might have been good to know about orthopnea, but even if present could be accounted for by the likely infectious process.
- *Acute coronary syndrome (ACS)?* Also unlikely, but this can be a tricky diagnosis. Should we have asked about family history or worsened SOB with exertion? Could an ECG have helped? Perhaps. But the general presentation does not suggest ACS.
- *Reactive airway disease?* Sounds like she has been treated for this in the past with albuterol and is even going to have PFTs performed, but, this patient has no wheezing on exam. This diagnosis seems unlikely.
- *Pulmonary embolism?* An elevated temperature has been described with PE and we don't actually know the patient's understanding of fever. Did she feel warm or actually take her temperature? Was there any history of thromboembolic disease. There was not ankle edema. Was lack of response to previous therapy a reason to test for PE? Without any other symptoms suggestive of PE, this diagnosis also seems unlikely.
- *Atypical infectious process?* Could the SOB be from an atypical infection such as pneumocystis, a fungal process, or tuberculosis? Seems unlikely but a little more detailed history could have been helpful.
- *Systemic process?* When the symptoms don't all fit, consider systemic causes of SOB such as anemia, thyroid abnormalities, even diabetic ketoacidosis; labs were done excluding many of these possibilities.

The data gathering so far is pointing to pneumonia. Were the items above considered? It seems like many of them were. Are there other aspects of the H&P which might have been helpful to hone down or expand this list?

✔ **Teaching point:** The HPI is one of the most important aspects of our data gathering.

**Risk Management/Patient Safety Opportunity #3:**

**Opportunity:** Poor correlation of past history and present complaint.
**Discussion:** It is always a delicate balance between being swayed by a diagnosis momentum from a previous encounter and gathering data from previous visits and testing. Though it was unknown to the clinicians treating the patient at the bedside, she had multiple previous visits to both primary care and to the emergency department. She had at least one documented heart rate of 114 bpm. She had received antibiotics and an albuterol inhaler. But she still presented to the ED on May 6th as her symptoms had not improved. Whereas pneumonia was a viable concern, could another cause of SOB have been occurring?

✔ **Teaching point:** Information from previous visits may be helpful for the current visit.

**Risk Management/Patient Safety Opportunity #4:**

**Opportunity:** Understand the limitations of testing.
**Discussion:** A CT brain scan 2 hours after stroke symptoms will be normal… an XR of the back does not have sufficient sensitivity to exclude a spinal epidural abscess, and a CXR with a "faint infiltrate" does not definitively prove pneumonia. Certainly, in the context of specific symptoms such as fever, cough, and shortness of breath, pneumonia is much more likely, but it is curious that the body of the report reads "faint infiltrate, probably pneumonia" and the impression is much more definitive: "Pneumonia, left upper lobe." The bottom line is that there are other causes of a pulmonary infiltrate in addition to

pneumonia. Following is a snippet of the examination of the defendant physician (a more expanded version follows later in the chapter):

**Q.** Can you have pulmonary infiltrates with pulmonary embolus?
**A.** Yes.

This is in no way proof of malpractice, but more a "caution" that we (the reader) need to correlate findings on imaging in the context of a patient's presentation and refrain from premature diagnostic closure.

✔ **Teaching point:** Understand the limitations of testing.

**Risk Management/Patient Safety Opportunity #5:**

**Opportunity:** Confirm patient's understanding of remaining diagnostic uncertainty.
**Discussion:** Was there "diagnostic uncertainty" remaining when the patient left the ED? Hard to say… but in patients where we have a consideration of other diagnoses, whether appendicitis in a patient with diarrhea or meningitis in a patient with viral symptoms, it is important that a patient understand what we have not ruled out.

✔ **Teaching point:** Our "last opportunity to get it right" is for the patient to return if their symptoms progress, change, or don't resolve.

## IV. The Bounceback

(From the opinion written by the EM plaintiff's expert):
The patient undergoes preoperative testing and then returns on May 19th for a hysterectomy. She was taken to surgery at 4:15 PM and the operation was completed at 7:00 PM. The following is the actual description of what occurred prior to her death.

> "Patient extubated at the end of case and saturation fluctuating 85% to 100%. After extubation patient alert complained of pain, tachypneic and tachycardic. Around 7:12 pm ABG sent, Fentanyl IV given to treat the pain. CXR done and patient moved to the stretcher. Pulmonary/critical care consults and requested ICU bed. Patient with supplemental oxygen and ready to be transferred RR then to ICU. Just after we left OR 4 patient became unresponsive – rush back to room – intubated immediately – right away connected to anesthesia machine with 100% oxygen. Full CPR started. EKG showed bradycardia, ventricular tachycardia and asystole during CPR. Epinephrine, defibrillation and atropine. Accordingly at 8:10 pm CPR stopped and patient pronounced."

**A nurse's note also states the following:**

"Surgery finished skin closed, vital signs maintained. 7:17 pm $O_2$ sat. fluctuated. ABG stat, chest X-ray done stat. Pt. started having labored and shallow breathing. Pt. coded at 7:27 pm. All resuscitation measures taken, CPR given. No responds [sic], pronounced death at 8:10 pm."

**Autopsy:**
**Cause of death:** "pulmonary thromboemboli due to bilateral lower extremity deep venous thrombosis complicating TAH for treatment of uterine leiomyomata." Microscopic examination states: "[h]istologic section of lung as noted above show pulmonary thromboemboli of various ages including those lacking sufficient organization (acute), organizing (subacute) and organized/recanalized (remote)."

**Author comments (Weinstock):** A lawsuit ensued…

## PART 2—LEGAL

**Author comments (Weinstock):** Before deposition and trial, a medical malpractice case starts with opinions of the plaintiff and defense experts. Below is the shortened opinion of the plaintiff's expert with predictable allegations; the PE should have been diagnosed and if it had been, the patient would still be alive. Opinions generally start with the experts' qualifications (I went to the best school ever and I am totally awesome) and with which documents have been reviewed (ED charts, hospital records, autopsy, photos, police/EMS reports, etc.)

Cast of characters (names changed, except where noted):
**The patient:** Barbara Noon
**Primary care doctor #1:** Dr. Shiland
**Primary care doctor #2:** Dr. Wolff
**EM doctor (attending):** Dr. Louis
**Resident EM doctor:** Dr. Chill
**Plaintiff's attorney:** Ms. Jeffries
**Defense attorney:** Ms. Jillian

## I. Opinion of Plaintiff's Expert Witness (shortened)

I am a physician licensed to practice medicine in the State of ____ and am Board Certified in Emergency Medicine and Internal Medicine. I have been the Chairman of [a] Department of Emergency Medicine. I have practiced emergency medicine for [decades] and I am fully familiar with the medical issues presented by this matter. I submit this affirmation in opposition to the motions for summary judgment made by defendant [Hospital]. The opinions set forth herein are all stated with a reasonable degree of medical certainty.

In my opinion, defendant Dr. Wolff [primary care physician who saw the patient at the second primary care visit] was negligent and departed from accepted medical practice in his care of decedent in that he failed to include pulmonary embolism in the differential diagnosis and failed to perform or prescribe diagnostic tests, including D-dimer, chest CT or V/Q scan, to rule out pulmonary embolism during his visits with decedent on April 29th and May 4th. In my opinion, if these tests had been performed, it would have resulted in the diagnosis of pulmonary embolism at that time. Once diagnosed, treatment of her pulmonary embolism at that time would have, with a reasonable of medical certainty, prevented decedent's death.

The basis for my opinion is [are] as follows: Pulmonary embolism (PE) is the obstruction of the pulmonary artery or one of its branches by material (blood clot, tumor, air or fat) that originated elsewhere in the body. Pulmonary embolism is a very common and, if not timely diagnosed and treated, is an often-fatal disease. Mortality can be reduced significantly with prompt diagnosis and appropriate treatment. Anticoagulation is the mainstay of therapy for acute PE and this therapy decreases the mortality rate from approximately 30% to between 2–8%. Other treatment modalities, depending on the patient's condition, include thrombolysis, inferior vena cava filters and embolectomy. And, given Mrs. Noon's presentation to Dr. Wolff's office on April 29th, accepted medical practice required that pulmonary embolism be included in the differential diagnosis. Decedent had several signs, symptoms, complaints and historical features that were consistent with pulmonary embolism. Additionally, she had an immediate past history of complaining of bilateral leg pain [at the previous primary care visit]. The notes from these visits were in the office chart and accepted medical practice required that Dr. Wolff review these prior entries in the chart when evaluating decedent; Dr. Wolff should have been aware of this history. Accepted medical practice required that Dr. Wolff include pulmonary embolism in his differential diagnosis in as much as decedent's complaints of shortness of breath, borderline tachycardia, coupled with the aforementioned history of leg pain, was suspicious for pulmonary embolism. And accepted medical practice required that further testing be performed to rule out PE. The fact that there were allegedly no complaints or findings with regard to decedent's calf/legs on April 30 does not exclude pulmonary embolism as a diagnosis.

In my opinion, the physicians at [the emergency department at the visit May 6th, detailed above] including [the attending emergency physician Dr. Louis and the resident(s)] were negligent and departed from accepted medical practice in failing to include pulmonary embolism in a differential diagnosis and in failing to perform necessary and indicated tests, including D-dimer, spiral CT of the chest, VQ scan or pulmonary angiography, to rule out pulmonary embolism. In my opinion, if these tests had been performed, it would have resulted in the diagnosis of pulmonary embolism. Once diagnosed, treatment of her PE on or about May 6th, would have, with a reasonable of medical certainty, prevented decedent's death. Accordingly, in my opinion, the negligence and malpractice of [the] Hospital was a substantial factor leading to Ms. Noon's death.

*Signed: EM plaintiff's expert witness*

**Author comments (Weinstock):** There are some pretty specific allegations, and the plaintiff has decided that there is a possible case here. They are paying for this "out of pocket" and often they get the opinion of an expert who does not suggest malpractice and decide not to take the case. However, with this situation, they proceed. Following is the deposition of the attending emergency physician, Dr. Louis.

## II. Deposition of EM Attending Physician (Dr. Louis) by the Plaintiff's Attorney (Ms. Jeffries)

My name is Ms. Jeffries. I represent the Plaintiff in this matter. If I ask you a question and you don't understand the way that I'm asking the question, please don't hesitate to tell me so and I'll be happy to try and rephrase it. Should you need a break or anything like that, don't hesitate. The only other thing I would ask is that, since you know the subject matter, you might anticipate the answer to a question that I'm asking, I would just ask that you try and allow me to get the full question out before you give your answer, and that's for the benefit of the court reporter.

**Author comments (Weinstock):** This is a pretty standard way that depositions begin; telling the defendant/witness to respond verbally instead of nodding (court reporter needs to record speech), inquiring about the credentials and training of the defendant/witness, and if this is a hired expert witness (hired by the plaintiff or defense) to ascertain their rates. For the sake of brevity, much of the 123 pages of deposition are condensed for ease of reading. To summarize, this defendant was the attending emergency physician who supervised the residents who saw the patient, was well trained, and was not paid.

**A. Recollection of the patient:**

**Q.** Now, Doctor, do you have any independent recollection of a patient by the name of Barbara Noon?
**A.** I don't have independent recollection of the case.

**Q.** When was the first time, other than the fact that your name is in the chart here — did you review this chart at any other time other than the day that you were in the emergency room or with your attorney?
**Defense attorney.** Objection!! But you can answer.
**A.** I reviewed the chart with my attorney for the purposes of this deposition.

**Q.** Okay. That's all I'm asking you. Is there anything in the chart that refreshes your recollection as to this particular patient, Barbara Noon?
**A.** My recollection is based on the chart.

**Q.** Understood. What I'm asking you is, does it give you a specific recollection, by reading the chart, of this particular [patient], Barbara Noon?
**A.** My only recollection in this case is predicated on what I have reviewed in the chart.

**Q.** Once you read the chart, did you recall this patient?
**A.** My only recollection is from the chart.

**Q.** It still doesn't answer my question. What I'm asking you is, I'm assuming, my assumption is that the name Barbara Noon in and of itself did not remind you of this particular patient; would that be correct?
**Defense attorney.** Objection!! Asked and answered.
**A.** I so apologize, I don't understand.

**Q.** All I'm asking you is, when you were going to be deposed and there was a patient by the name of Barbara Noon, did you know it was this particular patient that was in this particular chart?
**Ms. Jillian.** Objection!! Asked and answered. If you can answer.
**A.** The name means nothing, except that that was the name on the deposition.

**Author comments (Weinstock):** So, let's break this down a bit. To the casual observer, we might think the plaintiff's attorney is having a moment. Why are they asking the same question over and over! Looking more closely, the questions are slightly different, and they don't want anything to come up in trial that was not "discovered" during the depo. This line of questioning also demonstrates the importance of our documentation, as typically occurs with a busy emergency physician, if we don't have an "independent recollection" of the patient (as occurred in this case), what is documented in the chart is all there is to go on. What is the deal with all the objections? And then the advice from the defense attorney: "...but you can answer"? Well, the explanation is fairly simple; the attorney is "saving" these objections for trial and can call on these statements to be thrown out later.

**Author comments (Calvert/medical malpractice defense attorney – see detailed discussion below):** The attorney who is presenting the witness for deposition objects for a few different reasons.

1. The main one is that they view the question as legally flawed (e.g., misstates facts, assumes facts, vague, etc.) and they are preserving the right to bring it to the court's attention. If they do that down the road, the court will issue a ruling on the objection, and if the objection is sustained as being accurate, then the question may be struck from being played to the jury.
2. Specifically, in this case, these exchanges got a little chippy, and I sense that the defense attorney was both protecting her client and also letting the plaintiff's attorney know that she was going to engage her. This can slow down the opponent, distract, and potentially muddy the waters on the questions. It can also coach the witness, which is where the witness is influenced by the speaking objection and adjusts their answers.
3. The attorney taking the deposition can also object. Most frequently it is to the alleged non-responsive answer given by the witness. Sometimes that is accurate, and sometimes the objection is intended to push and pressure the witness. I have seen many witnesses get flustered and concerned with their answers being objected to, which can limit their focus and effectiveness. When I advise my clients prior to deposition and trial, I make it clear that the other side is going to object, and to not worry about it unless we take a break and I say otherwise, or if the judge makes a ruling at trial.

**B. Working with residents:**

**Author comments (Weinstock):** What is the culpability for an attending physician when the resident sees the patient? And does this absolve either of responsibility?

**Q.** Now, did Dr. Chill [EM resident physician] see the patient prior to you seeing the patient?
**A.** Yes.

**Q.** Dr. Chill was a resident?
**A.** Yes.

**Q.** Is Dr. Chill still at the hospital?
**A.** I don't know.

**Q.** Do you have any recollection of speaking to Dr. Chill?
**Ms. Jillian (defense attorney).** Regarding this patient or just ever?
**Ms. Jeffries (plaintiff's attorney).** Of course, regarding the patient, yes.
**Ms. Jillian.** He testified he has no independent recollection, so Objection!!
**Ms. Jeffries.** I can still ask him. I don't know if something is going to refresh it.
**A.** Sorry, I have no independent recollection, aside from what's in the chart.

**Q.** What information was inputted by Dr. Chill?
**A.** May I read?

**Q.** Absolutely. Just give us a page number and a reference; okay?
**A.** So on Page 2, I have a history of present illness, "42 year-old female"—

**Author comments (Weinstock):** Just as the defendant begins to read the resident's HPI, the defense attorney breaks in…

**Ms. Jillian.** Wait just for one second. You want him to read every note that the resident put into this record?
**Ms. Jeffries.** I didn't ask him that.

**Ms. Jillian.** What was the question?
**Ms. Jeffries.** I asked him what was the information that the resident inputted into the record, that's what I asked him. So, if he's telling me that the first thing he sees is the history of present illness, if I understand you correctly; is that correct, Doctor?
**A.** I'm sorry, can you repeat the question?

**Q.** That the first thing from the resident that was inputted was the history of present illness?
**Ms. Jillian.** You don't have to read the note. Just generally, if you can –
**Ms. Jeffries.** I might have him read the note, I don't know.
**Ms. Jillian.** Why would he need to read a note that's typewritten into the record of another doctor? You guys want to depose her anyway, I don't really see the point of him reading in a note of another doctor.
**Ms. Jeffries.** Well, because I might want to put it in there for the reference of other people who are using this deposition. When you have a deposition and you are preparing for trial and you have something that just refers to a point, as opposed to actually the statement, it doesn't make the deposition very helpful. So, in fact, I probably would have him read it.

**Ms. Jillian.** What is your question, Counselor?
**Ms. Jeffries.** I told him. I asked him what the question was. I don't know what you are talking about right now.
**Ms. Jillian.** Objection to the form of the question. If you can answer.

**Q.** Doctor, if you just read the first note in, that's all I'm asking for right now.
**A.** The first part of the note I see from the resident, Dr. Chill, is HPI, a history of present illness.

**Q.** If you would read the initial note.
**A.** "42 year-old female, denies any past medical history. Presenting with worsening shortness of breath for the last one week. As per the patient, for the first few days, she saw a PMD, ordered a PFT and PRN Albuterol. After a few days, patient had worsening shortness of breath, even at rest, no cough, subjective fevers, generalized malaise and body pains. travel history."

**Q.** Do you know if you spoke to her after that; would that be your custom and practice?
**Mr. Brown.** Spoke to who, Dr. Chill or the decedent?
**Ms. Jeffries.** I didn't hear what you said.
**Mr. Brown.** Spoke to who, Dr. Chill or the decedent?
**Ms. Jeffries.** No, Dr. Chill. Sorry.
**A.** My customary practice is the residents see the patient first, present, we discuss, and then I go independently talk to and examine the patient.

**Q.** So when you write this, what you are attesting to is that you actually saw the patient, evaluated the patient, and you agree with the resident's documentation; is that correct?
**A.** That's what I have written here, yes.

**Q.** Now, where it says, "Attending assessment and plan," was this inputted by you?
**A.** Yes.

**Author comments (Weinstock):** What is becoming clear is that the questions from an attorney are certainly different than the questions from an attending or a consultant… in a legal case it seems like every word can be sliced and diced and inspected as to its veracity. It is also becoming clear that a defendant needs coaching before going into a deposition; this is not what we learned in medical school! This physician is not giving the plaintiff any wiggle room.

### C. Correlation between attending and resident:

**Author comments (Weinstock):** Is the standard less for a resident (or a PA or NP) than the emergency physician? Not according to Wegman et al.[1] who reviewed 15 legal cases and 10 law review papers, finding that the standard is that of the treating emergency physician.

**Q.** Well, understood. But given the gestalt of the patient, is there any way of your telling from the chart that you did something or made a determination based upon this particular patient that would have been either your order or your order in conjunction with the resident or something that changed as a result of your evaluation? That's really all I'm trying to determine.
**Ms. Jillian.** Objection!! Asked and answered and to form.
**The Court:** You can answer.

**A.** From what I'm seeing on the chart, the resident's impression and mine was consistent.

**Q.** And what was the impression?
**A.** I'm going to move to my note on Page 9, so I have here a 42 year-old female, complained of shortness of breath for the past three days, worse today. And our plan to take from that point is to get the patient fluids, a chest X-ray, labs and a pregnancy test. And our plan was to observe and see the results of those tests and make further determination.

**Q.** When was the last time that you saw the patient?
**A.** I have a progress note on Page 8 at 17:58 in military time where I did my — right before signing out, we customarily round on the patients we're going to sign out, look at them again, and that's what that note was referring to.

### D. Results of CXR and how this factored into the MDM, diagnosis, and plan:

**Q.** Let's just go to the chest X-ray report.
**A.** Okay, the chest X-ray report, I see. Okay, I'm looking at a chest X-ray report on the bottom of Page 6 and the top of page 7. I'm sorry, is there a question?

**Q.** Yes, I said, I think it said there was a faint infiltrate.
**A.** The radiologist's report?

**Q.** Right. Is that right?
**Ms. Jillian.** Objection! to the form of the question. If you can answer that.
**A.** So the radiologist's report is "a faint infiltrate, probably pneumonia, is seen in the left upper lobe, there is no pneumothorax, the costophrenic angles are clear and the contour of the heart is normal. Impression: Pneumonia, left upper lobe."

**Q.** What is the significance, if any, Doctor, that the radiologist says "probably pneumonia"?
**Ms. Jillian.** What's the significance to him in treating the patient?
**Ms. Jeffries.** Yes, yes.
**A.** So a radiologist's report is based on two parts; they generally report all of the signs they see on an X-ray, and then based on their training, education and experience will make an impression, which is listed on the bottom of the report, that tells you what their feelings of the reading are.

**Q.** Can you have pulmonary infiltrates with pulmonary embolus?
**A.** Yes.

**Q.** Let me ask you this. Did Ms. Noon, Mrs. Noon also have signs and symptoms of pulmonary embolus?
**A.** I'm sorry?

**Q.** Did she have any signs and symptoms of pulmonary embolus?
**A.** You'll have to rephrase the question.

**Q.** I said, did the patient have any signs and symptoms of pulmonary embolus?
**A.** That's the same question.

**Author comments (Weinstock):** Yep, this witness is not giving the plaintiff's attorney any wiggle room…

**Q.** Right. You don't understand the question?
**Ms. Jillian.** He's asking you to rephrase the question.

**Q.** You don't understand the question?
**A.** I don't, I'm sorry.

**Q.** Okay. Let's do it this way. What were the signs and symptoms which she had which gave you the initial diagnosis of pneumonia?

**Author comments (Weinstock):** So now it's getting interesting; the allegation is a missed diagnosis of PE, but we all know that diseases can present in similar fashions, even to the point that fever can be present in BOTH pneumonia and PE. So, how does a clinician's incorrect diagnosis when made with appropriate data-gathering and logical medical decision-making, result in malpractice? Check out the exchange below while asking; was the care reasonable and was the diagnosis reasonable?

**A.** She had shortness of breath, fever, myalgias, she had vital signs of tachycardia, a fever and an oxygen saturation that's slightly below normal, and then she had an X-ray that confirmed that with the reading of pneumonia.

**Q.** So would it be fair to say that shortness of breath is also a sign or symptom of pulmonary embolus?
**A.** Yes.

**Q.** Is fever also a sign or symptom of pulmonary embolus?
**A.** It's not a common sign, but it can present that way.

**Q.** By the way, is 100.5 considered a fever in your institution?
**A.** 100.4 and above is considered a fever.

**Q.** Now, was there tachycardia?
**A.** The patient had vital signs with tachycardia during two of her four vital sign checks.

**Q.** I see three.
**A.** We consider greater than a hundred to be tachycardia.

**Q.** Oh, I see, so the hundred is the cut off, okay. So that's also a sign of pulmonary embolus?
**A.** Pulmonary embolus and pneumonia.

**Q.** And pneumonia, both, right. And the $O_2$ sats of 94, is that also a sign of pulmonary embolus?
**A.** Pulmonary embolus and pneumonia.

**Q.** Now, what's the significance of the fact that her O2 sat was 95 percent when she was on oxygen, two liters by nasal canula?
**A.** The possible significance is that the patient had a lower than normal oxygen saturation by a small amount.

**Q.** But the cut-off criteria has to be below 95 percent to be a sign of pulmonary embolus?
**Ms. Jillian.** Objection!!
**Q.** Usually, is that one of the clinical criteria?
**Ms. Jillian.** Objection! to the form of the question.
**The Court:** If you can answer it.

**A.** 95 percent and below is considered slightly below normal.

**Q.** Right, and a sign of pulmonary embolus or pneumonia right?
**A.** Yes.

**Q.** Now, you said she had myalgias?
**A.** Yes.

**Q.** Where do you see that she had myalgias; where do you get that from?
**A.** I'm looking at Page 2, under Dr. Chill's note, where she states body pain and generalized malaise.

**Q.** Well, the way I read it is, "no cough, subjective fevers, generalized malaise and body pains." So, I'm not sure if that says she has body pains, or it says that she doesn't have body pains. Can you ascertain which one is the correct interpretation?
**Ms. Jillian.** Objection!! What is your question to the doctor?
**Ms. Jeffries.** I'm asking him if that sentence, where it says, "after a few days, patient had worsening shortness of breath, even at rest, no cough, subjective fevers, generalized malaise and body pains," and

all I'm asking him is if that indicates that she did have body pains or she didn't have body pains, if he's clear about that.
**The Witness.** May I answer?
**Ms. Jillian.** Yes, you can answer.
**A.** I'm quite sure what it means is no cough, full stop, and then that the patient did have subjective fevers, generalized malaise and body pains.

**Q.** Okay.
**Ms. Jillian.** Just for the record, I'm going to object, also, to that line of questioning. Because you are asking him to interpret another doctor's note. You, again, are free to depose that witness.

**Ms. Jeffries.** Can I just say something?
**Ms. Jillian.** Of course.

**Ms. Jeffries.** Doctors have to interpret other doctor's notes all the time. That is the way medicine is practiced. So, to make that Objection! really doesn't make a lot of sense, but it's your Objection!!
**Ms. Jillian.** It is.

**Author comments (Weinstock):** OK, a bunch of attorneys arguing, then the witness breaks in with "can I answer?" and goes on to give a logical and most likely correct answer. Makes us proud! But it begs the question; if the wording was a little more precise initially, maybe this exchange didn't have to happen at all?

"After a few days, patient had worsening shortness of breath, even at rest, no cough, subjective fevers, generalized malaise and body pains"

Consider how clear your documentation is and try and avoid run on sentences or sentences where it is not clear if the answer is affirmative or negative. Not a huge point, but could pay dividends where a pneumonia diagnosis, turns out to be a PE.

## E. The WBC count:

**Author comments (Weinstock):** It is curious that there was an exchange about the elevated WBC count. After all, this supports the diagnosis of pneumonia. If it is to show that leukocytosis is consistent with a pneumonia diagnosis, it would be an argument for the defense. If it was to show that the WBC could be elevated in PE, it is bizarre.

**Q.** Now, what was the significance of the findings on the CBC, if any?
**A.** Would you like to know the abnormalities on the CBC?

**Q.** No. I can see them, because, very kindly, your institution tells me what's abnormal in their ranges. So, what I'm asking you is, what's the medical significance of those abnormalities? Not for you to read them to me, okay.
**A.** The patient had a slightly elevated white blood cell count and a slightly elevated seg count are the pertinent things that would stand out on the CBC.

**Q.** Can you also see that in pulmonary embolus?
**A.** It's a nonspecific finding, so yes. In any badness that happens to a patient, they can have a slightly elevated white count.

**Q.** Doctor, what is the significance, if any, that the infiltrate seen on the X-ray is in the left upper lobe?
**A.** I don't see any significance.

**Q.** How would you determine, in looking at an X-ray, if it's a sign of pneumonia or pulmonary embolus?
**A.** So the way we interpret any test and the chest X-ray in particular is we make a judgment based on the patient's presentation whether their signs and symptoms are consistent with an infection like pneumonia. And then, if we see a pneumonia on chest X-ray, that's a confirmation of what we suspected and it fits, it makes sense that a patient we suspected for a pneumonia then has a demonstrable pneumonia.

**Q.** But if those signs and symptoms are also consistent with a pulmonary embolus, how do you make the determination as to what it is; is it based, in part, on the fact that there's a much higher likelihood of the patient having a community-acquired pneumonia, as opposed to a pulmonary embolus?
**A.** So if we're already at the point in the patient's evaluation where the likelihood of pulmonary embolism is so low based on the patient's risk factors, signs and symptoms that that's not in part of the testing spectrum where we would consider it a test, then there would be no reason to look at the chest X-ray from the perspective of is this a pulmonary embolism.

**Q.** Well, let me ask you this, was there any differential diagnosis in this case, other than pneumonia?
**A.** There's always a differential diagnosis.

**Q.** So what is the differential diagnosis in this case?
**A.** From the recollection of the chart, it would include countless things, during our initial mental processing, and then as more and more evidence comes back, you begin to eliminate diagnoses that are below the testing threshold. So, in a patient like this with difficulty breathing, shortness of breath, we consider pulmonary embolism, we consider bronchitis, we consider pneumonia, we consider acute coronary syndrome, we consider air outside of the chest, the lung, like pneumothorax. Then as the tests come back, as we talk to the patient, we're able to keep things in or out, depending on whether there's enough likelihood to continue pursuing them.

**Q.** Well, you didn't do an ECG in this case; right?
**A.** There's no ECG on the chart.

**Q.** So you didn't see that there was any reason to take an ECG to rule out any acute coronary syndrome?
**A.** Patient had no risks, signs or symptoms that would lead us to think she had an acute coronary syndrome.

## F. How clinicians make a decision:

**Author comments (Weinstock):** When do we do a test? The "bird's eye" explanation is that we do a test when the risk of the test is less than the risk of missing the disease. We start with a broad differential on every patient, then gather data (H&P) to decide if we need further testing to rule in or out serious disease. This physician explains it well:

**Q.** When did you rule out pulmonary embolus?
**A.** We never are able to rule out a diagnosis. We get below a threshold where it's worth exposing the patient to the risk of testing.

**Q.** I'm very bad at statistics, so I understand basically what you are saying. But what I want to understand is, then, understanding you never rule anything out 100 percent definitively, when did you make a determination, maybe the better question is, a determination that you didn't need to test any further for pulmonary embolus?
**A.** At the time the resident and I discussed the case and then I independently examined the patient.

**Q.** And that's prior to the chest X-ray?
**A.** Correct.

**Q.** So what was the basis for making the determination that you didn't need to do any further testing to rule out or rule in pulmonary embolus?
**A.** So the patient had nothing in their clinical presentation that would make us go towards a diagnosis of pulmonary embolism.

**Q.** Well, when you say nothing in the clinical presentation, are you including the shortness of breath, the tachycardia, the oxygen saturation?
**A.** Those were all consistent with our initial leading diagnosis, which was an infection of the lungs.

**Q.** Which we have also, I think, discussed that it's also consistent with a pulmonary embolus, those signs?
**A.** Those signs can be. Right. But in a patient who comes with no risk factors, no preceding event, nothing in their presentation that would indicate they would be at risk of pulmonary embolism, we would not consider that to be a diagnosis that's worth the dangerous testing that goes into evaluating a pulmonary embolism.

**Q.** I understand what you are saying.

**Author comments (Weinstock):** Seems like they did a pretty good job of explaining. The plaintiff's attorney "understands" what they are saying... but agrees? Not sure we can go there just yet…

## III. The Verdict

This case went through depositions and then to trial.

The trial was going "very well," according to one of the participants and the attorneys, when an offer was made for settlement which was "substantially lower" than the threshold of the insurance company would have been expected to accept. Later the defense attorneys did an exit poll of the jury and every one said they would have voted for the defense.

## IV. The Legal Analysis

**T. Marc Calvert, JD**
Medical malpractice defense attorney with over 35 years of experience
Calvert, Leever & Ostler
Cypress, Texas

1. **If the patient recalls something different than the emergency clinician's documentation, which takes precedence in a legal action?**

As one can imagine, a patient remembering details which are different than the information contained in the medical records is not unusual; in fact, this is a given.

Which takes precedence? There are multiple considerations at play. First, unless there is a reasonable basis for doubting the contents of the record (e.g., there are confirmed errors or omissions in the record, there are indications of alterations, the clinician's record differs from the documentation of other staff such as nursing or social work), the written record should prevail. It was created at or near the time of the events, and there is a justifiable presumption that it is accurate unless shown otherwise.

A rule in law known as the "Best Evidence Rule" contemplates that the original of a document is preferred to a copy; the recordings which are memorialized in a medical chart (with and automatic date and time stamp) are the best evidence to what happened, until proven otherwise.

Second, it is common sense to appreciate that human memory is fallible, especially when a person is under duress or in pain. This often becomes quite visible during cross-examination. How can a patient accurately remember details of many hours in an ED when they have pain, fear, and have taken medications?

Finally, when someone has something to gain in their recitation of what happened, memory often seems to fit neatly with the theories of the claim, but this goes for both the plaintiff and the defendant. This pattern of inconsistency can be pointed out at various points in the trial, including closing argument. When money is being sought, it seems to greatly impact memory! But all things being equal, records trump memory. This is another reason for the records to be written well and contain what is important.

2. **What happens if there is a discrepancy between the documentation of the attending physician and the nurse or resident?**

When an attending physician has documentation which differs from another healthcare provider, such as a resident or a nurse, it can create issues. The ideal, of course, is for them to be similar in key areas of content; the next best thing is that the note made by the attending can address any differences. This could be done either directly (such as in the excellent made-up example by Dr. Weinstock above), by referring to the other note and clarifying, or by indirectly covering it with what is clearly a higher level of care entry. More focused, more robust, more experienced, more specific wins the race!

The problem, however, is that the attending note is often skimpier than entries made by others, which can be argued as a reflection of less time spent with and about the patient (though the reason is easy to understand; the clinician may be caring for 1–15 patients at a time). We know that the documentation is only that, information gathering, and care provided at the bedside is often not reflected in the documentation.

However, we should be cautious of actual discrepancies between the physician and the resident; key facts found in one and not the other raise questions. We do not want a circular firing squad between the attending and the resident, the primary care and the specialist, the nurse and the clinician. It is best when the story is consistent between providers. In a lawsuit, sometimes the approach is to refer to the documentation and studies ordered which support the attending, as well as confirming the attending's superior experience and judgment. If done carefully, the entries can be explained and often reconciled.

**Author comments (Weinstock):** OK. So, how about some specifics? At risk of redundancy, it is inevitable that it will occur, BUT the clinicians documentation should acknowledge that they have read the other documentation (for example the nurse triage note) and they have confirmed that their data gathering is accurate ("I have confirmed twice with the patient that their chest pressure is constant and has not resolved at all over last 4 hours"—or—"I addressed the 'sudden onset' of headache as documented by the triage nurse and spoke with the patient and they told me the headache started at 4:00 this afternoon and reached maximum intensity at 5:00." ). This specific approach to documentation is most reliable and believable and accurate.

**3. We all know the CXR cannot rule out PE, but it did suggest pneumonia – how does this play out at trial?**

The chest X-ray suggesting pneumonia appears to be the key crossroads to this case. The tug of war has been well described, and there are obvious arguments for both sides. For the doctor, a diagnosis of pneumonia fits with the clinical picture and the chest X-ray bolsters the argument for a pneumonia diagnosis. Further, pneumonia is the more common condition. This puzzle only comes together with the benefit of hindsight, which is inherently unfair.

For the patient's case, Dr. Delaney makes the point that the number of prior visits should have prompted a pause. Intercepting a bias from a repetitive diagnosis should be entertained with the occurrence of bouncebacks, the plaintiff's attorney will argue. This leads to the argument that the chest X-ray merely fed the diagnosis momentum, and what was really needed was testing to evaluate for a PE. The question will be: what is the downside to double checking and assessing for a condition which can suddenly kill? The response is that it is not standard of care to pursue testing which is not clinically indicated. How a jury will react to this penultimate debate is the rub!

**4. The WBC count: The WBC count can be elevated from pain/stress, steroids (prednisone), or can simply be a normal variation; a minimal elevation does not prove infection. How are unaddressed abnormal results used at trial?**

The sad truth is that any abnormal result can be used at trial to feed a story. The plaintiff's attorney wants to show that there was a lack of ordinary care provided by the defendant, and they will pounce on any abnormal results as clues that were ignored. The amount of emphasis will depend on the significance of the abnormal result. The argument can even be amplified to show that other aspects of the evaluation were not done in a complete or appropriate manner in order to show a pattern of substandard care. The abnormal and unaddressed WBC count helps add to the stack of evidence. The plaintiff will want to show that this "alarm bell" was ringing and ignored (i.e., not even addressed in an MDM note).

Countering this plaintiff tactic can be difficult. A note at the time which places the abnormal result in context is helpful, and so is moving to explaining the context and the big picture. If everything is an emergency, then nothing is an emergency. Showing a reasonable thought process as to why testing for a PE was not required is key.

At trial, stout expert support, helpful literature, and the defendant coming across as caring and competent are pivotal weapons to untangle the opponent's story of substandard care.

**5. Would you take this case for the defense and how would you defend it? What are the biggest weaknesses?**

I have great empathy for those in the trenches, who are trying their reasonable best. I would defend this case with that theme in mind. We are talking about human beings, imperfect but smart and talented and capable. Doctors take on the hard challenges and they want the best for their patients, and this doctor was trying hard. But medical problems do not play fair; they hide, they mimic, they deceive. I would argue at trial that this doctor's care met the standard of care, and it was reasonable to think horses when the hoofbeats were heard.

At trial, it is imperative that the doctor ooze caring and competence. I cannot say it enough. Reasonable explanations must be given, and the concern about the patient's repetitive visits can be countered with, "Pneumonia was the most likely diagnosis." Hindsight bias drives us to suspect a result that was not known when the care was provided.

The biggest weakness of this case is failure to assess for PE; it must be addressed directly by the defendant and the experts for the defense. Humility and empathy must be shown. A jury who sees a doctor distressed over these events, perhaps to showing visible emotion, is likely to view the doctor in a much better light than one who is callous and has a "you win some, you lose some" attitude.

## V. Medical Discussion—Evaluation of Shortness of Breath and Diagnosis of Pulmonary Embolism (PE)

**Matthew DeLaney MD, FACEP, FAAEM**
Associate Professor Department of Emergency Medicine
University of Alabama at Birmingham
Host of the podcast ERCast

Over the past several years I have been asked to review malpractice cases for both the plaintiff and the defense. It's become clear that most of these cases involve recurrent themes, which are also present in this case. Ultimately, the key issue is the failure to consider that a pulmonary embolism could be the cause of the patient's shortness of breath (SOB). Beyond this simple allegation of failure to consider, we have issues of possible diagnosis momentum in a patient who starts out with one diagnosis that seems to stick with her throughout her subsequent visits. Unfortunately, these issues merge and result in a bad outcome for everyone involved with the case.

**Failure to consider:**

The major issue here seems to be the failure to consider the diagnosis of pulmonary embolism (PE). While the vast majority of patients who present with SOB will not have an underlying clot, the incidence of PE is high enough that it must be on the differential. Freund et al. reported that the incidence of PE was 60 to 120 cases per 100,000 people/year noting that multiple studies have seen an increase in the overall incidence over the past decade.[2] While the strongest risk factors are (all with odds ratio > 10):

- fracture,
- hospitalization for heart failure or Afib (within the previous 3 months),
- hip/knee replacement,
- major trauma,

- myocardial infarction (within 3 months),
- previous venous thromboembolic event and
- spinal cord injury[3]

Per the International Cooperative Pulmonary Embolism Registry (ICOPER), 19% of patients will not have any notable risk factors.[4]

**Diagnosis momentum:**

This case suffers from diagnostic momentum[5] gone wrong! What starts as a fairly routine visit to the primary care office continues across four more interactions with the healthcare system including two emergency department (ED) visits before the patient's untimely demise. On the patient's initial visit, she does not report SOB but has lower extremity pain and is noted to be tachycardic. While this visit is otherwise unremarkable, it is notable that she returns 3 days later complaining of SOB, cough, and dizziness; on that visit her heart rate is 100 bpm. Her symptoms are attributed to anemia secondary to uterine fibroids and suggests she go to the ED. She presented to the ED a day later with "exertional shortness of breath for four days" which raises the question of whether she has been experiencing SOB preceding her initial visit to the primary care doctor. During this initial ED visit she has a chest X-ray and ECG, both negative, and blood tests which are unrevealing. She is diagnosed with "anxiety and bronchitis."

This is the point where the case gets significantly off track. It's just days later when she returns to the primary care office still complaining of SOB and wheezing where she is noted to be tachycardic. On this second visit to primary care, her dyspnea is attributed to her recent diagnosis of bronchitis/pneumonia. Interestingly, she receives prescriptions for pulmonary function testing, an echocardiogram, and beta-blockers for tachycardia, which raises the question as to how confident the primary care doctor was in their diagnosis.

We see the diagnostic momentum continue to pick up speed as she visits the ED again two days later (the visit which is the focus of this chapter); at this point she is complaining of SOB and is noted to be tachycardic with an oxygen saturation of 94%. An X-ray showed a faint infiltrate in the left lower lobe and after getting antibiotics and IV fluids she is discharged with Clarithromycin and a diagnosis of "shortness of breath and pneumonia."

It seems that there remained some degree of diagnostic uncertainty; making it natural to anchor onto a prior diagnosis. When she returns to the primary care doctor for a visit on May 4 she is given a nebulizer treatment for presumed bronchitis and is reported to have good results, this certainly muddies the water as we would not expect a pulmonary embolism to respond to nebulizers.

**Limitations of testing:**

Though in a patient with shortness of breath and an infiltrate, the most likely diagnosis arguably is pneumonia, there are certainly other causes including scarring, atelectasis, and PE; in fact the ICOPER registry found that 23% of patients with PE had an infiltrate on the CXR (other findings on CXR included cardiac enlargement (36%), effusion (30%), and atelectasis (24%)).[4] When a finding such as an infiltrate is seen on the CXR, consideration for correlation with the clinical picture is important; is there fever, productive cough, myalgias, or exposure to ill persons? In our patient, though there was no cough, there was a history of fever as well as a documented temperature in the ED of 100.5 degrees. Though not discussed specifically in the medical decision-making (MDM) note, this was likely confirmation that the shortness of breath was from a pneumonia – this was a tough case!

**Approach when a patient returns with ongoing symptoms:**

There are two approaches when a patient shows up with ongoing symptoms that are attributed to an existing diagnosis. First is the approach taken in this case; look for evidence to confirm the previous diagnosis. A second, and more helpful approach, is to pause and consider unexplored causes of the patient's symptoms. In this case it was initially reasonable to assume that the patient had bronchitis or pneumonia, but at some point, alternative diagnoses should have been considered, especially with a patient who seeks medical care on five separate occasions!

**The work-up:**

Working up SOB in the ED remains challenging as we see a large number of patients with signs and symptoms that could potentially be due to an underlying clot. Over the past two decades we have seen the development and validation of various tools and risk stratification systems for patients with a potential PE. Yet, this diagnosis is still missed initially in up to 20% of ED patients.[6] Despite the widespread prevalence of PE worldwide there seems to be substantial variation in the evaluation. Germini, et al. reported that in Europe ~25% of patients who were worked up for a potential PE had a positive diagnosis compared to only 8% of patients in the US. The authors suggest that these differences may be a result of differing thresholds regarding initiating an evaluation, rather than being due to using different diagnostic approaches.[7] In this case, as with other missed PEs, the key diagnostic error comes from failing to consider the diagnosis.

Ultimately, this is a tragic case where despite numerous interactions with the healthcare system the patient had a catastrophic outcome and we are left with numerous unknowns. Retrospectively, we have no idea if a D-dimer would have been helpful or for that matter if a CT angio would have given us an accurate and actionable answer that would have led to a different outcome. What does seem to be clear is that when once the diagnostic momentum began to pick up speed, the differential began to shrink and a common yet deadly condition remained undiagnosed. While it can be difficult to stop this speeding train, when we are faced with a patient who bounces back, we need to at least pump the brakes and think "What could we be missing?"

**Risk management pitfalls:**

There are several other common themes seen in malpractice cases. One of the glaring issues is the bounceback.[8,9,10] We have a 42 year-old female who over the course of less than two weeks has five interactions with the healthcare system. I am reminded of a quote that is often attributed to Greg Henry: "If somebody shows up in the ED more than three times, they are getting admitted, even if it is the pizza delivery driver!" While this may overstate the risk posed by bouncebacks, it does remind us that we should have a heightened level of concern.

In this case we see a glimmer of consideration during the second ED visit where the doctor documents, "May need to admit if she does not look better," but ultimately she is discharged. There are clearly situations where patients may inappropriately visit the ED repeatedly, but in this case we have an otherwise reasonable young patient who was not improving. While there is no reason to doubt the intentions of the teams that treated her, a plaintiff's lawyer would be quick to point out that the patient "Gave you five chances to get the diagnosis right." If she is discharged, documentation should state why alternative diagnoses are not thought to be occurring, and why the clinician feels discharge is safe.

The other big theme is the failure to consider PE. Moving beyond the specifics of HOW we work up patients with potential clots, is the bigger question of WHEN do we decide to initiate the evaluation.

**Visit #1:** There is no mention of shortness of breath during the patient's initial primary care visit. So, it is reasonable to not consider PE.

**Visit #2:** The primary care physician was correct to think about causes of SOB and ultimately refer the patient to the ED for further evaluation.

**Visit #3:** It is during the index visit to ED where we needed a strong consideration of PE as she was reporting exertional shortness of breath and with a negative work-up; there was not an alternative explanation. Could she have bronchitis and anxiety? Sure! But at this point other causes of SOB, most notably PE, should have been on the differential.

**Visit #4:** On the following primary care visit, the physician seems to put a good bit of thought into the patient's SOB and tachycardia to the point of giving her beta-blockers for tachycardia. Yet, there is no evidence that PE was at any point considered.

**Visit #5:** When she bounces back for a second ED visit she gets what looks like an extensive evaluation. Yet, there is not any clear consideration of possible PE. Did the presence of fever (temp of 100.5 degrees) lead them astray? Though fever is usually infectious, there are other causes of an elevated temperature,[11] including PE.

**Bringing it all together:**

Looking at the case retrospectively can certainly introduce the risk of bias, but in this case the patient has 4 visits where shortness of breath is a prominent feature, but PE is not considered. Not all patients with SOB need a PE evaluation, but given its prevalence and the risk of a missed diagnosis, I would argue that any patient in any setting who reports SOB should at least have PE included in the differential. Even a line in the chart saying, for example, "I considered PE and I think it is unlikely because…" would force us to think about the presence of a possible PE but also would give us some layer of protection from a patient safety and medico legal standpoint.

While this may seem like a wide net to cast, the literature suggests that when we use a structured approach to working up a potential PE, we are actually more accurate than when we rely on our bedside gestalt. In a retrospective analysis of over 1,500 ED patients, Medson et al. found that the "clinical hunch" or gestalt was associated with lower rates of PE diagnosis when compared to the PERC Rule, Wells score, revised Geneva score, and Years criteria.[12] When it comes to making the decision to work up a patient, a common concern is that if we apply clinical decision tools and tests like a D-dimer then we will end up unnecessarily testing a larger number of patients. While this certainly could occur, to date the literature suggests that using a structured approach to patients who could have a PE results in an increased rate of diagnostic accuracy rather than simply causing more downstream testing. Hoo, et al. found that the rate of CT angiograms that were positive for PE increased from ~3% to ~16% after the Well's score and D-dimer were incorporated into the electronic health record suggesting that this structured approach led to more appropriate use testing and imaging.[13]

## VI. Author Summary (Weinstock)

There is ongoing debate in the literature about the nuances of how to work up a potential PE, but as we see in this case, the big risk to both the patient and the clinician comes most often from failure to even consider the diagnosis, rather than a missed diagnosis as a result of using a particular risk stratification system or particular brand of D-dimer.

**Author comments (Weinstock):** I spoke with the physician about changes made as a result of this case. There is now a section in their MDM note which specifically states why they don't think a patient with pneumonia has a PE. This serves an important function; to have them think out of the box as to an atypical presentation of PE. We do this with other documentation, for example, in patients with stroke it is wise to state why thrombolytics are not indicated... (an area of high legal risk). This approach is a good example of the goals of this book: "Using legal outcomes to make patients safer."

## References


1. Wegman B, Stannard JP, Bal BS. Medical liability of the physician in training. Clin Orthop Relat Res 2012;470(5):1379-85. doi: 10.1007/s11999-012-2244-4. PMID: 22278849; PMCID: PMC3314772.
2. Freund Y, Cohen-Aubart F, Bloom B. Acute pulmonary embolism: A review. JAMA 2022;328(13):1336-45. doi: 10.1001/jama.2022.16815. PMID: 36194215.
3. Konstantinides SV, Meyer G, Becattini C, et al. 2019 ESC Guidelines for the diagnosis and management of acute pulmonary embolism developed in collaboration with the European Respiratory Society (ERS). Eur Heart J 2020;41(4):543-603. doi:10.1093/eurheartj/ehz405.
4. Goldhaber SZ, Visani L, De Rosa M. Acute pulmonary embolism: Clinical outcomes in the International Cooperative Pulmonary Embolism Registry (ICOPER). Lancet 1999;353(9162):1386-89. doi:10.1016/s0140-6736(98)07534-5.
5. Croskerry, P. Achieving quality in clinical decision making: Cognitive strategies and detection of bias. Acad Emerg Med 2002;9(11):1184-204.
6. Mansella G, Keil C, Nickel CH, et al. Delayed diagnosis in pulmonary embolism: Frequency, patient characteristics, and outcome. Respiration 2020;99(7):589-97. doi: 10.1159/000508396. Epub 2020 Jul 21. PMID: 32694258.
7. Germini F, Zarabi S, Eventov M, et al. Pulmonary embolism prevalence among emergency department cohorts: A systematic review and meta-analysis by country of study. J Thromb Haemost 2021;19(1):173-85. doi: 10.1111/jth.15124. Epub 2020 Nov 18. PMID: 33048461.
8. Sklar DP, Loeliger E, Edmunds K, et al. Unanticipated death after discharge home from the emergency department. Ann Emerg Med 2007;49(6):735-45.
9. Nunez S, Hexdall A, Aguirre-Jaime A. Unscheduled returns to the emergency department: An outcome of medical errors? Qual Saf Health Care 2006;15(2):102-8.
10. Gabayan GZ, Ash SM, Hsia RY, et al. Factors associated with short-term bounce-back admissions after emergency department discharge. Ann Emerg Med 2013;62(2):136-44.
11. Dutta A, March C, Weinstock M. When a fever is not a URI:If it's not in the differential, it won't be in the diagnosis. J Urgent Care Med 2022;17(2):13-16.
12. Medson K, Yu J, Liwenborg L, Lindholm P, et al. Comparing "clinical hunch" against clinical decision support systems (PERC rule, wells score, revised Geneva score and YEARS criteria) in the diagnosis of acute pulmonary embolism. BMC Pulm Med 2022;22(1):432. doi: 10.1186/s12890-022-

02242-1. PMID: 36414971; PMCID: PMC9682736.

13. Hoo GW, Wu CC, Vazirani S, et al. Does a clinical decision rule using D-dimer level improve the yield of pulmonary CT angiography? AJR Am J Roentgenol 2011;196(5):1059-64. doi: 10.2214/AJR.10.4200. PMID: 21512071.

# Case 8

## A 15 Year-old Girl with RLQ Abdominal Pain: It *is* an Appy ... Right?

**Primary case author:**
**David A. Talan**

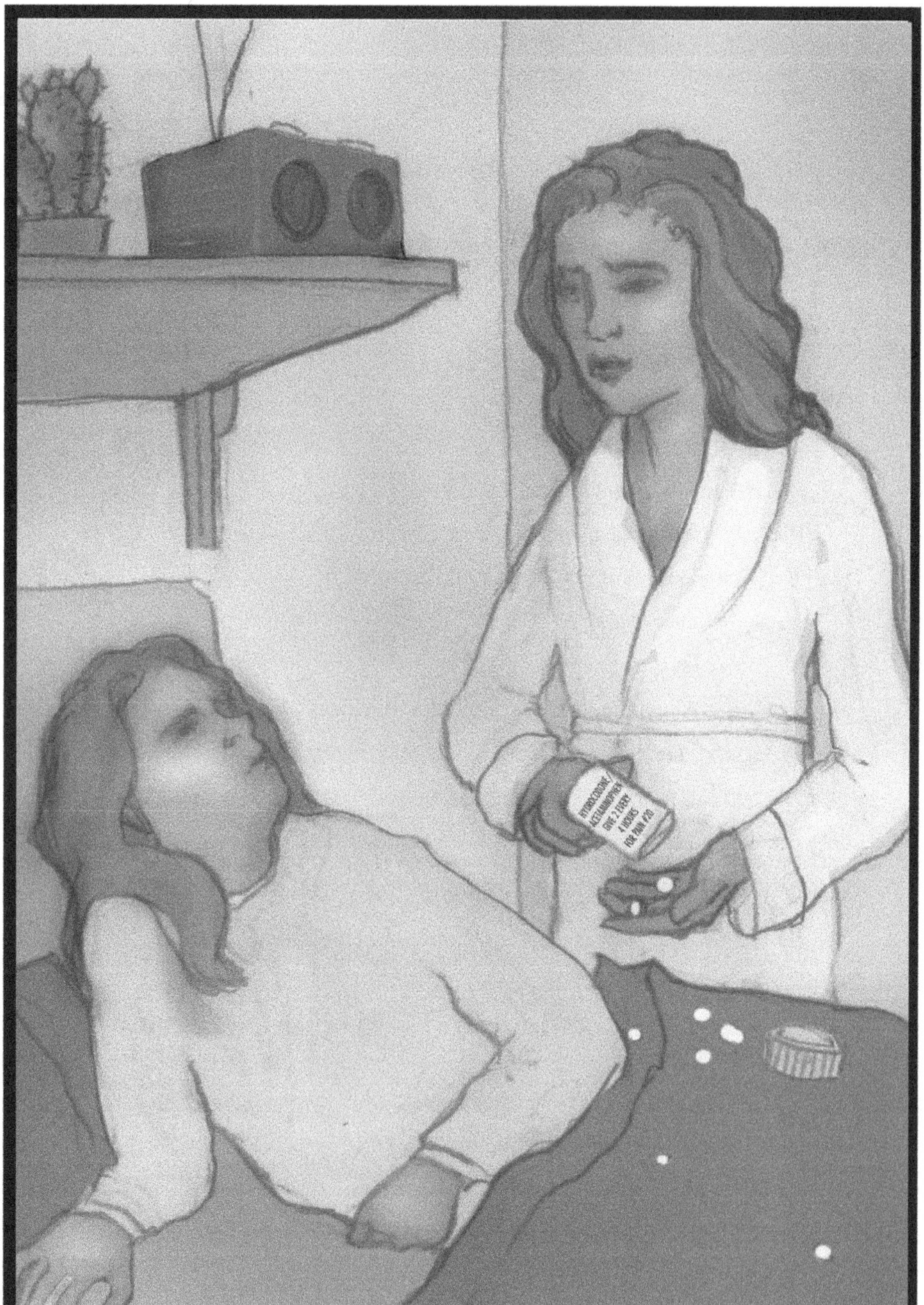
HYDROCODONE/
ACETAMINOPHEN
GIVE 2 EVERY
4 HOURS
FOR PAIN #20

# Case 8

## A 15 Year-old Girl with RLQ Abdominal Pain: It *is* an Appy ... Right?

One of the red flags for a missed diagnosis occurs when the primary complaint could be serious, and there is no alternative diagnosis. For example, in a patient with fever and headache and absolutely no other symptoms, how can we say it is not meningitis without doing a lumbar puncture? This patient had symptoms suggestive of appendicitis with a positive WBC count "kicker." Enter the alternative diagnosis ...

***Deep thoughts:***

1. *Does a 15 year-old girl with pelvic pain who is not sexually active need a speculum exam?*
2. *What is the real medical and legal risk with end-of-shift turnover of patients? Does the data suggest a method to decrease it?*
3. *Is there a legal risk in getting a WBC count when the results are ignored in light of more specific tests, such as a CT scan?*
4. *Why do patients decide to sue?*

**PART 1—MEDICAL**

## I. The Patient's Story

Ashley is a healthy, bright, and active 15 year-old girl; daughter and sibling, tons of friends. She enjoys movies, going to the mall, and is thinking of going out for cheerleading. But sometime in January or early February, like many 15 year-old girls, she was a participant in a seemingly innocuous event, a rite of passage. This action will have profound implications, not only for her, but for others in her community for years to come.

Our story begins on Monday, February 17 with nonspecific symptoms of fatigue, dizziness and abdominal pain. On Wednesday, February 19, Ashley goes to the school nurse and is sent home, but later in the evening the symptoms become unbearable. Her mother decides to take her to the hospital.

Close to midnight on Wednesday, February 19, Ashley and her mother present to the Emergency Department.

## II. The Doctor's Version (the following is the actual documentation of the provider)

**Date:** Wednesday, February 19 at 22:59

**Chief Complaint:** Abdominal pain

Vital Signs

| Time | Temp(F) | Rt. | Pulse | Resp | Syst | Diast | Pos. | Pain Scale |
|---|---|---|---|---|---|---|---|---|
| 00:12 | 99.8 | T | 124 | 18 | 100 | 64 | S | 10 |

**Triage (22:59):** "pt mother states abd pain, dizzy, fever, passed out at school."

**History of Present Illness (01:12):** The pt is a 15yo who is in good general health. No history of abd surgeries. No h/o ovarian cysts or endometriosis. LMP just finished. She states that she has had fatigue and dizziness in the past few days. Today the pt noted gradual onset of rlq aching which has worsened over the day. The pain is worse with movement and walking. + nausea without emesis. No diarrhea. No urinary sx. No vaginal bleeding or discharge. + fevers/chills. No earache, sore throat, sinus, cough, cold. No rash.
ROS: AOSN [all other systems negative]

**Past Medical History:**
**Allergies:** NKDA Meds: None PMH/PSH: Negative
**SH:** Non smoker, no alcohol

**Physical Examination (03:42):**
**Constitutional:** tired appearing; well nourished; A&O x 3, in no apparent resp distress.
**Throat:** Normal pharynx with no tonsillar hypertrophy. NECK: Supple; non-tender; no cervical lymphadenopathy. CARD: Regular rate and rhythm, no murmurs, rubs or gallops.
**Resp:** Breath sounds clear and equal bilaterally; no wheezes, rhonchi, or rales.
**Abd:** BS+, soft, Non-distended; + tenderness in the rlq, which is reproducible, no rebound, rigidity or guarding. No CVAT.
**Skin:** Normal for age and race; warm and dry; no apparent lesions.

**Emergency Department Course:**
**01:09** – Orders for CBC and triple contrast CT scan to r/o appy, plus pain and nausea medications.
**01:52** – Labs return: WBC count 17.2, Hb 11.6, plt 230. Urine pregnancy test and dip - negative.
**02:09 (RN)** – Pt. with about 600cc of emesis of food product. Dr. advised. Additional phenergan 12.5mg ordered. **Repeat VS: pulse 100, resp 24, BP 100/50**
**03:01 (RN)** – Pt. continues to c/o abdominal 6/10. Dr. advised.
**03:42** – Patient care transferred from DOC 1 to DOC 2. EMR records: "This chart has been electronically signed DOC 1. The receiving Physician accepted the transfer." At 3:58 DOC 1 orders another dose of pain and nausea medications.
**04:00 – (sometime just after 4AM):** CT results per radiologist: The appendix is normal in size without surrounding inflammatory change. Within the right adnexal area, there are several greater than 1 cm ovarian cysts visualized. The largest is about 3 cm in dimension with hazy attenuation suggesting a recent hemorrhage.
**04:59 – Repeat VS: pulse 88, resp 16, BP 98/48, pain scale 2/10**
**05:40 – Progress Note** *DOC 2*: "Patient resting comfortably. Family aware of results of CT scan for ovarian cysts on right. Will d/c with pain meds and f/u with GYN."
**Diagnosis Doc 2 (05:40):** Cyst – ovarian.

**After Care Instructions:** Follow-up with your physician in 2–3 days. Rx Vicodin #20, Phenergan PO and suppository. Instructions for ovarian cyst.

*Pamela Ramsey, MD*
*Kristen O'Donnell, MD*

## III. Risk Management/Patient Safety Opportunities (Weinstock)

**Author comments (Weinstock):** The evaluation and management of this case was actually well done. A young woman with short duration RLQ pain and a CT scan showing a normal appendix is reassuring. Additionally, there was an alternative diagnosis: hemorrhagic ovarian cyst. The patient felt better, and she was discharged with a reliable caregiver, her mom. Her vital signs had returned to normal, and there was every reason to believe the management of her cyst could be completed as an outpatient. But a few red flags were waving … not waving high … not waving strong … but still waving …

### Risk Management/Patient Safety Opportunity #1:

**Opportunity:** Not evaluating a documented chief complaint.
**Discussion:** I warned in Chapter one that we were going to be a "broken record"… and this is another example; the patient had a syncopal episode and there was nothing in the history or exam or MDM note which either acknowledges it or explores it further! Was this a primary process (arrhythmia/doubtful) or a secondary process (hypovolemia or vagal from pain??). Were there preceding symptoms, seizure activity, injury from the syncopal event, or other associated symptoms which would get us closer to a diagnosis?
✔ **Teaching point:** All chief complaints should be addressed.

### Risk Management/Patient Safety Opportunity #2:

**Opportunity:** Not appreciating the importance of fever in the history.
**Discussion:** Ashley didn't actually "give" us a diagnosis with her complaint of fever (as documented fever/chills), but in light of the final diagnosis of a "Cyst – ovarian," this does expose an inconsistency. First, did the patient actually have a fever? Perhaps the follow-up question could have been, "What do you mean by the term 'fever?' Do you feel warm or did you actually use a thermometer which read 100.4 degrees or higher?" If we become convinced of an actual fever, this is a game changer (as it was in case #2); there is no explanation in the MDM for her temperature elevation, which could possibly have been from an infection.
✔ **Teaching point:** When fever is present, consider infectious etiology, as well as less common causes of "fever;" including malignancy, rheumatologic disorder, medications/substances or metabolic.

### Risk Management/Patient Safety Opportunity #3:

**Opportunity:** Not repeating the abdominal exam before discharge.
**Discussion:** Abdominal pain is a high-risk complaint; we find a definitive diagnosis less than half the time. We are flying in the dark, using instruments (including our hands) to assess what is occurring in the abdominal cavity. Though many tests can "rule in" diagnoses, there are few tests short of surgery, which can definitively exclude life-threatening causes.[1] Ashley's CT scan showed ovarian cysts, but typically these cause symptoms mid-ovulation, not at the completion of menstruation. The radiologist noted findings "suggestive of" hemorrhagic ovarian cyst, but a definitive diagnosis remained just that, ***suggestive***. Repeating the abdominal exam prior to discharge would have gone a long way toward

confirming that a serious illness wasn't occurring, especially in a young patient who had received multiple doses of pain medications.

✔ **Teaching point:** Perform and document repeat focused examinations on all abdominal pain patients.

**Risk Management/Patient Safety Opportunity #4:**

**Opportunity:** Ignoring an abnormal test result.

**Discussion:** Current (and past) research is clear on the disutility of WBC counts, even suggesting that the mere act of obtaining a WBC count can lead doctors away from the correct diagnosis.[2,3] But if you do order a WBC count, an abnormal test result needs to be acted upon or explained in a progress note. Documenting a "real-time" progress note that the elevated WBC count was likely from stress demargination could have gone a long way toward explaining that a non-infectious explanation was suggested.

✔ **Teaching point:** It is easier to defend not ordering an inappropriate test, than not acting on an abnormal result.

**Risk Management/Patient Safety Opportunity #5:**

**Opportunity:** Not addressing documented complaints, i.e., syncope.

**Discussion:** This is a recurrent theme in malpractice cases as well as a recurrent theme in this book. Why would a patient tell the nurse about a symptom but fail to mention it to the doctor? It is not all the patient's fault; the patient feels that after medical information is conveyed to a medical-care team member, it is accessible to everyone on the care team, particularly in the age of electronic medical records (EMRs). The fallacy is that the doctor often doesn't spend the time sorting through the tremendous amount of extraneous material in a chart to find the pertinent information but is still responsible.

A good habit is to at least read the nursing triage note; it is hard to feign ignorance of this integral part of the chart. The nurse documented a syncopal episode, but this is not mentioned in the doctor's history, and a neurologic evaluation was not performed. Syncope is easily evaluated with a thorough H&P in a patient who is now alert and oriented, without current subjective or objective neurologic symptoms, and usually the only indicated testing is an ECG to evaluate for cardiac causes such as:

1. Brugada syndrome
2. Prolonged QT
3. Tachy- or brady-arrhythmia
4. Wolffe-Parkinson-White (WPW)/Lown-Ganong-Levine (LGL) syndrome
5. Hypertrophic cardiomyopathy (HCM)

Recognition of documented chief complaints does not necessarily require testing since many can be explored with H&P alone, and if a discrepancy exists, this can be documented in a progress note (e.g., it was documented that this headache patient had a fever, but I confirmed that their recorded temperature at home was 99.0° … stated to be "a fever for me.")

✔ **Teaching point:** Address all chief complaints documented by the nurse/triage.

**Risk Management/Patient Safety Opportunity #6:**

**Opportunity:** The patient's sexual history is just that, the ***patient's*** sexual history.
**Discussion:** For most patients, asking about sexual activity is a waste of time; can you imagine not doing a pregnancy test or a pelvic exam in an adult female patient with abdominal pain? A young patient who denies history of sexual activity presents a different issue. Is it appropriate to have a young girl's first pelvic exam done in a curtained room at 3 AM with an obscenity-shouting drunk hand-cuffed to the bed next door? This decision needs to be made with the patient and her parent(s). If they refuse, they need to understand the risk of misdiagnosis and the discussion documented. These doctors felt they had a cause when the CT returned a radiologic diagnosis of hemorrhagic ovarian cyst, but in light of recent sexual activity this would change the differential. Consideration should have been given to other causes:

1. Ovarian torsion (sudden onset of pain severe enough to cause syncope)
2. Pelvic inflammatory disease (PID) or tubo-ovarian abscess (TOA). Unilateral PID is unusual but not unknown and TOA can be diagnosed with an ultrasound (US).
3. Ectopic pregnancy is extremely unlikely with a negative pregnancy test. Consider heterotopic in patients undergoing fertility therapy, a history of PID or tubal ligation; none present with our patient.
4. Appendicitis missed on CT. Though the appendix was seen and noted to be normal, there remains a small percentage chance of false negativity for CT.

✔ **Teaching point:** If a pelvic exam is not done, document your recommendation and the risks of misdiagnosis. Document sexual history, particularly in young patients.

**Risk Management/Patient Safety Opportunity #7:**

**Opportunity:** Failure to inform the patient and her family that the diagnosis is not definitive.
**Discussion:** Patients like to be told a specific diagnosis, prescribed a specific therapy, and then get better; who wouldn't? Unfortunately, this is rarely possible in the ED setting. Over 90% of our chest pain patients turn out to have a non-cardiac etiology; even the ECG diagnosis of STEMI is not 100%. Abdominal pain is a hazy, swirling habitat of peristalsis and visceral pain in close proximity to "big red" and a couple of very important "beans." The pain is subjective and often linked to psychological stress, but frequently a sanctuary for a life-threatening process—clearly an area in which to "proceed with caution." When a patient with abdominal pain is discharged, these simple instructions may be helpful:

- "We think your pain was from [some bleeding into an ovarian cyst], but we're not a 100% certain."
- Return after 12 hours if you have any pain whatsoever.
- Return immediately with fever, worse pain, blood in the stool or any other concerning symptoms.

✔ **Teaching point:** Informing the patient of "diagnostic uncertainty" will encourage returning if symptoms worsen or do not resolve.

**Risk Management/Patient Safety Opportunity #8:**

**Error:** Not taking "ownership" of a hand-off patient.
**Discussion:** Cheung, et al., explored failures in a well-known high-risk area of emergency medicine, the patient handoff. This is discussed at length below. When a patient is accepted in a handoff, a focused exam and brief progress note will ensure that the initial physician's assessment was correct and that the patient's condition has not changed.
✔ **Teaching point:** Beware of handoff patients.

## IV. Guest Commentary—Patient Handoffs

**Ryan Longstreth, MD**
Co-author ***Bouncebacks! Emergency Department Cases: ED Returns***
Attending Emergency Medicine Physician

Patient handoffs in the ED are a fact of life, occurring between EM physicians to the inpatient team. Unfortunately, these "sign-outs" may lead to potential medicolegal liability.

A landmark publication by the Institute of Medicine, ***To Err Is Human: Building a Safer Health System***, concluded that Emergency Departments are susceptible to "high error rates with serious consequences." Errors in communication led to 70% of ED errors, while treatment delays were a direct result of poor communication 84% of the time. Nearly two-thirds of these treatment delays involved handoffs.[4,5]

Based on this IOM study, the Joint Commission (JC) established a list of patient safety goals, stating "The primary objective of a "handoff" is to provide accurate information about a [patient's] care, treatment and services, current condition and any recent or anticipated changes. The information communicated during a handoff must be accurate in order to meet [patient] safety goals." The JC's intent was to standardize the handoff process, making it clear and concise, allowing the opportunity for both providers to ask and answer questions.[6]

An article in the Annals of Emergency Medicine, ***Improving Handoffs in the Emergency Department***, also dissected the handoff process. The authors looked to provide "up-to-date evidence and collective thinking about the process and safety of handoffs." The authors noted that improper sign-outs were implicated in 24% of malpractice claims. The article addressed both legal issues and risk management concepts with the following recommendations:

- Reducing the number of unnecessary handoffs
- Limiting interruptions and distractions during the handoff
- Providing a succinct overview
- Communicating outstanding tasks, anticipating changes and conveying a clear plan
- Having information readily available for direct review
- Encouraging questions
- Having a clear moment of "transition of care" from provider number one to number two

The authors do acknowledge the fact that there are few studies addressing the handoff process and little data suggesting the key points of a good sign-out.[7,8] Thus, the JC's intent of standardization of the handoff process is difficult at the present time.

Could these concepts have improved the care Ashley received in the ED? During visit #1 at 03:42, there is a note stating care was transferred from ***DOC1*** to ***DOC2***. Unfortunately, it is unclear how well this transition was made since there was no note from the second provider as to when care was assumed and no repeat exam documented. A more delineated transition of care could have occurred with a phone consult to the PCP or GYN to review the work-up and ensure timely follow-up.

## V. The Bounceback

**Author comments (Weinstock):** The following excerpts allow us to trace the events in "real time." The story of Ashley's "bounceback" is told per interviews or deposition testimony by those involved in her care. To hear audio of these interviews, go to: www.embouncebacks.com.

**A. Ashley's mother, Linda Green:** (from deposition testimony)—Early Thursday morning Feb. 20 to Friday morning Feb. 21:

- "[When we got home] I tried to feed her soup. She didn't keep it down. She was sleeping all day. She was cold. She was freezing, wrapped up in a blanket like you wouldn't believe. I knew she was in pain. She said, 'Oh, my stomach hurts' She tried to get up and use the bathroom and she was just "uhhhh."
- "I slept with her through the night. She would wake up in pain and I would try to comfort her. I didn't want to give her the narcotics no sooner than 4–5 hour intervals. When she got up to get dressed I had to hold her up. She was not feeling well enough to do things on her own. I was holding her in the bathroom."
- "I called my [family practice] doctor Friday morning [February 21]. I was giving her Vicodin, you know, I thought maybe it was because the cyst ruptured, I really don't know. I told them, 'She's really sick, she's bad off. You can either get me in there this morning or I'm taking her to ER.' They came back on the phone and said to have her there by 11:00."

**B. Jim Alexander, family medicine resident:** at 11:00 AM Friday, February 21, 2003:

- "I was asked to see Ashley and had never seen her before. When she arrived, she was in a wheelchair, quite ill appearing. Her skin color was an off shade of grey, and her head was bobbing. She could barely hold it up. She had diffuse abdominal pain, which was not clearly rebound. I was not able to get her up to the exam table. She was writhing and moaning in pain."
- "She was clearly beyond outpatient management. I contacted the Emergency Department and let them know that she would be coming over. We are fortunate that the ER is right across the parking lot. She was wheeled over and left in the hands of the ER doc."

**C. Greg Decker, attending emergency medicine physician at ED #2:** at12:30 PM Friday, February 21:

- "I remember the details … I remember everything about this case; I can't get it out of my head. I was in there right when she arrived. I think I beat the nurse in the room. She was tender in the right lower quadrant, and I thought: should be a missed appendicitis. I figured we would get another scan and it would show a missed appendicitis. Didn't expect anything a whole lot worse. I'm sure we'll figure out what this is. The radiologist called me and she said, 'This is kind of strange. There is inflammation, but appendix looks OK. I don't know exactly what it is.'"
- "I figured I would do a pelvic exam. She had said she was not sexually active, and she was tender in the right adnexal. But there was no discharge or cervical motion tenderness (CMT) so we get an ultrasound (US) … it's got to be her ovary."
- "We did the US and really didn't come up with answer there either."
- "Her white count was low. I don't remember, maybe 2.5."
- "Looking at her now, she had been there for hours and was steadily worsening. I was watching this process happening in front of me, and I still don't have a good answer with all the medical technology I can throw at her. Something has to be done. So, I figured someone is going to have to open her up. I called surgery and OB."
- "The surgeons got there first and they said 'We don't think it's an appendix,' and I knew they

were going to say that because the [CT] scan showed it was normal. They wanted to watch her overnight. The OB/GYN residents said, 'We don't think it's a pelvic problem, we think it's her appendix. '"

- "Tom Harmon was the OB attending, and Tom stepped up to the plate. He said, 'I'll take her to surgery and if it turns out to be abdominal, surgery is going to be standing by. We'll see what's what.'"

**D. Tom Harmon, OB/GYN attending:** at 7:00 PM, Friday, February 21:

- "I was just getting ready to go off call when I got the call from Greg [Decker]. I told him I would come and look at her. Ashley was lying on the gurney and looked very sick, and there was no doubt she had diffuse peritonitis and needed to go to the OR for a diagnostic lap."
- "I had a moment of time with the patient and bent down and whispered in her ear and asked her if it was true she wasn't sexually active and she said that she was [active]."

**To the OR:**
**Friday, February 21 at 20:15** – [Blood pressure remains in the 80's–90's systolic]

- Per Dr. Harmon: "In the OR I started with a diagnostic lap, and pus just poured out through the trocars, and I realized there was no way I was going to do it laparoscopically, so I converted to an open lap. The most amazing amount of purulent material extruded through the surgical incision and in her pelvis. The right ovary was spewing pus and there were exudates over tubes bilaterally and the left ovary."
- "The decision was made to copiously irrigate. As she had just been put on ATB, my hope was that we would be able to salvage her pelvis."

**Author comments (Weinstock):** Postop, Dr. Harmon informs the family that she may need to go back for further surgeries but as the ATB had just been started, they would first give them a chance to work.

**Postop:**
**Friday, February 21 at 21:30** – PACU—Continued on broad-spectrum ATB including cefotan, doxycycline, flagyl and gentamicin. She continued to do poorly and remained hypotensive.
Pressors are started.

**Early the next morning:**
**Saturday, February 22 at 02:45** – Ashley is admitted to the ICU. Per her nurse, the family cannot be interviewed as "they were too emotional."
**07:15** – The family practice service is walking up the stairs to see the patient when a code is called overhead. They arrive in the ICU to find Ashley in full arrest with the father yelling, "No, no … this is wrong!"
Ashley is initially resuscitated and regains a pulse.
A few minutes later she arrests again and is unable to be resuscitated.
**07:45** – Tom Harmon (OB surgeon) arrives and speaks with the family.

**Final Diagnosis:** Ruptured ovarian abscess with sepsis and cardiopulmonary arrest.

## PART 2—LEGAL

## I. The Accusation/Cause of Action

Why sue? The answer seems obvious; two loving and engaged parents have lost their daughter. But every day brings adverse outcomes and deaths and not all the doctors are sued. In a sentinel study published in Lancet, Vincent, et al. found that the decision to take legal action was determined not only by original injury, but also by insensitive handling and poor communication after the original incident.[9] Four main themes highlight the reasons for litigation:

1. Standards of care: both patients and relatives wanted to prevent similar incidents in the future
2. Explanation: to know how the injury happened and why
3. Compensation: actual losses, pain and suffering or to provide care in the future for an injured person
4. Accountability: a belief that the staff or organization should have to account for their actions

Several factors likely accounted for the decision of Ashley's parents to sue. The initial doctors were not able to give an explanation after the bounceback visit, since the patient went to a different hospital for the second visit. Additionally, the family may have misinterpreted a discussion by the surgeon Tom Harmon at the second visit concerning the elevated WBC count at the first visit (see father's testimony below). Finally, an internet search by Ashley's mother found information which, taken out of the context, suggested that antibiotics would have saved her daughter's life.

**Following is deposition testimony of Ashley's father and mother (note: family names are changed).**

**Steve Smith (Ashley's father):**

**Q.** Did anyone ever explain to you, any health care provider at [ED #2] the cause of Ashley's death?
**A.** The only thing I recalled him [Tom Harmon] saying was, he said something about the infection, said if we would have caught it earlier, and I told him we had been at [ED#1] 2–3 days ago, and he seemed surprised, He called and had them fax him the information. I recalled him, I believe, responding that her WBC count was elevated, and the way I took it is he was upset that they didn't notice that she had infection, the way I took it.

**Q.** Did he say that any of the physicians at ED#1 did something wrong?
**A.** No. I don't recall.

**Q.** Has any health care provider told you that physicians at ED#1 did something wrong?
**A.** No, not that I'm aware of.

**Q.** And you feel that something more should have been done when Ashley was at ED#1
**A.** I do.

**Q.** And what do you feel should have been done?
**A.** [She] should have been kept overnight and watched and, if she had an infection, given antibiotics.

**Q.** Anything else?
**A.** No.

**Lucinda Smith (Ashley's mother)**
**Q.** Has any health care provider told you that the ER physicians at ED #1 did something wrong?
**A.** No.

**Q.** What prompted you to file this lawsuit?
**Plaintiff 's attorney:** Object. You're not to relate anything you learned from any of your counsel, me or anyone else in this office. But if you want to go ahead and answer, then that's OK.
**A.** Me and her father had discussed, you know, we talked a lot. "Do you think this should have happened," just conversations with other people. Boy, I had an ovarian cyst that ruptured and I was kept overnight and things like that and I kind of got to wonder if something else should have happened and that's just a concern I had.

**Q.** What kind of things do you believe should have happened?
**A.** I believe they should have kept her overnight.

**Q.** Anything else?
**A.** Knowing her white blood count level, I'm not a doctor or anything like that, but there's information "on-line," things like that that indicate to me that there was infection. I wish they would have just treated her with antibiotics. Of course, that's my belief.

**Q.** Do you recall what Web site?
**A.** I read it. I can always go back to it. It's right there.

**On October 12, 2004, approximately 1½ years after the initial visit, plaintiff's attorney Todd Stanley laid out his arguments and presented a demand to settle:**

Quite simply, given Ashley's presentation at ED#1 and with PID/TOA in the differential diagnosis, a pelvic exam should have been performed, which would have revealed adnexal pain and cervical motion tenderness which would have resulted in antibiotic administration and admission. Had this been done, it would have avoided this young lady from going into septic shock and she would have in all probability survived. While defendants claim they were led astray by a negative response regarding sexual activity (curiously the only piece of information in the case not charted) common sense would dictate not relying on such an inherently unreliable bit of information to rule out a potentially life threatening condition. I have conferred with both parents and have been authorized to communicate a [settlement] demand in the amount of $1.25 million.

**So, now the allegations are clear:**

1. The elevated WBC count should have prompted the initial doctor(s) to realize there was an infection and to start antibiotics.
2. Omitting a pelvic exam hampered the ability of the initial doctor(s) to make an accurate diagnosis.
3. She should have been admitted.

**Would you settle?**

Though honor and pride are at stake, many doctors will be surprised to find that their insurance company makes the decision to settle, not them. A contract signed just out of residency is forgotten 10 or 20 years into treating stab victims and sprained ankles.

**Author comments (Weinstock):** The defendants were surprised to learn that Tom Harmon, the gynecologist who cared for the patient at ED#2, was sitting across the table as a plaintiff's expert.

He fell into this role as one of his partners was a friend of the lead plaintiff's attorney and was asked to testify. To be clear, Tom is not a hired gun. I have personally known him for years, and he is honest, caring and extremely intelligent. He had never testified previously and has not since.

He described his feeling sitting across the table from the defendants, "I felt horrible. I realized these were two concerned doctors and I just felt horrible." He alleged that there was a delay in care and that a pelvic exam should have been done at the initial visit. Additionally, the patient did not have a firm diagnosis and should have been admitted.

## II. The Legal Analysis—Guest Interview

**Karen Clouse, JD (Interview continued after trial testimony)**
Partner with Arnold, Todaro & Welch, Columbus, Ohio
Defense attorney for this case

**Authors:** What factors played into the decision of settlement vs. trial?
**KC:** As in any case, there were a number of factors. We had two physicians-defendants who made very good witnesses in their own defense and could do a good job of explaining the decision-making process and treatment. We had good expert witnesses to defend their management. This was an unusual presentation which the subsequent treating ER physician and OB-GYN did not easily diagnose. Since they didn't recognize this as a tubo-ovarian abscess later in its evolution, part of the defense was that the standard of care didn't require our defendant doctors to suspect that "zebra" diagnosis when Ashley presented to the first ER. The entire defense team—attorneys, insurance company and physicians-defendants—were committed to defending the doctors' care rather than settling, and put in the time and resources necessary to do so.

**Author comments (Weinstock):** The plaintiff's settlement offer was refused and the case proceeded to trial.

## III. The Depositions/Trial (April)

The players: As Ms. Clouse, the defense attorney, previously discussed, the defendants decided to go to trial. It lasted two weeks and involved the testimony of many family members as well as expert witnesses. You may be surprised to learn that Tom Harmon (the gynecologist who cared for the patient in the second hospital) was one of them … for the plaintiff.

Cast of characters (names changed, except where noted):
**The patient:** Ashley Smith
**ED physicians defendants:** Pamela Ramsey and Kristen O'Donnell
**Plaintiff's attorney:** Todd Stanley
**Plaintiff's expert witness:** Tom Harmon, MD (OB/GYN) (Actual name)
**Plaintiff's expert witness:** Barbara Noonan, MD (EM)
**Defense attorneys:** Karen Clouse and Gail Arnold (actual attorneys)

**Author comments (Weinstock):** Let's jump right in with Dr. Harmon's testimony/allegations. Remember how relieved Dr. Decker (at ED #2) was to have a surgeon willing to assume definitive care of the patient? Whaaat??? Yes, he became a plaintiff's expert! Is an OB/GYN able to speak to a standard of emergency department care? That question will be answered by the jury.

The following is an interesting exchange by the attorney Mr. Stanley, who is revealing his plan to question the witness; the following is a colorful rhetorical comment by the defense.

**Mr. Stanley (plaintiff's attorney):** I intend to ask Dr. Harmon whether had Ashley been admitted and administered appropriate antibiotic therapy if she would have survived
**Ms. Arnold (defense attorney):** Do you believe if Kennedy hadn't been in a convertible he would be alive?

## A. Should the patient have had a pelvic exam and been admitted for observation?

**Cross-examination of plaintiff's expert witness Tom Harmon (OB) by defense attorney Gail Arnold:**
**Q.** (by defense attorney): … you have certain opinions critical of Dr. Ramsey and Dr. O'Donnell, is that accurate information?
**A.** Critical of them?

**Q.** Critical of their care.
**A.** That's fair to say

**Q.** What opinion do you have?
**A.** There were some things that I would have done that were not done in the emergency room.

**Q.** What?
**A.** Pelvic exam of the patient primarily.

**Q.** Anything else?
**A.** Observation of the patient for a longer period of time.

**Q.** How long?
**A.** Twelve to 24 hours.

**Q.** Anything else that should have been done?
**A.** Allowed to say in hindsight, empiric antibiotics would have been given provided that her pelvic exam would have confirmed pain and adnexal [tenderness].

**Q.** So you're saying there may be some conditional action taken depending on what findings were produced by the pelvic exam?
**A.** That's correct. The outcome might have been different if that had happened.

**Q.** What do you mean by that?
**A.** This young lady died from overwhelming sepsis, and I might—I believe I expressed the opinion that if antibiotics were started early, that might not have happened. I do believe this was a very complex case.

**Q.** When you say it was a very complex case, you mean the manner in which the patient presented was difficult to ascertain exactly what was going on?
**A.** Absolutely.

**Author comments (Weinstock):** Dr. Harmon is really not saying anything different than what we all know—the patient had an infection and antibiotics could have been helpful. He admits this is a tough case; however, this is a patient we see all the time. His experience with ED patients is selective, since he only sees patients ***when we*** decide to consult him, and these are not the average group of patients we see.

So how is his testimony refuted? The defense uses two main approaches. First, to show that the obstetrician is not trained in emergency medicine, so is not able to pass judgment on a different specialty.

### B. Can an OB/GYN speak for an emergency physician?

**Continued cross-examination of plaintiff's expert witness Tom Harmon (OB), by defense attorney Gail Arnold:**
**Q.** You are not an emergency medicine physician?
**A.** No, I'm not.

**Q.** You're not board certified in emergency medicine?
**A.** No, I'm not.

**Q.** Since completing your residency, have you ever practiced as an emergency room physician?
**A.** Definitely not.

**Q.** Have you even practiced in the context of an emergency physician other than doing a rotation when you were being trained?
**A.** Only as a consultant to the emergency department.

**Q.** As far as triaging patients in the emergency department, you have no clinical experience?
**A.** No, I do not.

**Q.** Are you familiar with the standards of care then that are expected of an emergency medicine physician in triaging teenage female patients?
**A.** Not directly.

**Author comments (Weinstock):** This is a clever line of questioning, since there is no other way he can answer. The questions are repeated in a slightly different fashion so the point is not lost by the jury. The second approach is to cajole Dr. Harmon into admitting that the diagnosis was so difficult to make that even upon entering the OR, a definitive diagnosis was not in hand:

**Q.**… you said sometimes it's difficult, and I was trying to ferret that out to determine whether or not her clinical situation really was that complex so as to not really know preoperatively which specialty would take her to explore. You're nodding your head. Does that mean you agree with what I've said?
**A.** There were questions even at the time we took her to surgery as to the exact cause of her condition.

**Q.**… you were surprised [with what] you found?
**A.** The extent of what I found, correct.

**Q.** Can you explain why you were that surprised? …her clinical presentation did not at all suggest the degree of severity of her actual condition?
**A.** That is correct.

**Author comments (Weinstock):** Another witness for the plaintiff was Barbara Noonan, a board-certified emergency medicine physician. Though she had been hired as an expert in the past, this was her first deposition and her first trial. The initial responses support the care of the ED physicians, subsequent ones do not. Some of her allegations are bizarre, others hit home. How effective was she?

## C. Should additional testing be done?

**Cross-examination of plaintiff's expert witness Barbara Noonan (EM) by defense attorney Gail Arnold:**
**Q.** Have you served as a medical expert witness in any other case prior to this one?
**A.** I have.

**Q.** On how many occasions?
**A.** Approximately six.

**Q.** You've been through this process which we're embarking upon today where there's a deposition taken to elicit your opinions?
**A.** I have never given a deposition in this circumstance.

**Q.** This is the first time you actually appeared to testify about a case?
**A.** Correct. I have been retained and asked for my opinions.

**Sexual history:**

**Q.** [Was it relevant whether she was sexually active]?
**A.** The history of sexual activity is well known to be unreliable, especially a young patient giving a history in front of her parents. It's probably not going to provide you with reliable information.

**Q.** Are you telling me that you don't trust what your patients tell you?
**A.** In this particular instance, we don't trust what our patients tell us. Patients are not always forthcoming and honest with that information.

**Q.** Is it below the standard of care for this patient's sexual history to not be documented in the record?
**A.** No, it is not below the standard of care.

**Transition of care:**

**Q.** Do you have criticisms of how the transition was handled?
**A.** The transition was handled as is typical.

**Q.** And was appropriate?
**A.** And it seemed appropriate.

**Additional testing:**

**Q.** [Was] additional testing indicated?
**A.** In my opinion, an ultrasound would have been the logical next procedure.

**Q.** Hypothetically, if the US had been done, do you believe that would rule out the need for a pelvic exam?
**A.** I think if a pelvic exam would have been done, it would at least be a reasonable certainty that PID would be diagnosed and she then would have received antibiotics.

**Q.** How would a pelvic exam be helpful in ruling out appendicitis?
**A.** It would be helpful to rule in other diagnoses, such as PID.

**Q.** By what findings?
**A.** Adnexal tenderness and cervical motion tenderness.

**Author comments (Weinstock):** Attorneys don't know about medicine? How about the this next zinger of a question?

**Q.** How would that diagnose PID as opposed to ovarian cyst, ovarian abscess, or ovarian hemorrhage?
**A.** Clearly there is some overlap amongst the conditions. However, the commonly held dogma is that a patient with PID would have bilateral symptoms and tenderness on exam. In a thin patient, you should be able to feel the size of her ovaries. You should be able to feel her fallopian tubes if she's thin enough.

**Q.** And tell me how a tubal ovarian abscess feels differently from a hemorrhagic ovarian cyst on pelvic exam?
**A.** It would be hard to distinguish the two. However, in a patient with PID, they're going to have bilateral, adnexal tenderness, which I wouldn't expect in the case of a unilateral, one sided ovarian cyst.

**Author comments (Weinstock):** Ever palpate a fallopian tube? Well, let's give the witness a break … this is her first deposition. The questioning continues:

**Disposition:**

**Q.** Should she have been discharged?
**A.** The patient should not have left the facility.

**Q.** And the reason specifically why the patient should not have left the facility is what?
**A.** I feel that the etiology of her pain and elevated WBC count was not fairly evaluated, and she should have been admitted for additional testing and consultation, which is the standard of care for a female with a WBC count of 17,000.

**Author comments (Weinstock):** The following is the defense again hammering home the disutility of the pelvic exam, and the plaintiff's witness standing his ground that the exam was "absolutely required." Maybe it would have been easier to just comment on the pelvic exam at the initial encounter …

## D. Would a pelvic exam have helped make the diagnosis?

**Continued cross-examination of plaintiff's expert witness Barbara Noonan (EM) by defense attorney Gail Arnold:**

**Q.** [Had it been done], what would the pelvic examination have showed?
**A.** Cervical motion tenderness.

**Q.** Would you expect to find cervical motion tenderness in the presence of a hemorrhagic ovarian cyst?
**A.** That's certainly possible, yes.

**Q.** So the physical findings don't really differentiate between cyst and [abscess], do they?
**A.** No.

**Q.** All right. But you still think, in your own words, a pelvic examination was "absolutely required?"
**A.** I believe it was.

**Q.** "Absolutely" is a harsh word, isn't it?
**A.** I think that [word is] accurate.

**Q.** I've heard that in medicine you never say never, and never say always.
**A.** I've heard that—I'm not talking about a general comment, I'm talking about a specific patient.

**Q.** So you don't think there's any reasonable discretion to allow for not doing a pelvic exam on this patient?
**A.** Not the way she presented. It is a reasonably uninvasive procedure that we do in any young lady with lower abdominal pain. Are there exceptions? Yeah. But this one I don't see as an exception.

**Author comments (Weinstock):** Let's drive this train into the station. Though the expert claims that all 15 year-old patients need a pelvic exam, that a fallopian tube could be palpated, or that an ultrasound could have been done at 3 AM seems far-fetched, it is hard to dispense with the fact that a repeat abdominal exam was not done and the patient was not informed of the lack of definitive diagnosis, likely prompting her mother to continue giving Vicodin every 6 hours through the night instead of bringing her back to the ED.

How about the legal strategy of trying both doctors together? After all, they did have different degrees of legal exposure. The interview with the actual defense attorney, Ms. Clouse, continues.

## IV. The Legal Analysis—Guest Interview

**Karen Clouse, JD (second half of interview)**

**Authors:** ***The two doctors were tried together. It would seem that the first doctor was placed in unnecessary legal jeopardy. Why did the defense make this decision?***
**KC:** Especially when the care of two defendants is closely connected, as in this case, plaintiffs' attorneys are often unwilling to settle with one defendant, fearing that the remaining defendant will then employ an "empty chair" defense and point the finger back at the defendant who has settled. We believed the better strategy was for both doctors to be fully engaged at trial, defending not only their care, but that of their partner. At trial, the jury was asked to separately determine whether each defendant had met the standard of care in the treatment each provided to Ashley, and to render a verdict in favor of each defendant ER doctor.

**Authors:** ***What was the defense strategy?***
**KC:** Our strategy was to repeatedly and consistently portray all phases of this ED encounter as thorough, caring and complete. Dr. Ramsey (ED doctor #1) took an appropriate history, did an appropriate exam and ordered the necessary and appropriate tests. Dr. O'Donnell (ED doctor #2) assimilated all of the clinical, laboratory and radiographic information in coming to a diagnosis and discharging the patient. The care met appropriate standards, and the diagnosis could not have been made at the time of the initial ED encounter, as reflected by the fact that it was not made when Ashley re-presented to ED #2 the next day. While we wanted to win on standard of care, causation was an important part of the defense.

**Authors:** ***How did you refute the allegations that an increased WBC count meant an infection was occurring?***
**KC:** We argued that the white count can be elevated for reasons other than infection, including stress and inflammation. There was not a left shift which tended to mitigate against presence of an infection and suggested the elevation was due to inflammation, i.e., from the hemorrhagic ovarian cyst. Plaintiffs tried to take that one value out of context to argue that the defendants should have diagnosed infection, while we argued the entire clinical picture, including normal discharge vital signs and an afebrile patient was not suggestive of infection.

**Authors:** ***What additional/different documentation would have helped you at trial?***
**KC:** Ashley's sexual history became a big issue in the case, with plaintiff's counsel arguing that the ED doctors mistakenly believed her history and failed to do an adequate exam. In reality, they didn't take her history at face value, as evidenced by the fact that Dr. Ramsey (ED doctor #1) did a pregnancy test, despite the history that she wasn't sexually active. It would have been helpful to have some documentation as to why a pelvic exam was not being done. Additionally, with the CT findings, it would have been helpful to have a progress note documenting that an alternate diagnosis had been discovered.

**Authors:** ***How can there be a "standard of care" for a one-in-a-million diagnosis?***
**KC:** That's why medicine is an art as well as a science. If there was just a cookbook or checklist of items to meet the "standard of care," medicine wouldn't be practiced by doctors, it could be practiced by technicians. The standard of care is how to treat the presenting clinical signs and symptoms. A heart attack may not always look like a heart attack, and cases may be defensible if that "garden variety" diagnosis presents in such an uncommon way that the ED doctor cannot reasonably be expected to make the diagnosis. In the same way, the ED doctor needs to use the standard of care of a reasonably-prudent

doctor in doing the necessary and appropriate exam and ordering the appropriate tests to try to come to the diagnosis or make the appropriate referral, but in the "one-in-a-million" diagnosis, that may not be possible.

**Authors:** ***Are there any colorful memories from trial or working with the defendants you would like to share?***
**KC:** The white count was something that became more of an issue as the case evolved at trial. The plaintiffs were permitted to call a pathologist who had not been previously identified or deposed as a rebuttal expert. He testified that the white count elevation was indicative of infection and not merely inflammation. We then tried to call a "sur-rebuttal" expert to refute the plaintiffs' pathology expert, but the court refused to allow us to do so. One of the keys to success in defending a case at trial is having engaged defendants. Both of ours played an active role both before and during trial discussing issues, brainstorming the approach to presenting medical concepts to the jury and attacking the plaintiff's theories.

**Author comments (Weinstock):** I have had several long discussions with the first ED doctor. She felt that her defense was augmented by sitting in on the depositions. This not only kept the experts "honest" but also helped to point out subtleties of the evaluation and management to the defense attorneys.

## V. The Verdict

Were the arguments effective in convincing "eight people who couldn't get out of jury duty?" A legal verdict is more than a simple up or down vote. The jury needs to find the physician not only breached the standard of care but that this breach was a direct and proximate cause of the patient's poor outcome/ death.

Though a "standards" defense is always preferable to a "causation" defense, the latter was an effective argument in this case. Even if the diagnosis had been made initially, it is hard to say if it would have changed the outcome. Additionally, even at the second ED, neither the pelvic exam nor ultrasound (two of the main allegations of the plaintiff) was diagnostic (in fact she had 3 pelvic exams in ED #2, with none showing discharge or cervical motion tenderness). An effective defense argument is that even if these had been done in ED #1, a diagnosis would have remained elusive.

**Instructions to the jury** (April)

Do you find by a preponderance of the evidence that Dr. Pamela Ramsey (ED physician #1) was negligent in failing to properly evaluate, diagnose and treat Ashley's condition as it was presented to her at ED #1?

- *8/8 jurors agreed "no"*

Do you find by a preponderance of the evidence that Dr. Kristen O'Donnell (ED physician #2) was negligent in failing to properly evaluate, diagnose and treat Ashley's condition as it was presented to her at ED #1?

- *8/8 jurors agreed "no"*

**Verdict:** Unanimous verdict for both defendants in less than one hour.

## VI. Motion for a New Trial

After a huge sigh of relief, the physicians are surprised to receive a letter on June 5. Plaintiff's counsel has filed a motion with the court for a new trial.
June 5

Plaintiff 's Motion for New Trial

To the Court, Your Honorable Judge Myron Bender:
As you may recall, the trial of the medical negligence and wrongful death action consumed a full two weeks, involved sophisticated concepts of medicine and science, and involved the testimony of five expert witnesses on behalf of the plaintiffs and six for the defense. Faced with ten days of trial and the testimony of 11 expert witnesses, the jury in this case got a carry out lunch and returned a verdict in one hour!

How eight people could deliberate and consider ten days of testimony and reach a decision in one hour is unfathomable. The simple answer is that they did not even seriously consider the evidence, and rushed their verdict in their haste to get out of the house on a Friday. It is respectfully submitted that this conduct constitutes "irregularity in the proceedings of the jury" and "misconduct of the jury" under Civil Rule 59A-1 & 2. Allegations for appeal:
Irregularity in the proceedings of the court, jury, magistrate, or prevailing party by which an aggrieved party was prevented from having a fair trial
Misconduct of the jury or the prevailing party
The judgment is not sustained by the weight of the evidence

Respectfully,
*Todd Stanley*
Todd Stanley, Esq.

**Defense response:**

Response: Defendants Memorandum Contra Plaintiff 's Motion for New Trial

While understandably disappointed with the jury's verdict against them, Plaintiff fails to present this Court with any legitimate grounds for granting a new trial. Plaintiff were given a full and fair opportunity to present their evidence.

Plaintiffs suggest that a new trial must be granted because of an irregularity in the proceedings as the jury deliberated for only one hour to reach its verdict. First, there is no mathematical formula mandating the jury deliberate a certain number of minutes per witness or days spent in trial. Second, although there were many witnesses, a number of common themes were addressed repeatedly. Third, the trial did span two weeks, but actual trial days were ten, of which the first was spent in jury selection and last in closing arguments. Additionally, six days started late or ended early. Given that the jury decided the defendants were not negligent, the jury did not need to consider testimony related to subsequent care at ED #2 or evidence on any proximate causation issues. Finally, the jury received the case for deliberations at 10:45 in the morning and had the entire afternoon to deliberate—they were not under time constraints. None indicated any conflicts or difficulties with deliberating as long as necessary to find a verdict. They consulted amongst themselves and were able to reach their verdict without long deliberation.

Sincerely,
*Gail Arnold*
Gaily Arnold, JD

**Author comments (Weinstock):** There were other arguments … but you get the point …

**Trial Court's ruling:** On July 20, the judge dismisses the Motion for New Trial.

So who won? The defendants won the trial, but at the expense of four years of worry, endless hours of depositions and review of documents and likely subclinical PTSD. Who won? You be the judge.

## VII. Medical Discussion—Evaluation of Pelvic Pain/Diagnosis of Tubo-ovarian Abscess (TOA)

**Guest Author:**
**David A. Talan, MD, FACEP, FIDSA**
Emeritus Professor of Emergency Medicine and Medicine/Infectious Diseases
The David Geffen School of Medicine at UCLA
Department of Emergency Medicine, Ronald Reagan UCLA Medical Center

Dr. Talan is board certified in emergency medicine, internal medicine, and infectious diseases. He has written and researched extensively on the intersection of infectious diseases and emergency department care. He serves on the editorial board of the Annals of Emergency Medicine and has numerous publications in high-impact journals, including The New England Journal of Medicine and the Journal of the American Medical Association.

*************

I am primarily an emergency physician, but have training and practice experience as an infectious diseases specialist. For over 30 years, through my research and teaching, I have focused on the diagnosis and treatment of infectious diseases in the ED. I am frequently asked to review medical-legal cases involving infectious disease issues during the course of ED care.

This case comes down to whether or not the emergency physicians on Ashley's first visit should have suspected and treated pelvic inflammatory disease (PID) and tubo-ovarian abscess (TOA). The clinical diagnosis of PID is imprecise and many episodes go unrecognized with consequences of tubal infertility and chronic pelvic pain. Therefore, it is recommended that clinicians rely on more sensitive and less specific diagnostic findings and err on the side of over-treatment. This strategy is emphasized in the Centers for Disease Control and Prevention's (CDC) Sexually Transmitted Infections Guidelines, last published in 2021.[10] In this regard, the 2021 guidelines are similar to those of 2002,[11] which were applied at the time of this case. These guidelines state, "Empiric treatment of PID should be initiated in sexually active young women and other women at risk for STDs if the following minimum criteria are present and no other cause(s) for the illness can be identified: uterine/adnexal tenderness or cervical motion tenderness."

In this case, the diagnosis of PID/TOA should have been an initial consideration in an adolescent girl with a history of fever/chills and lower abdominal pain and tenderness. One criticism was that the charting did not indicate whether or not Ashley was sexually active. When she bounced back, she denied being sexually active so it is likely that she would have answered similarly at the first visit. The recorded history that Ashley denied vaginal discharge supported the doctor's assertion that she asked about intercourse and suggested that he considered PID. The fact that a pregnancy test was done at the first visit indicated that they were not naive to the possibility that she might not be fully forthcoming about sexual activity. Alternatively, this acknowledged their skepticism and potentially implicated their incomplete evaluation, which did not include a pelvic examination. While it is possible for a virgin to get PID, it is so rare that it nearly qualifies as a religious miracle.[12]

Ultimately, if PID is somewhere on our radar, it cannot be reasonably excluded without conducting a pelvic examination. Note the legal standard is "reasonably excluded," not ruled out to the nth degree. Imaging may mostly exclude other conditions, like appendicitis, but even when imaging identifies a possible TOA or pelvic free fluid, these findings still require clinical correlation. I have never seen a vaginal ultrasound report comment on cervical motion tenderness or vaginal discharge!

We should also acknowledge barriers to conducting a pelvic examination. A pelvic examination can be psychologically traumatic to a 15-year-old girl and requires their assent, and since the time of this case in 2002, there is increased sensitivity to respecting a patient's personal boundaries to being touched, particularly when it comes to examination of the genital area. Besides a chaperone, a pelvic examination takes time to set up, optimize positioning, and requires special lighting and equipment. On the other hand, when a pelvic examination is indicated, such as when PID and TOA are reasonable possibilities, we have to do our best convince the patient of its need and work through these barriers. A less invasive exam with a single finger or small speculum can also be offered.

In this case it was unlikely that a pelvic examination would have added determinative diagnostic information. Ashley denied vaginal discharge, and when a pelvic examination was done during the second ED visit, neither discharge nor cervical motion tenderness were found. A study of female ED patients 14–20 years old published in 2018 found that pelvic examination findings did not increase accuracy of detection of confirmed gonococcal, chlamydial, or trichomonal infection compared to history alone, although as many as half of PID cases are not associated with these infections.[13] Regardless, documenting that a pelvic examination was considered and justifying why it was not done (i.e., denied sexual activity and vaginal discharge, and a diagnosis was found on imaging) would have helped in the emergency physicians' defense.

It was contended that the elevated while blood cell count of 17,200/mm$^3$ should have led to suspicion of PID/TOA. Interestingly, an elevated white blood cell count is not among the more specific findings (including other inflammatory markers) listed for the diagnosis of PID in the CDC's 2002 or 2021 guidelines, which include the following:

- oral temperature >38.3°C (>101°F),
- abnormal cervical mucopurulent discharge or cervical friability,
- presence of abundant numbers of WBCs on saline microscopy of vaginal fluid,
- elevated erythrocyte sedimentation rate,
- elevated C-reactive protein, and
- laboratory documentation of cervical infection with *N. gonorrhoeae* or *C. trachomatis*.

During her first ED visit, Ashley did not have a fever; her measured temperature was under 100°F. However, since she gave a history of fever and chills and had a very elevated white blood cell count, infection should have been strongly considered. While generally true that an elevated white blood cell count is non-specific for bacterial infection, as the elevation increases, so does the specificity. When combined with a history of fever and rebound abdominal tenderness, it could be contended that a white blood cell count of 17,200/mm$^3$ was far more consistent with TOA than a hemorrhagic ovarian cyst. Here's the thing about tests from a legal perspective; when you order it, you own it. So, if the result is very abnormal, you are obligated to reconcile it, and it's best to do that in your charting.

Here's a couple more subtle issues. Our "normal" temps have a diurnal variation.[14] We are warmest in the afternoon and coldest in the wee hours of the morning, with a variation of about one degree Fahrenheit. Ashley's temperature measured at 0012 was 99.8°F, which while not strictly considered a fever, was high for the early morning and consistent with her reporting fever. Also, her history of syncope and low diastolic and mean arterial pressure (MAP) when her vital signs were repeated—98/48 mmHg (normal diastolic 14–18 year-old, 50–80 mmHg; her MAP was slightly below 65), even for a 15 year-old, even though not tachycardic, might have suggested broader laboratory testing, including lactic acid, to evaluate for sepsis and organ dysfunction. SIRS sepsis criteria, which were met in this case, had been proposed but not promulgated until the Surviving Sepsis Campaign in 2003 and then through to the 2015 CMS SEP-1 bundle. Now, this is a common litigation theme. Whether SIRS are screening criteria allowing a response based on clinical judgment vs. a rule mandating testing and treatment for presumed bacterial infection typically gets debated among opposing experts.

Since 2003, nucleic acid amplification testing for chlamydial and gonococcal infections has been introduced, including with the capability for rapid turnaround in the timeframe of ED care. Self-inserted vaginal swab specimens have been shown to be as accurate as those obtained from the cervix by pelvic examination and point-of-care (POC) tests have been shown to vastly improve the accuracy of ED STI treatment compared to our usual empirical approach.[15, 16] Although not commented upon, if this case was among most PID associated with chlamydial and gonococcal infection, and occurred in 2022 at the small number of hospitals that offer POC testing, then a patient could self-collect a specimen for rapid testing before a pelvic examination was considered.

The radiologist's interpretation of the contrast CT scan was critical. He noted that the appendix was normal without inflammatory changes, and there were right ovarian cysts, the largest 3 cm, with some hazy attenuation suggestive of recent hemorrhage. Note that there was no mention of inflammation around the cysts. The radiologist's read led away from the diagnosis of PID and TOA since it provided another explanation for Ashley's presentation, and the absence of inflammatory changes mitigated against suspicion for infection suggested by other findings. Had the radiologist's impression of the first CT scan been "probable hemorrhagic cyst with surrounding inflammatory changes, cannot rule out TOA," then the emergency physicians would have been obligated to consider TOA and consult a gynecologist. It's hard to believe that there were no signs of inflammation with contrast enhancement around the cysts. We do not know Ashley's weight, but a main cause of false-negative CT scans for appendicitis is paucity of intra-abdominal fat. And it is unclear if ultrasound would have added anything in this case, although it would have helped exclude ovarian torsion and cholecystitis. Had I consulted on this case, I would have strongly recommended that the CT scan be reviewed by a radiologist. Otherwise, this was a difficult case because Ashley denied sexual activity and lacked many of the characteristic clinical findings of PID, (i.e., measured fever, vaginal discharge, and cervical motion tenderness), while her adnexal tenderness had another apparent explanation.

Of note, the CT scan done two days later did show inflammatory changes but no "cyst" and, in retrospect, indicated rupture of the TOA. The defense argued that Ashley's diagnosis was difficult since it was also not immediately clear on the second visit. However, this was in part related to the fact that the abscess had ruptured and the radiologist was not able to compare the second CT scan to the first one.

Negligence is ultimately not about the standard of documentation, examination, or diagnostic consideration, it is about violating the standard of care (i.e., treatment). The 2021 CDC STI guidelines state, "Diagnosis and management of other causes of lower abdominal pain (i.e., ectopic pregnancy, acute appendicitis, ovarian cyst, ovarian torsion, or functional pain) are unlikely to be impaired by initiating antimicrobial therapy for PID." Note the mention of the diagnosis of ovarian cyst. The parenthetic example diagnoses in 2002 CDC guidelines were more limited—"ectopic pregnancy, acute appendicitis, and functional pain," and did not include ovarian cyst. Otherwise I suspect that the plaintiff's attorney would have blown up the caption the size of a courtroom wall and perhaps it would have changed the verdict.

Ashley could have been given intramuscular ceftriaxone and a prescription for oral doxycycline and metronidazole, the currently recommended outpatient treatment for PID, as well as next day instead of 2–3 days follow-up just in case this represented a TOA and not a hemorrhagic ovarian cyst. Also, CT with contrast misses about 5% of appendicitis cases, so that remained a possibility.[17] Some of my own research has focused on nonoperative treatment of uncomplicated appendicitis with antibiotics, including outpatient management, which has been demonstrated to be safe and effective.[18] Also, while urinary symptoms and costovertebral angle tenderness were not described, pyelonephritis is among the alternative diagnoses found when appendicitis is first suspected and not confirmed by CT in women.[20] When in doubt—CYA—Cover the patient (and Yourself) by giving Antibiotics.

Note that Ashley vomited and was treated with an anti-emetic but there was no documentation that she was given and passed a PO challenge before discharge, violating the basic emergency care "road-test" tenet and supporting the plaintiff's argument that hospitalization was required. So, it was not clear if she could have even taken oral antibiotics. The 2002 and 2021 CDC STI guidelines do not endorse routine hospitalization of adolescents with PID, but both list TOA as an indication for hospital admission and parenteral antibiotics.

Death from PID/TOA is rare, particularly in young healthy women. Ashley's abscess was 3 cm, relatively small, and in most instances would be successfully treated with antibiotics alone and no drainage. Most mortality associated with PID, rare as it may be, is related with TOA rupture, which in some even previously healthy individuals can elicit an exuberant and catastrophic inflammatory response.[19]

No studies exist in which patients with suspected life-threatening infections are randomized to immediate or delayed therapy and then followed for their outcome. Therefore, causation is largely expert opinion based on known outcomes of disease in general, the health of the host, their condition and extent of the infection at the time of the possible earlier diagnosis, the virulence and susceptibility of the infecting organism(s), and the time between the possible earlier and actual treatment.

Had Ashley been started on antibiotics about 3 days sooner than she was and hospitalized (or discharged with closer follow-up) at time of the first ED visit, it could be contended that she would have survived for the following reasons:

- Mortality in treated TOA in a young healthy individual is rare.
- Had she not initially responded or worsened, she could have had drainage prior to rupture.
- Had the abscess ruptured, she could have received earlier operative and hemodynamic support.

A causation defense strategy is that earlier antibiotics would not necessarily have prevented abscess rupture and its inflammatory consequences.

## VIII. Author Summary (Weinstock)

What can we learn from ***this*** tragic case?

1. It is easier to defend not ordering an inappropriate test than not acting on an abnormal result. We said this in a previous case and it is true here also.
    - Getting a WBC count was destructive to the doctors at ED #1 from a legal standpoint since they had to defend against several allegations that an infection was missed.
    - When she presented to ED#2, the WBC count was 2.5, prompting the surgeons to recommend admission for observation of gastroenteritis, delaying her care. If you are ordering a WBC count because you think the surgeon will want it (a very charitable thing to do), ask the surgeon first if he/she will testify for you when you send home a "gastroenteritis" patient with an elevated WBC count who ends up having appendicitis or a 15 year-old girl with an elevated WBC count who you think has a hemorrhagic ovarian cyst. Would guess the answer would be "No."
2. When accepting a handoff patient, plan on accepting the patient as your own.
3. Perform a repeat abdominal exam.
    - Before ED discharge reassess at bedside with a documented repeat abdominal exam. This will serve to pick up progression of disease and to allow for additional discussion time to complete the "big close."
4. Inform the patient and family/friends about diagnostic uncertainty.
    - If Ashley's mother understood the radiologist's reading was suggestive of hemorrhagic ovarian cyst and not diagnostic, she may have returned earlier to be re-evaluated … and this chapter would never have been written.

**Author comments (Weinstock):** Thanks to both of the initial ED doctors for making this information available and discussing the intricacies of the case, as well as to the multiple subsequent physicians who cared enough to remember the patient and take the time to explain their thoughts. This case was an EM RAP segment including interviews with multiple physicians who cared for Ashley.

## References

1. Rosen MP, Siewert B, Sands DZ, et al. Value of abdominal CT in the emergency department for patients with abdominal pain. European Radiology 2003;13(2):418-24.
2. Snyder BK, Hayden SR. Accuracy of leukocyte count in the diagnosis of acute appendicitis. Ann Emerg Med 1999;33:565-74.
3. Silver BE, Patterson JW, Kulick M, et al. Effect of CBC results on ED management of women with lower abdominal pain. Am J Emerg Med 1995:13(3):304-6.
4. Committee on the Quality of Health Care in America, Institute of Medicine. To Err Is Human: Building a Safer Health System. Washington, DC: National Academies Press 2000:36.

5. WHO Collaborating Centre for Patient Safety Solutions. Communication during patient hand-overs. Patient Safety Solutions 2007;1:Solution 3.
6. Joint Commission. 2006 critical access hospital and hospital national patient safety goals #2E. Available at: http://www.jointcommission.org/PatientSafety/ NationalPatientSafetyGoals/06_npsg_cah.htm
7. Cheung DS. Improving handoffs in the emergency department. Ann Emerg Med 2010;55:171-80.
8. Apker J, Mallak LA, Applegate EB 3rd, et al. Exploring emergency physician–hospitalist handoff interactions: development of the handoff communication assessment. Ann Emerg Med 2010;55(2):161-70.
9. Vincent Young M, Phillips A. et al. Why do people sue doctors? A study of patients and relative taking legal action. Lancet 1994;343(8913):1609-13.
10. Workowski KA, Bachmann LH, Chan PA, et al. CDC. Sexually transmitted infections treatment guidelines, 2021. MMWR Recomm Rep 2021 70(4):1-187.
11. CDC. Sexually transmitted diseases treatment guidelines 2002. MMWR Recomm Rep 2002;51(RR-6):1-78.
12. Cho HW, Koo YJ, Min KJ, et al. Pelvic inflammatory disease in virgin women with tubo-ovarian abscess: A single-center experience and literature review. J Pediatr Gynecol 2017:30(2):203-208
13. Farrukh S, Sivitiz AB, Onogul B, et al. The additive value of pelvic examinations to history in predicting sexually transmitted infections for young female patients with suspected cervicitis or pelvic inflammatory disease. Ann Emerg Med 2018;72(6):703-712.
14. Refinetti R. The circadian rhythm of body temperature. Front Biosci 2010;15(1):564-594.
15. Lunny C, Taylor D, Hoang L, et al. Self-collected versus clinician-collected sampling for chlamydia and gonorrhea screening: a systemic review and meta-analysis. PLOS One 2015;10(7):e0132776
16. Gaydos CA, Ako MC, Lewis M, Hsieh YH, Rothman RE, et al. Use of a rapid diagnostic for Chlamydia trachomatis and Neisseria gonorrhoeae for women in the emergency department can improve clinical management: report of a randomized clinical trial. Ann Emerg Med 2019:74(1):36-44.
17. Rud B, Vejborg TS, Rappeport ED, Reitsma JB, et al. Computed tomography for diagnosis of acute appendicitis in adults. Cochrane Database Syst Rev 2019;2019(11):CD009977
18. Talan DA, Moran GJ, Krishnadasan A, et al. — The CODA Collaborative. Analysis of outcomes associated with outpatient management of nonoperatively-treated patients with appendicitis. JAMA Netw Open 2022;5(7):e2220039.
19. Mickal A, Sellmann AH, Beebe JL. Ruptured tuboovarian abscess. Am J Obstet Gynecol 1968;100(3):432-6.
20. Pooler BD, Lawrence EM, Pickhardt PJ. Alternative diagnoses to suspected appendicitis at CT. Radiology 2012;265(3):733-742.

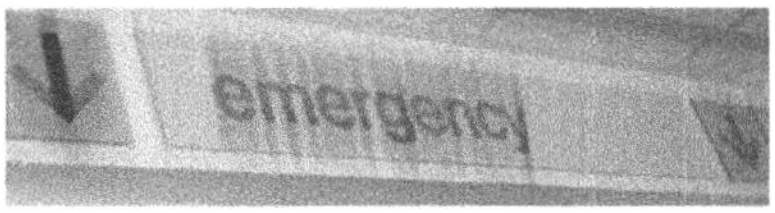


# Case 9

## A 46 Year-old Male with Neck Pain: Pounding a Square Peg into a Round Hole

**Primary case authors:**
**Thomas Blackwell**
**Stephen Colucciello**

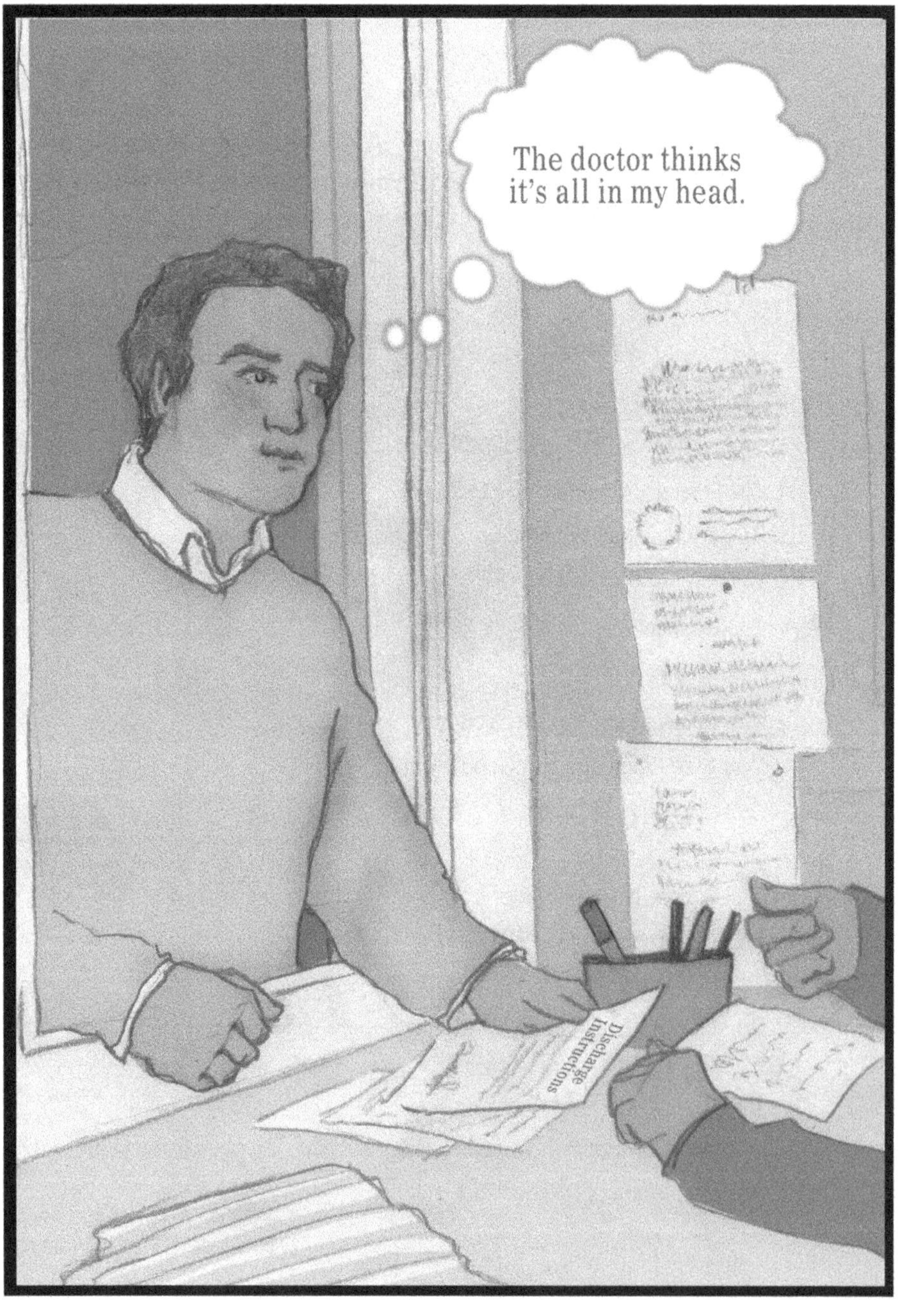
The doctor thinks it's all in my head.
Discharge Instructions

# Case 9

## A 46 Year-old Male with Neck Pain: Pounding a Square Peg into a Round Hole

The eye does not see what the mind does not know.

We are a proud bunch. Bizarre findings are often converted to a more plausible diagnosis, such as anxiety. The approach, "If I don't understand your pathology, chances are that it isn't real," leaves us with the "spackle" (the putty used for filling holes in dry wall) to fill the gaps in our knowledge. Of these spackling diagnoses, one of the most frequent is "anxiety."

***Deep thoughts:***

1. *Is the resolution of neurological symptoms reassuring?*
2. *Does diaphoresis suggest a more serious illness?*
3. *When we hear hoof beats, when is it time to go zebra hunting?*
4. *What constitutes adequate documentation of informed refusal (against medical advice/AMA)?*

**PART 1—MEDICAL**

## I. The Patient's Story

Steven Heller is a 46 year-old man who lives in a rural community. His daily commute is long; 90 minutes each way to the mill, where he works performing skilled heavy labor. He is happily married to Lauren with two children, an 11 year-old son and a 14 year-old daughter, Zach and Carolyn.

While driving home from work one warm, end-of-summer evening, Steve develops neck pain, a feeling his hands are not coordinated and a shaky feeling. Feeling unsafe to drive further, he pulls over to the side of the road and dials 911. While waiting for the medics to arrive, he also calls his wife.

At home with their kids, Lauren receives Steve's call. He is scared—this is not like him. She quickly gets the children in the car and drives them to her mom's house. On her way to the hospital she receives another call from Steve; dialing from the back of the squad. He says simply, "I think I'm dying."

At 9:02 PM, the paramedics arrive at the emergency department:

## II. The Doctor's Version (the following is the actual documentation of the provider)

**Date:** September 6

**Chief Complaint:** Severe left neck pain, blurry vision, loss of coordination both upper extremities
**Nurse note (21:10):** While driving home from work, the patient experienced an onset of severe neck

pain, shakiness and uncoordinated hands. He pulled over and called 911. Now, without symptoms.

**History of Present Illness (21:32):** 46 year-old male was brought in by ambulance after a frightening episode while driving home from work. He has never had a similar episode. He was fine earlier in the day. He was driving home when he felt hot, felt a sharp pain in left side of his neck, got shaky and felt frightened and uncoordinated. He then pulled to the side of the road, called 911 and was transported to the hospital. His symptoms improved during the ambulance ride. Now he feels normal. He reports no pain or weakness. No fever. However, he did report diaphoresis while in the car.

**Past Medical History:**
**Allergies:** NKDA Meds: None PMH/PSH: Negative
**FH:** Both parents had cancer
**Soc Hx:** ½ pack per day tobacco use and occasional alcohol use

**Physical Examination (21:34)**

Vital Signs

| Time | Temp(C) | Rt. | Pulse | Resp | Syst | Diast | Pos. | $O_2$ sat | RA Pain |
|---|---|---|---|---|---|---|---|---|---|
| 21:10 | 37.1 | 0 | 76 | 18 | 160 | 90 | U | 98% | 10 |

**Constitutional:** Alert and oriented, speaking and answering questions normally. No distress
**Throat:** Normal pharynx, no swelling or exudate
**Neck:** Supple; non-tender; no cervical lymphadenopathy, Full ROM and no JVD
**Cardio:** Regular rate and rhythm, no murmurs, rubs or gallops
**Resp:** Breath sounds clear and equal bilaterally; no wheezes, rhonchi, or rales
**Abd:** BS+, soft, Non-distended
**Skin:** Normal for age and race; warm and dry; no apparent lesions
**Neuro:** Symmetrical motor and normal sensation, CN 2-12 WNL, gait normal

**Emergency Department Course:**
**21:45** – The patient's wife arrives in the ED
**22:00 to 24:00** – Testing:

- **ECG** – NSR @ 90 bpm, no acute st-t changes, no ectopy, early repolarization
- **CXR** – No acute disease, no pneumothorax
- **CT head** – No intracranial bleed, disease or abnormality (read by tele-radiologist)
- Laboratory results including CBC, BMP, and troponin are all normal

**Medical Decision-Making Note:** Patient ambulatory without signs and symptoms of CVA or cardiac disease. Patient prefers to go home and follow up with his doctor.

**Diagnosis: (00:15)**
Neck pain of undetermined etiology – suspect musculoskeletal
Stress related anxiety reaction
Situational stress at work
**Plan:** Follow up with Dr. Abby Macerolla in 2–3 days if any recurrence of symptoms. Rx for Ativan 1 mg at bedtime (avoid if driving or at work). Return to ER if any symptom worsens.

*Jim Carozza, MD*

## III. Risk Management/Patient Safety Opportunities (Klauer)

**Author comments (Weinstock):** Though the ultimate diagnosis is not always found at the first encounter, we feel compelled to provide the patient with a final product, a diagnosis. All good things, including ED visits, must come to an end, but that does not mean the evaluation is completed. The art is recognizing when a diagnosis is premature, and when our testing does not have adequate sensitivity to exclude the disease we are looking for.

**Risk Management/Patient Safety Opportunity #1:**

**Opportunity:** Inadequate history.
**Discussion:** Read the HPI again; it is mostly a restatement of the triage chief complaint, then a bunch of stuff that is obvious. Unless of course it was dictated at the end of the shift and not much was remembered. "The patient was well until he had symptoms" (really?). "The symptoms brought him to the ED" (really?) "and now the symptoms are better." OK. Additionally, the ROS are a bit brief: "he reports no pain or weakness." What's our differential here?
✔ **Teaching point:** Now at Case 9, we can't even apologize for being a broken record, so we will be succinct: "History is king."

**Risk Management/Patient Safety Opportunity #2:**

**Opportunity:** Inadequate neurological examination.
**Discussion:** Many cases which proceed to litigation have only a cursory explanation of the chief complaint. A good rule of thumb is to document by focusing on the question the patient's presentation is asking, as if we expect a misdiagnosis to occur—the billing/coding requirements should be secondary. For instance, in undifferentiated abdominal pain in a 12 year-old male patient, an independent physical examination for testicular torsion and appendicitis needs to be performed. These are questions the RLQ pain patient's presentation is asking. In head injury cases, the neurological examination should be performed and at times, repeated.

In cases of neurological complaints, we should be focused on diagnoses of key clinical entities such as stroke, TIA, subarachnoid hemorrhage, neck artery dissection. The examination should reflect consideration of these life-threatening entities.

"Symmetrical motor and normal sensation, CN 2–12 WNL, gait normal" as was documented in this case, might be enough for an ankle sprain or GU complaint. However, when the presentation is neurological, a neurological examination is required. Items such as mental status, cranial nerve assessment, motor strength, sensation, and cerebellar function should be included.

"Can I claim a thoughtful, careful evaluation and documentation for the possibility of serious neurological pathology?" This doctor could not.
✔ **Teaching point:** The history and exam should focus on the area of chief complaint.

**Risk Management/Patient Safety Opportunity #3:**

**Opportunity:** Lack of recognition of serious neurological symptoms.

**Discussion:** Until we have been humbled by an unusual vascular distribution for ischemic stroke or TIA, we are often quick to dismiss nonspecific neurologically-based symptoms. "Failure to diagnose" results in loss of the end-game before we even get started.

Unfortunately, the complexity of stroke syndromes is nearly endless. We have two choices:

- Learn every possible variation
- Recognize the complexity of the issue and our limitations

Both need to be done while resisting the temptation to explain away what we do not recognize as lacking a vascular distribution. It is the variation in presentations resulting from perforating vessel occlusion, watershed infarcts (often including the borders of multiple vascular regions), leptomeningeal artery (terminal end artery) infarcts and other partial vascular distribution strokes that are overlooked by the inexperienced or busy physician.

Adding further to confusion is carotid or vertebrobasilar dissection. These dissections often result in embolic phenomena, prompting symptomatology along the distribution of the dissecting vessel. A differentiating factor is pain, rarely present in traditional ischemic strokes or TIAs.

Although this patient didn't have a headache, his initial symptom was severe neck pain; such pain, followed by neurological symptoms, should prompt serious consideration for dissection. Do the neurological symptoms fit a potential vascular distribution of the vessels known to dissect in the neck? We may be able to discount the patient's report of "shakiness" and fright as too non-specific. However, upper extremity incoordination makes sense from a posterior/cerebella circulation perspective.
✔ **Teaching point:** If there is a question about unexplained neurological symptoms, consider admission.

**Risk Management/Patient Safety Opportunity #4:**

**Opportunity:** Overreliance on normal tests.
**Discussion:** A common error made in diagnostic data analysis is to assign more value to a test than is deserved. An excellent example is the white blood cell count (WBC) used in the decision-making process for the evaluation for appendicitis; how is a test which is only about 50% sensitive (and less in children) helpful?[1-3] Many of our surgical colleagues have assigned unwarranted importance on a normal WBC count. We've all heard the response on the other end of the phone, "Their white count is normal. They can't have appendicitis." Absurd!

Making dispositions for patients with neurological symptoms on the basis of a normal CT scan is similar. In TIA patients the CT would be expected to be normal. Even the MR is not 100% sensitive.
✔ **Teaching point:** Normal neuroimaging study does not rule out TIA/Stroke and should not factor into disposition decisions.

**Risk Management/Patient Safety Opportunity #5:**

**Opportunity:** Using the diagnosis of anxiety without clinical basis.
**Discussion:** Diagnosing anxiety should make us anxious, even though it is such a significant part of our practice. Sometimes we pound these square diagnoses repeatedly until they fit into the round hole we are working with. Here's one for Bartlett's book of quotations, "Everyone dies, even if they have anxiety." Here's another, "Are there any patients in the process of dying who do ***not*** feel anxious?"

How can we avoid this? First, when considering an anxiety diagnosis, put the hammer away. If the diagnosis doesn't fit, then don't force it:

- If a patient doesn't have a previous anxiety diagnosis with history of similar symptoms in the past, use caution in initiating this diagnosis.
- If a patient isn't reporting the symptom of anxiety prior to the somatic symptoms, it is unlikely that anxiety provoked the event.
- Inform patients that we do not have definitive objective testing for anxiety, so if somatic symptoms progress or change, a return visit is mandatory.

When there is an adverse outcome, the use of the diagnosis "Anxiety" is likely to weaken the defense's case. Juries do not take kindly to assigning a psychiatric diagnosis to a plaintiff with real pathology. To the lay juror, this is the equivalent of the doctor saying, "It's all in your head."(See cartoon at the beginning of this chapter!)
✔ **Teaching point:** Unless a patient has a known history of anxiety and has experienced previous similar symptoms, resist the temptation to attribute the symptoms to anxiety.

**Risk Management/Patient Safety Opportunity #6:**

**Opportunity:** Poor medical decision-making.
**Discussion:** The first diagnosis is: *Neck pain of undetermined etiology—suspect musculoskeletal.* Now flip back to the neck exam: *Supple; non-tender; no cervical lymphadenopathy, Full ROM and no JVD.* … you do the math.
✔ **Teaching point:** It is hard to explain neck pain as musculoskeletal when the exam documents a neck which is non-tender with palpation and full range of motion.

**Risk Management/Patient Safety Opportunity #7:**

**Opportunity:** Not formally recommending admission.
**Discussion:** Should our patient be admitted? Though that question can be debated, one point cannot: it is not up to the patient to make the diagnosis and decide the disposition. What's the deal with the phrase, "the patient prefers to go home?" Unless the patient has subjective pain with ureterolithiasis, the doctor should decide if the patient needs a "room at the inn."
✔ **Teaching point:** If a patient requires admission, document your recommendation.

**Risk Management/Patient Safety Opportunity #8:**

**Opportunity:** Not obtaining an informed refusal.
**Discussion:** The doctrine of informed consent includes informed refusal. Just as patients need to have the capacity to consent to treatment or a procedure, they must also possess the capacity to refuse. If a patient is not oriented to person, place, time and situation and is not of the age of majority (18–21 years-old, depending on the jurisdiction), he or she doesn't have the capacity to consent or refuse. Use of the term "capacity" is not incidental or casual, but it is a legal term which is differentiated from "competence," assigned by legal proceeding, not healthcare providers.
✔ **Teaching point:** Casual conversations about admission to "buff the chart" are ill advised, as reflected in the following exchange.

In this case, it is curious that the physician's documentation includes a statement that the patient would "prefer to go home." Admission was not specifically offered. Reading between the lines, the physician is hedging his bet. He may not feel admission is warranted, but he also finds reassurance that the patient would prefer discharge. Herein lies the problem; this is a dangerous tight rope to walk. Any good plaintiff's attorney, worth the price of his penny loafers, will trap a physician in his or her own web in less than ten minutes:

**Attorney:** So Doctor, you discussed admission with the plaintiff.
**Defendant:** Yes, I did.

**Attorney:** So you must have felt that admission was warranted.
**Defendant:** Well, it was one option.

**Attorney:** So, Mr. Jones refused admission?
**Defendant:** Not exactly. He said he would prefer to go home.

**Attorney:** Doctor, can you advise the jury what the elements are of an informed refusal?
**Defendant (option 1):** No. I can't.

**Attorney:** Then it is clear that you could not have obtained an informed refusal from my client.
**Defendant (option 2):** Yes. I can. The patient must have the capacity to refuse, must be old enough to consent or refuse, and must understand the risks and benefits of the proposed treatment, any treatment alternatives and the option of no treatment at all.

**Attorney:** Did you go through this process with Mr. Jones?
**Defendant:** No, I did not.

## IV. Against Medical Advice (AMA) Documentation (Weinstock)

The seminal decision "Against Medical Advice" (AMA), sometimes called "The Cardozo Doctrine," was made by Justice Benjamin Cardozo (1870–1938), subsequently appointed to the United States Supreme Court by President Herbert Hoover to succeed Justice Oliver Wendall Holmes; "Seldom in the history of the Court has an appointment been so universally commended." (***New York Times***, February 16, 1932, p. 1)

The case was ***Schloendorff v. Society of New York Hospital***. The plaintiff, Mary Schloendorff, was admitted to New York Hospital in January 1908 suffering from "some disorder of the stomach." She consented to being examined under ether, but not to have surgery. The surgeon found a fibroid tumor and, while Mary was under the effects of the ether, proceeded to remove it. She suffered from infection and developed gangrene of her fingers with ensuing amputation and severe pain. The non-profit hospital was sued with the intention to hold the institution responsible for the actions of its employees.

The New York Court of Appeals (1914), in an opinion written by Justice Cardozo, found the action constituted medical battery. The decision established principles of informed consent and ***respondeat superior*** (legal obligations of an employer for the actions of its employee) in U.S. law. Per Cardozo: "Every human being of adult years and sound mind has a right to determine what shall be done with his own body; and a surgeon who performs an operation without his patient's consent commits an assault, for which he is liable in damages. This is true except in cases of emergency where the patient is unconscious and where it is necessary to operate before consent can be obtained."

Of note, the Schloendorff Rule was another byproduct: A non-profit hospital could not be sued for the actions of its employees. This was eventually overruled in 1957 in ***Bing v. Thunig.***

Five items to document when a patient leaves against medical advice (AMA):

1. Patient is adult or emancipated minor.
2. Patient is of sound mind (Documentation can include specific questioning of each component of A&OX3 and/or that the patient does understand/comprehend the implications of her or his actions).
3. Patient has been informed of potential consequences of non-treatment.
4. Family, friends and/or the patient's physician have been involved in the decision-making process.
5. There is a signature on the AMA form of patient, family member, physician and nurse.

## V. The Bounceback

After discharge from the ED, Steve leaves his car on the side of the road and drives home with his wife. They plan to get up early and for Lauren to drop him at his car so he can drive to work and she can return home to get the kids to school.

The alarm rings early. Sluggish from a 5 AM arousal, Lauren rolls over to wake her husband, but he is unresponsive. Through her panic, she dials 911. The paramedics arrive and take Steve to the closest hospital, a small rural ED about 30 minutes from their home:

**ED visit #2**

Presents to ED per medics at 06:03.

- Physical examination: Temp 36.6, pulse 70, RR 10, BP 150/70, sat 95%. His extremities are flaccid. He can open his eyes but is unable to speak.
- Testing: Brain CT—normal.
- A decision is made to transport to tertiary care center. Intubated prior to transport.
- He is flown to the regional tertiary care facility (the same ED where he was originally seen).

**Tertiary care hospitalization:** The patient maintains stable vitals, is unresponsive and all four extremities are flaccid.

- He is seen by vascular surgery, neurology and cardiology.
- Advanced imaging reveals a left vertebral artery dissection with brainstem infarct. There is no flow in right vertebral artery.
- The patient is admitted with prolonged hospital stay. There is only minimal improvement of motor and cognitive function.
- A G-tube is placed, and a tracheostomy is performed.

**Final Diagnosis:** Quadriplegia secondary to brainstem infarct, left vertebral artery dissection with non-patent right vertebral artery.

**Disposition:** He is discharged with need for extensive convalescent care, including ventilator support.

# PART 2—LEGAL

## I. The Accusation/Cause of Action

- Failure to admit.
- Failure to obtain consultation or transfer for further evaluation.
- Failure to recognize TIA or stroke in evolution.

- Failure to perform a complete diagnostic evaluation that would have identified the dissection.

At deposition, Steve's wife, Lauren, told a powerful and heart-rending story. She described how the children were now in middle and high school. They didn't go to the hospital and never got to speak with their father again.

## II. Witness Statements and Depositions (summary)

**Deposition of the initial ED physician:**

- The patient was observed for over three hours in the Emergency Department.
- The patient had a very stressful event with his employer at work, which he did not document in the medical record.
- The symptoms were best explained by stress and an anxiety reaction.
- His tests were all normal and he had no signs or symptoms of stroke or TIA while in the ED.
- There was no need for admission.

**Deposition of Lauren Heller (patient's spouse):**

- She and her husband knew something was wrong, since he never asks for help.
- The fact that he pulled over while driving and called 911 was evidence that something out of the ordinary had occurred.
- She was "scared" to take him home, since they lived 1½ hours away from the hospital.
- She described how the loss impacted their children.

**Deposition of defense expert:**

- Really tough case.
- Very easy with hindsight bias to say what should have been done during ED visit #1. Unfortunately, patient presented after a profound event while driving, and rather than listening to his wife or taking into consideration the rural location and difficult access to further medical care, the ED physician chose to attribute the event to social stress and anxiety.
- If the patient had been admitted to hospital #1 for observation, he most likely would have had the same outcome.

## III. What Would Greg Do (WWGD)?

**Greg Henry, MD**
Past president of The American College of Emergency Physicians (ACEP)
Past Professor of Emergency Medicine at the University of Michigan

Greg discusses diagnosis of vertebral artery dissection, differentiation of functional vs. organic complaints, settlement vs. trial and his two pet peeves.

**"If you call an organic process psychiatric, we have another name for you—the defendant"**

This case allows me to speak about two pet peeves: The first is the psychiatric diagnosis. If you call a psychiatric process organic, it's hard to go wrong. However, if you call an organic process psychiatric, we have another name for you—the defendant. It's interesting we have a gentleman with no psychiatric history who is given the diagnosis of anxiety when he presented with symptoms which are referable to one anatomic area. Can I find a single anatomic location for this patient's symptoms? Absolutely, it's in the posterior fossa, involves either the upper part of the vertebral and or basilar artery. It is perfectly explainable. The fact that the symptoms waxed and waned should be supportive of a transient ischemic attack (TIA).

When a patient presents with an obvious anatomic location, referable to a specific vascular pattern, we need a specific vascular diagnosis. The tendency to call it psychiatric means that we have decided to blame the patient for the illness. No matter how anxious the patient looks at any one moment in time, the better part of valor is to assume an organic condition. This approach rarely gets anyone into trouble.

The second pet peeve is the exam. Whenever a diagnosis is potentially neurological, a neurological exam should be on the chart. I know I sound like a broken record on this issue, but nothing beats a real examination. The process forces you to think anatomically about the regions in the nervous system that may be supplied by certain vascular territories.

A negative CT scan means just that, there is not obvious disease on the film at this time. The performance of a CT scan seems to be more religious ritual than a scientific pursuit of information, similar to believing if you stay under the covers the monster under the bed can't eat you. We do not expect positive CT findings with a TIA.

Regarding settlement, it definitely needs to be explored and pursued. This case is not defensible on a standards basis; if a patient is diagnosed with TIA, the standard of care is to pursue the work-up of TIA. Check the ECG for dysrhythmias. Arrange an ECHO and carotid study. Start antiplatelet therapy, such as aspirin or Clopidogrel. A great plaintiff's expert, who actually knows how to speak to a jury, could finish this physician off in a nanosecond.

The real question of worth in this case is: was the outcome inevitable? This is very difficult to say because there is only minimal proof that anticoagulation helps in the posterior fossa for prevention of further disease. But all of this science needs to be put aside—this will be tried in front of a jury which believes that you are better off in medical hands when bad things happen.

I would push for settlement.

## IV. Trial/Settlement

What did the defense decide to do? They settled following the wife's deposition. Clearly, any jury would view the plaintiff and his family sympathetically. Although the adjudication of any case should be carried out fairly without bias, a jury of the patient's peers, not the physician's, will judge the facts presented. When the jury can relate to the travails of the plaintiff and the financial need is obvious, jurors often side with plaintiff compensation rather than minimizing financial impact to the physician (which will just be paid by the insurance company anyway, right?). Many view a medical malpractice policy as a "patient compensation fund" for those who have experienced a bad outcome.

Dissecting this case and assessing the likelihood of a defense verdict reveals several additional weaknesses:

- The symptoms suggest a neurological etiology; unfortunately the physician placed too much weight on resolution of symptoms and a normal CT scan. Additionally, the neurological examination was minimal, allowing the plaintiff's attorney to discredit the physician by asserting an incomplete evaluation was the basis for misdiagnosis.

- A cursory discussion about admission occurred, implying the physician considered it and then dismissed it. He recorded that the patient preferred to be discharged, but an informed refusal was not obtained. They would contend that if the patient was told that he may have had a TIA with potential for ensuing severe neurologic consequences, he would have preferred admission.

**Outcome:** A non-disclosure agreement was signed at the time of settlement, therefore the exact amount is unknown, but it is estimated to have been between $100,000 and $200,000.

## V. What Would Greg Do (WWGD)? (Further discussion now that he knows the legal outcome)

I was not surprised that this case was settled by the defense; but I am surprised that the ***plaintiff*** was willing to settle. A case such as this could have tremendous value depending on the stupidity of the physician, the likeability of the family and the amount of rage that can be created in a jury. For the insurance company to obtain an indemnity payment of only $100K and $200K speaks to its brilliance. To try the case would have cost $100K, so the extra amount is minimal—this had the best possible outcome for the physician.

For the plaintiff to win at trial, the key is teaching the jury the anatomic basis of diagnosis. This disease entity is often referred to as the Count of Monte Cristo syndrome. As it turns out, the Count of Monte Cristo didn't actually have this syndrome, but in the novel a character is described as "a corpse with living eyes"— a posterior fossa syndrome affecting the basilar artery and everything including the pons. Since the lowest cranial nerve that is functioning is the third cranial nerve, this "corpse" was able to look up and down but not side to side since that would involve the sixth nerve nuclei.

As the case progressed, the plaintiff's counsel would merely quiz the doctor as to the fact that such cases have been known for over 150 years. He could then have the doctor draw out the posterior fossa anatomy showing where the vertebral arteries joined to form the basilar artery and the posterior communicating arteries and describe how those symptoms are generally not right-or left-sided. There are other ways that this can be presented, but in all of the scenarios, the physician loses.

The defense strategy is simple: admit to stupidity regarding the anxiety diagnosis up front and concentrate on the proximate cause relationship between missing the diagnosis and the ultimate locked-in syndrome; basically saying that even if the diagnosis was made, it would not have changed the outcome.

## VI. The Legal Analysis—Guest Interview

**Jennifer L'Hommedieu Stankus, MD, JD**
Emergency Medicine physician
Former medical malpractice defense attorney and military magistrate

**Authors:** *Should the defense have settled this case?*
**JS:** Without question, this case should have been settled at the earliest possible juncture. It would not be

defensible in court, and the trial costs alone are close to the settlement amount. Frankly, I'm amazed that the family settled for so little. I don't know what was going through their minds; perhaps they simply wanted an acknowledgement by the physician that there was a major failing, even gross negligence. Sadly, failure to recognize dissection is not an uncommon malpractice occurrence; when things don't add up, go back and re-examine. If there are any signs of focal neurologic deficits, at any point, something more needs to be done, be it a consult, a CTA of head and neck—something. To rule out TIA/CVA with a noncontrast CT is completely inappropriate, amounting to malpractice.

**Authors:** *How would you defend the case?*
**JS:** With a Hail Mary. The only way to defend this case is causation; the outcome would have been the same regardless of timely and proper diagnosis; failing to meet the standard of care did not affect the outcome. An expert could be found to argue both sides, but it's a crap shoot. Who would the jury believe? They will almost always side with the more sympathetic party, which is the grieving family, not the "rich doctor."

**Authors:** *What could have been done differently at the initial ED visit to make the case more defensible?*
**JS:** Be very careful about diagnoses on discharge, particularly when it is unclear. Labeling this as anxiety is inappropriate at best. The patient has no history of anxiety, so you are telling the jury that you thought this was "all in his head." The funny thing is ... this was all in his head, but in a very organic way. [Authors' note: see illustration at the beginning of this case.] Nothing will turn a jury's angry eye onto you faster than labeling the patient or making judgments in the medical record, particularly without foundation. In this case, it made the physician look careless, foolish and dismissive. It is true that when patients experience the symptoms of a dissection pulmonary embolism (PE) or ACS, they often feel anxious or like they are going to die. Yes, a sensation of impending death is anxiety-provoking.

**Authors:** *If the case had proceeded to trial, how would the plaintiff approach the questioning?*
**JS:** Consider these potential questions from the plaintiff's attorney:

- "And clearly, doctor, you didn't even do a thorough neurologic exam." What vascular causes should one think of in a hypertensive male when there are focal neurologic deficits?
- Aren't emergency medicine doctors trained to recognize the most life-threatening problems? Isn't vertebral artery dissection such a problem?
- And tell me, doctor, why you ordered a CT scan of the head? Was it to rule out a stroke or TIA? Can you enlighten the jury on what percentage of the time this scan would be helpful in making that diagnosis?
- "I see ... so you sent Steve Heller, a husband and father to two loving children, home with a new diagnosis of 'anxiety,' on the basis of a CT scan which misses a stroke most of the time."

**Authors:** *How should this encounter been documented?*
**JS:** Even if not explicitly stated in a progress note, your differential should be reflected in the HPI and ROS. As emergency physicians, we are trained to rule out the bad things first. It is impossible to know what this physician was thinking from his scant notes, but it appears from the record and the decision to image that TIA or stroke was on the list. If that was true, the patient should have been admitted.

## VII. Medical Discussion—Evaluation of Neck Pain, Diagnosis of Vertebral and Carotid Artery Discussion

**Thomas Blackwell, MD**
Carolinas Medical Center
Emergency Medicine Physician

**Stephen Colucciello, MD**
Clinical Professor Emergency Medicine Wake Forest Medical School
Vice Chair Emergency Medicine Carolinas Medical Center

Introduction

- Remember one thing... Neck pain plus neurological symptoms = Dissection.
- If you are to remember a second thing, think dissection if a young person presents with an apparent stroke.

For you overachievers, there are a few more things to remember (not nearly as important as the first two):

- If the neurologic complaint is unilateral limb weakness, it's often (but not always) anterior circulation (carotid).
- If symptoms are bilateral, facial, vary between right and left, are accompanied by dizziness or nausea, or are just plain confusing, it's posterior circulation (vertebral).

**Brief look at the demographics and pathophysiology:**

Dissections of the carotid and vertebral arteries are rare with a combined incidence of only about 3 cases per 100,000; however, they do account for about 25% of all ischemic strokes in the young (30 to 45 years of age). Carotid dissections are about 3 to 5 times more common than vertebral artery dissections.[1]

The anatomy of any artery consists of three layers from inner to outer; the intima, the media, and the adventitia. A dissection occurs when the wall of the artery is compromised and blood collects between the layers of the wall and causes vascular occlusion as it expands in the intramural space.

The clinical presentation is typically an acute onset of unilateral neck pain often with a neurologic deficit. Confusingly, neurological symptoms are often delayed or not present at time of the initial evaluation. However, a neurological deficit will manifest in about 70% of dissections at some point during their progression.[2] The deficit might be permanent (stroke), or could be transient (TIA). Unfortunately, the transient deficits are often labeled as "anxiety-related" especially if the brainstem was compromised.

Complications of dissections include, but are not limited to, cerebellar and brainstem infarction, subarachnoid hemorrhage, and pseudoaneurysms which can cause a mass effect and compress nearby structures such as cranial nerves. Thrombi can also form and shower the brain with clots leading to infarctions. This embolic "shower" can result in apparently "non-anatomic" complaints since multiple and even bilateral territories can be involved.

Causes of cranio-cervical dissections can be from trauma including extreme neck positions or can be spontaneous. Since neurological symptoms might be a late presentation, patients might not even remember the inciting event. Precipitants may be as innocuous as quickly turning their head to parallel park, or prolonged neck extension while painting a ceiling. Of course, a trip to the chiropractor is the most infamous event leading to a dissection.

**Evaluation of neck pain:**
As with all emergency complaints, we need to quickly determine the age-old question, "sick or not sick?" An initial assessment should focus on "red flag" symptoms including major trauma, fever or chills, neurological symptoms, anterior neck pain, history of IV drug use, or unexplained weight loss. Any of these symptoms (plus a few more) should automatically raise your suspicion that someone could fall into the "sick" category.

The physical exam can often narrow your differential and help determine what imagining modalities or what interventions are indicated. Range of motion, muscle palpation, and most importantly, a detailed neurological exam to evaluate for weakness, paresthesias, or exacerbation of symptoms with specific movements/positions can refine your differential diagnosis.

Imaging of patients with a chief complaint of neck pain may be warranted with a history of trauma, progressive neurological findings, constitutional symptoms like fever and chills, infectious risk, history of malignancy, or persistent severe pain that prohibits daily activities. The most common forms of imaging in neck pain are plain radiography and MRI. CT scan is preferred in patients with a history of major trauma. MRI is the best study to evaluate the spinal cord, nerve roots, bone marrow, discs, and other soft tissues while plain X-rays can evaluate fractures, joint space narrowing, and osteoarthritis. A discussion on dissection imaging is below.

**Vertebral and carotid artery dissections:**
Carotid artery dissections are usually less of a diagnostic challenge than that of a vertebral artery dissection. They often occur in a patient who sustained trauma to the neck, and complains of pain of the head or face, with a neurological deficit contralateral to the pain. Unfortunately, the diagnosis is more difficult when the neurological symptoms resolve before presentation to the emergency department. Interestingly, some patients describe a "whooshing" noise in their ear which can actually represent their own carotid bruit. The physical exam may reveal a partial Horner syndrome; however, this is present in less than 50% of cases; assess for lid lag, a small pupil, ptosis, and miosis. Anhidrosis is rare. The physical exam findings may also be transient, confusing the diagnosis. If trauma-related, especially for patients involved in motor vehicle collisions, look for a seat belt sign to the neck. However, the vast majority of patients with a cervical seat belt sign do not have a carotid artery dissection. A seatbelt sign of the neck associated with a clavicular, cervical or facial fracture is more likely to be associated with a carotid injury than a seatbelt sign alone.

Vertebral artery dissections will usually present with neck pain and headache which is often times located in the occipital-cervical area. Minor trauma often precedes the pain. About 70% of patients will describe some type of neurological deficits which may present later in the progression if the disease.

Neurologic symptoms may include:

- Recent major or minor trauma (twisting neck, chiropractic manipulation)
- Occipital headache, often with neck pain
- Brainstem symptoms, such as:
    - ◊ Nausea and vomiting
    - ◊ Ataxia or clumsiness
    - ◊ Facial numbness, pain, or weakness
    - ◊ Vertigo
    - ◊ Visual complaints including double vision
    - ◊ Trouble swallowing or speaking

Physical exam findings can include:

- Posterior bruit
- Cranial nerve deficits
- Cerebellar findings (past pointing, truncal or limb ataxia)
- Motor deficit
- Problems with fine motor movement and proprioception

Imaging: The two most common imaging modalities are a CT or MR angiogram. If there is concern for intracranial blood such as a subarachnoid hemorrhage (SAH), first obtain non-contrast images of the brain (CT best) followed by the contrasted studies of the head and neck. An acute SAH is best seen on non-contrasted studies. Because of the difficulty of obtaining a STAT MRI, CT and CTA are often the first investigations obtained. CT scans can demonstrate ischemia or hemorrhage while the "A" in "CTA" can help identify any irregularities in the vascular lumen or thickening of an arterial wall. An MRI can detect an intimal flap and luminal thrombosis and any hyperintensity of the vessel wall visualized on T1-weighted imaging is considered pathognomonic. If both of those tests are unavailable at your facility, vascular duplex scanning can detect abnormal flow in about 95% of patients. However, it is only specific to dissection in 20% of patients so it is usually not recommended. In general, if you do not have either CTA or MRA/MRI, it is time to transfer the patient!

**Functional or organic?**

Distinguishing between anxiety and organic pathology is an important skill. How can we avoid confusing anxiety with serious neurological issues? If in doubt, assume organic disease but there are a few clues which increase the chance that the anxiety-related presentations are actually from anxiety:

a. Long history of recurrent anxiety-related complaints. The first visit to an ED for a supposed functional problem is a red flag (at least a pink flag).

b. Younger age of onset—It is less common to first develop an anxiety disorder in middle or advanced age; only about 15% of patients develop an anxiety disorder after age 40.

c. Classic anxiety-related complaints include:

- Shortness of breath
- Palpitations
- Light-headedness
- Trouble swallowing
- Chest pain
- Paresthesias (Of course these can also be symptoms of MI, PE or TIA)

d. Patients with organic complaints that are mistaken for anxiety are often middle-aged or older and have no prior history of anxiety-related complaints. Paralysis, ataxia, clumsiness, unilateral weakness, visual field cuts, diplopia and (especially) incontinence are not typical anxiety-related complaints. Although all of us have seen a case of hysterical paralysis, this diagnosis is made on the basis of covert observation, serial exams or neuroimaging. Any patient with hard neurological findings should be considered to have organic disease until proven otherwise, especially if neck pain is present!

e. Also remember that patients with anxiety disorders do get sick; functional illness does not protect against organic disease. You may have heard some cynical physicians profess that "Every turkey has their Thanksgiving."[3]

Many medical processes can present with psychiatric symptoms.[4] One study of 1,340 patients admitted to a VA psychiatric unit found that 2.8% of patients had psychiatric symptoms attributed to a medical disorder with factors contributing to a misdiagnosis including failure to obtain appropriate history (34%), inadequate physical exam (44%), failure to obtain necessary labs (34%), failure to address abnormal vitals (8%), failure to obtain indicated neuroimaging (3%), and lack of a mental status exam (all).[5] Some common medical emergencies that can present with psychiatric symptoms include coronary artery disease, pulmonary embolism, hypoglycemia, neurosyphilis, neuroendocrine tumors, and thyroid disorders. One study showed that in a cohort of low risk chest pain patients, 47% reported abnormal anxiety symptoms which lead to a high rate of re-presentation to the emergency department and a low rate of medical diagnoses.[6] Before assuming a patient's presentation is all psychiatric in nature, make sure organic disease can be safely ruled out.

**Treatment:**
Extracranial carotid and vertebral artery dissections are important to consider in patients who present with stroke-like symptoms, especially in younger patients. Like with anything in medicine, once a diagnosis is made, what's next? How are these patients treated? Carotid and vertebral artery dissections have been associated with a high risk of recurrent stroke. Markus, et al. used a randomized prospective parallel design study to assess if antiplatelet treatment or anticoagulation is a superior treatment option for these patients; 250 patients were assessed and after a twelve month follow-up period, there are no significant differences in either treatment arm when it came to prevention or stroke, or residual stenosis and occlusion when comparing antiplatelets or anticoagulation.[7]

Is there a role for tPA? Skepticism for the use of tPA remains high among clinicians when considering potential risks in these dissection patients. Risks considered include intramural hematoma extension, intraluminal thrombus dislocation and embolization, or development of a subarachnoid hemorrhage. Tsivgoulis et al. determined IV thrombolysis does not adversely affect dissection related ischemic stroke patients any more than regular acute ischemic stroke patients.[8]

The decision to administer IV thrombolytics after a confirmed dissection should be made between the emergency medicine provider and the neurology or neurosurgery team together.

Reperfusion rates after endovascular repair have also been studied. Hoving, et al. reviewed 16 studies that showed favorable clinical outcome and successful reperfusion in patients with a proximal intracranial occlusion and concomitant ICA dissection; they used a 90 day NIHSS and found that majority had a favorable outcome.[9]

**Diagnosis aids:**
The Denver and Memphis Screening criteria for blunt cerebral vascular injury (BCVI), can be used to help screen for vertebral and carotid artery dissections.[10]

## VIII. Author Summary (Weinstock)

Anyone who presents to the emergency department with a chief complaint of neck pain and any neurological symptom should have dissection on the top of the "can't miss" diagnoses. Obtain imaging quickly and call a specialist for help if the diagnosis is made.

## References

1. Lee VH, Brown RD, Jr., Mandrekar JN, et al. Incidence and outcome of cervical artery dissection: A population-based study. Neurology 2006;67:1809-12.
2. Rao AS, Makaroun MS, Marone LK, et al. Long-term outcomes of internal carotid artery dissection.

Vasc Surg 2011;54(2):370-75.
3. Tucci V, Siever K, Matorin A, et al. Down the rabbit hole: emergency department medical clearance of patients with psychiatric or behavioral emergencies. Emerg Med Clin North Am 2015;33(4):721-37.
4. Yeager-Cordial E, Ison J, Becker R, et al. Psychiatric manifestations of organic disease: Don't get fooled! J Urgent Care Med 2022;16(11):11-15.
5. Reeves RR, Parker JD, Loveless P, et al. Unrecognized physical illness prompting psychiatric admission. Ann Clin Psychiatry 2010;22(3):180-5. PMID: 20680191
6. Musey PI Jr, Patel R, Fry C, et al. Anxiety associated with increased risk for emergency department recidivism in patients with low-risk chest pain. Am J Cardiol 2018;122(7):1133-41. doi: 10.1016/j.amjcard.2018.06.044. Epub 2018 Jul 5. PMID: 30086878
7. Markus HS, Levi C, King A, et al. Cervical artery dissection in stroke study (CADISS) investigators. antiplatelet therapy vs anticoagulation therapy in cervical artery dissection: The cervical artery dissection in stroke study (CADISS) randomized clinical trial final results. JAMA Neurol 2019;76(6):657-64. doi: 10.1001/jamaneurol.2019.0072. PMID: 3080S1621; PMCID: PMC6563567
8. Tsivgoulis G, Alexandrov A, Chang J, et al. Safety and outcomes of intravenous thrombolysis in dissection-related ischemic stroke: An international multicenter study and comprehensive meta-analysis of reported case series. J Neurol 2015;262(9):2135-43. doi: 10.1007/s00415-015-7829-x. Epub 2015 Jun 25. PMID: 26108410
9. Hoving JW, Marquering HA, Majoie CBLM. Endovascular treatment in patients with carotid artery dissection and intracranial occlusion: A systematic review. Neuroradiology 2017;59(7):641-47. doi: 10.1007/s00234-017-1850-y. Epub 2017 Jun 3. PMID: 28580530; PMCID: PMC5493704
10. Kim DY, Biffl W, Bokhari F, et al. Evaluation and management of blunt cerebrovascular injury: A practice management guideline from the Eastern Association for the Surgery of Trauma. J Trauma Acute Care Surg 2020;88(6):875-87. doi: 10.1097/TA.0000000000002668. Erratum in: J Trauma Acute Care Surg 2020;89(2):420. PMID: 32176167

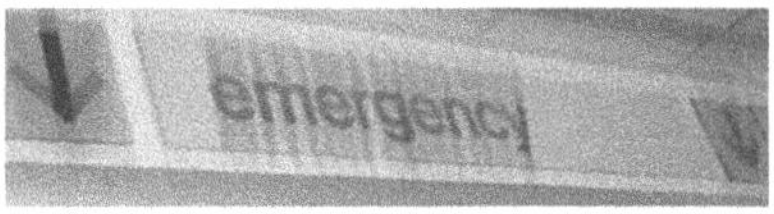


# Case 10

## A 26 Year-old Woman with Weakness & Falls: A Rough Life, a Tough Prognosis

**Primary case author:**
**Jason Adler**

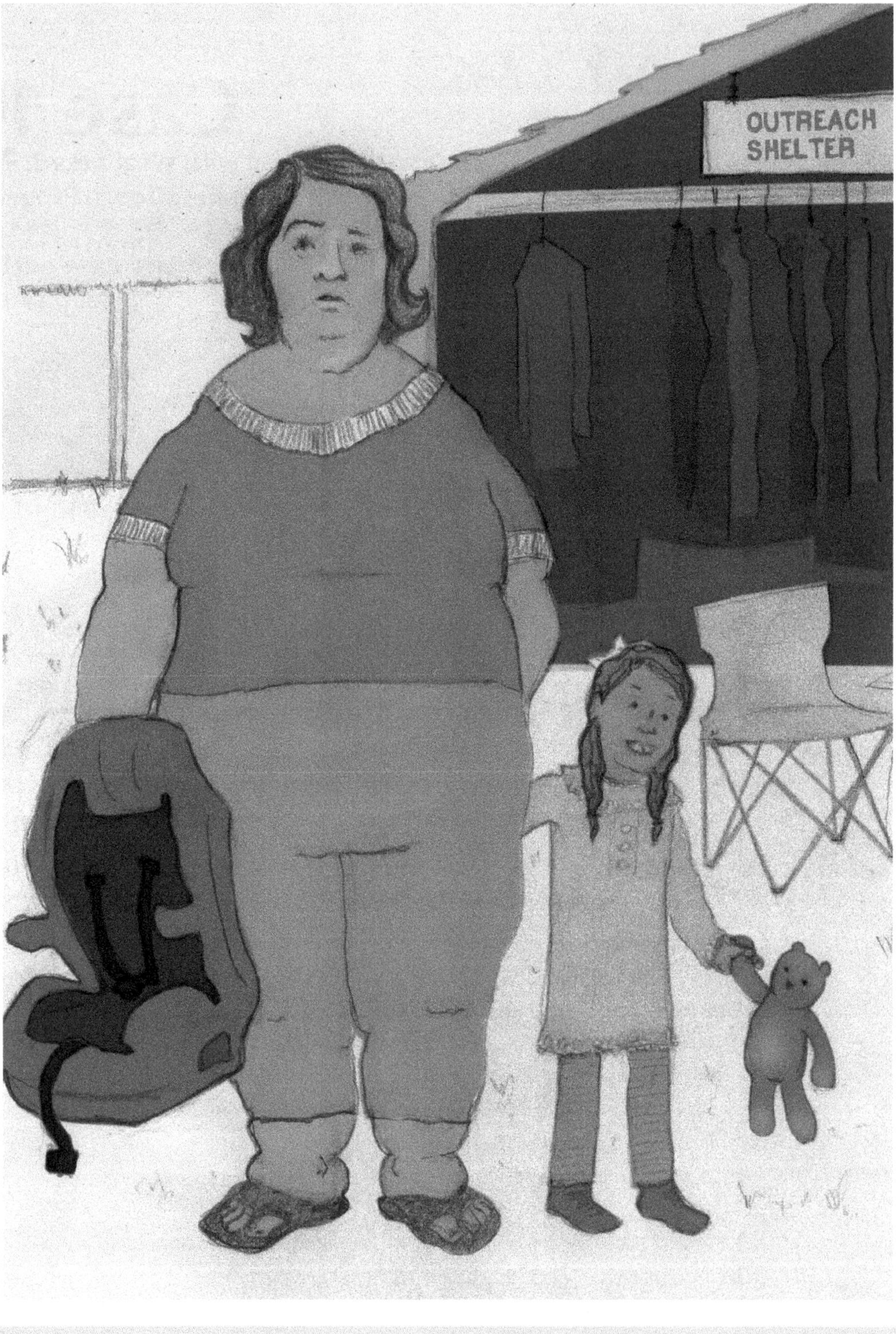
OUTREACH
SHELTER

# Case 10

## A 26 Year-old Woman with Weakness & Falls: A Rough Life, a Tough Prognosis

How come we complain when a patient returns the next day, but the small business owner never does? "You're back again? Why didn't you buy everything you needed yesterday?" Ever heard of a "punitive wait?" "If not, you are about to" ...

***Deep thoughts:***

1. *How far should we go in evaluating transient, non-specific symptoms?*
2. *What role do risk factors play in the decision-making process?*
3. *When two providers care for a patient, how is responsibility divided when there is a bad outcome?*
4. *Why is it called a waiting "room" and an emergency "department?"*

**PART 1—MEDICAL**

## I. The Patient's Story

Crystal does not have it easy. At the age of four, her father moves her to Louisiana. She is only to see her mother again briefly. Becoming pregnant in the 12th grade, she drops out of school and moves in with the soon-to-be father. Her pregnancy is complicated by anemia so severe that she requires a blood transfusion, but she delivers a healthy daughter by caesarian section.

It is not long before she becomes pregnant again, and on August 12, delivers another healthy daughter. Her boyfriend leaves, and Crystal moves into a mobile home, all the while working as a housekeeper at the Shifting Sands Resort Hotel. He returns and moves in next door, but they are not able to stay together due to "too much arguing." At one point, she is arrested for smashing his windshield and slashing his tires.

Crystal and her two daughters move out of the mobile home shortly after the floor in the bathroom falls through. She can now see the ground below the trailer. Bad goes to worse as she is fired from the hotel due to a misunderstanding about vacation. She wanders from job to job, first working in another hotel then in a children's daycare. Times remain rough; there is a 45-minute commute each way, and she quits work when her car breaks down.

Two years later, her children go to live with their father. Crystal is soon pregnant again; it is during this pregnancy that she learns of her mother's sudden and untimely death. Depression sets in. She is admitted to a mental health facility for almost 10 days, but no medications are prescribed since she is pregnant. A third C-section results in a healthy baby girl at Cape Hope Hospital. Crystal names her Joy.

With a new child, she attempts to get her two oldest children back, but their father refuses. She has a new boyfriend and finds work as a cashier at the Icy Penguin service station. One night she arrives home to find her apartment building surrounded by EMS vehicles and is told her boyfriend has burned it down.

She remembers an argument from earlier in the day:

He said, "I'm moving and going to Florida." I said, "Go ahead. Then he got mad." The boyfriend is subsequently charged with arson and sent to jail.

Several years later, Crystal is stopped for a traffic violation and the police notice that her child is not in a car seat; she is cited. She does not show up for the court date, and her driver's license is revoked. She now receives government assistance with food stamps and is placed on Medicaid. With no way to get to work and a young child to care for, she moves into a shelter.

On **March 9**, she goes to a clinic across the street from the shelter with complaints of heavy menstrual cycles, sinus pain, and tension in her neck. Vitals show BP 128/70 and weight of 279 pounds (down from 331 after taking Adipex a few years earlier). She has lab work which shows a WBC count of 11.8, Hb 6.8 (MCV low at 58), and platelet count 513. She is started on Septra and Flexeril with recommendations to get a pelvic US and see a hematologist. She returns to the clinic two weeks later and is started on iron. Surgical therapy is recommended. The diagnosis: Severe anemia and menorrhagia.

**Saturday, April 7** is Joy's third birthday, and the shelter helps by throwing a party at Chuck E Cheese's. While there, Crystal develops a headache which persists through the weekend.
**Tuesday, April 10**—Crystal is at the shelter and reaches for her daughter's car seat to put her into the daycare van. Crystal has a sudden onset of a hand cramp, then falls to the floor and cannot get up for three minutes. "[I was] standing and just fell." She calls for help but then finds that she is able to walk. There is no head trauma. She is driven to the ED.

## II. The Doctor's Version (the following is the actual documentation of the providers)

**Date:** April 10 at 09:58

**Chief Complaint (per RN):** "Fell/numbness to leg"

**Physical Examination:**

Vital Signs

| Time | Temp(C) | Rt. | Pulse | Resp | Syst | Diast | Pos. | Pain Scale | Pulse ox |
|---|---|---|---|---|---|---|---|---|---|
| 10:10 | 98.5 | 0 | 62 | 16 | 122 | 83 | S | 0 | 100% |
| 15:00 | | | 60 | 18 | 140 | 60 | | | |

**Triage:** Acuity 3–green. Pt ambulatory, tearful stating she fell last PM and this morning. Stating leg numbness. Pt. sounds congested. Equal hand grips bilaterally.

**History of Present Illness: (11:15)** (note: all documenting, ordering, and treatment per PA): Right leg and arm numbness last night and today with fall x 2 – denies previous or current injury. Severity mild-moderate. Weakness RUE and RLE which is new. Numbness x 2 episodes, approx. 1 minute each. No problems with vision, impaired speech, difficulty swallowing confusion. She has approximately half of her prescription for Septra remaining which she says "makes me sick." Pt. reports prior Hb was 6.7 but is "taking iron."

**Past Medical History:**
**Allergies:** NKDA
**Meds:** Septra, Zyrtec, Flexeril
**PMH:** Anemia
**PSH:** C/S x 3
**FH:**
**SH:** Smoker > 2 PPD, alcohol – none, drugs – none

**Physical Examination:**
**Psych:** Mood and affect are normal.
**Eyes:** PERRL.
**Throat:** Normal pharynx with no tonsillar hypertrophy.
**Neck:** Supple.
**Card:** Regular rate and rhythm, ht. sounds nl.
**Resp:** No respir distress, breath sounds nl.
**ABD:** Nontender, no organomegaly.
**Skin:** Color nl, no rash. Warm and dry.
**Neuro:** Cranial nerves normal as tested. EOM's intact, PERRL, cerebellar normal as tested. No motor or sensory deficit. Reflexes normal.
**MS:** Non-tender, normal ROM, no pedal edema.

**Emergency Department Course:**
**11:15** – Orthostatic VS: Lying BP 130/43 and pulse 65–Standing 145/80, pulse 56
**12:15** – Tylenol 975mg PO—Note: Pt. refused. "I've already tried Tylenol and Motrin"
**13:00 (per RN)** – X-ray tech informed me pt removed IV "because it hurt"—documented on AMA (pt. was asked to sign AMA form showing knowledge of risks of removing IV)

**Testing:**
WBC 9.2, Hb 7.6, plt 1,342,000
Lytes, BUN/creat – WNL, LFTs WNL, glucose 92, pregnancy test – negative
**CT scan head** – Indication: Head Pain
**Interpretation:** Normal per radiologist
**Urine toxicology screen:** Positive for marijuana
**Diagnosis (14:45):** Sinusitis, substance abuse, paresthesias, anemia
**Discharge (15:15):** Per RN: Discharge instructions given. Verbalized understanding. Discharged home. Rx doxycycline 100mg Q12 hours #20, Motrin 800mg q8 hours PRN pain, F/u with PCP ASAP for recheck and further Tx, return with increased symptoms or problems

*Scott Davidson, PA*
*Afram Aminah, MD*

## III. Risk Management/Patient Safety Opportunities (Adler)

**Author comments (Weinstock):** When we are faced with one problem at a time it is usually not too difficult to arrive at a diagnosis. Chest pain and diaphoresis in a 50 year-old man or sudden onset of flank pain and hematuria are good examples. When symptoms are nonspecific in a patient with numerous medical, psychiatric, and social problems, the complexity increases.

**Risk Management/Patient Safety Opportunity #1:**

**Opportunity:** Poor history of present illness (HPI).
**Discussion:** A common theme throughout this book: great "review of symptoms," but minimal HPIs. Our patient has concerning symptoms of numbness and weakness on one side of her body, but it is likely that her young age moves stroke down or off the differential. This type of presentation requires the provider to sit down and get a thorough story. What was the exact onset and duration of the symptoms? Has this occurred in the past? Were there any associated signs or symptoms? Did this become a legal issue? You betcha! The following is the physician answering a question from the plaintiff's attorney:

**Q.** (Plaintiff's attorney): Doctor, when you reviewed Ms. Johnson's chart, did you note her history of right-sided leg and arm numbness and the fact that she had fallen within the previous 12 hours?
**A.** (Doctor Aminah) Well, in terms of the fall, sir, I need—I need more information to make any assessment because it was not clear from the history about the fall as to why she fell. From [the history] she did fall twice, he [the PA] said. Whether she lost her balance, whether she was dizzy, you know, and did she actually hit the ground or just lose her balance, I don't know. So that fall, I could not make any conclusion, because she—she said that she didn't injure herself. So, whether she didn't actually hit the ground and just lost her balance, I cannot make any conclusions about that fall. The doctor was left to defend an incomplete evaluation performed by someone else.
✔ **Teaching point:** The diagnosis is only as firm as the data obtained to confirm it.

**Risk Management/Patient Safety Opportunity #2:**

**Opportunity:** Not evaluating risk factors.
**Discussion:** The inclusion of risk factors supports the complexity of care while demonstrating risk stratification. The chart had a section for family history, but it was left blank. Crystal's later deposition revealed what should have been included there: history of stroke in her 16 year-old sister and in both of her parents.
✔ **Teaching point:** Risk factors matter.

**Risk Management/Patient Safety Opportunity #3:**

**Opportunity:** Not asking for help.
**Discussion:** This case is a good lesson for all emergency clinicians whether a seasoned emergency physician, a resident, a PA or an NP; sometimes we need help. Examples may include needing another set of hands with a crashing patient, an interventional cardiologist for the STEMI patient, a call to a consultant with the "unusual illness" patient (lupus, methemoglobinemia) and the patient with an uncertain diagnosis. In this specific instance, the relationship between a physician and a PA/NP, should be fully explored and defined before clinical work begins. In some EDs all PA/NPs are directly supervised, with every patient being seen by a physician. In others, the PA/NP may function autonomously without direct supervision. This decision involves a balance between cost, efficiency, safety and risk. According to the Emergency Department Benchmarking Alliance (EDBA), ED APP staffing increased from 23% of EDs in 2010 to 62% in 2016.[1]
✔ **Teaching point:** The PA/NP-physician partnership should be a team effort.

**Risk Management/Patient Safety Opportunity #4:**

**Opportunity:** Unaddressed contradiction in chart.
**Discussion:** The brain CT indication states "head pain," but this is not mentioned in the HPI. Did she really have head pain or was the PA forced to pick from a list of indications? If she did have head pain, questioning about onset and other symptoms, such as fever, would have been helpful. If she did not have head pain, documenting such in the context of other neuro symptoms was essential.
✔ **Teaching point:** All patient complaints need to be explored in the H&P.

**Risk Management/Patient Safety Opportunity #5:**

**Opportunity:** Over-reliance on testing.
**Discussion:** It seems most likely that the brain CT was done to evaluate for TIA or CVA, not headache. During the PA's deposition (see below), he admitted that his understanding was that a negative CT excluded TIA or CVA. Would anyone be reassured with a negative back X-ray when evaluating for spinal epidural abscess? How about a normal CBC when evaluating for appendicitis? Reliance on a negative CT alone in the context of ischemic stroke/cerebrovascular disease is a misapplication of data. The non-contrast head CT can be rapidly obtained and is widely available. The role of a non-contrast head CT in the evaluation of acute ischemic stroke is to rapidly exclude intracranial hemorrhage and identify potential eligibility for reperfusion therapy.[2] A non-contrast head CT has a low sensitivity for acute ischemic stroke: 12% for acute ischemic strokes less than 3 hours-old, 16% for ischemic strokes greater than 12 hours-old, and an overall sensitivity of 16%.[2]
✔ **Teaching point:** Understand limitations of testing.

**Risk Management/Patient Safety Opportunity #6:**

**Opportunity:** Not recognizing the dangers of thrombocytosis.
**Discussion:** Thrombocytosis is an uncommon diagnosis, and its acute management would exceed the bounds of most emergency physicians. However, it does not take a brain surgeon (or hematologist) to recognize that when the platelets are three times the upper limit of normal, there may be extra clotting. Faced with an overweight patient with new onset unilateral arm and leg weakness, the thrombocytosis tips the scales in favor of an acute neurologic event.[3,4] Case studies in the literature have demonstrated a relationship between thrombocytosis and stroke in younger patients.
✔ **Teaching point:** If you order testing, be prepared to address abnormal results.

**Risk Management/Patient Safety Opportunity #7:**

**Opportunity:** Unclear documentation surrounding the cognitive process of the evaluation.
**Discussion:** The medical decision-making section is an opportunity to document your thought process and rationale for including/excluding diagnoses, ordering studies, interpretation of studies, and reassessment/progress notes. In this case, there is sparse documentation of the medical decision-making (MDM). We see the test orders, results, and brief comments about the AMA discharge. The diagnosis isn't aligned with the work-up; we know a CT was ordered, though unclear why. We see the diagnosis of sinusitis, but that isn't addressed anywhere in the chart.
✔ **Teaching point:** By using a pause before signing your note, you have the opportunity to review what you have done and written and ask yourself, does this line up?

**Author comments (Weinstock):** If you were the attending, would you want to see this patient yourself? If you were the PA/NP, would you want to bounce this off the attending? Reading the history, I don't have a good idea what is going on. Why and how did she fall and was this related to the paresthesias? Why was a CT done, looking for bleed, mass, TIA/CVA—was a normal CT supposed to be reassuring? What's the deal with a diagnosis of substance abuse? (Did the clinician think she smoked some dope behind the pews before sending her daughter to preschool, then was so "stoned" she fell and had unilateral numbness which resolved within minutes?) The "feel" of this chart is an ED staff at odds with their patient. After all, who has a patient, soon to be discharged, sign an AMA form because her IV hurts and she refuses Tylenol?

## IV. The Bounceback

Crystal is asymptomatic after leaving the ED on Tuesday, but at 3AM the following morning, Wednesday April 11th, she wakes to go to the bathroom and, "I just start falling." She gets back to sleep, and then per routine is awoken by the church at 6AM. After she gets her daughter off to daycare she is driven to the Rocky Fork Department of Social Services building. While waiting to be seen, she experiences "sweat pouring down my face ... I can't see nothing ... slurry speech and real bad headache." Medics are called:

**EMS report:**
**09:23** – Dispatched to Social Services building, 1236 Wahalla Street. Reason for dispatch: Breathing problems.
**09:32** – Arrive on scene.
**09:35** – Vitals: pulse 74 regular, Resp 20, BP 126/70, sat 100%, ECG NSR. Signs and symptoms: Headache. GCS normal.
**10:15** – Arrive at Cape Hope ED:
**(EMS final report):** 26 y/o female complaint headache with burning sensation across her nose. Pt. was seen at Cape Hope yesterday and treated for sinusitis. Patient requests transport to ED for evaluation again today. Patient transported w/o incident or delay to lead charge nurse and then to triage.
**ED Visit #2, Wednesday, April 11, 2006:**
**10:32** – (RN #1): Triaged and placed in waiting room.

- "Pt. here via EMS with c/o HA. States seen here yesterday and Dx with sinusitis and given Rx for same but has been unable to get filled. Pt. A&O x 3. NAD."

**10:48** – (RN #2): One episode emesis. Pt. comes to triage desk stating, "I feel sick" and not answering detailed questions.

- "Pt. Dx with sinusitis yesterday and has not taken Rx. Pt. vomited in triage, clear, frothy emesis, resp easy, skin W/D." Returned to waiting room.

**11:49** – (RN#2): Comes back to triage desk stating, "I feel really sick."

- Per RN: "Resp easy, skin W/D, no more episodes of vomiting, pt. stable." Returned to waiting room.

**13:56** – Name is called and she is placed in an ED room (3 hours 23 minutes after arriving by EMS).
**14:45** – Initial exam by physician assistant (PA) Adam Thompson:

- HPI: "Pt. was at social services today and had syncopal episode. Came to ED c/o HA and not feeling well. Had another flaccid episode. Pt. has been aphasic and right-side paralysis."

- PE – Pt. is aphasic, will only moan. Unable to test strength due to slow or no response to commands. Will withdraw right arm from deep pain 2/5 strength.
- The staff now responds quickly: Brain CT - Acute CVA left middle cerebral artery distribution.

**Diagnosis:** Acute CVA with aphasia and right-hand hemiparesis.

**Hospital Course:**

- **Neuro consult:** She is awake and alert but not cooperative. At times, she will move her arm in a nonspecific fashion, but most of the time has neglect. She is mute without the ability to repeat or comprehend speech. She has global aphasia.
- **Impression:** "Suspect stroke is secondary to the thrombocytosis and related hyper viscosity syndrome."
- **In-hospital testing:** reveals 90% left carotid artery stenosis.
- **Disposition:** On April 19, after eight days in the hospital, she is discharged for outpatient rehabilitation.

**Outcome:** Crystal now lives with her 7 year-old daughter, Joy. With rehab, her condition has improved, and she is able to walk her daughter to the bus stop across the street but cannot walk her as far as the park. Her speech is not clear, and her thought processes have not returned to baseline. She is embarrassed to be seen, spending most of her time at home. There are no family contacts and few friends. A nurse's aide visits the house for several hours three times a week to help with basic activities of living.

At a five-hour deposition on February 16 (3 years later), she stated that the last contact with her first two daughters was 5 months ago. She tried to call at Christmas, but the phone was not in service and has not been connected since.

## PART 2—LEGAL

**Author comments (Weinstock):** Crystal's hard life just got harder. In addition to all her previous problems, she now has difficulty with speech and no use of her right upper extremity. Could her TIA have been diagnosed at the initial visit? If she had been admitted, would it have changed the outcome?

## I. The Accusation/Cause of Action

- Failure to diagnose
- Failure to initiate preventive therapy for management of TIA
- Failure to recognize thrombocytosis as risk for CVA
- Failure to manage increased platelets
- Failure to arrange appropriate and timely follow-up for evaluation of TIA and prevention of CVA

## II. How Does the Plaintiff's Attorney Decide if There is a Case?

**Author comments (Weinstock):** When a patient is initially pursuing litigation, the case is brought to the attention of the plaintiff's attorney by the patient. However, the attorney has only superficial medical expertise. So, medical experts are needed to give advice as to whether negligence occurred.

The following is the abbreviated letter from the retained plaintiff's expert, Dr. Redd, the ED physician who reviewed the case. He later was an expert witness at the legal proceeding (more below). Often, the plaintiff's attorney will have three to four "experts" review a case. They want objective information, since the plaintiff's attorney (and client) get nothing if they lose, which occurs about 85% of the time if the case goes to trial. The plaintiff's best opportunity for a financial reward is through pretrial settlement.

Michael C. Redd, MD, FACEP
ED Medical-Legal Expert
353 E. Torrence Rd.
Boca Raton, FL 33433

Catherine LeFort, Esq.
LeFort, Johnson & Pruitt
Telemark Square
Summersville, NC 28451

Dear Ms. LeFort,

I had the opportunity to review the medical records of Crystal Johnson. I feel that the care and treatment provided to Ms. Johnson on 4/10 was below the accepted standard of care.

[Omitted here are 5 paragraphs summarizing the case]

When a patient presents to the emergency department with episodic hemiparesis, weakness and two episodes of falling, the first diagnosis in the differential is TIA. Ms. Johnson's risk factors of obesity, smoking and a hypercoagulable state due to her extreme thrombocytosis make this diagnosis more likely. TIA is the diagnosis that needs to be considered first.

Since a significant number of patients who experience a TIA will have a CVA within the first week, it is imperative to treat them immediately upon presentation. In fact, many institutions admit all patients presenting with TIA symptoms, especially ones presenting with their first TIA. The extremely elevated platelet count should have raised a red flag as to both the diagnosis and need for immediate intervention.

A diagnosis of sinusitis does not make clinical sense. A normal brain CT, which likely showed a significant view of the sinuses, with right-sided numbness and falling, makes it very difficult to justify a diagnosis of sinusitis. The falls, numbness and headache were not adequately explained, when in fact a diagnosis of TIA should have been the first consideration. Reading the chart, it would seem that the diagnosis of TIA was never seriously considered. A normal exam and CT scan cannot rule it out. It is a diagnosis based upon presenting signs, symptoms and risk factors; Ms. Johnson had [all three].

She did not receive any intervention with the typical medications to prevent CVA, such as aspirin. She also had a very treatable condition that was a major risk factor for her, the extreme thrombocytosis of 1.3 million. This was more than 3 times the highest acceptable number of platelets on this lab's test normal range. This level would increase the risk for stroke significantly and was easily treatable within the time frame between this visit and the next day, when she had the left middle cerebral artery infarction. Unfortunately, she was discharged.

On her return visit to the ED, she arrived by squad with significant complaints and was sent to the waiting room after being triaged. She came to the triage nurse twice and each time was sent back to the waiting room. This seems inappropriate for someone who has come in by squad, is a return from the day before (which should be a red flag) and for someone with her symptoms.

In summary, I do feel that the care and treatment provided to Ms. Johnson did not meet the standard of care. If I may be of any further assistance in the case, please do not hesitate to contact me.

Sincerely,
*Michael Redd*
Michael C. Redd, MD, FACEP

## III. Guest Interview—Confessions of a "Hired Gun"

**Michael Redd, MD, FACEP**
ED Medical-Legal Expert
Boca Raton, FL

**Author comments (Weinstock):** I found Dr. Redd, the plaintiff's expert, and he agreed to a brief telephone interview. I asked him some uncomfortable questions and he was honest and forthcoming. I also spoke with his co-workers, and they uniformly agreed, from paramedics to nurses to physicians, that he was one of the best doctors they had ever worked with: engaged, caring, smart and nonjudgmental.

**Authors.** *How did you get involved in testifying?*
**MR.** A friend of mine founded a company which supplies experts for legal cases. He asked me if I would do it and I agreed. That was many years ago.

**Authors.** *How many cases have you done? Have you worked for both sides?*
**MR.** Well, all the cases don't go to trial, so I have looked at probably 100 total. Many are just to give the attorney an opinion about the care received in the ED. Sometimes it involves just an ED chart and sometimes includes hundreds of pages of hospital records. Of the 100, I have been deposed on 15 or 20 but only six have actually gone to trial. Of all my cases, about 90% were for the plaintiff and the rest for the defense.

**Authors.** *How much do you charge for your services?*
**MR.** For general record review I charge $500 per hour with a two-hour minimum. Depositions are $700 bucks an hour and it's $5,000 for a trial. Of course, if I have to go out of town, travel is also paid. I like to get a retainer up front because sometimes it's difficult to get paid. Some firms don't know what to look for, small firms, looking to hit it big—they want the information but don't always have the resources to pay for it.

**Authors.** *What types of cases have you been involved with?*
**MR.** PEs are a big one. Cardiac. MIs ... a few. Abdominal pain, appendix. Pelvic problems. One case where the nurse asked further about evaluating for the compartment syndrome and the doctor said no. A number of strokes and TIAs. No missed foreign bodies, but they say this is common. One case was a patient with a splenectomy with a temp of 103 and unknown source. Poor documentation and no vaccine documented. The patient came back next day septic and died. Documentation: Unless you document it, the court says you didn't do it. I've had at least two cases where the doctors went back and documented after they found the outcome; if we can't even trust you to not change the record, how can we trust anything you say?

**Authors.** *What does it feel like having the defendant emergency physician across from you?*
**MR.** Not good. The first deposition I was at, the attorney was harassing and belligerent. One of their objectives is not to see what you know but to see if they can intimidate you on the stand. They want to know this up front. They will bring up things to make you look bad, to try and get you flustered. If you stay calm and say "I don't know about that," it's much easier. Don't let 'em get to you. Depositions are easy. Being on the stand is painful and anxiety provoking. All the jurors are looking at you. People in the seats are looking at you. The defendant physicians are the ones who you feel bad for. If they tried to change records, I don't feel bad, but if they made a mistake, I do feel bad for them. You have to be careful in what you say. Try and not to trap yourself. Memorize the chart.

**Authors.** *Do you know what percentage you won?*
**MR.** That's the interesting part. Most are settled and I never found out what actually happened. Of the ones that went to court, five of the six went for the defense. I remember at one of them [I heard] the defense lawyer say, "I can't believe we won this case." One was a missed appy. Most could have gone either way. I don't remember the one that was won by the plaintiff, not offhand.

**Authors.** *Do you remember the deposition in this case, Crystal Johnson?*
**MR.** I do. It was a video conference; the defendant physician was not there. The entire deposition took four hours; it was kind of painful. They asked me about my credentials, my medical malpractice record, my childhood, all trying to discredit me as a witness. The defense attorney was combative, he didn't have a case so tried to trick me into admitting I reviewed the record for a different case. He was grasping for straws. I called it Cape Valley Hospital and not Cape Hope hospital. It was miniscule and totally irrelevant to the case.

**Authors.** *You read the defendant physician's testimony. How would you have answered the questions?*
**MR.** Well, that was the problem! At the point of the deposition, it was beyond fixing; he really didn't have an argument. As far as the PA, he was not well trained. He didn't know about thrombocytosis; he didn't even know what it meant. He thought you could rule out a TIA or stroke with a CT scan.

**Authors.** *Do you work with PA's? How do you avoid getting in the same situation as this doctor?*
**MR.** The biggest problem with this case is not realizing that everyone with these findings needs to be seen by the physician. This patient passed out, has paresthesias, an elevated platelet count. I would have seen the patient—that's the responsibility of the physician. The PAs need to be trained to talk to the doctor when these symptoms are present.

**Authors.** *Have you ever been deposed or sued?*
**MR.** Yes, about [10 years ago] I received a 180-day letter. From the minute I got the letter I was distraught. It was on my mind every day. After three months they dropped the case.

**Authors.** *Do you remember the case?*
**MR.** Yeah, the patient was seen initially by a PA. It was a baby with a cold and the vitals were fine. They were asked to see the pediatrician the next day. I later found out that the child went home and vomited and aspirated and went into respiratory arrest before they could follow up. He expired a few days later. I remember the kid, the bed number and everything. The case was dropped as they couldn't find a witness. Nothing wrong was done.

**Authors.** *If you had such a bad experience, how can you testify against other doctors?*
**MR.** One reason is that it causes me to look at certain disease patterns from someone else's mistakes. Some experts will take a case for anybody, I only take cases for the plaintiff where it is pretty clear there was malpractice. It's improved the care of my patients. I'm a better physician because of the legal work I've done.

## IV. The Legal Analysis—Plaintiff's Attorney

**Mark Kitrick, JD**
Plaintiff's attorney, President of Kitrick, Lewis & Harris Co., L.P.A., Columbus, Ohio
Past President of the Ohio Association of Trial Lawyers

**Author comments (Weinstock):** The following is commentary by plaintiff's attorney Mark Kitrick (not involved with the case) discussing how cases are selected. Later, we will hear from Rich Milligan, a medical malpractice defense attorney discussing the defense strategy in this case.

### How a Plaintiff's Attorney Decides if There is a Case

**Initial review—the patient contacts the attorney:**
A plaintiff's lawyer initially analyzes three aspects of a potential medical malpractice case.

- Is there a strong liability case against the possible defendants?
- What are the claimant's damages?
- Is there adequate malpractice insurance coverage or are there collectible defendants' assets?

In conjunction with this review, we must also consider practical business considerations:

- The firm's advancement of costs and anticipated time prosecuting the claim
- The state's statutory caps on damages for pain and suffering and economic losses
- The reputations and likeability of the potential defendants
- What subrogation amount must be reimbursed
- Past jury verdicts and settlements in the relevant locale

By the time the case is filed, the trial lawyer will need to know the medicine, be prepared to spend $50,000–$150,000 (the range on this case) and will have retained the appropriate expert witnesses, including an EM physician for the standard of care, a stroke expert and medical economists to estimate the damages. Most importantly, the lawyer must be highly impassioned for the client's cause. Of the many cases lawyers review, relatively few survive this vetting process.

**Liability (was there negligence in this case?):**
Assuming the reviewing physician opines favorably for the plaintiff, one main fact tilts the scales toward representation: The deadliest cause of Ms. Johnson's complaint was not excluded and the doctor did not pursue further investigation. Such an approach resonates with juries because it demonstrates more than negligence; it suggests intentional or gross negligence. From a juror's perspective, such behavior is more actionable and unforgivable.

First, when the defendants treated Ms. Johnson, they did not take a detailed history. Everyone knows this is a basic failure. For example, Ms. Johnson's family history of stroke was a crucial fact, and it was ignored; one cannot separate people from their bloodline. As well, the events surrounding the fall were not adequately explored. Further, her headache history was missed. Finally, the defendants should have recognized her extremely high platelet count and compared it to results from March 9 [the clinic visit one month before the ED visit].

Second, whether true or not, most people believe that if a stroke is diagnosed early on, it can be readily treated. Though the defendants did a head CT, there was no solid analysis of the unilateral numbness. A sharp trial lawyer will make it seem obvious that Ms. Johnson was at high risk for a stroke, based on risk factors and weight, smoking two packs a day and noncompliance. Of note, all this may not convince a plaintiff's attorney to take her case since a good defense attorney can use her conduct against her.

Third, Ms. Johnson was the recipient of government assistance. Most people believe that someone on assistance receives less personal attention and fewer "expensive" tests, primarily because the doctors and hospitals don't receive as much reimbursement. A three-hour wait on return, among other facts, may cause the jurors to question whether she was the victim of the defendants' presumed prejudice.

**Liability insurance coverage:**
It is noteworthy that no one seemed to be truly in charge. There did not seem to be a hospital protocol for a responsible party; discovery may uncover whether the communication failure was widespread. A concerning byproduct for the defense is that plaintiff's counsel is forced to sue more doctors, employees and agents because no one can determine who is responsible. This approach may be advantageous to the plaintiff when one defendant points a finger at another or tries to blame an "empty chair."

**Author comments (Weinstock):** The empty chair defense is used by the defendant to place the blame on a party which is not part of the suit or no longer a part of the suit. It was used successfully in Case 6.

**Damages:**
The defendants' combined negligence caused Ms. Johnson to suffer serious, permanent conditions, which require significant, long-term medical care. Her economic costs, even if a portion are paid back to the government vis-a-vis its statutory subrogation claim, drive up the settlement or verdict. Because of this patient's major damages (some of which will not be subject to state caps) and the jury sympathy/empathy that exists, it is more likely that a lawyer will take her case.

**Conclusion:**
For plaintiffs to prevail, it helps if a jury is outraged with the defendants. The most successful plaintiff strategies allow the jurors to think about themselves and their family and how the defendants' actions have put them in jeopardy. They should be made to feel that their verdict sends a message to the defendants and society at large. In other words, if plaintiff's counsel demonstrates that this case is not just about Ms. Johnson, but about protecting the community, a significant plaintiff's verdict is likely to follow.

## V. The Legal Proceedings—The Depositions

**Author comments (Weinstock):** This case presents significant difficulties for the defendants; both the PA and physician were named. The PA testified that he discussed the case with the attending, but there was no notation of that on the chart. Despite signing the chart, the attending did not have any recollection of the discussion.

| |
|---|
| Cast of characters (names changed, except where noted):<br>**The patient:** Crystal Johnson<br>**ED defendant doctor:** Dr. Afram Aminah<br>**ED physician assistant (PA):** Scott Davidson<br>**Plaintiff's attorney:** Alan Krause, Esq.<br>**Plaintiff's expert witness:** Michael Redd, MD (Board certified emergency medicine)<br>**Defense attorney:** Randall Scoville, Esq. |

**Author comments (Weinstock):** Watch how the plaintiff's attorney plays the PA off the attending physician.

## A. Who is responsible for the patient's care, the doctor or the PA?

**Deposition of physician assistant Scott Davidson by plaintiff's attorney Alan Krause:**
**Q.** Was there always during your tenure at Cape Hope, was there always an emergency physician in the emergency department?
**A.** Yes, sir.

**Q.** All right, sir. And do I understand that always you would discuss the care and disposition with the emergency physician prior to the patient being discharged?
**A.** Every case.

**Q.** And as it pertains to Crystal Johnson, who did you discuss her care with?
**A.** Dr. Aminah.

**Q.** And you discussed her care with Dr. Aminah before Crystal was discharged?
**A.** That is correct.

**Q.** Why did you do that?
**A.** That's what I do. That is the requirement we have—that I have with the supervising physicians. I discuss every patient with them. They are in charge and, therefore, I discuss all patients with them.

**Author comments (Weinstock):** What do you think the physician had to say about it?

**Deposition of ED defendant doctor Afram Aminah by plaintiff's attorney Alan Krause:**

**A.** (Dr. Aminah): Yeah. To the best of my recollection, sir, I don't remember Scott Davidson (PA) speaking to me about Ms. Johnson. If he did, I don't remember what he said.

**Q.** All right, sir.
**A.** That's to the best of my recollection.

**Q.** Doctor, were you in charge of Crystal Johnson's care while she was in the emergency department on April 10th?
**A.** To the best of my recollection, sir, I—I never did see Ms. Johnson. That's to the best of my recollection.

**Q.** So were you in charge of her care?
**A.** Well, I was a backup physician for [the PA] Scott Davidson, but to the best of my recollection Scott Davidson never did discuss Ms. Johnson. If he did, you know, I don't remember and also I did not see Ms. Johnson.

**Q.** So that I can make sure that your answer is clear—
**A.** Yes, sir.

**Q.** —I understand then the answer to my question to be no, you were not in charge of Crystal Johnson's care while she was in the emergency department on April the 10th. Is that correct?
**Defense attorney Mr. Scoville:** Objection.
**A.** I was—

**Defense attorney, Mr. Scoville.** You can answer.
**A.** I was the backup physician, sir, and I think to the best of my recollection Scott Davidson never discussed with me Ms. Johnson. And if he did, I don't remember, sir.

**Author comments (Weinstock):** Ouch! Who hasn't in the course of a busy ED shift forgotten a conversation which occurred or not occurred? Who has signed charts, previously dictated/documented, without reading the whole chart? I have; we all have. Does this place us in legal jeopardy? The answer would have to be "yes," but like all of medicine, there are shades of gray. It may be one thing to fail to discuss a case, but does signing the chart of a patient you never saw or discussed ramp up the risk?

**Continued deposition of ED defendant doctor Afram Aminah by plaintiff's attorney Alan Krause:**

**Q.** Given that your initials [are] on her chart, you do believe you signed off on her chart?
**A.** Yes, sir. Yes, sir.

**Q.** Doctor, are you familiar with the provisions of [your state's] administrative code as to your duties as a backup supervising physician?
**A.** No, sir, I'm not aware of that, sir.

**Author comments (Weinstock):** This may seem unusually harsh, but how many of us are aware of the administrative codes in our states? The grilling continues:

**Q.** Is that your signature there, Dr. Aminah?
**A.** Yes, sir.

**Q.** All right. To your knowledge, does your signature appear, initials, anywhere else in the chart, other than on this particular page?
**A.** My signature is on the following page after that.

**Q.** Are you able to tell from looking at the chart what date and time that you would have signed off on the chart?
**A.** The date, I mean, was the 10th, but the time, sir, I'm not able to say what time, sir.

**Q.** Are you able to say by looking at the chart whether you signed off on the chart before or after Ms. Johnson's discharge?
**A.** As to my understanding, sir, that hospital policy and regulation requires that before a patient is discharged a physician must sign off on the chart, sir, and I think we follow that policy.

**Q.** All right, sir. My understanding from your testimony is that you did not have any discussions with Mr. Davidson about Ms. Johnson on April 10th of 2006. Is that correct?
**A.** That's the best of my recollection, sir.

**Author comments (Weinstock):** Is this doctor taking care of patients, or just following a hospital policy to sign charts? Of course, there is a reason that there is a policy to sign charts, to take responsibility for the patients under your care. The onslaught continues:

**Q.** So who was in charge of her care on April 10th?
**A.** My understanding is that physician assistants are licensed, you know, health providers, and they follow the hospital policy and procedures.

**Q.** And so would the answer to my question be that the PA in this case, Scott Davidson, was the one that was in charge of Crystal Johnson's care on April 10th?
**A.** Yeah. That's my understanding, sir, because they're licensed health providers, and they follow the hospital policy and procedures governing their work. I didn't know anything about Ms. Johnson, sir, and the first time I knew anything was when I got that lawsuit in the registered mail.

**Author comments (Weinstock):** Could this actually be true? A patient "bounces back" one day later with a horrible outcome and the doctor doesn't find out about the outcome until a letter arrives in the distant future? In our ED, it seems like you are assaulted when you walk through the double doors: "Do you remember that lady you saw yesterday in Room seven with the numbness? Well, she came back today with a stroke." Not that it has ever happened to me; I've just heard stories.

Did the doctor and PA discuss this case upon learning of the stroke diagnosis? Were there accusations at that time? This question is almost routine in a deposition; "Doctor, with whom did you discuss this case upon learning of the 'bad outcome'?" Oh, to be a fly on the wall.

When I was a kid, I would sometimes go fishing at a trout farm. Ever been to one? Ours had a small, stone-lined pool where the fish would come to be fed. It wasn't really fair; my dad paid a few bucks, and we threw in a line into the pool and instantly caught a healthy trout. Even through my childhood eyes, I never deluded myself into thinking I was a great fisherman, but sometimes a real fisherman will throw a line into the ocean and catch a big fish.

### B. Do past legal actions matter?

**Q.** All right, sir. So other than the claim that was made against a bunch of physicians at Cook County, no other—no other claims have ever been asserted against you?
**A.** No. No. Because the other one I mentioned in interrogatories.

**Q.** Yes, sir. Tell me about that.
**A.** Yeah. This was a patient who had chest pain for 24 hours. The patient was seen at the urgent care and was referred to our emergency department and the patient was followed by—by a PA, and then we followed the patient. The patient's chest pain had gone by then. And since the patient's pain had been gone for 24 hours, we wanted to evaluate to find out, you know, when did the patient's ischemia begin? The claim was that there was a delay in—in care of that patient and there—I was named. Physician assistant was named, hospital was named, and it was settled.

**Q.** And do you know who the PA was that was involved in that matter?
**A.** The PA has passed away, sir.

**Q.** Did you ever see, physically see, that patient while that patient was in the emergency department?
**A.** No, sir.

**Q.** All right, sir. Were you a backup supervising physician for that PA?
**A.** Yes, sir.

**Q.** Did you sign off on that patient's chart?
**A.** I discussed the patient. I discussed—the PA discussed the case with me from the beginning, so I was involved in the care of that patient from the beginning. I saw all the results and everything. Yes, sir.

**Q.** And—and to the best of your knowledge, that's different than the situation involving Crystal Johnson, correct?
**Defense attorney Mr. Scoville.** Objection.
**Plaintiff's attorney Mr. Krause.** You may answer the question.
**A.** Yeah. To the best of my knowledge, I never did see Ms. Johnson and I do not remember Scott speaking me to about Ms. Johnson. If he did, as I said, I don't remember.

**Author comments (Weinstock):** Well, the doctor's favorite song is now in our heads like a broken record. His strategy is to continue to deny that he ever saw the patient, though that strategy seems a bit questionable while watching the plaintiff's attorney "reel in" the big one.

Depending on state law, scope of practice regulations, and local hospital bylaws, there is significant variation in PA/NP supervision requirements and policy. Is the "to the best of my knowledge I never saw Ms. Johnson ..." approach the correct way to go? To find out, we asked Rich Milligan, a medical malpractice defense attorney and trial lawyer with over 25 years of experience.

## VI. The Legal Analysis

**Rich Milligan, JD**
Defense medical malpractice attorney
Health and Medicine Practice Group, Buckingham, Doolittle & Burroughs, LLP, Canton, Ohio

**ED doctor bails out on his PA:**
The way this physician responded in deposition was a disaster! I am not sure if it is his lawyer's fault or his own; I suspect both. His testimony not only damages his defense, but that of the PA.
As a defense lawyer, I want a doctor that a jury likes, one who steps up to the plate and takes

responsibility. The medicine is secondary. If the jury starts out by thinking you are ducking your professional responsibility, the benefit of the doubt is going to be with the patient. Medicine is complicated; jurors respect the difficulty of diagnosing conditions. If you were on a jury, would you believe that this physician has no responsibility for the care because he merely signed the chart and didn't see the patient or review the record? I don't think so!

This case presents a very difficult problem. The PA, who is required to work under physician supervision, arguably made a mistake. The ED doctor, in signing the chart, did not pick up the mistake. It can only be detrimental to the entire defense for the ED doctor and PA to point an accusatory finger at each other.

**Defense strategy:**
As a defense lawyer, my job is to figure out how the facts can best be reconciled so the testimony is supportive, not accusatory. Part of my strategy would be for the ED doctor to accept responsibility for his role:

- "I work with Scott Davidson regularly."
- "He is a very competent PA. I trust his skills and judgment."
- "I don't remember seeing Crystal Johnson or seeing her chart."
- "As part of my standard practice, when I sign off on a chart for a patient that I have not seen, I look at the chart to make sure I am comfortable with the care that was given by the PA. If I have questions, I will talk to the PA. I may also see the patient. If necessary I will do additional testing or order different therapies."

By answering in this way, the ED physician is only admitting what he must, that he doesn't remember and that in his standard practice he would do what is reasonable, at a minimum to look at the chart. In most states, a physician is not required to see the patient or even discuss the case with the PA. But you must supervise! If you don't, you can be held legally liable.

The only option is for the doctor to acknowledge what he doesn't remember and fall back on his standard practice, likely within the standard of care for a board-certified emergency medicine physician. Great athletes sometimes win games with horrible coaching, but one thing is true in both the sporting world and lawsuits: Neither poor athletes nor bad witnesses win without good preparation. Here, we have a terrible witness, poorly prepared. To the extent that the testimony reflects a "strategy," it is a bad one, horribly executed. The witness comes off as dishonest and dismissive of his obligations as a physician.

## VII. The Legal Proceedings—The Depositions (continued)

**Author comments (Weinstock):** The physician was obviously not coached by our two attorneys. Was he coached at all?

**C. How discrepancies between clinicians are used by a plaintiff's attorney.**

**Continued deposition of ED defendant doctor Afram Aminah by plaintiff's attorney Alan Krause:**
**Q.** From your review of her chart, would you have included TIA in your differential?
**A.** Well sir, to me, I'll have to see a patient, evaluate and, you know, see what the past medical history is, what treatment they received, what's the current treatment, and review their studies, and then I can formulate, you know, an opinion as to what is the problem.

**Q.** Yes, sir. But you've reviewed Ms. Johnson's chart of April 10th, correct?
**A.** Yes, sir.

**Q.** And you've reviewed it thoroughly, correct?
**A.** What do you mean by "thoroughly," sir?

**Q.** Well, you've been sued, doctor. I mean, I assume you've reviewed Ms. Johnson's chart given the allegations that have been made against you. I assume that you've reviewed it thoroughly, have you not?
**A.** I have—

**Defense attorney Mr. Scoville.** Objection. At the start [of the deposition] you asked him if he didn't understand the question to let you know and he told you he didn't understand "thoroughly," and so I object to your lecturing the witness.

**Q.** Well, do you understand the term "thoroughly?"
**A.** I've reviewed Ms. Johnson's chart, sir.

**Q.** All right. Based upon your review of her chart, would you have included TIA in her differential had you been the medical professional who saw her?
**A.** As I said, sir, there are a lot of conditions that cause transient neurologic symptoms and TIA is one of them.

**Q.** Yes, sir, and I understand that's what a differential is all about. My question is, had you seen Crystal Johnson on April 10th, would you have included TIA in your differential? And if you can answer the question with a yes or no, please answer it with a yes or no and then please feel free to explain.

**Defense attorney Mr. Scoville.** Objection. And if you can't answer it with a "yes" or "no," you can also tell him that.

**A.** As I said, sir, when I evaluate the patient, sir, I have to take a history, do, you know, a physical exam, review the medications, review the past history, past treatment, and then I can formulate an opinion as to what is the problem. And that's the normal and customary way that I follow a patient. And that's the best answer I can give you, sir.

**Q.** Okay. So—so my understanding is that Ms. Johnson's chart contains a history, correct?
**A.** Yes, sir.

**Q.** It contains her complaints, correct?
**A.** Yes, sir.

**Q.** It contains what medications that she was taking, correct?
**A.** Yes, sir.

**Q.** All right, sir. So, my understanding is all of the things that you would do in the work-up of a patient were done with Ms. Johnson? Doctor, you've been a teacher before, correct?
**A.** Yes, sir.

**Q.** All right. And you—you do case presentations to students when you teach, correct?
**A.** Yes, sir.

**Q.** All right, sir. Now, all of the things that you indicate that would be done in the work-up of a patient, do you believe that they were done in the work-up of Crystal Johnson?
**A.** Yeah. Reviewing the charts, sir, Ms. Johnson was evaluated, history was obtained, personal history was obtained and those studies were done.

**Author comments (Weinstock):** OK. Due to my benevolent nature and my pity on you, the reader, I have omitted the next several pages of testimony, which includes this question being asked again in slightly different format about 20 more times. I can attest that it is painful to read. Imagine how painful it was for those around the table. Did the plaintiff's attorney let him off the hook?

**Q.** Doctor, let me just say this. I don't have to be anywhere until tomorrow, and I want to see if I can get an answer to this question. It's a hypothetical question, based upon your having— being a board-certified emergency physician and someone who's been involved in teaching. And so, my question is, based upon your review of this chart, what would you have done—I know you didn't see her—but what would you have done had you seen this patient based upon your review of this chart?
**A.** As I said, sir, from my review, Ms. Johnson had transient neurologic symptoms which resolved. As I said, there are many causes of that. TIA is one of them.

**Author comments (Weinstock):** So, he finally admits that TIA is in the differential ... or does he? How about hypercoagulable conditions?

**Q.** Now, do you know what I mean by the term "hypercoagulable condition?"
**A.** Yes, sir.

**Q.** What does that mean?
**A.** It means that something that can clot easy, readily.

**Q.** Did Ms. Johnson have a hypercoagulable condition when she presented to the emergency department on April 10th of 2006?
**A.** Not to the best of my knowledge, sir.

**Q.** All right, sir. To your knowledge, is there any relationship between an elevated platelet count and stroke?
**A.** To the best of my knowledge, sir, there's no correlation between the level of the platelet count and neurologic symptoms. That's to the best of my knowledge, sir.

## VIII. Medical Discussion—Evaluation of Neuro Complaints and Timely Diagnosis of Stroke

**Jason Adler, MD, FACEP, FAAEM**
Clinical Assistant Professor
University of Maryland School of Medicine

This case is just so unfortunate. I can't imagine what Crystal was feeling from the moment she was driven to the emergency department through the end of her hospitalization.

What do we know about the first visit? The triage note focuses on two falls and leg numbness. There is an observation of congestion. Grip strength was tested and symmetric. The HPI acknowledges both falls, with right arm and right leg numbness described as "new," with no new injury. There is a past medical history of anemia, and social history consistent with smoking two packs per day. No abnormalities were noted on the exam above the neck (sinuses), and the neuro exam is documented as cranial nerves and cerebellar function being normal "as tested," with no motor or sensory deficit. There is an indirect suggestion she may have had a headache based on the indication written on the CT and the order for Tylenol.

**A differential diagnosis at this point may include:**

- A thromboembolic event from a TIA or Acute Ischemic Stroke (AIS)
- Hemiplegic migraine
- Metabolic derangement
- Seizure
- Syncope

Even though the HPI lacks some context and sequence of events, most of us would be thinking about a TIA or acute ischemic stroke. Yes, it would be helpful to ask if Crystal's arm and leg went numb and weak prior to and leading to the fall, and if the same occurred around the time of the second fall. Were there any prodromal symptoms? Did the symptoms completely resolve between episodes? Did Crystal have a headache at some point? Has she felt sick lately? Sinus pressure?

Two of the medications noted (Zyrtec, Flexeril) don't align with past medical history stated. Why was she taking them? What is the family history? What does "as tested" mean on the neurological exam and was gait assessed? None of these questions are clearly answered based on the available documentation. The initial orders include orthostatics, a CBC, chemistry, pregnancy test, toxicology screen and head CT. The head CT is particularly interesting. The indication on the record mentions "head pain." There is no mention of a headache on the HPI. Whether for a headache or concern for TIA/AIS, the CT was performed, negative, and Crystal was discharged (or left AMA without any indication of a plan for admission).

**Key Point–"What the brain doesn't look for, the eye won't see:"**

There was enough information after the history and exam, despite their limitations, to have a high suspicion of TIA or AIS and consider keeping her in the hospital.

She experienced two episodes of weakness and numbness; keying in on those symptoms, they are both negative or ablative phenomena, which is suggestive of ischemia. Mimics, such as migraine or seizure, are often associated with positive symptoms such as paresthesias. The latter was included in the diagnosis but not mentioned anywhere else in the record. In this case, her symptoms also correlated to a vascular territory which should have heightened concern for an ischemic event. The occurrence of two discrete episodes may suggest some instability or evolution in process. Symptoms as brief as 10 seconds have been associated with an ischemic stroke.[5]

Assuming the exam is normal as documented, also with limitations, the rationale for keeping Crystal in the hospital is that stroke is preceded by a TIA in 12%–30% of patients, with the highest risk in the first 24 hrs. [6,7] Her symptoms were consistent with TIA until proven otherwise.

Had Crystal stayed in the hospital, she likely would have had advanced diagnostic imaging and continued neurological assessments. Based on the most recent recommendations,[8] a CT angiogram of the head and neck and/or CT perfusion would have been performed to evaluate a causative vascular lesion and delineate ischemia respectively. These studies can be rapidly performed and are used to support decision making related to thrombolysis or thrombectomy. MRI studies are the gold standard diagnostic test for acute ischemic stroke, but not always immediately available in the context of the ED evaluation.

There are a number of risk stratification tools to evaluate for a TIA, include ABCD2 and the Canadian TIA score, each have limitations and the position of the American College of Emergency Physicians (ACEP) most recent clinical policy[9] suggest risk stratification scores not being used as a sole determinant of who is safe for discharge.

Having known about the family history of strokes in multiple relatives and recognizing the thrombocytosis would only heighten your concern. That said, the minimum threshold to pursue a TIA/AIS evaluation had already been exceeded.

The diagnostic work-up and evaluation do not appear to be consistent with a concern for a TIA. If never considered, it will never be discovered.

**Key Point—"What the eyes may see, the brain may too:"**

What was the rationale for ordering a toxicology screen? A young patient comes in after two discrete episodes of unilateral upper and lower extremity weakness with subsequent falls. How does the toxicology screen support or refute any pathology on the differential diagnosis? She also has a history of mental illness, not discussed in the chart, but noted in the prologue of this chapter. Is it possible the diagnostic evaluation was influenced by something subconscious during the encounter?

The head CT was negative. Cognitively, we missed the first opportunity by either assuming a negative head CT cleared a TIA or moved past it too quickly. The final diagnosis was sinusitis, substance abuse, paresthesias, and anemia. The first three diagnoses were never mentioned in the chart or evaluated, and the last doesn't explain her presentation. Was there premature closure? We may never know.

There may have been an opportunity to course correct prior to signing the patient out against medical advice. I doubt the PA who wrote this chart thought others would be reading it years in the future. And therein lies the opportunity. As we work through a clinical encounter, interpreting new information as it comes in, reassessing, we can ask ourselves, "does this make sense?" The medical decision-making section is an opportunity to wrap everything together. There isn't much medical decision-making documented here, but cognitively, had that question been asked, perhaps the opportunity may not have been lost.

**D. The thrombocytosis: continued deposition of ED defendant doctor Afram Aminah by plaintiff's attorney Alan Krause:**

**Q.** When you signed off on this chart, I assume that you saw that Ms. Johnson's platelet count was a million, three hundred and forty-two thousand, didn't you?
**A.** Scott Davidson did not discuss Ms. Johnson with me, sir.

**Q.** Yes, sir, but you looked at her chart and you signed off on it. Did you see that her platelet count was a million, three hundred and forty-two thousand?

**Defense attorney Mr. Scoville.** Object to the form of the question.
**A.** As I said, sir, Scott Davidson never discussed Ms. Johnson with me, sir.
**Q**. Dr. Aminah, that wasn't my question. My question was, when you signed off on her chart, did you see that she had a platelet count of a million, three hundred and forty-two thousand?

**Defense attorney Mr. Scoville.** Objection.

**A.** As I said, sir, Scott Davidson never discussed Ms. Johnson with me, sir.

**Q.** Yes or no, when you signed off on her chart, did you see that she had a platelet count of a million, three hundred and forty-two thousand?
**A.** Scott Davidson never discussed the case with me, sir.

**Q.** So the answer to my question would be no, you didn't see that?
**A.** As I said, sir, Scott Davidson never discussed the case with me, sir.

**Q.** I know, Dr. Aminah. When you signed off on this patient's chart, did you see—did you look at her CBC?
**A.** Scott Davidson never discussed the case with me, sir.

**Q.** That wasn't the question I asked you, Dr. Aminah. The question I asked you is whether or not when you signed off on this patient's chart you noted that she had a platelet count of a million, three hundred and forty-two thousand, yes or no? It's a simple question. Yes or no, did you note it?
**A.** Scott Davidson never discussed the case with me, sir.

**Q.** So the answer to my question would be no, you didn't note it?
**A.** All I can tell you, sir, is that Scott Davidson never discussed the case with me, sir. That's my answer.

**Q.** Yes, sir. So, your answer to the question of whether you noted it in her chart at the time you signed off on it, your answer to that question is: Scott Davidson never discussed the chart with me.
**A.** That's my answer to you, sir.

**Q.** Okay. So, did you look at her chart before you signed off on it?
**A.** I looked at the diagnosis and I signed off.

**Q.** Did you look at the CBC?
**A.** No, sir.

**Q.** Why not?
**A.** Scott Davidson never discussed the case with me, sir.

**Author comments (Weinstock):** Seems clear at this point that the doctor was coached to answer all questions the same way. Does this absolve him of responsibility? How damaging is the previous case he had with a PA where the patient died? His answers remain consistent until the end when he finally admits he did not see the platelet count. Did the plaintiff's attorney wear him down? Did his strategy crack?

**E. Collaboration between the physician and the PA:**

**Q.** Do you wish he had today? As you sit here today, do you wish that Scott Davidson would have said, Dr. Aminah, I've got a patient that has transient neurologic symptoms and has a platelet count of a million, three hundred and forty-two thousand? As you sit here today, do you wish that Mr. Davidson had told you that?
**A.** As I said, Scott Davidson is a licensed physician assistant and follows hospital policy and procedure.

**Q.** Well, let's play "what if." What if he had?
**A.** As I said, sir, I would have gone to see the patient sir, examined the patient, take the history and go through what I've described, sir, and then formulate an opinion as to the diagnosis and management.

**Author comments (Weinstock):** Three and a half hours and over 100 pages of deposition testimony later, the doctor finally admits that if he knew the specifics of the case, he would have evaluated the patient himself. Would he have discharged her?

**Q.** You said you did not know whether you would have discharged her because you didn't have a chance to examine her?
**A.** Ms. Johnson had transient symptoms which are resolved. The discharge was reasonable for her.

**Q.** You said that you never even looked at [the platelet count which was] a million three, correct?
**A.** Yes, sir.

**Q.** I understood you to tell me previously that if you had noted that her platelet count was a million, three hundred thousand-plus, my understanding is that you told me that you personally would have looked in on this patient, that you personally would have gotten more detail about the circumstances surrounding her fall. Do I understand you correctly to say that you personally would have gone to Ms. Johnson and gotten more information?
**A.** Yes sir.

**Q.** All right. That's all the questions I have.

**Author comments (Weinstock):** There was an additional allegation regarding thrombolytics at the second ED visit. Remember the visit where the patient had a stroke in the waiting room? Not my fault, says the ED doctor. Not my fault, says the paramedic. Not my fault, says the triage nurse. Not my fault, says the hospital.

**F. Was she a candidate for thrombolytics? We switch gears to the deposition of the plaintiff's emergency medicine expert, Dr. Michael Redd (the same physician who wrote the initial letter alleging negligence) by plaintiff's attorney Alan Krause:**

**Q.** Was she a tPA candidate?
**A.** On the first visit, no. On the second visit, possibly.

**Q.** And what was it that makes it possible versus [the fact that] she was a candidate?
**A.** Time frame of when the stroke actually started. But I can't tell when exactly it was.

**Q.** Back then, it was how long before?
**A.** Three hours.

**Q.** Now, back in 2006, was that the standard in terms of what would have been done?
**A.** Well, 2006 was right on the cusp of when that was happening. They would have been doing inter-arterial tPA by sending her to another hospital. If the stroke happens immediately, you have a time frame in which to intervene. If you don't know when it started, you don't want to give [tPA] because that can cause a bleeding in the stroke area. So, if you know a stroke started exactly at noon, and you can see the person, they suddenly have right-sided weakness and numbness and other issues that become obvious that it's a stroke, you have a time frame to get it fixed.

**Q.** As of 2006, then, it's your testimony that tPA and retrieval could have been done?
**A.** It could have been done, yes. That certainly was an option.

**Author comments (Weinstock):** Before reading what happened next, consider:

- Could this happen in your practice?
- If it did, would you proceed to trial or settle?

If you are an emergency physician, would you have seen this patient?
If you are a physician assistant or nurse practitioner, are there mechanisms in place to easily discuss difficult cases with the physician?
If you are a nurse working in triage, would you have "treated" this patient with a "therapeutic wait?"
If you are a hospital administrator, does your current policy account for this scenario?

## X. The Decision—Settlement vs. Trial

This case did not go to trial but was settled for an extremely large sum; enough to provide for life-long care of the patient, estimated to be in the millions of dollars.

Envisioning a trial, it is hard to see how the defense would proceed, particularly when faced with two providers who disagree about who had responsibility. It would be easy to play them off each other. Would a jury sit patiently as Dr. Aminah continued to evade answering the questions? Since the PA has already admitted he was not aware a TIA could have occurred in the face of a normal CT, this would be easily rebutted with expert witnesses.

## XI. Thrombolysis in Stroke—Legal Considerations

This is a CVA case, the hottest of hot-button issues in Emergency Medicine. Though it turns out the patient was not a tPA candidate (partially due to the prolonged amount of time spent in the waiting room), doctors have lost suits where they gave tPA and where they failed to give tPA.

Stroke litigation can be divided into five broad categories:

- Failure to give tPA with absence of a specific hospital protocol (i.e., the hospital does not have a protocol for giving tPA or for rapid transfer to facility that does)
- Failure to offer tPA (i.e., patient arrives within "window" and is not offered tPA)
- Misdiagnosis of stroke (i.e., Dx of vertigo, migraine, anxiety/panic) or failure to recognize stroke in evolution
- Complications of therapy/failure of informed consent (i.e., complication for which the patient was not aware)
- Hemorrhagic stroke after informed consent (known but unintended consequences of treatment)

## XII. Medical Discussion (Adler continued)—Evaluation of Neuro Complaints and Timely Diagnosis of Stroke

The discussion surrounding the safety and efficacy of tPA for acute ischemic stroke has been ongoing for decades. The ECASS III study,[10] assessed the clinical efficacy of tPA randomized patients to a 3–4.5 hour from time last known well. The 4.5-hour window, utilizing strict inclusion criteria, is currently supported by American Heart Association/American Stroke Association,[11] American College of Emergency Physicians, American College of Cardiology, European Stroke Organization, National Stroke Foundation, and National Institute for Health and Care Excellence. tPA is approved by the FDA up to a 3-hour window.

From a medicolegal standpoint, there are several studies that suggest most litigation involves failing to give tPA or failing to give tPA timely. Ganti, et al.[12] reviewed closed cases from 1996-2020, finding 100% were related to failure to give tPA or a delay in giving tPA. Additional published studies support the most common reason for litigation involving a failure to treat, a failure to treat timely, or failure to treat with thrombectomy, as opposed to complications from its administration. However, it's important to recognize that although this may be statistically true, sampling bias results in many more patients who haven't received tPA than those who have. This creates a larger pool of potential plaintiffs in the non-tPA recipient group.

## XIII. Guest Interview—Medical

**Evie Marcolini, MD**
Associate Professor of Emergency Medicine
Dartmouth Geisel School of Medicine

**Authors.** *What is your impression of Crystal's initial visit—two episodes of right-sided numbness which resolved?*
**EM.** From what is written, Crystal had a sudden onset of R hand weakness, then fell and couldn't get up for 3 minutes, all of which resolved spontaneously. Looking at this retrospectively, it is an unprovoked

episode, with a neurologic deficit (unable to move) that resolved. Of course, we know the end of the story, so this looks obvious that it is a TIA. When reading the chart, I have to ask, "what would I have done in this situation?" How many times do we have an impression of the patient (reliable vs. unreliable, accurate vs. exaggerating) and let that sway our evaluation and actions? Crystal had a transient neurologic deficit, which is by definition TIA, in the setting of multiple risk factors for stroke (family history, tobacco use, elevated platelet levels).

**Authors.** *How would you approach this patient?*
**EM.** From the documentation, and by definition, TIA is in the differential, but it leaves me wanting more of the story. Did this ever happen before? Did she have any pain? When did it start? What other symptoms were present during the event? I don't see a review of systems – what was she experiencing prior to the event? How did she feel afterward? What prompted her to come into the emergency department? The triage note states that she "sounds congested" and is tearful. Does she have complaints of congestion, headache or sinus-related symptoms? There may have been more to this story, but it is not documented. Let's be honest – we all have patients that don't strike us as reliable in the first moments. If they have complaints that fall into a risky category such as TIA or stroke, we should be hypervigilant in proving to ourselves that this is not the case. Similar to the intoxicated patient who complains of headache (and is later found to have a subdural hemorrhage after they "dry out") – we have to convince ourselves that the patient does not have a TIA or stroke.

**Authors.** *If your primary consideration is stroke or TIA, is there a low-risk group that can be sent home?*
**EM.** The scoring tools are not in and of themselves a way to decide on whether to send the patient home. If the patient has multiple risk factors, I want to know if they have the optimal risk mitigation in place.

1. Are they taking aspirin or another anticoagulant?
2. Are they taking a statin or do they have a recent LDL that shows it is not indicated?
3. Do they have a recent echo confirming that there is no cardiac abnormality which increases the risk for stroke (atrial fibrillation, valvular problems, wall motion abnormality, etc.)?
4. Do they have neurology follow-up?

If they have all these in place, they don't require admission. If they don't have these in place, I would admit under observation status to obtain these risk mitigation studies. Finally, does the patient have a support system? Do they live with family or friends who will notice whether they have stroke-like symptoms in the next week? If they are unhoused, they will be very unlikely to have a reliable witness over the following week; this is not strictly an indication for admission, but it certainly increases my concern that they need to have optimization for safe discharge. An observation admission gives us the chance to educate the patient, check all the risk mitigation boxes, and get them set up with a neurology follow-up.

**Authors.** *Should our patient have been hospitalized?*
**EM.** Yes, this patient was not on aspirin or statin, and it is unlikely that she had a recent echo. She would have benefitted from all of the above, including education about stroke.

**Authors.** *How do the elevated platelets play into your decision model?*
**EM.** Elevated platelets certainly increase my suspicion for TIA, based on the physiology of platelets, clot formation and stroke. I can't see how we get a result of 1.3 million platelets and we would not want to know more – Why does she have thrombocytosis? What is causing this? If my initial differential includes TIA, the elevated platelets stick out like a sore thumb and push me to gather all the data, which then supports the diagnosis of TIA: transient neurologic deficit, family history, tobacco use, elevated platelets, and lack of risk mitigation for subsequent stroke. The rest is protocol.

**Authors:** *To throw out a hypothetical, assuming the patient had not been placed in the waiting room, but seen immediately by the ED doctor with a CT confirming CVA, can you walk us through some of the pros and cons of thrombolytic therapy?*
**EM:** The picture of stuttering symptoms with no current deficits, and a CT confirming CVA indicates that the stroke has completed (since it is visualized on a non-contrast CT), but there is certainly risk of another subsequent stroke. Thrombolytics are not indicated with a normal neurologic exam and completed stroke. I would want vascular imaging to see if she has a dissection, atherosclerosis or critical stenosis as etiology of the emboli, and a full workup for the etiology of her stroke.

## XIV. Author Summary (Weinstock)

When two providers see a patient, who is medically and legally responsible? It is safe to say that if the attending could have seen the outcome in a crystal ball, he would have taken more ownership of the patient. If the PA had recognized he was left with diagnostic uncertainty exceeding his training or comfort level, he would have asked for help. When he told the plaintiff's attorney that he spoke with the attending and he knew this because he always speaks with the attending, it was clear the case was lost. Now the plaintiff's attorney is not fighting against two providers alone, but is assisted in his battle since they are also fighting against each other.

This case was featured on the podcast Risk Management Monthly (RMM), resulting in a lively discussion. One point hammered home by one of the panelists, John Rockwood, an amazing PA that I have had the pleasure of working with for many years, is that this is a team effort; we are all working together and need to be available for consultations if needed.

**Take home points:**

- Use caution in ordering tests which do not have a good chance of establishing the diagnosis. An unrecognized false positive can be misleading. An unrecognized true positive can be devastating.
- When a patient is discharged without a clear diagnosis, a plan must be in place for completion of the evaluation. Though Crystal could have been discharged from the ED, but only with the understanding of the potentially worst diagnosis, and definitive plans for further testing the next day, the safest approach would have been admission.
- One approach when thrombolytics are an option is to present the patient and family with the risks and benefits and let them make the decision (of course, with your guidance). If lytics are not used, specifically document why they were not given.
- The last summary point for this case also applies to all the cases in this book; though we have the most advanced technology in the world at our fingertips, history is still king!

## References

1. Augustine JJ. More advanced practice providers working in emergency departments. 2017. [Accessed March 1, 2023]. Available at: http://www.acepnow.com/article/advanced-practice-providers-working-emergency departments/?singlepage=1.
2. Chaela JA, Kidwell CS, Nentwich LM, et al. Magnetic resonance imaging and computed tomography in emergency assessment of patients with suspected acute stroke: A prospective comparison. Lancet 2007; 369(9558):293-98
3. Basak R, Chowdhury A, Fatmi L, et al. Stroke in the young: Relationship with iron deficiency anemia and thrombocytosis. Mymensingh MJ 2008;17(1):74-77. Accessed March 20, 2023.

4. Williams B, Morton C. Cerebral vascular accident in a patient with reactive thrombocytosis: A rare cause of stroke. Am J Med Sci 2008;336(3):279-81. doi:10.1097/MAJ.0b013e3181862556
5. Siket MS, Silver B. The 10-second stroke: A case report. J Stroke Cerebrovasc Dis 2015;24(6):e133-4. doi: 10.1016/j.jstrokecerebrovasdis.2015.01.024. Epub 2015 Apr 25. PMID: 25920752.
6. Johnston SC, Gress DR, Browner WS, et al. Short-term prognosis after emergency department diagnosis of TIA. JAMA 2000;284(22):2901-6. doi: 10.1001/jama.284.22.2901. PMID: 11147987.
7. Chandratheva A, Mehta Z, Geraghty OC, et al. Population-based study of risk and predictors of stroke in the first few hours after a TIA. Neurology 2009 Jun 2;72(22):1941-7. doi: 10.1212/WNL.0b013e3181a826ad. PMID: 19487652; PMCID: PMC2690971.
8. Powers WJ, Rabinstein AA, Ackerson T, et al. American Heart Association Stroke Council. 2018 Guidelines for the early management of patients with acute ischemic stroke: A guideline for healthcare professionals from the American Heart Association/American Stroke Association. Stroke 2018;49(3):e46-e110. doi: 10.1161/STR.0000000000000158. Epub 2018 Jan 24. Erratum in: Stroke 2018;49(3):e138. Erratum in: Stroke 2018 Apr 18: PMID: 29367334.
9. American College of Emergency Physicians Clinical Policies Subcommittee (Writing Committee) on Suspected Transient Ischemic Attack: Lo BM, Carpenter CR, Hatten BW, et al. Clinical policy: Critical issues in the evaluation of adult patients with suspected transient ischemic attack in the emergency department. Ann Emerg Med 2016;68(3):354-70.e29. doi: 10.1016/j.annemergmed.2016.06.048. Erratum in: Ann Emerg Med 2017;70(5):758. PMID: 27568419.
10. Hacke W, Kaste M, Bluhmki E, et al.; ECASS Investigators. Thrombolysis with alteplase 3 to 4.5 hours after acute ischemic stroke. N Engl J Med 2008;359(13):1317-29. doi: 10.1056/NEJMoa0804656. PMID: 18815396.
11. Powers WJ, Rabinstein AA, Ackerson T, et al. Guidelines for the early management of patients with acute ischemic stroke: 2019 update to the 2018 guidelines for the early management of acute ischemic stroke: A guideline for healthcare professionals from the American Heart Association/American Stroke Association. Stroke 2019;50(12):e344–e418.
12. Ganti L, Kwon B, George A, et al. Tissue plasminogen activator and patients with acute ischemic stroke: The litigation landscape. J Am Coll Emerg Physicians Open 2022;3(1):e12646.

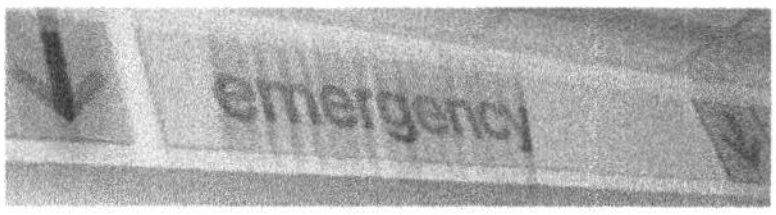


# Case 11

## A 43 Year-old Man with Leg Pain: Settle or go to Trial?

**Primary case authors:**
**Michael Pallaci**
**Nicholas LaFountain**
**Brock Landrum**

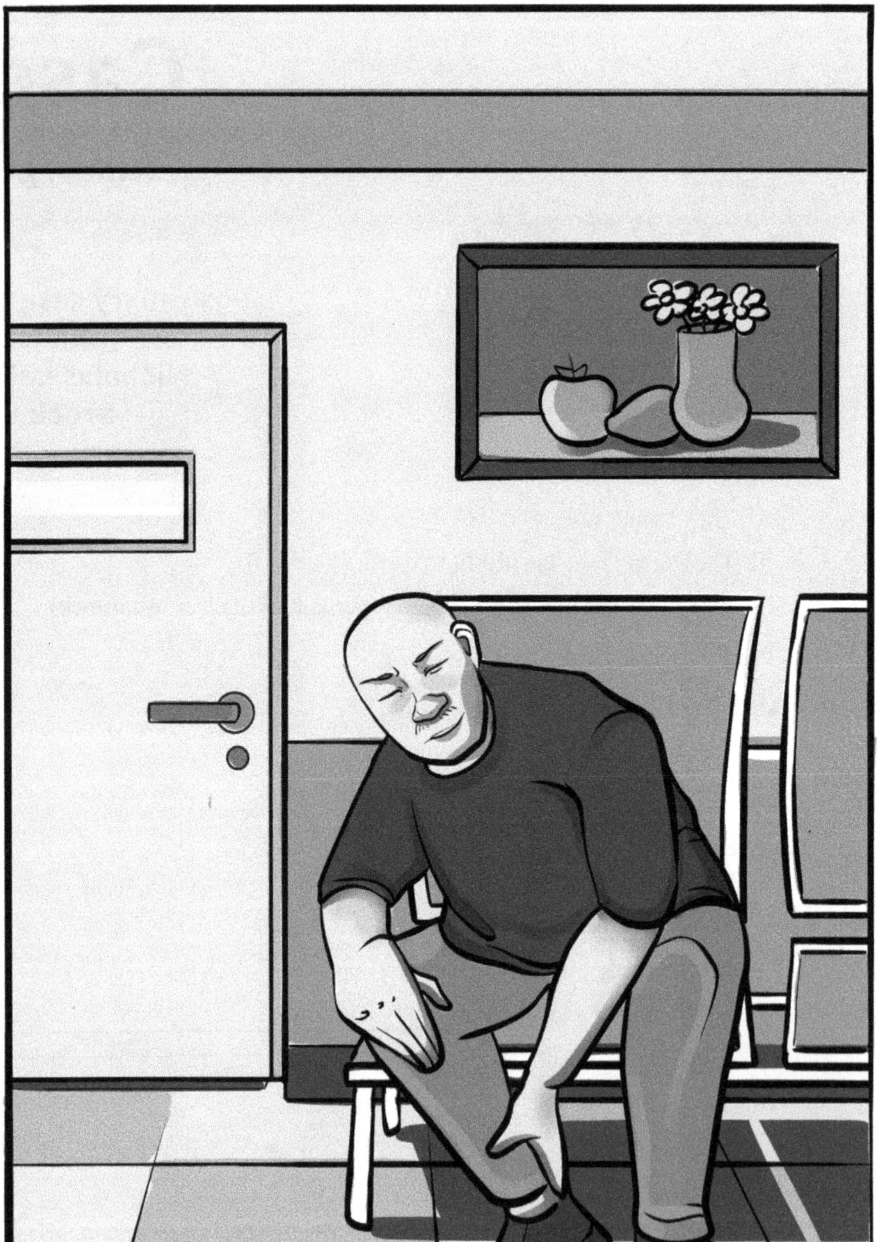

# Case 11

## A 43 Year-old Man with Leg Pain: Settle or go to Trial?

Why is it that patients don't come in with a chief complaint of "pain out of proportion to exam?" It would make life so much easier…

***Deep thoughts:***

1. *How much investigation and how much documentation is enough to discharge a patient who is tachycardic?*
2. *What is a "curbside consult" and how does it affect the legal outcome when there's a bad medical outcome?*
3. *What goes into the decision to settle or go to trial, and what are your options when you don't agree with your insurance carrier?*

## PART 1—MEDICAL

### I. The Patient's Story

Tom and Kim Green met at a small college in the rural Midwest in the late 90's. Tom was studying electronics, while Kim was studying fish and wildlife management. They enjoyed each other's company and quickly became good friends, eventually falling in love and getting married.

Kim took a job as a professor at another small rural college in the Midwest close to where she and Tom went to school, and Tom worked for a local tech company, but his real passions were family and music. He played drums while he was in college, and still played on occasion while his son Sean and his daughter Sadie danced, making movies and laughing. He did everything with the kids: Painting, magic tricks, playing songs, and cooking dinner.

One afternoon, Kim noticed some swelling on 5 year-old Sean's chin. She took him to the Emergency Department (ED), where the provider was concerned enough to have him transferred to the children's hospital to be admitted for IV antibiotics. He was discharged two days later with a diagnosis of cellulitis due to a combination of Strep and Staph.

Tom left work early the following Friday because he wasn't feeling well. When Kim got home, he left the kids with her and drove himself to an urgent care. His temperature was 102°F, and he was experiencing body aches, congestion, and a mild cough. He had a negative rapid Strep and a negative flu screen, but the urgent care provider prescribed Tamiflu based on clinical suspicion. Over the weekend, Kim did her best to bring him back to health. Soup, essential oils, over-the-counter meds, homemade juice, herbal teas, whatever she could think of. He seemed to do a little better Saturday, but on Sunday he stayed in bed all day. Sunday night, he developed pain in his leg.

## II. The Doctor's Version (The ED Chart) (the following is the actual documentation of the providers)

**Chief Compliant (at 19:40):** Right Lower Extremity Pain

**History of Present Illness (per Tara Mudge, PA at 19:40):** pain rated at a 10/10 to his posterior right knee x 3 days. Pt. states that he was Dx with the flu 4 days ago and has been bed ridden for the past 4 days. He is drinking fluids well and taking Tylenol and ibuprofen to help with his pain. Pt. denies active or recent cancer. Calf swelling, leg swelling, localized tenderness along DVT system, pitting edema, recent immobilization of leg, previous DVT, redness or swelling. Pt. denies CP, SOB. No other complaints.

**Past Medical History/Triage:**
**PMH:** Negative
**PSH:** Negative
**Medications:** None
**SH:** No alcohol or drug use

Vital Signs

| Time | Temp(F) | Pulse | Resp | Syst | Diast | Sat (room air) |
|---|---|---|---|---|---|---|
| 19:41 | 98.2 | 114 | 18 | 105 | 63 | 100% |

**Physical Examination (at 19:50)**
**General:** Alert, mild distress
**ENT:** Normal inspection, pharynx normal, no signs of dehydration
**Resp:** Chest nontender, no respiratory distress, normal breath sounds
**Card:** Regular rate and rhythm
**Abd:** Non-tender, normal bowel sounds
**Back:** Normal inspection
**Skin:** No embolic lesions, color normal, no rash, warm dry and intact
**Extremities:** Non-tender, full ROM, no pedal edema
**Neuro:** Oriented x4, motor normal, sensation normal

**Orders:** BMP, Magnesium, D-dimer, Hydromorphone 1mg IM, Hydrocodone-APAP 5-325 mg PO, Ondansetron 4 mg PO ODT, Enoxaparin 77 mg SQ, Mag-Oxide 400 mg PO

**Results (at 20:17):**

| | | | |
|---|---|---|---|
| **NA** | 132 | | (130-142 MMOL/L) |
| **K** | 3.6 | | (3.8-5.0 MMOL/L) |
| **Cl** | 95 | L | (101-111 MMOL/L) |
| **$CO_2$** | 23 | | (21-31 MMOL/L) |
| **Bun** | 15 | | (7-18 MG/DL) |
| **Creat** | 1.4 | H | (0.40-1.20 MG/DL) |
| **Cal** | 9.1 | | (8.4-10.2 MG/DL) |
| **D-DIMER** | 1140 | H | (0-599 NG/ML) |

**Progress Note (at 21:10):** Pt continues to deny SOB/ CP. Pt. scheduled to return for outpatient US for DVT ro tomorrow. Pt given lovenox sub q prior to discharge home for the evening

**Diagnosis:**
Leg pain
Elevated D-dimer

**Disposition:** Discharge home in stable condition

*Tara Mudge, PA*
*Dr. Michael Beretta*

## III. Risk Management/Patient Safety Opportunities (Pallaci, Weinstock)

**Risk Management/Patient Safety Opportunity #1:**

**Opportunity:** Recognize the significance and importance of discharge tachycardia.
**Discussion:** At the patient's initial encounter, vital signs included an elevated heart rate of 114 bpm. While the physician assistant's physical exam states "regular rate and rhythm," a repeat set of vitals is not recorded, and tachycardia is not addressed in the MDM. Unexplained tachycardia, especially at time of discharge, is a finding that warrants re-evaluation, as well as consideration for alternative acute pathology (i.e. PE, sepsis, etc.). In a patient with isolated leg pain who will undergo a delayed work-up for DVT, persistent tachycardia should raise suspicion for pulmonary embolism (PE) if symptoms of PE are present (tough in this case due to the lack of chest pain and shortness of breath is documented both in the HPI and on re-evaluation).
✔ **Teaching point:** Be wary of tachycardia on discharge, especially if there is not a good explanation.

**Risk Management/Patient Safety Opportunity #2:**

**Opportunity:** Have a heightened awareness for patients complaining of severe pain. Is this pain out of proportion (POOP)?
**Discussion:** At their initial visit, the patient reported "10 out of 10 calf pain" and was documented to be in mild distress. The treating physician felt that the patient's pain was significant and treated with 1 mg of IM hydromorphone followed by hydrocodone/acetaminophen. However, there was no documentation regarding response to treatment or re-evaluation. While patients may not explicitly report "pain out of proportion," severe refractory extremity pain warrants consideration for limb ischemia, compartment syndrome, and necrotizing soft tissue infection.
✔ **Teaching point:** If the patient's level of pain is out of proportion to the suspected diagnosis, alternative diagnoses should be considered.

**Risk Management/Patient Safety Opportunity #3:**

**Opportunity:** Return instructions should specifically state why to return.
**Discussion:** At the initial encounter the patient was discharged following treatment with Lovenox with a plan for outpatient follow-up for doppler US. While this is a common protocol for DVT work-up when ultrasound is unavailable, there remains diagnostic uncertainty at the time of discharge. This scenario especially warrants a discussion and emphasis on return precautions, including signs and symptoms that suggest alternative pathology (i.e., infection), as well as potential complication of DVT (i.e., pulmonary

embolism or phlegmasia). This patient was instructed to return to the ED immediately for severe or refractory pain, thus prompting their return visit.

✔ **Teaching point:** Provide action and time specific discharge instructions accounting for serious disease.

**Risk Management/Patient Safety Opportunity #4:**

**Opportunity:** Avoid a catastrophic missed diagnosis by not anchoring or prematurely stopping the work-up.

**Discussion:** The chief complaint of (unilateral) "leg swelling" is common in the ED; often patients have already done their "Internet research" and concluded that they might have a DVT. This situation can easily lead to anchoring bias, including exclusively focusing the history and physical exam on risk factors and features of a specific diagnosis, such as DVT. However, it is important to maintain a broad differential; in the case of unilateral limb swelling/pain, consider vascular disease, infectious processes or trauma.

✔ **Teaching point:** Avoid anchoring bias and premature closure.

**Author comments (Michael Pallaci, Nicholas LaFountain and Brock Landrum):** The patient had significantly worsening pain and swelling of his right lower extremity prompting him to call EMS and arrive at 0525 the next morning, despite an appointment scheduled at 0800 for his DVT ultrasound.

## IV. The Bounceback

**Chief Compliant (at 0525):** RLE pain, swelling

**History of Present Illness (Per Dr. Michael Beretta at 0545):** Seen here last night for RLE pain, d-dimer elevated, given instructions for O/P doppler today. Got sq Lovenox prior to d/c. Returns by EMS for doppler. No cp/sob. No fever. No trauma/injury.

Vital Signs

| Time | Temp(F) | Pulse | Resp | Syst | Diast | Sat (room air) |
|---|---|---|---|---|---|---|
| 05:25 | 97.5 | 124 | 18 | 122 | 90 | 96% |

**Physical Examination:**
**General:** Well developed, well-nourished lying in bed who appears nontoxic
**Eye:** Sclera anicteric
**ENT:** MMM
**Respiratory:** No respiratory distress
**Skin:** Warm and dry. No appreciable rash
**Neuro:** Awake and alert with normal speech and mental status, moves all extremities equally, no focal deficits or lateralizing signs
**Psych:** Very anxious
**MS:** Unilateral leg swelling and tenderness. No erythema or warmth
**Orders (at 0545):** Hydromorphone 2 mg SQ, Venous Duplex RLE

**Transition of care progress note (per Dr. David Sharpe at 0750):** [I have assumed care in a patient that was] signed out [to me] for further management. Markedly tender right lower extremity, especially in calf but extending from ankle to mid-thigh, with swelling. Some discoloration/mottling of medial malleolar region. Patient notes symptoms have worsened since arrival in ED.

**Orders per Dr. Sharpe (at 0756):** BMP, Blood Culture x2, CBC w/diff, Creatine Kinase, Urinalysis w/ culture, Lactic Acid, CT Right Lower Extremity W Contrast, Venous Duplex Ultrasound Right Lower Extremity, X-ray chest portable 1 view, X-ray Right Tibia-Fibula 3-view.

**Results:**

| | | | |
|---|---|---|---|
| **WBC** | 2.82 | L | 4.50-11 .00 K/MCL |
| **Hemoglobin** | 16.2 | | 13.5-17.5 G/DL |
| | | | |
| **NA** | 127 | L | 130-142 MMOL/L |
| **K** | 3.7 | | 3.6-5.0 MMOL/L |
| **$CO_2$** | 18 | L | 21-31 MMOL/L |
| **Gluc** | 143 | H | 70-99 MG/DL |
| **Bun** | 35 | H | 7-18 MG/DL |
| **Creat** | 2.7 | H | 0.4-1.2 MG/DL |
| **Anion Gap** | 17.7 | H | 5-11.5 |
| | | | |
| **CPK** | 6403 | H | 22-238 U/L |
| | | | |
| **Lactate:** | 6.9 | H | 0.5-2.2 MG/DL |

**X-Ray Right Tibia/Fibula 3-Views:**
**Radiologist Impression:** Negative X-rays of the right tibia and fibula. No stress reaction or fracture of the tibia or fibula. No soft tissue gas collection or foreign body. The ankle mortise is normally aligned.

**Venous Duplex Ultrasound Right Lower Extremity:**
**Radiologist Impression**
No evidence of acute deep or superficial thrombosis in right lower extremity.

**Progress Note (at 0845):** Throughout the morning, the patient remained awake alert, with tachycardia noted. IV fluids were given. Additional work-up was ordered, which demonstrated a significant lactic acidosis. An X-ray of the leg was also obtained, which did not show any subcutaneous air or acute bony changes. There was concern for a possible compartment syndrome, and surgery was consulted. Surgery stated that this appeared to be a myositis and not compartment syndrome, recommended CT of the lower extremity for further evaluation. CT was subsequently obtained (full read below) which did demonstrate myositis. Creatine kinase results noted, confirming the presence of a rhabdomyolysis. IV fluids continued and a sodium bicarbonate drip was ordered.

**CT Right Lower Extremity With Contrast:**
1. Diffuse subcutaneous and intermuscular fascial edema involving all compartments of the right lower extremity, most compatible with myositis. The possibility of compartment syndrome is unlikely based on multicompartmental involvement; however, compartment syndrome is not a CT diagnosis.
2. Intramuscular edema is noted in the adductor magnus muscle, biceps femoris muscle, soleus muscle, peroneal muscles, and deep posterior compartment muscles of the leg. No focal intramuscular fluid

collection to indicate abscess or hematoma.
3. No acute osseous abnormality identified.
4. Small joint effusion in the knee.
5. Mild lymphadenopathy in the distal right iliac chain and groin.
6. Although not a dedicated angiographic study, the femoral arteries and veins appear grossly patent.

**Summary Of Emergency Department Course:** Patient lost peripheral IV access and right internal jugular central venous catheterization was attempted. He became more agitated and tachycardic during the procedure and was unable to tolerate placement of the central line.

**14:07:** He then developed bradycardia and subsequent PEA cardiac arrest requiring initiation of CPR. Intraosseous access was obtained, and femoral central venous access was attempted during CPR. Patient had return of spontaneous circulation after 22 minutes of CPR with epinephrine, sodium bicarbonate, calcium gluconate administration. Patient was intubated during CPR and was started on IV fluids, IV Vancomycin and Levaquin. Initial arterial blood gas showed a pH less than 6.8 with a $pCO_2$ of 107 mm/Hg.

The decision was then made to transfer to higher level of care. Transfer was delayed due to multiple area hospitals being unable to facilitate transfer due to bed availability and due to not having adequate care resources for the patient's medical condition. Eventually, an outside hospital ICU accepted transfer once patient was considered more stable, specifically a pH greater than 7.0. The patient had three total cardiac arrests prior to transfer. He received multiple blood product transfusions as well as vasopressor support and IV fluid resuscitation. His leg was noted to become more ecchymotic and swollen throughout his ED course.

**21:30**: He was transferred and admitted to outside hospital ICU in critical condition.

**Hospital Course:** Upon arrival to the outside hospital, general surgery and orthopedic surgery performed operative debridement and right hip disarticulation with findings consistent with necrotizing soft tissue infection. At the time of debridement, the infection had extended into his thorax. After his operation, he continued to develop worsening septic shock with multiorgan failure including poor neurologic examination with fixed dilated pupils and the decision was made to withdraw care. He was pronounced dead one day after transfer.

**Final Diagnosis:** Necrotizing Soft Tissue Infection Resulting in Septic Shock with Multiorgan Failure and death.

## PART 2—LEGAL

## I. The Accusation/Cause of Action

Multiple accusations were made in this case.

- Negligence of the Emergency Medicine providers resulting in failure to diagnose, physical suffering, and wrongful death.
- Negligence of the surgeon resulting in failure to diagnose, physical suffering, and wrongful death.
- Loss of consortium.
- The hospital was sued for the acts and omissions of the defendants.

There were multiple defendants: The Emergency Medicine providers including two physicians (Dr. Beretta, the doctor who cared for Tom on both initial presentations, as well as Dr. Sharpe, who relieved Dr. Beretta at 7:00 AM at the second visit), Tara Mudge (the physician assistant who did the initial evaluation on the first visit), Dr. Felipe Rodriguez (the orthopedic surgeon), and the hospital. The accusation of negligence toward the EPs emphasized the lack of bloodwork and imaging on the initial visit as well as the lack of consideration of an infectious process or identifying sepsis.

## II. The Depositions

**Author comments (Weinstock):** The emergency providers (Mudge, Beretta and Sharpe) were all employed by the same contract management group, and therefore, were represented by the same counsel. Dr. Rodriguez (ortho) was an employee of the hospital. So, he and the hospital were jointly represented by separate counsel.

Before the depositions, the hospital and Dr. Rodriguez (ortho) settled for $4.5 million. This left only the emergency providers as defendants. There were approximately 56 hours of deposition testimony.

There were fireworks; some of the depositions became quite contentious and nasty. Multiple topics were covered, but we will focus on the four issues discussed in the risk management section above (discharge tachycardia, pain out of proportion, return precautions and anchoring bias) as well as the timing of the surgical consult/diagnosis and the concept of a curbside consult.

Cast of characters (names changed, except where noted):
**Defendant PA:** Tara Mudge, PA (defendant PA who saw pt at the first visit)
**Orthopedist defendant:** Dr. Rodriguez (orthopedist defendant)
**Plaintiff's expert:** Dr. Vandelay (Chairman of Prestigious Academic ED)
**Plaintiff's expert:** Dr. Kennedy (EM)
**Defense expert:** Dr. Thomas (Double Boarded in EM and ID)
**Defense expert:** Dr. Ingram (Trauma and General Surgery)

### A. Discharge tachycardia:

**Author comments (Weinstock):** The discussions regarding tachycardia mostly focused on the cause and whether it was reasonable to discharge the patient with persistent tachycardia.

**Cross-Examination of plaintiff's expert Dr. Vandelay (Chairman of Prestigious Academic ED) by defense attorney:**

**Q.** Does pain cause tachycardia?
**A.** It can, I think it is possible that pain can cause transient tachycardia but it doesn't cause prolonged tachycardia or persistent tachycardia that doesn't go away. So, in this case there's no explanation for this tachycardia.

**Q.** And can dehydration cause tachycardia?
**A.** Dehydration can but usually it's severe dehydration that is responsible, especially resting tachycardia can be caused by severe dehydration but it doesn't persist typically, and I don't think there's any evidence that this patient had severe dehydration.

**Cross-Examination of defense expert Dr. Thomas (Double Boarded in EM and ID) by plaintiff's attorney:**

**Q.** Do you believe it's within the standard of care to discharge from the emergency department a patient with tachycardia the cause of which is undiagnosed?
**A.** It's too general but I think in this case…it was reasonable to discharge Mr. Green with his elevated pulse.

**Cross-Examination of plaintiff's expert Dr. Kennedy (EM) by defense attorney:**
**Dr. Kennedy:** In short, we've got a guy here…(who) went home with no explanation for his tachycardia except dehydration…when a patient comes for care and abnormalities are found, they should be either explained or mitigated. And all I'm saying is we have a set of vital signs here that are not normal, and I don't see an explanation that definitively satisfies why they are the way they are, I'm not saying we should never discharge a patient with a heart rate of 114 or even a tachycardic patient, I'm saying that we should have a substantial reason why and a DVT does not count…what we have is a patient that's tachycardic, recurrent leg pain that went home, without an explanation and without correction…I don't think a prudent group of my peers in this state at the time this occurred would send a patient home tachycardic, hypotensive with an empiric diagnosis of right lower extremity DVT with a D-dimer of 1140.

**Author comments (Weinstock):** The patient's presenting blood pressure of 105/63 (MAP 77) on the first visit, while below normal, obviously does not meet any definition of hypotension. As this discourse continued, Dr. Kennedy made an interesting concession:

**Q.** And by the way, can pain also cause tachycardia?
**A.** Pain can cause tachycardia.

**Cross-Examination of Dr. Beretta (Defendant physician/both visits) by plaintiff's attorney:**

**Q.** Does a DVT cause a patient to have an elevated temperature?
**A.** It can.

**Q.** Typically, does it?
**A.** My recollection of what I've read on this is that it causes fever 10 to 20% of the time.

**Q.** Does a DVT cause a patient to have tachycardia?
**A.** The DVT itself wouldn't typically cause the patient to have tachycardia, but fever or pain could cause the patient to have tachycardia.

**Q.** When the patient is discharged, had you diagnosed the cause of the tachycardia?
**A.** Not definitively.

**Q.** Had you treated the tachycardia?
**A.** I had treated one of the potential causes for the tachycardia, his pain.

**Q.** And then did you wait to see if the pain medications decreased his tachycardia?
**A.** I waited to see what effect the pain medication had on the overall patient.

**Q.** What was the lowest pain value that he gave you that evening?
**A.** I believe the lowest we have documented is 6.

**Q.** Okay. And that's with what kind of pain medicine on board?
**A.** He had received a half milligram of Dilaudid, which is a relatively light dose early on. And then later on, a one milligram dose, which is a more standard starting dose. So, I'd have to look specifically at the time line as to at what point along that continuum the pain score was documented.

**Q.** Do DVTs cause tachycardia even with the administration of pain medicines?
**A.** DVTs don't directly cause tachycardia. They can be associated with tachycardia if there's an associated pulmonary embolism, if there's associated pain, or if there's associated fever.

**Cross-Examination of defense expert Dr. Ingram (Trauma and General Surgery) by plaintiff's attorney:**

**Dr. Ingram.** Of course, tachycardia is related to a whole host of different issues, including simply being sick enough to come in to the hospital and being in front of a physician or a health care provider. So, there is a wide range of things that can give you tachycardia…it can be one of the markers of an infection of any sort including an NSTI.

**Q.** When Tom Green was sent home on the night of the 18th, had the cause of the tachycardia been diagnosed?
**A.** He was given a presumptive diagnosis of a DVT, and could that presumptively diagnosed DVT and the fact that he was in pain and the fact that he was in a hospital have resulted in the tachycardia? The answer is yes.

**Q.** But the tachycardia could have also been caused by an infection at that time, couldn't it?
**A.** Yes. There are a whole host of things that could have caused that tachycardia, so yes.

**B. Pain out of proportion:**

**Author comments (Weinstock):** This was a topic that was discussed surprisingly little during the depositions given the ultimate diagnosis.

**Cross-Examination of Dr. Beretta (Defendant-physician) by plaintiff's attorney:**

**Q.** Do DVTs cause the type and severity of pain that Tom Green was experiencing?
**A.** They can.

**Q.** Is it usual or unusual?
**A.** I wouldn't say that it's either. I've seen it several times. It's not every time, but it's happened. I've seen patients with that level of pain with DVT multiple times.

**Cross-Examination of Dr. Ingram (Trauma and General Surgery expert for the defense) by plaintiff's attorney:**
(Reviewing an article written by Dr. Ingram on NSTI):

**Q.** And so that tells me that if you have pain out of proportion, that is a significant risk factor of a necrotizing soft tissue infection, isn't it?
**A.** Correct.

**Q.** And he had pain out of proportion on the evening of the 18th, did he not?
**Defense attorney.** Objection.
**A.** He did.

**Author comments (Weinstock):** Counsel will frequently object during a deposition, but since a judge is not present, the objection is not ruled on and the witness answers the question. Counsel does this to get their objection on the record, and it can be dealt with during the trial. This is a surprising admission by the defense expert, considering that the defendant himself stated that he did not consider the patient to have pain out of proportion. This really comes down to what we consider to be "pain out of proportion," out of proportion to what? If we are thinking about pain out of proportion to the physical exam, then Dr. Ingram is correct. He had a benign physical exam with severe pain. So, it is reasonable to say that his pain was out of proportion to his exam. However, Dr. Beretta answered in terms of whether the pain is out of proportion to the suspected diagnosis, which in his experience with patients with DVT was not the case.

**Cross-Examination of plaintiff's expert Dr. Vandelay (Chairman of Prestigious Academic ED) by Defense attorney:**

**Q.** Is there some way to quantify what pain out of proportion is to a caregiver, to a physician who is examining a patient?
**A.** It's a subjective term. Pain out of proportion really means more pain than we would expect based on the physical findings. So, for example, a patient says I have excruciating leg pain, but you palpated it, it doesn't seem to be that tender and you look at it and it doesn't seem to have many physical findings but they're complaining of this very heightened level of pain, then that would be sort of consistent with pain out of proportion.

**C. Return precautions:**

**Cross-Examination of Dr. Beretta (Defendant) by plaintiff's attorney:**
**Q.** Did you review those discharge instructions before Tom left the hospital?
**A.** Did I review them on the chart or did I review them with Tom?

**Q.** Well, let's go first on the chart, and then with Tom.
**A.** Okay. I would have been very unlikely to have reviewed them on the chart, because I would have reviewed them verbally with Tara [the PA] and she's very reliable and capable of putting the discharge instructions in that I ask for. And I almost certainly would have reviewed them with the Greens.

**Q.** What do you recall with respect to your discharge discussion with Tom and his father?
**A.** I recall almost no details of the discussion of the instructions. But it's my common practice to go through and review what the plan is, what I want them to do, you know, what activities they can and can't do, what medications to take. In this particular case, what the thought process was and why we were giving the Lovenox injection and what the plan was for coming back to have the doppler done in the morning.

**Author comments (Weinstock):** This answer illustrates a common technique when testifying, namely describing your "common practice." It is understood that we are not going to remember everything that we did and didn't do years later, but it is acceptable (and encouraged) to state that you are highly confident that you did or did not do something because it is your common or customary practice.

**Q.** What's the significance to an emergency room physician of a bounceback patient within eight hours?
**Defense counsel.** Objection.
**A.** That really depends on the clinical situation. Sometimes patients bounce back because we tell them to bounce back specifically, either for a scheduled visit or if certain criteria are met. Sometimes they bounce back because something changed or something got worse or they weren't able to manage symptoms at home. There's a lot of reasons for a patient to bounce back.

**D. Anchoring bias:**

**Cross-Examination of defense expert Dr. Thomas (Double Boarded EM and ID) by plaintiff's attorney:**

**Q.** On the evening of the 18th, what would have been in your differential diagnosis of Mr. Green?
**A.** I think I would have thought about deep vein thrombosis in someone who has been described as bedridden and not feeling well. So, I think that would have been primary among my considerations. I would put infection on the list at the beginning but I think then in the absence of other findings of a skin and soft tissue infection, it wouldn't have been high on my list. So, I would have done the same thing. I would have pursued the diagnosis of deep vein thrombosis and arranged for an ultrasound and in this circumstance they couldn't get it right away, and giving Lovenox is fine.

**Cross-Examination of plaintiff's expert Dr. Kennedy (EM) by defense attorney:**
**Q.** So, it's reasonable based on everything you've seen in the chart from the 18th that a provisional diagnosis of DVT is reasonable as of the 18th in the evening?
**A.** I think a DVT is in the differential diagnosis; I don't think it's reasonable to prematurely narrow the differential diagnosis to a clot at all, because DVTs don't typically cause isolated pain without swelling or some risk factor that would cause a DVT in this particular patient.

**Author comments (Weinstock):** This is a curious answer from the plaintiff's expert on several levels. First, while DVTs do typically cause swelling, it is not universal. Second, isolated pain is not at all uncommon with DVT, and third, the patient was bedridden for the previous four days, which would certainly be considered a risk factor for DVT.

**Cross-Examination of defense expert Dr. Ingram (Trauma and General Surgery) by plaintiff's attorney:**

**Q.** So, I'm just saying at 5:25 AM included in the differential for a physician with these changes would be infection, correct?
**Defense counsel.** Objection.
**A.** Just with a change in the location of pain in this specific patient, the answer would be no, I still would not enter this in as part of the differential.

**Q.** When would a potential NSTI have been included in a physician caring for Tom Green's differential diagnosis to be within the standard of care?
**A.** By the time the physical exam was done where there was spreading of the erythema edema and skin changes, the mottling of the skin in and around the ankle area, at the time that all of that was occurring, the diagnosis of NSTI should have been part of the standard differential diagnosis.

**Cross-Examination of plaintiff's expert Dr. Vandelay (Chairman of Prestigious Academic ED) by defense attorney:**

**Q.** With Mr. Green on the 18th, there was no suspected source of infection was there? For example, he didn't have any cellulitis or any open wound on the 18th, correct?
**A.** Well sure there was, I mean, so he had leg pain, now we don't know off the bat that that leg pain is due to, as they thought, a DVT or something else, but it was yet to be determined, that source of infection.

**Q.** Was it reasonable to entertain a diagnosis of DVT on the evening of the 18th for Mr. Green?
**A.** Yes, but not only DVT. I think it's appropriate to consider that he had a DVT in the face of other evidence. So, for example, I would say that subjectively DVTs are not nearly as painful as things like a deep tissue space infection, so having such significant pain is unusual for DVT.

**Q.** So just to summarize regarding your opinions on the 18th, it's your opinion that Mr. Green was providing evidence of potentially sepsis, correct?
**A.** Yes.

**Q.** And that required to be worked up separately, presumably you would have recommended admission to the hospital at that point?
**A.** Yes…I think this patient required admission and further investigation as to a source, potential source of infection.

**Cross-Examination of Dr. Beretta (Defendant physician) by plaintiff's attorney:**

**Q.** When you were involved in his care on the 18th, did you create, formally or informally in your mind differential diagnoses for Tom Green?
**A.** I infrequently form a formal list of differential diagnoses, but every time I see a patient, the process of, you know, what diagnoses do I need to consider in this patient? Which diagnoses can I rule out by history and physical exam alone? Which diagnoses do I need further testing to rule in or rule out? And then which diagnoses are most likely? That process goes through my head on every patient. Although I rarely, if ever, sit down and either write on a piece of paper or list in my mind, these are the ten or twenty or thirty things that are in the differential. That's not really part of my thought process on a patient by patient basis. But again, informally that thought process goes through my mind in every patient.

**Author comments (Michael Pallaci, Nicholas LaFountain and Brock Landrum):** This exchange highlights the dilemma that we frequently face regarding whether or not to document a differential diagnosis in the chart. There is no universal agreement on this issue. From a medicolegal perspective, the advantage is that it shows what diagnoses were considered and demonstrates your thought process. The disadvantage is that it could be medicolegally disadvantageous if there is a bad outcome and the eventual diagnosis is not listed, or if you state that you considered a diagnosis but did not fully evaluate for it or did not include a sufficient explanation as to why you thought it wasn't present. [Pallaci Mike, Markowski Kevin, Weinstock Mike, Adler Jason. Emergency Medicine Documentation (US). In: Mattu A and Swadron S, ed. CorePendium. Burbank, CA. CorePendium, LLC. https://www.emrap.org/corependium/chapter/recXKF8nep5mkJcI3/Emergency-Medicine-Documentation-US#h.sbdtapuifka. Updated January 5, 2023.]

**Q.** And what was your thought process with respect to Tom Green on the night of the 18th?
**A.** My thought process was that he had been immobile for four days, had isolated lower extremity pain with a risk factor for DVT given the immobility. Had a presentation that was consistent with that and that was, in my mind at that point, the most likely diagnosis and was my working diagnosis. There, of course, are other possibilities, but given the totality of the clinical picture, as I evaluated the patient, looked at his leg, did an exam, took the history, heard how this had developed, and put all that together, at the top of my differential diagnosis was DVT.

**Q.** Okay. And what did you do to rule in or rule out an infectious process with Tom on the evening of the 18th?
**A.** It would be the history and physical exam. He had no breaks in the skin, had no erythema, had no warmth, had no fluctuance that would suggest an underlying abscess or anything like that. And he had an alternative diagnosis that was a far more likely explanation for his constellation of findings.

**Q.** Okay. So, is it fair to say that all the possible things that could have been at work with Tom to bring him to the hospital were that constellation of symptoms? With you–in your mind's eye and your thought process that night as the emergency room physician, you were 99 or 100% DVT and everything else was a 0 or a 1?
**A.** No.

**Q.** Okay. So, can you tell me what percentages of probability you assigned to DVT versus other causes?
**Defense attorney.** Objection. Go ahead, Doctor.
**A.** No, I can't tell you that. I can tell you that at the time that Mr. Green left the emergency department I thought that the most likely diagnosis was DVT, and that the ultrasound would potentially confirm that in the morning. And if it didn't, then we could pursue the others.

**Q.** In your comment, you don't have any reference to possible compartment syndrome, do you?
**A.** No.

**Q.** You don't have any reference to possible infectious process, do you?
**A.** No.

**Q.** So, when you leave the hospital at 7:00 or so in the morning of the 19th, your thought process is, Tom Green has a DVT?
**A.** No. When I leave the hospital at 7:00 in the morning, my thought process is Tom Green's most likely diagnosis is DVT.

**Q.** Okay. Most likely diagnosis is DVT. Did you have any other possible, not remote, but other possible diagnoses that would be applicable to him?
**A.** Sure. It was all the same ones that we discussed before that were going through my thought process the previous night, but my impression was still that DVT was the most likely diagnosis.

**Q.** Why didn't you order any labs on the morning of the 19th?
**A.** Because my impression from the night before hadn't really significantly changed and the test that I thought was likely to rule in the diagnosis that was most prominent on my differential was going to be completed in about an hour's time. And if I was correct about what my suspected diagnosis was, there wasn't any lab testing that would be indicated. And then if it was not present, then we can have the lab testing at that point.

**Author comments (Weinstock):** This is one of the key exchanges, addressing a central issue that will decide the outcome. Did Dr. Beretta miss this diagnosis because of premature closure, or does his explanation adequately demonstrate a reasonable thought process that meets the standard of care, what a reasonable and prudent physician with similar training would have done in a similar circumstance?

**E. Timing of surgical consult/diagnosis:**

**Author comments (Weinstock):** Dr. Ingram, the surgical defense expert witness, pulled no punches in his testimony. He placed the responsibility for the delay in diagnosis squarely on the shoulders of the surgical consultant, Dr. Rodriguez (the surgeon). The plaintiff's counsel continuously tried to nail down the defense experts and especially the defendant himself regarding when Tom Green was past the point of no return.

**Cross-Examination of defense expert Dr. Ingram (Trauma and General Surgery) by plaintiff's attorney:**

**Q.** From your review of the medical records, when was that first diagnosable?
**A.** The diagnosis of this disease in this specific case would have been confirmed intraoperatively at surgical exploration…So to answer you, although it's a difficult one to ascertain with any definitive time, I would answer it being the moment that CT scan was done, resulted, and looked at by the surgeon. That would be my best guess as to when the diagnosis ought to have been made…once the surgeon saw the leg, he now owns this consult and he didn't pick up the diagnosis of the necrotizing soft tissue infection…once we have the results of the CT scan, it really now becomes important and incumbent upon Dr. Rodriguez to look at the results of the CT scan and put it together with the physical findings.

**Q.** So, the only thing from the CT scan that's within the realm of necrotizing soft tissue infection that you say Rodriguez should have picked up on was this fascial layer, correct?
**A.** Correct. And the fact that there's muscle edema. But I think that the finding that certainly caught my eye and I suspected would catch the eye of most surgeons that take care of these patients is that fascial edema.

**Q. (Reading from an article on NSTI).** "The predominant challenges in the early management of NSTI are related to delayed clinical diagnosis resulting frequently in delayed treatment" – do you see that?
**A.** I do.

**Q.** And you would say that that was in part because of Dr. Rodriguez, correct?
**A.** Correct.

**Q.** And you would agree that that was in part because of Dr. Sharpe, wouldn't you?

**Defense attorney.** Objection.
**A.** Again, it is the responsibility of Dr. Rodriguez, the surgical consultant, to make the diagnosis. So, did Dr. Sharpe (EP who accepted transition of care on visit #2) not make the diagnosis? That's a true statement. But the responsibility for making the diagnosis really rests squarely with the surgical consultant.

**Cross-Examination of defense expert Dr. Thomas (Double Boarded EM and ID) by plaintiff's attorney:**

**Q.** Doctor, can you list for me all the opinions which you anticipate giving at the trial of the action?
**A.** Sure. With regard to standard of care, I think the emergency providers in the ED on the 18th and 19th met the standard of care…and with regard to whether earlier treatment might have made any difference, I think on the 18th had Tom Green been admitted and started on antibiotics in the hospital, I don't think any surgeon would have operated on him and I expect he would have had a similar course as he did when he came back to the emergency department on the morning of the 19th. I don't think antibiotics either on the 18th or the 19th alone would have affected his outcome. Group A Strep necrotizing fasciitis requires surgical debridement or amputation for the person to survive. I think on the 19th there was an opportunity in the morning for amputation. If it had been done, maybe a hip disarticulation, there was a chance that Tom Green might have survived. I don't know that. I would say that's speculative. But otherwise after, let's say about 10:00 or 11:00 when his blood pressure dropped, I don't think any different treatment would have saved his life unfortunately…this is a tragic case. I feel very sorry for everyone involved, particularly Mr. Green's family, but unfortunately I don't think his disease could have been reasonably diagnosed sooner than it was such that it would have affected his outcome, which must be a hard thing to hear but that's my opinion.

**Cross-Examination of plaintiff's expert Dr. Kennedy (EM) by defense attorney:**

**Q.** So, the infection's not going to go away with just antibiotics, it needs surgical debridement, fair?
**A.** I can't say that the infection's not going to go away, but I think any prudent person reviewing this case and having seen 20 cases of nec fasc and lost limbs would agree that just treating with antibiotics and waiting to call the orthopedic surgeon in case something else needed to be done would not be a prudent course of action. And for the orthopedic surgeon to look at it and go, let's just wait and see, would not be a prudent course of action. So, I don't know when we should have saved a limb or a life, but I do know the earliest we could have started doing things is the evening of the 18th and definitely by 8:00 on the morning of the 19th.

**Cross-Examination of Dr. Beretta (Defendant physician ) by plaintiff's attorney:**

**Q.** As you sit here today, do you have any opinion as to whether, if Tom Green had had a debridement procedure and been administered broad spectrum antibiotics, was there a time at which…let's start with his leg. That his leg would have been saved?

**Defense attorney.** Objection. Go ahead.
**A.** It's possible that there is, but there's no way to know when that would be.

**Q.** Okay. So…is there a time by which you believe his life would have been saved when he was a patient at your hospital?

**Defense attorney.** Objection.
**Hospital's attorney.** Objection.

**A.** There's no way for me to know when it was too late for Tom Green. But considering the way that he presented and how this condition hid itself…he had a disease that was awful, that progresses rapidly, where early diagnosis is critical and often difficult. In this case, I think early diagnosis was impossible.

**Q.** Do you hold any opinions as to whether or not Tom Green would have survived had he been transferred or seen at a tertiary referral hospital on the evening of April 18th?
**A.** I believe if he was seen at a tertiary referral center on the evening of the 18th that they very likely, probably, almost certainly would have taken the same course that I took.

**Q.** Do you hold any opinions as to whether if Tom Green received broad spectrum antibiotics on the evening of the 18th, if he would have survived?
**Defense attorney.** Objection.
**Hospital's attorney.** Objection.

**A.** It's pure speculation, but if you're asking my opinion, my opinion is no.

**Q.** Okay. Do you hold any opinion if he would have received broad spectrum antibiotics before noon on the 19th, would Tom Green have survived?

**Defense attorney.** Objection.

**A.** I think that it's unlikely. Antibiotics are an adjunct to treatment of necrotizing soft tissue infections. What he really needed was surgery.

**Q.** Well, that's where I was going next. Do you have an opinion as to whether if Tom Green had received a surgical debridement of the necrotizing tissues on the morning of the 19th, together with adjunct broad-spectrum antibiotic therapy, if he would have survived?

**Hospital's attorney.** Objection.
**Defense attorney.** Objection.

**A.** I think we've kind of covered this before and that there certainly was a point of no return. Identifying when that is impossible, and really trying to put your finger on a specific time, I think, would be irresponsible. It's just guesswork.

**F. Curbside consult:**

**Cross-Examination of Dr. Rodriguez (Surgical Consultant; Dismissed from Suit) by defense attorney:**

**Q.** Do you have a recollection of how you first became involved in the care of Mr. Green?
**A.** Sure. I was operating on the day Mr. Green was consulted to me. I got a phone call from Dr. Sharpe and at the conclusion of my first scheduled case of the day, I went in to go see Mr. Green when he had been in the emergency department. The reason for the consultation was curbside for the evaluation of a preliminary diagnosis of compartment syndrome. I stopped what I was doing and I went to go see Mr. Green in between cases.

**Q.** You mentioned the word "curbside." What do you mean by "curbside"? Is that a consultation?
**A.** Yeah, it is a consultation as a quick evaluation to help figure out a differential diagnosis.

**Q.** Okay, I'm just wondering about the term. Is "curbside" an actual term of art, is it a slang term for the type of consult? I've heard the term used before, but I'm just wondering how you're using it.
**A.** Curbside consults happen a lot of the time in medicine where you have a colleague or a friend call you for a quick thought process on something, whether it's foot pain or shoulder pain or…so it's a…it is a curb…I don't know, it's a curbside consult.

**Q.** So, as we discussed at the beginning of your deposition, you did not write a consult note regarding your consultation with Dr. Sharpe regarding Mr. Green, correct?
**A.** That's correct.

**Q.** Why didn't you write a consult note?
**A.** I was going to finish the curbside consult at the end of the day and when I had spoken to Dr. Sharpe and he didn't look good, at some point I realized that it was not dramatically going to change his plan, and truthfully, I just forgot.

**Cross-Examination of defense expert Dr. Ingram (Trauma and General Surgery) by plaintiff's attorney:**
**Q.** When did you form an opinion that Dr. Rodriguez had breached the standard of care?
**A.** I was very concerned when I first read the packet of documents that were sent to me because there was a striking lack of documentation from the surgical consultant. And so right from the get-go I wanted more information on what the surgeon was thinking, what the surgeon did, because there was simply no documentation…but the first time I was sure that he had breached the standard of care was when I read his deposition.

**Q.** Okay, so let's talk about your hospital a little bit. Do you have surgical curbside consults?

**Defense attorney.** Objection.

**A.** No.

**Q.** What was the practice at this hospital with respect to curbside consults between surgeons, including orthopedic surgeons and emergency room physicians, what was that practice?
**A.** At the hospital that Mr. Green was seen at, I do not know what the practice is, but I'll tell you as a general principle, we should not be doing "curbside consults."

**Q.** If it was a practice and sometimes they got more detailed consultations, if that was their practice and a requesting physician wanted a more detailed consult, it would be incumbent upon that physician to ask for that, wouldn't it?
**Defense attorney.** Objection.

**A.** I can't answer that question because I'll tell you this, this was not a curbside consult as we know curbside consults. In a situation like this, we should never be getting a curbside consult. So, I really can't answer your question.

**Q.** Okay. And so, Dr. Sharpe should have called for a full consultant, is that your testimony?

**Defense attorney.** Objection.
**A.** The answer is yes, and that's what occurred in this situation to the best of my understanding from reading the medical record.

**Q.** Dr. Rodriguez testified he would have expected Dr. Sharpe, the way they practiced medicine at this hospital, to give him more information.

**Defense attorney.** Note my objection, lack of foundation. Go ahead.

**A.** I think the answer to your question is that may be how they did things there, but again, it wouldn't meet the standard of care on either side. The responsibility of the consultant is to start right from scratch, get a history, do a physical exam, check all the past medical records, and then formulate a diagnostic plan.
**Q.** If that was the pattern of practice in at this hospital at the time that Tom Green presented, Dr. Rodriguez would have been acting within accordance with that understanding or a curbside consulting physician, wouldn't he?

**Defense attorney.** Objection. Go ahead.

**A.** I can't give you an opinion on that because this whole concept of a curbside consult really falls below the standard; and the consult that he did, as best as I can tell from his deposition because he did not document, which is also a failure, that as best as I can tell from his deposition would constitute a full consultation. He saw the patient. He spoke to the patient. He examined the patient. He took part in the ordering of the imaging and then he followed up with that patient. And so, in my opinion, that would be a consultation.

**Cross-Examination of plaintiff's expert Dr. Vandelay (Chairman of Prestigious Academic ED) by Defense attorney:**

**Dr. Vandelay.** The use of the term "curbside" is challenging because…it's not official. But a lot of times it happens, an orthopedist or a surgeon comes down and gives an opinion…

**Q.** In this case you would agree that what Dr. Rodriguez did in terms of consulting on this patient was not a curbside consult, correct?
**A.** Yeah…again, that is a slang term used for someone who just happens to be in the area and you ask them something. I'll leave it to him to have his own definition, but my understanding if a consultant comes down to evaluate a potential surgical condition and I ask them to do that, then I am treating that as a consult.

## III. The Negotiations

All defendants wanted to go to trial and so did their insurance company. As he stated in his deposition, Dr. Beretta, the defendant physician, felt that Tom Green had a disease that progressed rapidly when early diagnosis is impossible. However, even had he suspected an NSTI when he felt there was no evidence of it on the evening of the 18th, ordered a CT and consulted Dr. Ingram, nothing would have changed. All of those things happened the next day, after the disease process had progressed for 12 hours, and Dr. Ingram still declined to take him to the OR. He certainly wouldn't have taken him 12 hours earlier. Dr. Sharpe felt that he did everything that he could have done. He initiated a work-up after the doppler was negative, consulted the surgeon, provided excellent care when he deteriorated, and spent hours trying to resuscitate him and get the tertiary care center to accept him in transfer. The antibiotics were a miss, but as most of the experts stated in their depositions, they are an adjunct. Without surgery, Tom didn't stand a chance, and that was not Dr. Sharpe's decision to make.

Plaintiff's counsel offered early on (well before depositions) to settle the case for policy limits, $1 million. This was immediately rejected by the defense. Both sides felt that they were in a strong position after deposition testimony was provided. The case was scheduled for trial.

## IV. The Twist

As the trial approached, Dr. Beretta began to have second thoughts. He was a mid-career physician with three kids, two in college, and a wife who had sacrificed a lot over the course of their marriage and was very much looking forward to retirement, hopefully sooner than later. He consulted with a personal attorney with malpractice defense experience, and they discussed his exposure. While he felt as confident as ever that they were in the right and met the standard of care, he recognized that this was going to be a very emotional case. The patient's wife, Kim, was a very sympathetic plaintiff, and the jury might have a hard time getting past the emotion of a young widow and two kids growing up without their father. It might not be too difficult to convince a jury full of lay persons that the doctors must have done something wrong.

They concluded that the likelihood of losing was very low, maybe 10–15%. More importantly, the likelihood of a judgment beyond policy limits was even lower, but also not zero. While juries are typically unlikely to grant awards that threaten physicians' personal assets, this is the type of case where it could happen. A tragic case, involving a very sympathetic family.

After much consideration, Dr. Beretta changed course. He had his personal attorney send a "hammer letter" to the insurance company demanding that they settle within policy limits. While they were not legally required to comply with the demand, they knew that it was never a good idea to have an unhappy witness who didn't want to go to trial on the stand. And they also knew the legal ramifications of the hammer letter. If the jury ruled for the plaintiff and returned a judgment above policy limits, their refusal to comply with Dr. Beretta's demand to settle opened the door for Dr. Beretta to sue them for personal assets that he lost in the judgment. As the trial date approached, Dr. Beretta placed more and more pressure on the insurance company to settle and made it clear that his intent was to sue if any of his personal assets were lost. A few days before the trial was set to begin, a settlement was reached for $500,000.

## V. The Legal Analysis

**T. Marc Calvert, JD**
Medical malpractice defense attorney with over 35 years of experience
Calvert, Leever & Ostler
Cypress, Texas

**1. What is the legal risk to PA and the doctor?**
Under the doctrine of respondeat superior, an employer may be liable for the acts of an employee or agent when such acts are in the course and scope of the employment or agency. Here, it does not appear that the PA is employed by or the agent of the doctor, and it sounds like the PA is employed by the hospital. The plaintiff's attorney may well press that the triage process was not done correctly and routed the patient to be initially evaluated by the PA. So, the hospital may be required to defend their policies and procedures. I would argue that the PA should be held to the standard of care which would be provided by a reasonable PA in that circumstance, and not the standard that would apply for a doctor. It would depend on state law, and the judge, regarding how successful that argument would be.

**2. How does the legal risk play out when care is transitioned to the day shift doctor?**
I view the process of seeing this patient as similar to a relay race; for each leg of the race, did the provider run it reasonably based on what they knew at the time? The return to the ED, a new evaluation, and then the day shift doctor taking over all have aspects which will be scrutinized. The famous questions of, "What did they know and when did they know it" will be studied. Thus, there are risks for both doctors. Anchoring bias has been discussed, and both have to be aware of being swept up in that natural tendency. The notes from both need to be clear and thorough. Their testimonies should be supportive of each other, if possible. The opposing attorney will most definitely attempt a divide and conquer approach and will try to get them to criticize the other, or to damn with faint praise (e.g. "I don't think I would have done it that way, but I can see why it was done"). There is legal benefit to taking the high road and supporting each other and avoiding the devastating approach to throw the other clinicians under the bus.

**3. Would you recommend to settle or go to trial?**
**Standard of care:**
Without the benefit of seeing and hearing the main players, it is difficult to say for sure, but I think this is one to consider taking to trial. Why? Over the decades, I have been taught by physicians about truisms in the ED: Common things are common, hoofbeats are usually horses, not zebras, and it takes time for conditions to manifest. This man's disease process seems to be exceedingly rare, was arguably not likely to be detectable early, and was not likely reversible once diagnosed. There was no intentional act, there was no lack of care. Rather, if anything, it was a rabbit that needed to be pulled out of a hat. We cannot punish human beings, albeit very smart and capable human beings, who are trying to help others but who cannot always defy nature and the odds. The reasonable care provided is not always what hindsight would prescribe; that is not negligence.
**Causation:**
On top of that, it seems very questionable that causation can be shown. That is, the evidence seems to indicate that when it was reasonably able to be discovered, it was not curable. That makes it hard to prove to a jury, and even harder to prove to an appellate court. I would recommend loading up with a herculean expert line-up and the best of the literature on the issues.

**4. Is there a concern for a judgment which exceeds policy limits?**
I have sympathy for Dr. Beretta; his analysis of the legal puzzle is reasonable. When there is a legitimate risk of an excess verdict (one that exceeds insurance money and could put personal assets at risk), it is not uncommon for a doctor to ask the insurance company to settle. Using something like a "hammer letter" is one approach. State laws likely vary widely on the details as to the level of responsibility of the insurance company in this situation. It should not be viewed as a given that the case will be settled just because the doctor wants it settled, even if a hammer letter is sent. The objective exposure of the defendant, based on the evidence, along with the amount that it can be settled for, are among the variables that are considered by all involved.

**5. How important are the experts?**
This is the type of case which underscores the importance of having elite experts. Not just smart, accomplished people, but experts who come across well to lay people and who can skillfully handle tough cross-examination. The mantra should be that this was a giant curveball, and nothing could have stopped it once it was able to be diagnosed. Sincere testimony from the physician and PA defendants are also essential, showing that they gave it their reasonable best, will positively impact a jury of decent people.

**Final thoughts:** Just because the diagnosis was missed, does not mean it was malpractice. Consider all the first responders who rushed to the Twin Towers on 9/11. Arguably they failed but would anyone dare say they were negligent?!

## VI. Medical Discussion

**Michael Pallaci, DO**
Professor of Emergency Medicine, Northeast Ohio Medical University
Adjunct Clinical Professor of Emergency Medicine, Ohio University Heritage College of Osteopathic Medicine
Medical Director, Virtual Care Simulation Lab and EM Residency Core Faculty, Summa Health System

**Nicholas LaFountain, MD**
Clinical Assistant Professor of Emergency Medicine
Northeast Ohio Medical University Clerkship Director and EM Residency Core Faculty
Summa Health System

**Brock Landrum, MD**
Administrative Chief
Wright State University
Boonshoft School of Medicine

**Why was this diagnosis missed?**
Was it the delay and/or failure to diagnose necrotizing soft tissue infection (NSTI) that ultimately led to septic shock and the patient's demise? Was the differential diagnosis too narrow, failing to consider an infectious etiology? Did Dr. Beretta anchor on the deep vein thrombosis (DVT) diagnosis and ignore important symptoms and signs, or was this an atypical presentation of a difficult diagnosis that hid itself until it was too late?

**The differential:**
At the patient's initial presentation, the working discharge diagnosis was DVT versus an unspecified benign etiology for "leg pain." Once the doppler was negative, even at the time of surgical consultation, the diagnosis most prominently considered was compartment syndrome, which would not have explained the patient's fever, shock or alteration in mental status. An earlier diagnosis could have saved Tom Green's life, but when was it reasonable to expect the physicians involved to make that diagnosis? (1) On the first visit? (2) When the doppler came back negative and skin changes began to be seen? (3) When the CT read came back? or (4) When the patient went into shock? That's what the jury would have been tasked with deciding had the parties not come to a settlement prior to trial.

The differential diagnosis of leg pain includes:

- Injury (fracture, strain or tear of the ligaments or musculature, cartilaginous injury)
- Acute limb ischemia
- DVT
- Infection (cellulitis, erysipelas, NSTI, abscess, myositis)
- Rhabdomyolysis
- Electrolyte abnormalities (especially potassium and calcium derangements)
- Compartment syndrome

Many of these can be ruled out effectively with a good history and physical exam. Infectious etiologies and DVT, however, can be difficult to differentiate with history and physical exam as they both typically present with redness, swelling and pain. This is commonly referred to as the "red leg dilemma."[1] Cellulitis of the leg is a challenging diagnosis due to many mimics such as venous stasis, DVT, lymphedema, contact dermatitis, and other inflammatory dermatoses. One study found 31% of patients diagnosed with lower extremity cellulitis in the ED were given a different diagnosis prior to discharge from hospital or within 30 days of discharge from the ED.[2] Not only do Emergency Physicians (EPs) struggle with diagnosing cellulitis of the leg, we also struggle differentiating it from a DVT. One study found that 17.4% of patients diagnosed with leg cellulitis ended up having a positive duplex ultrasound for DVT on outpatient ultrasound.[3] This case highlights the need to consider infection and DVT together in the differential diagnosis of leg pain.[4]

**The work-up:**
At the patient's initial visit, work-up was limited to a D-dimer and BMP. In hindsight, and knowing the outcome of the case, was there a role for additional laboratory evaluation, specifically CBC, ESR and/ or CRP? Unfortunately, leukocytosis will not help distinguish cellulitis or infection from DVT, as it is a famously non-specific marker and both etiologies can cause leukocytosis of similar degrees. One study found a higher mean WBC with DVT than with cellulitis of the leg.[3] Even worse, the sensitivity of leukocytosis in cellulitis and erysipelas was only 50%.[5] CRP and ESR elevation are associated with both DVT and cellulitis of the leg, but have similarly poor specificity[5,7] CRP/ESR elevation is positively correlated with both acute DVT and cellulitis of the leg.[5,8] The same issue is again seen in the use of D-dimer in an attempt to distinguish between DVT and infection. D-dimer elevation, even when combined with an elevated Wells DVT score, is seen in both DVT and lower extremity cellulitis.[9] The patient in this case had an elevated D-dimer likely due to infection and not DVT, given his negative duplex ultrasound on the second visit, which shows the potential danger in using a D-dimer to differentiate between these etiologies.

While history, physical exam, and lab work were unlikely to have been helpful in this case, point-of-care ultrasound could have been useful; compression ultrasonography for evaluation of DVT has been shown in multiple studies to have sufficient sensitivity and specificity for evaluation of DVT in patients in the ED, especially when performed by an attending physician with ultrasound training.[10,11,12,13,14] It is especially important to consider if the ED does not have 24/7 radiology coverage for lower extremity ultrasound, such as in this case. A bedside ultrasound would have likely shown no evidence of DVT, which may have prompted the EP to consider other etiologies, including infection. Bedside EP point of care ultrasound can also show findings of soft tissue infection including cobble stoning in cellulitis and fluid collections in abscesses.[15] Unfortunately, point of care ultrasound was not an option at this facility on the night Tom Green presented, as the machine was out of service and in need of repair.

Tom Green not only had an infection that is very difficult to diagnose due to its vague presentation and low incidence, but also one in which early diagnosis is critical to avoid catastrophic outcomes. One study showed that only 15% of admitted patients found to have necrotizing fasciitis had the diagnosis at time of admission.[16] The LRINEC score was developed to help identify NSTI, with a score greater than 6 concerning for NSTI.[17] Subsequent meta-analysis, however, showed the LRINEC score to be only 68.2% sensitive and 84.8% specific.[18] Because of these poor text characteristics, these authors recommend against the use of LRINEC in the evaluation of possible NSTI.

Other signs, symptoms, and tests also show poor sensitivity for NSTI. Fever (46%), hemorrhagic bullae (25%) and plain films (49%) all identify fewer than half of NSTI cases when used in isolation.[18] If gas is seen on plain films it may help make the diagnosis, but a normal plain film does not rule out the presence of soft tissue gas, let alone NSTI.

NSTIs can be either monomicrobial or polymicrobial, and only those infections that involve anaerobic bacteria cause soft tissue gas. The most common cause of monomicrobial NSTIs (and the cause in this case) is Group A Strep (Strep pyogenes), which is an aerobe that would not present with gas in the soft tissues.

MRI is a very effective diagnostic tool with a sensitivity >90%. However, it also has a false positive rate of 39%.[19] MRI is also less practical in the ED due to limited availability as well as delay in surgical evaluation and management, the gold standard of treatment. Point of care ultrasound has been suggested by some to be useful in the diagnosis, but to date the literature is scant and a combination of ultrasound findings to either rule the diagnosis in or out has been elusive. CT with contrast remains the best initial imaging modality in the ED with a sensitivity between 80–97%,[20] but it is important to remember that less than 36% of NSTIs on CT imaging will show soft tissue gas.[20]

Could this diagnosis have been made earlier and the outcome have been changed? These authors feel that diagnosing this condition on the initial presentation would have been difficult to say the least. However, an expanded differential and early surgical intervention on the return visit could have possibly altered the outcome. The fact that the surgical consultant was still not convinced that the patient required surgical intervention after several additional hours had passed, after the physical findings began to show themselves and after the CT had been completed means one of two things: Either someone should have made the diagnosis earlier (certainly Dr. Rodriguez, possibly Dr. Sharpe, and maybe even Dr. Beretta), or this was an atypical presentation of a lethal disease that hid itself until it was too late.

## VI. Author Summary (Weinstock)

- Be wary of tachycardia on discharge, especially if there is not a good explanation.
- If the patient's level of pain is out of proportion to the suspected diagnosis, alternative diagnoses should be considered. Documentation that the pain is not out of proportion to the exam and/or the suspected diagnosis can be helpful if the suspected diagnosis turns out to be incorrect.
- Be careful to avoid anchoring bias and premature closure.
- It can be difficult to differentiate infection from DVT with history and exam, consider imaging.
- Necrotizing soft tissue infection is an extremely difficult clinical diagnosis that cannot be ruled in or ruled out using the LRINEC score, any specific lab, or imaging. Maintain a high index of suspicion and have early surgical consultation if NSTI is prominent in the differential diagnosis.
- Curbside consults are medicolegally dangerous. If a consultation is required, the consulting provider needs to make clear what their expectations are, and the consultant needs to do an evaluation and document their findings/recommendations.

**Conclusion:** Perhaps the most important take-home point is non-medical. As Dr. Beretta discovered by going through this process, the decision of whether to settle or go to trial is an incredibly difficult, individualized decision that must be made based on the risk tolerance, confidence, values and priorities of the physician. While the ultimate power frequently does not lie solely with the physician, most of us don't realize that we have significant leverage to influence that decision. If a provider wants to settle and the insurance company doesn't, a "hammer letter" can be used to demand settlement within policy limits, and can open the insurance company up to a lawsuit if there is a judgment beyond policy limits. However, this is a double-edged sword. If you don't want to settle and they do, you could be the recipient of such a letter and subsequently subject to a bad faith claim.

## References


1. Patel M, Lee SI, Thomas KS, et al. The red leg dilemma. A scoping review of the challenges of diagnosing lower-limb cellulitis. Br J Dermatol 2019;180(5):993-1000. doi: 10.1111/bjd.17415.
2. Weng QY, Raff AB, Cohen JM, et al. Costs and Consequences Associated With Misdiagnosed Lower Extremity Cellulitis. JAMA Dermatol 2017;153(2):141-46. doi: 10.1001/jamadermatol.2016.3816.
3. Rabuka CE, Azoulay LY, Kahn SR. Predictors of a positive duplex scan in patients with a clinical presentation compatible with deep vein thrombosis or cellulitis. Can J Infect Dis 2003;14(4):210-4. doi: 10.1155/2003/675682.
4. Criado E, Burnham CB. Predictive value of clinical criteria for the diagnosis of deep vein thrombosis. Surgery 1997;122(3):578-83. doi: 10.1016/s0039-6060(97)90131-8.
5. Lazzarini L, Conti E, Tositti G, et al. Erysipelas and cellulitis: clinical and microbiological spectrum in an Italian tertiary care hospital. J Infect 2005;51(5):383-9. doi: 10.1016/j.jinf.2004.12.010. PMID: 16321649.
6. Lapić I, Padoan A, Bozzato D, Plebani M. Erythrocyte Sedimentation Rate and C-Reactive Protein in Acute Inflammation. Am J Clin Pathol 2020;153(1):14-29. doi: 10.1093/ajcp/aqz142.
7. Roumen-Klappe EM, den Heijer M, van Uum SH, et al. Inflammatory response in the acute phase of deep vein thrombosis. J Vasc Surg 2002;35(4):701-6. doi: 10.1067/mva.2002.121746.
8. Bucek RA, Reiter M, Quehenberger P, et al. C-reactive protein in the diagnosis of deep vein thrombosis. Br J Haematol 2002;119(2):385-9. doi: 10.1046/j.1365-2141.2002.03886.x.
9. Maze MJ, Skea S, Pithie A, et al. Prevalence of concurrent deep vein thrombosis in patients with lower limb cellulitis: A prospective cohort study. BMC Infect Dis 2013;13:141. doi: 10.1186/1471-

2334-13-141.
10. Crisp JG, Lovato LM, Jang TB. Compression ultrasonography of the lower extremity with portable vascular ultrasonography can accurately detect deep venous thrombosis in the emergency department. Ann Emerg Med 2010;56(6):601-10. doi: 10.1016/j.annemergmed.2010.07.010.
11. Pomero F, Dentali F, Borretta V, et al. Accuracy of emergency physician-performed ultrasonography in the diagnosis of deep-vein thrombosis: A systematic review and meta-analysis. Thromb Haemost 2013;109(1):137-45. doi: 10.1160/TH12-07-0473.
12. Pedraza García J, Valle Alonso J, Ceballos García P, et al. Comparison of the accuracy of emergency department-performed point-of-care-ultrasound (POCUS) in the diagnosis of lower-extremity deep vein thrombosis. J Emerg Med 2018;54(5):656-664. doi: 10.1016/j.jemermed.2017.12.020.
13. Lee JH, Lee SH, Yun SJ. Comparison of 2-point and 3-point point-of-care ultrasound techniques for deep vein thrombosis at the emergency department: A meta-analysis. Medicine (Baltimore) 2019;98(22):e15791. doi: 10.1097/MD.0000000000015791.
14. Canakci ME, Acar N, Bilgin M, et al. Diagnostic value of point-of-care ultrasound in deep vein thrombosis in the emergency department. J Clin Ultrasound 2020;48(9):527-531. doi: 10.1002/jcu.22892.
15. Chau C, Griffith J. Musculoskeletal infections: Ultrasound appearances. Clin Radiol 2005;60(2):149-159. doi:10.1016/j.crad.2004.02.005
16. Wong CH, Chang HC, Pasupathy S, et al. Necrotizing fasciitis: Clinical presentation, microbiology, and determinants of mortality. J Bone Joint Surg Am 2003;85-A(8):1454-60.
17. Wong CH, Khin LW, Heng KS, et al. The LRINEC (Laboratory Risk Indicator for Necrotizing Fasciitis) score: A tool for distinguishing necrotizing fasciitis from other soft tissue infections. Crit Care Med 2004;32(7):1535-41. doi: 10.1097/01.ccm.0000129486.35458.7d.
18. Fernando SM, Tran A, Cheng W, et al. Necrotizing soft tissue infection: Diagnostic accuracy of physical examination, imaging, and LRINEC score: A systematic review and meta-analysis. Ann Surg 2019;269(1):58-65. doi: 10.1097/SLA.0000000000002774. PMID: 29672405.
19. Malghem J, Lecouvet FE, Omoumi P, et al. Necrotizing fasciitis: Contribution and limitations of diagnostic imaging. Joint Bone Spine. 2013;80(2):146-54. doi: 10.1016/j.jbspin.2012.08.009.
20. Zacharias N, Velmahos GC, Salama A, et al. Diagnosis of necrotizing soft tissue infections by computed tomography. Arch Surg 2010;145(5):452-5. doi: 10.1001/archsurg.2010.50. PMID: 20479343.

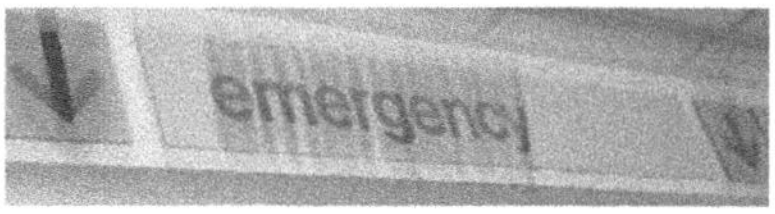


# Case 12

## A 27 Year-old Woman with Neck Pain: Bounce, Bounce, Bounce, Bounce, Bounce, Bounce, Bounce, Bounce, Morgue

**Primary case authors:**
**Christopher San Miguel**
**David Chang**
**Colin G. Kaide**

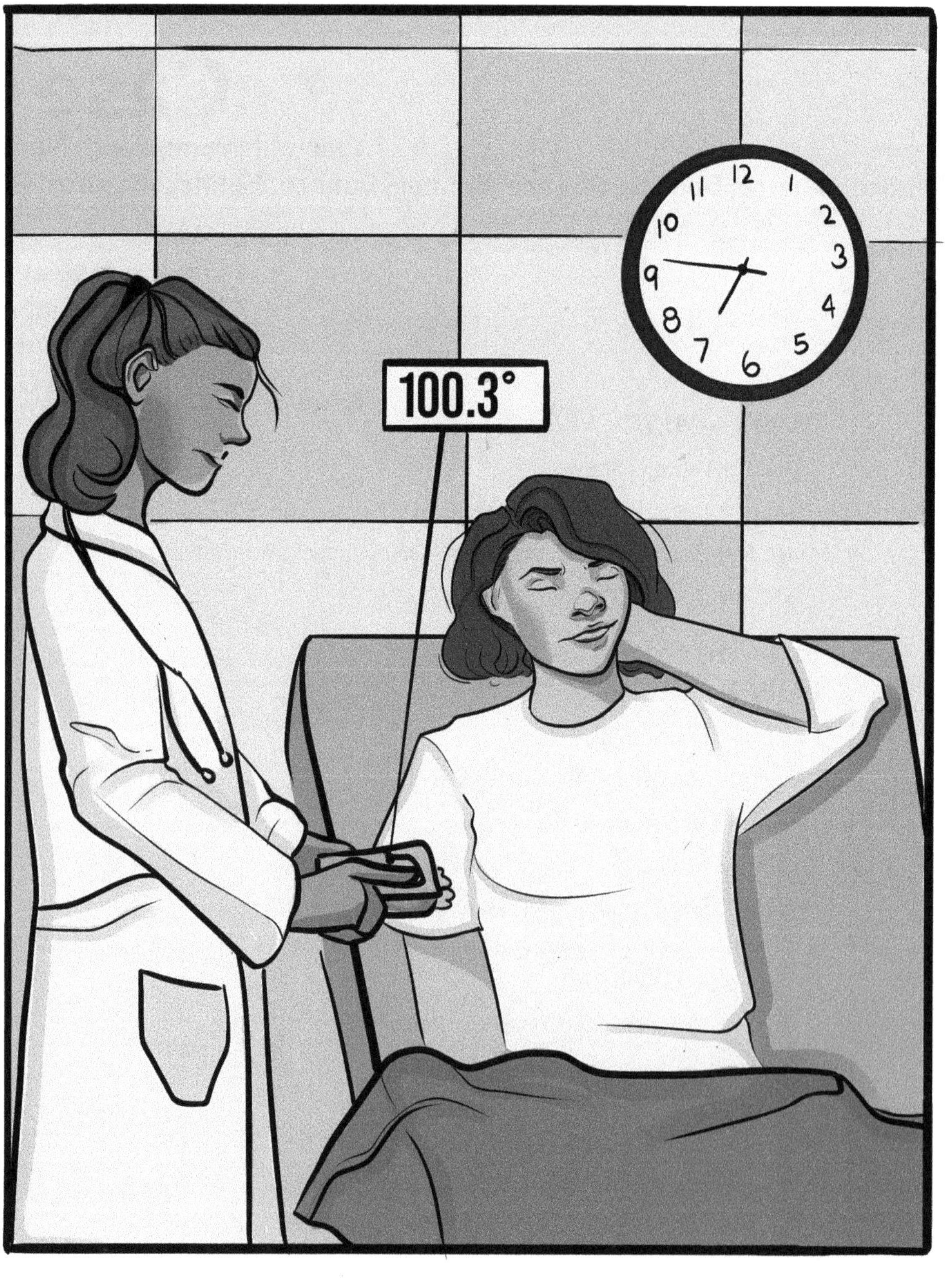
100.3°

# Case 12

## A 27 Year-old Woman with Neck Pain: Bounce, Bounce, Bounce, Bounce, Bounce, Bounce, Bounce, Bounce, Morgue

***Deep thoughts:***

1. *Multiple visits to the ED for the same complaint is a harbinger of bad outcomes; how did 6 visits, some with tachycardia still present at discharge and with progressive symptoms, slip past multiple clinicians?*
2. *The patient had 2 CT scans of the cervical spine. When is "the donut of truth" really "the donut of half-truths?"*
3. *How does the history of a recent MRSA abscess figure into subsequent visits?*
4. *How might prior treatment with trimethoprim/sulfamethoxazole confuse the presentation of MRSA sepsis?*
5. *What are "anchoring bias, confirmation bias, diagnostic momentum, premature closure, Yin Yang Out and Zebra Retreat" and how do they play into this case?*

**PART 1—MEDICAL**

**Author comments (Weinstock):** This case demonstrates some unique teaching points, including multiple bounceback visits, multiple providers, multiple EDs… and a final diagnosis which is unclear even at time of the legal action. It is a good example of why we should be cautious of diagnosis momentum, to consider the limitations of exam and testing, and how a case is defended when the etiology of the outcome is not clear.

## I. The Patient's Story

Missy M is a 27 year-old woman who had a complicated life as a teenager, becoming pregnant at age 14, dropping out of high school, and suffering from bouts of depression and multiple suicide attempts. She was diagnosed as bipolar in her early 20s. She uses marijuana recreationally but has never used injectable drugs. After finishing high school, she gets her State Tested Nursing Assistant certificate. She currently has 3 children. Our story starts when she presents to the ED for a "spider bite."

## II. The Doctor's Version (the following is the actual documentation of the provider)

**Visit #1: Seen at Hospital A, January 21st** (initial ED visit)

Missy M was seen in the ED for what she called a "spider bite" on her left hip. She had a 2 x 3 cm area of redness without fluctuance. She was diagnosed with cellulitis and discharged on cephalexin and TMP-sulfamethoxazole (Bactrim). She was given instructions to follow up in 48–72 hours.

**Chapter author comments:** There are no problems with this ED visit. The diagnosis, treatment, and follow-up are all appropriate for cellulitis.

**Visit #2: Seen at Hospital A, January 25th** (4 days after initial visit)

**Chief Complaint:** Buttocks abscess

**History:** Missy M is a 27 y.o. female who presents to the Emergency Department for the evaluation of abscess. Patient states that she was seen in the department [4] days ago and was diagnosed with a spider bite to the left buttocks. She states that the area has gotten larger and more painful since the visit. She reports pain in the area rated 10/10 in severity. She denies any fever, chills, nausea, vomiting, or diarrhea. Patient reports that she does have a history of recurrent boils. Nursing note and vitals reviewed.

**Physical Exam:**
Skin: Skin is warm and dry. No rash noted. [There is a] 2 cm x 3 cm indurated abscess on the left buttock.

**Procedure Note:** An abscess was visualized on the lateral aspect of the left hip, approximately 2 cm x 3 cm in size. There is approximately 4 cm of surrounding cellulitis. The area was cleansed using Betadine solution. Local anesthesia was achieved using approximately 6 mL of 1 % lidocaine with epinephrine utilizing the field block technique. A 1 cm incision was made in the center of the abscess, with immediate release of copious quantities of purulent material. An aerobic culture was obtained and sent to the laboratory. The abscess was thoroughly expressed, with significant drainage of material. Loculations were disrupted via hemostats. The abscess was packed using quarter inch iodoform gauze packing. The patient tolerated the procedure well without immediate complication.

**Medical Decision-Making:** After the abscess was drained, the patient was given instructions for follow-up with her primary care provider and return for increasing symptoms. She was discharged with additional cephalexin and TMP-Sulfamethoxazole to continue for the next 5 days.

**Chapter author comments:** There are no issues with this visit. The patient was continued on an appropriate antibiotic regimen after the infectious source was controlled by the bedside incision and drainage.

**Visit #3: Seen at Hospital A, January 29th** (4 days after last visit)

**Chief Complaint (per triage RN):** Neck Pain

**History of Present Illness:** This patient is a 27 y.o. female who presents with neck pain that started 2 days ago and gradually has gotten worse. It [started] in the L periscapular region and spread to involve her left neck. [Also] radiated into her L arm. She has tried ibuprofen [with] minimal effect.

**Physical Examination:**

Vital Signs

| Time | Temp (F) | Pulse | Resp | Syst | Diast |
|---|---|---|---|---|---|
| | 98.3 F | 86 | 18 | 125 | 72 |

**Constitutional:** She is oriented to person, place, and time.
**Neck:** At rest cervical spine is held at lateral bending 10° left rotation 10° right motion. Rotation was from 10° right to 45° right. From 10° right to 10° left with pain. Lateral bending: From 10° left to 30° left from 10° left to 0°: To the right.
She is tender to palpation of the left sided SCM muscle, trapezius and rhomboids. No neck adenopathy
**Neurological:** She is alert and oriented to person, place, and time. No weakness of arms or legs. Light touch intact.
**Skin:** Skin is warm and dry. Abscess left buttock region is not indurated. The packing is out. There is no drainage and I think it's healing well.

**Testing: CT cervical spine without contrast:** Cervical spine straightening but no fracture or dislocation.

**Emergency Department Course:** Nursing notes reviewed. The patient received hydromorphone (Dilaudid) for pain along with orphenadrine (Norflex) IV. She was improved and moving her neck much better. Her left buttock abscess did grow MRSA that was sensitive to Bactrim. Plan is to discharge home with instructions to return if worse and follow up with her primary doctor. She should complete her Bactrim to help her abscess heal.

**Diagnosis:** Torticollis, Healing buttocks abscess

**Chapter author comments:** The documentation for this visit was excellent. There is a detailed exam that supports the writer's conclusion that the neck pain is muscular. It also includes a re-examination of the abscess site. Furthermore, the clinician acknowledges the patient's current treatment and comments on the appropriateness of her antibiotic based on the culture. At this point, the clinician appears to have arrived at a reasonable conclusion based on the medical reasoning. Perhaps the only thing which could have been added would have been an explicit discussion on whether the clinician thought the previously diagnosed infection was related to the patient's current neck pain.

**Visit #4: Seen at Hospital A. January 30th** (1 day after last visit)
*Dr. Zulu*

**Chief Complaint (0830):** Worsening neck pain

**History of Present Illness (PA):** Missy M is a 27 year-old female who presents with complaints of left sided trapezius pain that began 2 days ago when she woke up. She was seen in the ED last night and had a CT scan of her cervical spine that was negative. She had IV Hydromorphone and muscle relaxers with improvement. She was discharged home on cyclobenzaprine (Flexeril) and hydrocodone/acetaminophen (Norco) prescriptions. She states her father lost her prescriptions and her paperwork on the way home.

**Physical Examination:**

Vital Signs

| Time | Temp (F) | Pulse | Resp | Syst | Diast |
|---|---|---|---|---|---|
| 0830 | 97.7 F | 100 | 20 | 112 | 82 |

**Neck:** Tender left trapezius. Good strength and sensation upper extremities
**Note:** Other aspects of the physical exam were documented as normal (this is shortened by the author for readability).

**Medical Decision-Making:** The patient was given methylprednisolone (Solu-Medrol) 125 mg IM and Norflex 60 mg IM. The patient was also given a dose of diazepam (Valium) and Hydromorphone IM. The patient will be discharged home with a limited prescription for Norco and Flexeril.

**Supervising Physician Documentation:** She was seen by PA and myself. Apparently, she was here during the night and said that she had a stiff neck that was progressing to the point that she is unable to move it in any direction. She states that she does see a chiropractor and had her neck manipulated couple of weeks ago. A diagnosis of torticollis was made. She was given a prescription for hydrocodone as well as intravenous hydromorphone. She returns crying stating that she is no better and to make things worse, her father lost her prescriptions on the walk home last night. In any event, patient does have a tender trapezius on the left. She does have palpable spasm. She does have limited range of motion in all directions. She was given Norflex IM as well as Solu-Medrol. Additionally, she will be given IV diazepam and hydromorphone. On recheck, she is more comfortable. She will be discharged with instructions for alternating ice and heat, Norco 5 mg and Flexeril. She should follow-up with her PCP.

**Diagnosis:**
1. Torticollis
2. Tobacco abuse
3. History of bipolar disorder

**Chapter author comments:** The patient's first real Bounceback visit occurred less than 24 hours after she was diagnosed with torticollis. It appears that diagnosis momentum likely played a role; these authors feel that the previous diagnosis was reasonable as it is documented she has pain with range of motion and has her head turned to the side. However, the PA in the current visit documents a normal range of motion. The physician's documentation is a bit more detailed and notes limited range of motion in all directions along with palpable spasm. Torticollis can be quite painful, but typically once the spasm is broken the patient experiences only mild soreness. In this case, the patient has returned with pain so severe that it requires Norflex, Solu-Medrol, Valium, and Hydromorphone, which is unusual after breaking the original spasm. However, with improvement in her symptoms, her overall presentation is not too much different from her original visit.

**Visit #5 Seen at Hospital B, January 31st** (1 day after last visit)

**Author comments (Weinstock):** This is one of the two visits in which the physician is later named: *Defendant Dr. Charlie*

**Chief Complaint:** Neck pain radiating to L upper back

**History of Present Illness (0530):** 27 y.o. female presents to ED via EMS with complaints of neck pain, radiates shoulder and back of neck, The patient states she was seen at Hospital A a week ago, given IV medication and discharged home with pain medication. The patient states she returned to Hospital A two days ago for same symptoms and discharged home with Flexeril. The patient states she's also experiencing chills and sweats.

**Past Medical History:** Depression; Migraine; Chronic back pain; and Bipolar affective
**Allergies:** None
**Medications:** Cephalexin, cyclobenzaprine, cyproheptadine, acetaminophen/hydrocodone, ibuprofen, lurasidone, mupirocin, ondansetron, sertraline, trimethoprim/sulfamethoxazole, trazodone
**Surgical history:** Tubal ligation, Cesarean section
**SH:** Positive for marijuana use. Positive for tobacco use. Negative for alcohol use or injectable drug use

**Physical Examination:**

Vital Signs

| Time | Temp(F) | Pulse | Resp | Syst | Diast |
|---|---|---|---|---|---|
| | 98.8° F | 107 | 18 | 147 | 104 |

**Patient presentation:** Alert. Well appearing, No apparent distress
**ENT Exam:** Pharynx normal, Neck supple. Moist mucous membranes
**Cardiovascular Exam:** Regular rate and rhythm, No edema
**Pulmonary Exam:** Lungs clear, No respiratory distress, Chest non-tender
**Gastrointestinal Exam:** non tender, Soft, Non-distended
**Musculoskeletal Exam:** Reproducible pain over her left trapezius
**Skin Exam** Intact, Warm, dry, No rash, No lacerations
**Neurological Exam:** Alert, Oriented x 3, No motor deficits, No sensory deficits. Oriented to person, oriented place and time, usual mental status, speech normal, cranial nerves normal, sensory exam intact
**Cranial nerves:** Normal

**Testing:**
WBC 15.3 78% Neutrophils

**Contrast Enhanced CT Neck: Impression**
1. Unremarkable enhanced CT examination of the soft tissues of the neck.
2. Significant acute sinusitis of the frontal and ethmoid sinuses as discussed.

**Ddx:** considered but not limited to abscess, blood clot, muscle spasm, meningitis, epidural abscess/ hematoma.

**Medical Decision-Making:** Patient presents with neck pain. The patient has reproducible pain over her left trapezius. She was given valium for muscle spasm. We obtained the patient's records from Hospital A for the last 2 days for the same thing. She had an additional CT cervical spine with contrast today that was normal. She was given Norco and Flexeril to go home on 2 separate occasions. The patient had Solu-Medrol while at Hospital A that likely caused her leukocytosis. The patient had a CT neck with contrast that was normal. The patient became verbally assaultive with staff. The patient was discharged home and she can continue her medications written yesterday.

**Clinical Impression:** Torticollis

**Chapter author comments:** This is the first truly problematic visit. In addition to her severe neck pain, she is now complaining of chills and cold sweats. She is also tachycardic. In addition, her work-up reveals an elevated white count. The clinician attributes it to the steroids from the day prior; this is not an unreasonable conclusion, except it doesn't explain her subjective chills and sweats. This clinician is anchoring on the diagnosis of torticollis causing them to ignore or downplay signs and symptoms which do not support this original diagnosis. The challenge with any bounceback patient is to simultaneously assess their clinical picture from a new unbiased lens while also considering the previous evaluation and test results. The clinician does not have immediate access to her previous record (she is now at hospital B and had been at hospital A) and reasonably orders a CT scan of the neck with contrast. Presumably this was out of concern for a potential soft tissue abscess or infection. However, the read becomes problematic for the clinician. While finding no abnormalities in the neck, the radiologist did include acute sinusitis in the impressions. The clinician does not acknowledge this. This certainly could be contributing to the patient's subjective fevers and white count, with consideration of a different antibiotic regimen. Alternatively, if there are no clinical signs of sinusitis, it may be unrelated to her complaints, as the CT findings are not specific for sinusitis. Either course of action could be reasonable, but by not acknowledging, we are left to wonder whether the physician didn't see the second impression or just ignored it.

**Author comments (Weinstock):** This is a really nice time to take a breather… Wow, not only has the patient been seen 5 times in 11 days, but 3 of those visits are for a complaint of neck pain. It is true that some of these symptoms, such as chills and sweats, are nonspecific and there is a wide ddx, but in fact there are not tons of bad things that can still be going on after a negative contrast CT... but there are a few! The trick is to make sure that there is adequate bedside data collection (H&P) and to understand the limitations of testing (contrast CT neck).

## III. Risk Management/Patient Safety Opportunities (Weinstock)

**Risk Management/Patient Safety Opportunity #1:**

**Opportunity:** Asking a follow-up question.
**Discussion:** It is common that patients and clinicians have a different understanding of medical (or nonmedical) terminology. What did this patient mean by chills and sweats; on the surface it seems that a concern could be infection. However there are many reasons for chills (simply they are cold) or sweats (Hodgkin's disease or TB)… but with such a wide range of possible etiologies, we need to define what the patient actually means by chills and sweats. If they mean fever (or had a recorded temperature 100.4 degrees or above), this would be a game changer.
✔ **Teaching point:** Clarify ambiguous information.

**Risk Management/Patient Safety Opportunity #2:**

**Opportunity:** Obtaining past records.
**Discussion:** Though it is understandable that hospital B might not know what occurred at hospital A, one

person who might know… is the patient! Though the allegation in this med mal action is not radiation poisoning from too many CTs, there is minimal utility in wasting time repeating a test which was just performed and came back negative.

✔ **Teaching point:** Previous testing is often known by the patient or can be obtained by reviewing a previous visit.

**Risk Management/Patient Safety Opportunity #3:**

**Opportunity:** Tachycardia.

**Discussion:** Unexplained tachycardia is a common theme in these cases and has been shown to be present in 71% of "possible error" patients who died within a week of their ED discharge.[1] But what do we do with a well-appearing patient who is tachycardic and ready to go home? These 4 tips can help to avoid a misdiagnosis:

Confirm that the chief complaint correlates with the final diagnosis

Ensure that the Ddx accounts for less common diagnoses (especially with a bounceback visit)

Rechecking the patient

Repeating the vitals

Finally, if the tachycardia is thought to be from the patient's pain, state this in the documentation.

✔ **Teaching point:** Reasons for unexplained tachycardia should be addressed and the pulse repeated.

**Risk Management/Patient Safety Opportunity #4:**

**Opportunity:** Consider referred pain.

**Discussion:** Consider that neck pain could be from the chest (acute coronary syndrome) or the lungs (Pancoast tumor) or the ears (otitis media) or the larynx (mass), or the esophagus (esophagitis/candidiasis/mass), or from the back of the throat (peritonsillar abscess/PTA or retropharyngeal abscess/RPA) or even from globus hystericus.

✔ **Teaching point:** When testing to the affected area is negative, consider referred pain.

**Risk Management/Patient Safety Opportunity #5:**

**Opportunity:** Understanding limitations of testing.

**Discussion:** The contrast neck CT covers a lot of things in the differential, but there are certain diagnoses which are not reliably seen such as osteomyelitis, a herniated disc, or a spinal epidural abscess (SEA), with 2 studies finding that it is only seen 6–18% of the time (See Section IV. Medical discussion, below).

✔ **Teaching point:** All tests do not have the same sensitivity for serious disease.

## IV. The Doctor's Version (the following is the actual documentation of the provider)

**Visit #6: Seen at Hospital A, January 31st** (same day, later in the morning)

**Summary of visit (for space considerations):** This is a similar visit to the previous with pain on palpation of the neck. She is given morphine, hydromorphone and valium IV which improve her symptoms. The diagnosis is again torticollis.

**Chapter author comments:** It is unclear as to why this physician was left out of the lawsuit. It may be because during this visit she denied fever or chills according to the HPI, or perhaps it was overlooked by the attorneys. Given the patient's statement that she lost her Norco prescription, the seed of wariness may have been planted in the mind of the doctor, causing her to think the patient may have been drug seeking. It seems unlikely that the physician knew the patient had just been discharged from hospital B. The patient has once again jumped from one health system to another, making it more difficult for the bedside clinician to see details of the previous visit(s), but also raising concern for possible secondary gain/malingering.

**Visit #7: Seen at Hospital A, Feb 1st** (one day later) – The PA who saw the patient on this visit was also named in the action.
Defendant PA-C Tango

**History of Present Illness (0356):** Missy M is a 27 y.o. female who presents with complaint of bilateral muscular neck pain. Patient reports that she has had pain in the neck for 2 weeks. She has been seen and evaluated here in the ED multiple times. She reports that the pain is throbbing in both sides of the neck and is worse with turning the neck. She reports some radiation of the pain into the bilateral upper extremities. She denies any numbness, weakness, tingling in the distal upper extremities. Patient has received Norco, Dilaudid, Flexeril, and [lorazepam] Ativan for her pain symptoms in previous visits. She does currently have Norco and Flexeril at home which she states is not strong enough for her pain symptoms. She denies any current headache, blurred vision, speech impediment, numbness, weakness, tingling in the upper and lower extremities bilaterally, right knee or other focal neurological deficit.

**Physical Examination:**

Vital Signs

| Time | Temp(F) | Pulse | Resp | Syst | Diast |
|---|---|---|---|---|---|
| | 97.7° F | 118 | 20 | 137 | 88 |

**Constitutional:** She is oriented to person, place, and time. Well-developed and well-nourished
**Head:** Normocephalic and atraumatic
**Mouth/Throat:** Oropharynx is clear and moist. No oropharyngeal exudate
**Neck:** Normal range of motion. Neck supple. She has no cervical adenopathy
**Cardiovascular:** Normal rate, regular rhythm, normal heart sounds and intact distal pulses. No extrasystoles are present. Exam reveals no gallop, no distant heart sounds and no friction rub. No murmur heard
**Pulmonary/Chest:** Effort normal and breath sounds normal. No respiratory distress. No wheezes, no rales
**Abdominal:** Soft. Normal appearance and bowel sounds are normal. She exhibits no distension and no mass
There is no hepatosplenomegaly. There is no tenderness. There is no rigidity, no rebound, no guarding, no CVA tenderness, no tenderness at McBurney's point and negative Murphy's sign. No hernia
**Cervical back:** She exhibits tenderness (Tenderness along the musculature of the neck bilaterally) and spasm. She exhibits normal range of motion, no bony tenderness, no swelling and no deformity
**Thoracic back:** Normal
**Lumbar back:** Normal

**Neurological:** She has normal strength. She displays no tremor. No cranial nerve deficit or sensory deficit. She exhibits normal muscle tone. Negative Rovsing's and Kernig signs
**Skin:** Skin is warm and dry. No rash noted. No erythema. No pallor

**Medical Decision-Making:** Patient remained stable here in the ED. Patient's and physical examination findings were all reassuring. Upon re-evaluation, the patient is feeling better with a benign repeat examination. Patient was comfortable with the plan of discharge home to follow up with the primary care provider in the next 2 days. The patient is instructed to return to the ED for any worsening of their symptoms. Patient was discharged in good condition with all questions answered.

**Diagnosis:** Torticollis, unspecified.

**Chapter author comments:** This is now the 7th visit and the 5th visit for the same complaint. The patient describes pain radiating into both arms which seems to be a progression from previous visits. Similarly to Visit #6, Visit #7 ended with no further diagnostic testing and a final diagnosis of torticollis. Although he doesn't explicitly discuss them in his MDM, the PA does document negative Kernig and Rovsing's signs; presumably he meant Brudzinski rather than Rovsing's given the context of the physical exam. This shows some consideration for meningitis. The PA's conclusions in his MDM are based on his assessment that the patient's exam was reassuring. It would be helpful if he had explicitly stated what was reassuring. Was it it the normal neurological exam? However, in retrospect, I would argue with this PA that the patient's HR is too elevated for safe discharge home. In fact, if you plot the presenting heart rate by ED visit, it has been climbing from her original measured HR of 86 at visit #3. These chapter authors feel that the tachycardia along with the intractable pain, should have prompted a more extensive work-up.

**Visit #8: See at Hospital B. February 1st** (same day)
*Defendant PA-C Bravo*

**Stated Complaint:** NECK PAIN/HA/FEVER

**History of Present Illness (19:47):** 27 y/o F presents to the ED c/o neck pain that began a week and a half ago and has not subsided since onset. The pt also c/o a headache, nausea, and fever that has been ongoing over the course of the past 2 days. The pt denies any vomiting and any other acute symptoms.

Vital Signs

| Time | Temp(F) | Pulse | Resp | Syst | Diast |
|---|---|---|---|---|---|
| | 100.3° F | 146 | 20 | 132 | 72 |

**Physical Exam** (shortened for chapter readability).
Alert, oriented x 3, Normal mood affect, Normal process, Normal Content, Normal speech
**Musculoskeletal:** Other - cervical paraspinal tenderness
**Skin:** Intact, Warm, dry, No rash, No lacerations
**Neurological:** Alert, Oriented x 3, No motor deficits, No sensory deficits
**Mental Status:** Oriented to person, place and time, usual mental status. Normal speech. Cranial nerves normal. Gait normal. Sensory exam intact

**Medical Decision-Making:** Patient resting comfortably. She received the following: Norflex injection and oxycodone (Percocet, 2 each). Reports mild improvement. Plan is for discharge and follow-up with her provider. Return precautions given for worsening or persistent symptoms.

**Clinical Impression:** Strain of neck muscle.

**Chapter author comments:**This is the patient's penultimate ED visit. The documentation is quite sparse, which does not work in the PA's favor. There is no differential diagnosis, no explanation of thought processes, and the presented plan and impression only address the neck pain. In the history, the PA clearly documents that the patient has reported a fever. Coupled with the wildly abnormal vital signs, the reported fevers should have prompted an infectious work-up, even if the patient hadn't been a bounceback. In fact, in this case, we would venture to say that this patient's bounceback status caused her to get less of a work-up than she normally would. Every subsequent provider sees that she has already received a fairly extensive work-up, with few objective findings, and therefore reasons that if significant pathology were present, it would have been found already. The only problem with this logic is that it assumes the patient has received all the tests necessary to assess their condition! In this case, spinal epidural abscess (SEA) has to be a consideration with severe neck pain, fever, and possibly some radicular pain. It's true that the patient has had two CT scans; but neither of these tests are sensitive for SEA; she required an MRI of her spine. (see discussion and reference in the medical section below) These chapter authors believe previous providers and this PA were falsely reassured by the negative diagnostic studies.

**Visit #9 for Neck pain and altered mental status. Hospital A. Feb 3rd (2 days later)**
*Dr. Foxtrot*

**History of Present Illness (08:30):** Missy M is a 27 year-old female who presents to the Emergency Department by EMS for the evaluation of altered mental status. Per EMT, they were called to the patient's home this morning due to her neck and back pain. They believed that she may have taken too many of her prescription drugs because she was showing symptoms of altered mental status. Patient was recently seen in the ED for back and neck pain and was given Flexeril. This did not help her pain so she then went to Hospital B and received a prescription for Valium. She reported that she only took Norco at home around 5:30AM, but told the EMS that she had taken two Valium today. Patient says that she is in continuous pain due to her neck and back, but there is no pain radiation. There are no modifying factors. She has associated slowed speech, dry mouth, headache x 3 days, weakness, intermittent fever, and trouble swallowing. She denies drug or alcohol use. She says she is supposed to be taking medication for her bipolar disorder, but says she has not for the past year.

**Physical Examination (shortened for chapter readability):**

Vital Signs

| Time | Temp(F) | Pulse | Resp | Syst | Diast |
|---|---|---|---|---|---|
| | 100.8° F | 139 | 30 | 102 | 57 |

**Neck:** Decreased range of motion (second to pain) present. No tracheal deviation present.
**Cardiovascular:** Normal rate, regular rhythm. Exam reveals no gallop. No murmur heard.
**Pulmonary/Chest:** Effort normal. No strider. No respiratory distress. She has no decreased breath sounds. She has no wheezes. She has no rales.

**Neurological:** She is alert and oriented to person, place, and time. She has normal strength. She is not disoriented. No tremor. No cranial nerve deficit or sensory deficit. No seizure activity. Coordination normal.
**Psychiatric:** She has a normal mood and affect. Her behavior is normal. Her mood appears not anxious. Her affect is not angry and not inappropriate. Her speech is slurred. She does not exhibit a depressed mood. She exhibits an altered mental status.
**Imaging:**
WBC: 13.1
Segs Absolute 12.3
Lymphocytes absolute 0.3
Hgb: 11.3
Plt: 126

**Gas (15L NRB):** pH 7.15/66/124

**CSF:**
Color and character: CSF LIGHT YELLOW and CLEAR
RBC: 40
WBC: 680
Segs 89, Lymphs, CSF 2, Monocytes, CSF 9
Protein: 415
Glucose: 53

**Electrolytes and renal function:**
Sodium 142
Potassium 4.5
Chloride 107
$CO_2$ 19
Glucose 69
BUN 37
Creatinine 2.8

CRP 33 (H)
Sed rate 71 (H)
Procalcitonin 12.83 (Ref range 0.05 - 0.09)

**Urinalysis:** WNL except glucose (100) and blood (moderate) and WBC (15-25)

## V. Hospital Course

**Blood Culture (Resulted next morning):** Staph aureus (MRSA)

**CT Head w/o contrast:** Partial opacification of the R frontal sinus, new from previous exam. Opacification of one of R anterior ethmoid air cells, stable from previous study. IMP: R frontal sinus disease, new from study of 1-29.

**CT Chest w/ contrast:** Clinical Info: Chest pain and SOB. IMP: Multiple patchy and nodular densities scattered throughout both lung fields, consistent with multifocal pneumonia or septic emboli.

**Medical Decision-Making:** Patient was examined, and laboratory work was obtained. Patient was confused and lethargic and a lumbar puncture was obtained suggesting meningitis. CT scan of the head showed opacification of the sinuses as noted, and a CT scan of the chest was concerning for multiple opacities, possibly septic emboli. Patient was given 2 g of Rocephin and a gram of vancomycin IV. She was admitted to the ICU with the diagnosis of meningitis and sepsis.

**Infectious Disease Consultation:** With the caveat that the history and exam are limited, based on them, imaging and the CSF studies, the best unifying explanation would be that she had MRSA bacteremia (possibly from the skin and soft tissue abscess) which could have caused a possible right-sided endocarditis with septic emboli (based on the CT chest findings). An epidural abscess with parameningeal CSF pleocytosis (most probably cervical given the neck pain) which would be hard to pick up on CT neck. The unilateral chemosis and eye swelling with restricted extraocular eye movements could be from a septic cavernous sinus thrombosis which will also be difficult to pick up on a CT head. Isolated meningitis from Staph aureus in a community acquired setting is unusual.

**Hospital Course:** Patient was admitted to the ICU and continued to deteriorate. She was electively intubated without complication. Plan is to add additional imaging. Given her history she will be transferred to a tertiary referral hospital, Hospital C, for further management.

**Transfer to Tertiary Referral Hospital (Feb 4th):** Prior to presentation here, she was s/p PEA arrest in the elevator secondary to severe ARDS with refractory hypoxemia, severe, metabolic acidosis and septic shock with multisystem organ failure. On arrival to the MICU she was in PEA arrest and cyanotic. CPR was initiated with return of spontaneous circulation. Downtime with CPR was about 4 to 6 minutes. However, the patient remained hypoxic post arrest and required bag mask ventilation with PEEP valve for almost 1.5 hours because she was unable to tolerate mechanical ventilation with precipitous desaturation. She went into Afib with RVR. Unsynchronized cardioversion was attempted but she reverted back to Afib then was started on amiodarone drip. She was sedated and paralyzed. Started on CVVHD for renal failure. She had no neurological response post arrest. On day four, CT brain showed signs of severe anoxic brain injury. The family made the decision to change code status ta DNR-CCA on 2/8. Later that evening the decision was made to withdraw care. The patient was pronounced deceased at 12:15am on 2/9/15.

## PART 2—LEGAL

## I. The Depositions—The following is actual deposition testimony, condensed from over 5,000 pages

Cast of characters (names changed, except where noted):
**The patient:** Missy M
**The clinicians:**
Dr. Charlie—ED physician-defendant, at Visit #5 Seen at Hospital B, January 31st
PA-C Tango—Physician assistant-defendant, at Visit #7: Seen at Hospital A, Feb 1st
PA-C Bravo—Physician assistant-defendant, at Visit #8: Hospital B. February 1st, (same day) **The experts:**
**Defense expert witnesses:**
Dr. Alpha—Infectious disease
Dr. Golf—Infectious disease
Dr. Sierra—Emergency Medicine
Dr. Delta—EM, IM, ID
**Plaintiff's expert witnesses:**
Dr. Hotel—ID
Dr. India—EM, IM, CC
Dr. Kilo—EM

**Author comments (Weinstock):** Imagine this was your case; a tough diagnosis for sure! Now, consider how using legal outcomes can make patients safer (yes, the theme of this book). Imaging yourself as the "defendant" clinician. As you sit in a chair being questioned by a plaintiff's attorney, was there a way to improve the data gathering (history and physical or testing), expand the differential or to better explain in an MDM note as to why you did think your diagnosis was occurring, and why you did not think the patient had an SEA? This is how we can learn from cases to improve patient safety and decrease legal risk to prospectively address these issues before a patient is discharged on your next shift!

Here is how these clinicians responded:

**Depositions of clinicians:**

**Doctor Charlie MD (at Hosp B) – Visit #5, Jan 31st**
What was her differential?

- She was considering potential causes of Missy's neck pain being abscess, blood clot, muscle spasm, meningitis, epidural abscess, and hematoma. She considered SEA but didn't think it was the cause.
  - Did not believe epidural abscess was causing Melissa's neck pain because she had no signs of systemic infection (i.e., no fever or sore throat). Denied IV drug use. No neuro deficits. She did acknowledge the patient described chills and sweats which could have represented a fever.
  - She did not believe meningitis was a cause of the symptoms because Missy had no systemic signs of infection and no neurological deficits.

Was she aware that the patient had a past history of a recent MRSA infection?

- She was aware Melissa had been diagnosed with MRSA infection when received records from Hospital A.

How do you diagnose SEA?

- When she suspects epidural abscess, usually does an MRI. She is not aware of any other way to definitively rule out an SEA other than MRI.

- She agrees her WBC of 15.3 was high and she had a left shift, but attributes it to steroid use.
- She agrees unrelenting neck pain can be red flag for SEA.

**PA-C Tango PA-C (at Hosp A)–Visit #7: Seen at Hospital A, Feb 1st**

Should infection be in the differential?

- Depending upon patient's history or PE, infection should creep up on radar if the patient has evidence of fever or complaints of HA even if symptoms had been brief in onset or with a history of IV drug use. More concerning would be if altered mental status or a focal deficit was present.
- He believes infection as cause of neck pain is something that needs to be considered if a patient has a recent diagnosis of any type of infection, MRSA or otherwise, if they complained of severe neck pain in the weeks following the diagnosis. He did not know she had a MRSA abscess within 2 weeks of the visit. He did not look at prior visits.

Was SEA on the Ddx and how do these patients present?

- He does not believe M was in much distress when he saw her between 3:30 and 3:45. She did not exhibit any of the things you would expect to see with somebody in severe pain.
- The only pulse recorded in chart is 118 bpm. She was recorded as tachy, but when he examined her, he did not find her to be tachy and he didn't note a number. He noted she was not tachy on PE. Under cardiovascular he states normal rate, regular rhythm, normal heart sounds.
- The patient told him she had been to ED several times for severe neck pain and she said it was throbbing on both sides of the neck, sometimes worse with turning. The patient reported radiation into both UES, but denied numbness weakness, tingling. He explained meds she had been on from previous visits and that she still had continued pain. The patient complained of HA, but denied blurred vision, speech problems, numbness or weakness in extremities or any focal neuro deficit making SEA less likely.

Why was additional testing not ordered?

- The reason he didn't order blood work or MRI or other testing was because she didn't complain of fever, nausea, or neuro complaints and he also believes the history and exam did not match an infectious picture.
- He believes you evaluate things to the best of your ability, with the understanding that all disease changes over time and every clinical picture changes and there is no way to completely rule out any disease process.
- The patient did not have the classic triad of pain, fever and neurologic symptoms so he didn't think about SEA.

How does torticollis present?

- He defines his diagnosis of torticollis as a spasming of the anterior musculature of the neck and that was more of an agreement with the previous provider's evaluation.

**PA-C Bravo PA-C (at Hosp B)–Visit #8: Hospital B, Feb 1st, (same day)**

Do you remember how the patient presented?

- It was a busy day in the ED and Missy was brought back to a care room with complaint of neck pain. She evaluated her in the presence of a medical scribe and felt she had a pretty basic complaint of neck pain with paracervical tenderness. She didn't appear toxic, skin was warm and dry, was talkative, and able to move about the room. She went back to desk and ordered a med that she felt was appropriate.
- She saw other patients while meds were given. The nurse came to her and she had a plan in mind that if this med worked they would d/c her. Nursing said her neck was better but she was upset she did not get pain medications. So, she ordered a low risk dose of oral pain meds and printed the d/c instructions.

- Melissa said she didn't want to talk again and just wanted her d/c papers. PA-C Bravo acquiesced and returned to her work station.
- From initial assessment and nursing report that she was feeling better, and then seeing her up and ambulating in hallway, felt d/c was appropriate at that time. If meningitis was on the differential, would normally do lumbar puncture.

How do you explain the abnormal vital signs?

- She believes a temp of 100.3 that was taken would not constitute a fever. Her training was anything 100.5 and above is a fever, so she would not consider 100.3 to be febrile.
- She agrees pulse of 146 is tachy, but when she assessed M and put stethoscope to her chest she didn't believe the pulse was that markedly elevated. Can't say it was less than 100, but can speak to using stethoscope up to 60 times a day and when she evaluated M her pulse was not markedly tachy.

How would you have ordered testing if SEA was on the differential?

- If spinal abscess on differential, would order MRI, CT, and L spine to rule it out with IV contrast.

Disposition:

- She offered the patient the chance to be reevaluated and to talk to her again, but the patient wanted her to be discharged. If she thought it was unsafe for Melissa to leave she would have advised her of that and made note of that in the chart.
- Her only understanding of M's improvement came from the nurse who indicated she was moving her neck more and that her neck was better. Also, her assessment of her condition at the coffee stand.
- She didn't see any evidence that concerned her or would suggest IV drug usage and M denied it in her history. She thought that torticollis made sense based on her observation and impression.

**Author comments (Weinstock):** And now here come the experts… but this case is a little different from the others, as we do not have an autopsy defined cause of death. The experts not only need to allege malpractice, but convince the jury that the patient had a likely SEA. Seems like a high bar, but they do make some good points, especially with the subsequent visits.

**Experts Weigh in:**

**Plaintiff's experts:**
**Dr. Hotel, MD (ID)**

1. He thinks M had an infection and it was a spinal infection in her neck. She had that on Feb 1 but doesn't think she had meningitis at that point. He thinks she developed bacterial meningitis sometime between Feb 1 and Feb 3.
2. He thinks it spread from her bloodstream to her neck, and then, because of its proximity to the meninges, subsequently spread to her meninges.
3. He thinks it is more likely than not, the source of the MRSA came from the buttocks abscess.
4. He believes the patient was bacteremic on the 31st when seen by [defendant] MD Charlie (visit #5). Should have ordered blood cultures. Not doing so was below standard of care (SOC).
5. He believes there was discitis or SEA on the 29th.
6. He believes that when the patient was seen on Feb 1st by PA-C Tango (visit #7), she had an SEA. He specifically does not draw a distinction between epidural abscess and epidural infection.
7. He believes that lung involvement was because of endocarditis.
8. PA-C Tango fell below the SOC by not pursuing a diagnosis of epidural or spinal infection within the neck. There was evidence that should have led him to suspect it:
   - The patient had returned several times to the ER within the prior few days.

- He should have known the patient had a MRSA infection roughly one week earlier. Missy was on Bactrim, which was enough of an indication that she was being treated for infection.
- The patient described radiation which increases the risk of SEA.

9. If MRSA bacteremia or MRSA infection in spine had been identified, treatment would have been admission to the hospital for IV antibiotics. SOC would have involved a spinal surgeon be involved along with an ID doctor.
10. PA-C Bravo (visit #8) was required by SOC to have sent for blood cultures and an MRI. Had she ordered blood cultures would've come back positive as MRSA can grow as quickly as 6 hours; range is 6–18 hours.
11. If MRI had been performed would've shown abnormalities within the neck that were consistent with infection.
12. The history is sufficient to support the finding of SEA. Prior records from each previous ER visit were suggestive, WBC of 15,000 on Jan 31st was suggestive, report of fevers when PA-C Bravo (visit #8) evaluated her along with fever of 100.3 and HR of 150 were also sufficient.
13. He can't tell when she developed the endocarditis but he can say that on Feb 3rd the CT of her chest suggested septic emboli. He would estimate roughly 24-48 hours before the septic emboli, but one can have varying degrees of any process.
14. Believes she would have survived if aggressive care was initiated on Feb 1st and also by Feb 3rd.
15. SOC required spinal tap by PA-C Bravo (visit #8) on Feb 1st. The first thing would have been to check labs, including cultures, and then do cervical MRI. He believes the diagnosis would've been made with MRI, in which case the tap would not have been necessary. However, had the MRI been normal, which he highly doubts, a tap would have been the next step. The diff Dx would have been made with cervical spine infection leading the list and meningitis after that.
16. SOC required Doctor Charlie, PA-C Bravo, and PA-C Tango to do an MRI of the neck and blood cultures. He believes M would've survived if SOC had been met and had a full recovery.

**Dr. India MD (EM/IM/CC)**

1. There were two possibilities of source of MRSA, either it came from buttocks abscess and spread or she was just predisposed to getting Staph infections to start with and that lead to hematogenous spread which led to her having the septic PE and parameningeal infection.
2. When Doctor Charlie (visit #5) saw her on Jan 31, the diagnosis was most likely MRSA meningitis or MRSA SEA. A paraspinal infection at some point starts in the soft tissue. When it gets to the point where there is a pocket of pus, that's an abscess.
3. She thinks she had SEA when PA-C Bravo (visit #8) saw her on Feb 1and a Staph bacterial infection. They remember the blood showed Staph. Mother said clinic told her she didn't have meningitis but there was an infection, an epidural abscess.
4. When PA-C Bravo (visit #8) saw Missy on Feb 1 she had either SEA or meningitis. Specifically, which one he cannot say. She had a Staph related infection of the paraspinal region of the spinal cord and bacteremia. She had evidence of systemic signs and symptoms of a bacterial infection within all reasonable likelihood attributable to MRSA, which was spread hematogenously from a skin infection to the spinal/paraspinal region.
5. PA-C Bravo did a very cursory neurologic exam on Feb 1. The documentation includes a standard exam; she has them grip her hands. She said she saw Melissa up walking to get a beverage. She admits that the note does not indicate that there were any neurologic compromises at that time.
6. On Feb 1, Melissa presented to PA-C Bravo with neck pain, HA, fever; she is basically presenting with a little red flag waving, "Hi, I have meningitis." PA-C Bravo evaluated the patient and was aware the temp was slightly elevated. M was presenting with a fever and if you look on med list there are meds that can interfere with ability to fight infection including hydrocodone/APAP and

prednisone. Symptoms were concerning for meningitis or SEA.

- The exam that was done was not adequate. She was required to check orientation, pupillary responses, cranial nerves, neck suppleness, and can they bend chin down to chest? Check bending the knee up and straightening it out. Check strength in arms and legs, sensation in arms and legs.
- Melissa needed further evaluation including lab work including CBC, Chem 7, blood cultures, CSF for gram stain and culture, bacterial antigens if the hospital does it, cell count and differential, glucose and protein and she would then need to contact the supervising physician.
- Discharging the patient without this information was a breach in the standard of care. Further, if the patient had gone to have that testing done, you would get blood cultures and lab work in the meantime.
- She disregarded fact that Melissa presented with a HR of 149 bpm suggesting there is a severe process going on, more than you would expect from just someone having neck pain from muscle spasm.

7. If a thorough evaluation had been done, meningitis would have been found. He intends to opine that PA-C Bravo departed from SOC for a PA.
8. If you're evaluating a patient for fever, HA, and neck pain who has likelihood of meningitis then prescribing outpatient prednisone for treatment is inappropriate. They admit that patients with Strep pneumonia causing meningitis do better if they get IV steroids. However, to send someone home on outpatient prednisone for neck pain when you should be considering meningitis or SEA does not meet the standard of care.

**Dr. Kilo, MD (EM)**

1. The patient had an infection in her cervical spine that may have actually manifested in the thoracic spine first. The thoracic location is based on the exam provided by the physician during the first visit.
2. The origin of this infection was more likely than not a seeding of the aforementioned areas from a previously diagnosed and treated MRSA abscess of the hip.
3. Sinusitis is unlikely to be the originating site of infection.
4. The patient likely did not have a primary bacterial meningitis but may have developed a meningitis-like clinical picture later in the course of her hospitalization.
5. The clinical picture became identifiable as a diagnosable life-threatening condition on or about January 31st when the patient was seen by Dr. Charlie (visit #5) at Hospital B.
6. PA-C Tango (visit #7) fell below the standard of care in his treatment of Ms. M. He had sufficient evidence (more likely than not) to have performed testing including but not limited to lab work, MRI, and LP, or involved in attending physician.
7. During the visit at Hospital on February 1st (visit #8) PAC Bravo should have performed an MRI of the cervical and thoracic spine. If these studies were negative, she should have performed an LP.

**Author comments (Weinstock):** Pretty critical, and pretty definitive of the diagnosis of SEA… the defense has a different theory. How does the defense respond?

**Defense experts:**

**Dr. Alpha, MD (ID)**

1. She had MRSA in her blood. He doesn't think she had an epidural abscess. We'll never know if it was right-sided endocarditis. He thinks she had a complication of the frontal sinusitis. At the last encounter (visit #9 on Feb 3rd), she had very unusual appearance of her left eye seen in intracranial

thrombophlebitis. The critical illness was a suppurative complication of frontal sinusitis which would lead to what is probably a suppurative thrombophlebitis.

2. When she went to Tertiary referral Hospital C, she was seen by an ID doc who speculated as to whether she might have an epidural abscess. They commented she only had a non-contrasted CT but she had a contrasted CT of the neck a couple of days before (around the 29, 30, 31st maybe). A contrasted CT of the neck is a pretty good study for an epidural abscess. This is not as good as MRI, but fairly good.
3. She saw several providers and impression was this was torticollis or a spasm. Dr. Alpha thinks the time course would be a little unusual for an epidural abscess due to MRSA. It's pretty aggressive for neck pain going on a couple of weeks especially when you combine her clinical course with the imaging.
4. ID doc at Hosp C also mentioned intracranial septic thrombophlebitis as one of the reasons she presented so ill. Having more info than that doc did, don't think it was an epidural abscess. Dr. Alpha thinks it was septic thrombophlebitis.
5. CSF findings are more consistent with a parameningeal infection than a primary MRSA meningitis. For primary MRSA meningitis, you would likely have a positive culture. It doesn't rule it out if she was on the vancomycin when they did the LP, but thinks the LP wasn't done too long after she got the antibiotics. MRSA is just the kind of bug you'd expect to see on a culture. Dr. Alpha thinks the CSF could be consistent with an SEA, even though he thinks it is more consistent with suppurative thrombophlebitis.
6. He also thinks it was sinusitis, frontal or otherwise, because she had more than just frontal, that led to an intracranial complication such as septic thrombophlebitis.

**Dr. Golf, MD (ID)**

1. Thinks it was an unusual case of MRSA sinusitis initially in the frontal sinus and then the ethmoid sinuses. This was a regional infection that worsened and may have been an obstructive component to it; the radiologist said there was blockage of the frontal and ethmoid sinuses. Dr. Gold thinks she had severe MRSA sinusitis, essentially "pus under pressure." Sinusitis was there on a scan on Jan 31, suspects it was there smoldering for several days before that, then there was an intracranial component of the disease, so in the vascular structures that are immediately next to that sinus there was thrombophlebitis with secondary MRSA bacteremia. She worsened from there and had SIRS or sepsis from that condition.
2. He admits patient did not complain of sinus pain, discharge, fullness or pressure.
3. He doesn't think the CT on the 29th showed evidence of sinusitis because it hadn't obstructed at that point. There was some thickening of the mucous membranes but no air fluid levels, no confluence of fluid, at that point. He thinks as the sinusitis got worse, it obstructed and there was blockage of the fluid coming out and that's when "this thing got really bad" on the 3rd.
4. He does not believe she had an SEA at any point.
5. She only had meningitis in the sense she had parameningeal focus of infection that resulted in abnormal spinal fluid when they did the spinal tap. She did not have meningitis in the way we think about it. It was a secondary phenomenon.
6. He believes on Feb 1st the temperature of 100.3 was significant for fever.
7. Never any conclusive evidence that it was a SEA, which tends to begin either in the bone disc interface of the spine or in what we call the facet joints. The contrast CT that was done on the 31st got a good look at the bones and the disc and joint and the soft tissue, and there was no pus in there.
8. He believes source of neck pain on 1st was part and parcel of the whole presentation and worsening sinus infection. Why her neck pain seemed to be such a focal point of her symptomatology is not exactly clear, but he thinks it was all a continuum of the gradually worsening sinus infection with a general systemic effect. He admits that he "isn't real sure how it all connects there."

**Dr. Sierra, MD (EM)**

1. His opinion is M died of sepsis, and that is really all he can say.
2. He has no opinion as to what caused her sepsis, except that the organism was probably MRSA. The same organism was cultured from the boil on her hip. He believes it seeded into her blood causing sepsis.
3. The patient died of organ failure and definitely had lung involvement. It didn't come from the cardiac valves. Thinks it either came from the boil or it was the same organism she was harboring in her system. It is well known that people who are carriers of MRSA, which she was as demonstrated by recurrent boils, harbor MRSA innocently in their nose.
4. She did not have bacterial meningitis but may have had viral meningitis as an unrelated clinical picture, but he can't say for sure. His basis of opinion is that bacterial meningitis, if it was going on for 2 weeks and was the cause of her neck pain, she would've gotten sicker more quickly. When they did the spinal tap on Feb 3rd the fluid was slightly yellow but basically clear. There were only 640 segs.
5. He can't say she had an SEA to a probability because there was never an MRI. That, coupled with her symptoms, which he thinks were classic torticollis for two weeks, he sees no evidence definitively that she ever had an SEA.
6. The classic hallmark of SEA will be worsening pain becoming unbearable. These things don't usually take several weeks, it is usually within 3–4 days the patient seeks medical attention because the pain is so unbearable. More importantly, it starts impinging on the cord and you get neurological symptoms which is what brings them in because they can't walk or become incontinent.
7. She reported to her sister the only thing that gave her relief was hot showers. Hot showers relieve muscle spasm and gets more flow going. You get better venous return and less congestion. That all fits with torticollis, as did the exams. Has no doubt she was suffering from torticollis.
8. It is very hard to say exactly when her septicemia started. The bacteremia might have started at the beginning of February, not much before that. He doesn't believe septicemia was present until the 3rd when she had an altered level of consciousness (one of the hallmarks of septicemia). You start getting organ failure and one of the organs that starts failing is the brain. Could she have had some bacteria in her blood when she saw PA-C Tango?
9. The fact she was on Bactrim could account for a smoldering course for her sepsis.

**Dr. Delta, MD (EM/IM/ID)**

1. He thinks an undiagnosed neck infection was occurring, and SEA is a possibility.
2. He read the ID specialist's deposition. He disagrees that Staph originated from sinus and caused venous thrombosis in the brain and that was the cause of death. She possibly had right-sided endocarditis. There was some suggestion she may have had septic emboli and that happens with Staph bloodstream infections. There's no doubt she had Staph in her bloodstream and that alone would be enough to kill somebody, and he thinks it did.
3. He believes it was a MRSA Staph that may have been from her abscess and is probably related because of proximity in time. She had documented MRSA documented on Jan 21 and within a week or two seemed to have the same type of organism in her bloodstream.
4. He later admits that SEA is the most likely cause.
5. She was first diagnosed with bacteremia on the 3rd, but hard to say when it started. With a Staph bloodstream infection, patients are extremely ill, and he doesn't think she demonstrated that before Feb 3rd.
6. Some of her complaints may have suggested infection sooner. Looking back, there was probably some infection brewing, but people who die from a Staph blood infection are not ambulatory and do not appear very well. He doesn't think she was bacteremic during previous visits.
7. When she first developed her butt abscess, some of the Staph got into the bloodstream. Staph tends

to go places and "set up shop" as an abscess where it is protected from the immune system and from antibiotics somewhat. What isn't protected is when bacteria are in the blood and it can be gobbled up after it initially occurs by the immune system. Also, she got treated with Bactrim on the 21st that could further assist to clear it from the blood but wouldn't always clear it from wherever it set up shop. Once she stopped taking antibiotics around the 31st, she was very sick with the expected presentation when the Staph is no longer suppressed and then breaks into the bloodstream.

8. The reason the SEA is among the possibilities is she complained of neck pain and she had a Staph infection, but there are many parts of her presentation that prospectively wouldn't suggest SEA. She had consistent findings of tenderness in her muscles, and that wouldn't be expected with SEA. On the other hand, looking back, it makes you wonder if there was something undiagnosed deeper in her neck contributing to her neck pain besides the pain that seemed to be localized in her muscles.
9. Skin and soft tissue infections with MRSA are very rarely the cause of SEA.
10. Although SEA can't be definitively ruled in or out at this point, the one thing that makes it less likely is all the providers were able to demonstrate muscle tenderness, spasm, and that would not be consistent alone with an SEA.

## II. The Verdict

The case returned a verdict for the plaintiff in the sum of $350,000.

## III. The Legal Analysis

**T. Marc Calvert, JD**
Medical malpractice defense attorney with over 35 years of experience
Calvert, Leever & Ostler
Cypress, Texas

**Initial thoughts:**
When multiple healthcare providers have seen the same patient, each provider needs to be able to satisfactorily run their leg of the relay race, that is, to offer reasonable explanations for the care provided within the window of time that they saw the patient. Now, given the fact that there were prior visits, it will be necessary to touch on what consideration was given to that fact, and to the details of those visits. The attorney will need to question the patient, possibly depose the prior providers, review the prior records including ED and primary care, and tease out who has the most responsibility.

Some of the things that are mentioned do raise questions; her father losing the prescriptions and paperwork as they walked home from the hospital seems to be an unusual circumstance. Most people don't walk to the emergency room, and losing paperwork in that manner seems to indicate a certain level of confusion or even chaos. Her mental health history will be assessed, and one of the documented instances of her becoming very verbally combative, also raise questions as to whether these things influenced, or reasonably misled, the providers and how they evaluated her.

The biggest legal danger is the catastrophic outcome, particularly for such a young patient. Lay people will wonder why specialty consultation and hospitalization did not occur earlier. Therefore, it is imperative that each provider be able to explain, and justify, their actions within the treatment puzzle. If those steps can be shown to be reasonable, based on the persuasive and compassionate testimony of the defendant as well as support from good experts, and the literature, it can be a game changer.

**How could the documentation have been improved?**
In general, for a note in the records to be effective, it's not necessarily the length of the note, but the quality that matters. It's obviously easier to assess once we know the outcome. However, with every patient, there are some hot issues and questions which require attention, and perhaps, explanation.

Tachycardia is obviously one of those issues. Even a brief note, offering an explanation as to the possible cause, could been helpful. The documentation not only indicates that it was appreciated, but that there is a possible legitimate explanation (i.e., pain, fever, or dehydration). More detail concerning the history from the patient would also be helpful to the defense; this is particularly important given the unique number of visits to the ED. At some point, a provider is going to have to sit down and try to connect the dots and chronicle how this condition has changed and evolved.

**How does lack of an autopsy (definitive diagnosis) affect the legal proceedings?**
Since the burden of proof is on the plaintiff, the lack of an autopsy here poses a potentially huge hurdle for their ability to prove what caused the death. This is pivotal to the question of what could have been done to possibly prevent the death. The plaintiff needs to show what the likely cause of death was with reasonable medical probability. That is usually interpreted "more likely than not." However, starting with the United States Supreme Court case of Daubert v. Merrell Dow in the early 1990s, the law requiring reliable science to prove causation has become more stringent.

Thus, defendants can rightly bring up an array of possibilities which trigger doubts that a different course of action would have made a difference. Was there some underlying heart condition which caused her death? How can it be proven that a sooner diagnosis or more aggressive treatment plan would have altered the course and outcome? Is there any literature on these issues? Without an autopsy, it can be argued that the plaintiff's lawyers are simply speculating and cannot sustain their burden of proof with the required quality of evidence. This situation typically features a hot debate between experts, with literature and studies at the core.

**Do the 3 defendants share responsibility equally?**
Legal responsibility greatly depends on how each defendant comes across to a jury. Displaying the combination of caring and competence, along with humility and likeability, can make a huge difference. The doctor will likely be held to a higher standard than the advanced practice providers in the minds of the jurors. Ultimately, the pivotal point is how well they come across.

Finally, as set out above, causation could be a major area of battle in this matter. In this case, the defendant who saw her earliest may be more vulnerable since it may be argued that earlier diagnosis afforded an opportunity for the treatment to be more successful. The argument that it was probably too late to make a difference is less effective for the earlier treater.

**Would the defendants all have the same attorney, or different attorneys?**
No, the potential of a conflict of interest between the defendants would require separate counsel. I would recommend that there be unity and cooperation, and with this approach, there is a potential for better results. Three skilled defense attorneys all pushing in the same direction can be formidable.

**Would you push to settle or try to go to trial?**
Whether to settle or go to trial would depend on the strength of the client in terms of being able to effectively testify in addition to the caliber of our expert support. Given the number of ED visits, I would probably encourage mediation and that consideration be given for a reasonable settlement. Because

there are some real questions on causation, based on no autopsy, this leverage could result in a reasonable settlement.

**Were you surprised by the small judgment?**
Yes. If they truly felt there was negligence, it should have been higher. However, I think the amount could be an indication that the jury saw some context or traits with this patient which made things extra challenging. Also, it might reflect that they did not really blame the defendants, per se. They just felt obliged to provide some level of compensation to the family. This is a relatively common compromise that some juries make.

**A personal aside:**
By way of brief personal experience, I tried a shoulder dystocia case many years ago. The child suffered a brachial plexus injury during delivery and was 6 years old when we tried the case. He was very sympathetic. We had strong expert support and felt that the trial had gone our way. To our surprise, we lost.

Despite evidence that the child would never be able to use his right arm, and it would greatly impact his work and his activities of daily living for his whole life, the jury returned a verdict of $170,000. The plaintiffs' attorney had asked for millions. If they really felt there was negligent care, why the low amount of damages?

In talking to some of them after the verdict, they felt a lot of sympathy for the child and felt that he needed something. However, they also recognized that the obstetrician had tried his best, and they did not feel anger or antipathy towards him. They did not want to ruin him. It was a tough situation, and they just decided to provide something for the family to help them out.

The moral of the story is that a lot of juries think like that, and so the idea of mediating and pointing out significant strengths like no autopsy, and therefore the possibility of an appeal, could yield a settlement that is not exorbitant and which folks on both sides can live with. There are a fair number of cases which fall into that category.

## IV. Medical Discussion—Evaluation of Neck Pain in the Setting of Fever

**Christopher E. San Miguel, MD**
Clinical Associate Professor of Emergency Medicine
The Ohio State University Wexner Medical Center

**David K. Chang, MD**
Emergency Medicine
Kaiser Permanente
Fontana Medical Center

**Colin G. Kaide, MD**
Clinical Professor of Emergency Medicine
The Ohio State University Wexner Medical Center

It is difficult to conjecture the exact sequence of events that led to the unfortunate death of this young mother of three. A lack of autopsy restricts us to careful examination of the timeline, documentation, diagnostic tests, and expert testimonies. However, every emergency medicine curriculum will emphasize a handful of critical presentation patterns that should raise red flags for emergent evaluation and management. The classic triad for spinal epidural abscess is

- fever,
- localized back pain, and
- neurologic deficits,

but simultaneous presentation is seldom seen in early presentation.[1] Therefore, any fever with localized back pain should raise concern for spinal epidural abscess. This is seen with our patient who presented with persistent debilitating neck pain since 1/27, report of subjective chills/sweats on 1/31, and temperature of 100.3°F on 2/1. The patient was also potentially taking antipyretic-containing medications (the acetaminophen in Norco) which could have masked the fever and would have been important to know. It is unclear why this critical diagnosis was overlooked; anchoring or confirmation bias to a musculoskeletal etiology are possibilities. Spinal epidural abscesses are a rare etiology for back pain, are often missed initially, and frequently require multiple presentations before diagnosis and management.[2]

Epidural abscesses come in two flavors. There are intracranial epidural abscesses (IEA) and the more common, but still relatively rare, spinal epidural abscess (SEA). A SEA forms between the dura mater and vertebral bone. While the dura is adherent to the bone above the foramen magnum, it exists as a true space below this level and containing vessels and fat. The combination of rich vasculature and fatty space makes it an ideal location for abscess formation. In one study, hematogenous spread from a skin infection/soft tissue infection was the 2nd most common source (22% of cases) and was only surpassed by unknown etiology (30% of cases). Other potential sources include spinal procedures, IV drug use, osteomyelitis, sepsis, abdominal, and intravascular catheter associated (in descending order of frequency).[3–7] Additional risk factors include being immunocompromised, malignancy, alcohol use, diabetes, CKD, and recent spinal fracture.[4,8] Our patient's recent history of MRSA abscess and skin infection should have been a significant clue and risk factor early in the diagnostic work-up and likely the etiology of a SEA given later positive blood cultures for MRSA.

*Staphylococcus aureus* is the primary culprit for up to 70% of cases of SEA.[5,9] Other common pathogens include *Staphylococcus epidermidis* (often associated with device infection), Streptococcal species, and gram-negative bacteria such as *Escherichia coli* (often associated with UTI) and *Pseudomonas aeruginosa* (often associated with IVDU). Mycobacteria, fungi, and parasites are rare but possible.[6,10]

The most common location for SEAs is the lumbar or thoracic spine due to their larger space and venous plexus. Cervical SEAs occur less frequently at 5–20% of occurrences but carry a higher mortality and neurologic sequalae.[6,4,10, 11] Neurologic dysfunction can be a consequence of direct compression of the spinal cord but can also be secondary to ischemic effects on compressed vasculature or septic thrombophlebitis.[6,10]

Interestingly, our patient did not have any documented neurologic deficits despite our suspicion of cervical SEA. Plaintiff's expert Dr. India criticized PA-C Bravo's neuro exam as being "very cursory" and "inadequate," but it is hard to say that a better exam would have helped with the diagnosis. Of note, SEAs more commonly occur in the T/L spine which was not imaged and could have been missed (as alluded to by Dr. Kilo 's concerns). The latter does not explain why a T/L spine SEA would cause cervical pain; however, neurological dysfunction was only seen in 68.4% percent of cervical infections and in general, only 8% to 37% of patients demonstrated the classic triad of back pain, fever, and neurologic dysfunction. [6,5,10,11]

Lab work when SEA is suspected should include a WBC which often demonstrates a leukocytosis. This was elevated to 15.3 (78% Neutrophils) in our patient but was unfortunately not drawn until the patient's 3rd visit for neck pain on 1/31. ESR, CRP, and 2 sets of blood cultures are also recommended as part of the work-up[6,10] but were delayed until the patient appeared critically ill during her 7th ED visit from onset of neck pain on 2/3. ESR and CRP would turn out to be elevated to 71 and 47 respectively, and blood cultures would grow MRSA. Lumbar punctures are generally discouraged for routine suspicion for SEA as cultures are often negative and the procedure itself may risk traversing the abscess and seeding a meningitis or subdural infection.[6,10] Gram stain will typically present negative, cultures are positive < 25% percent of the time, [12] and other abnormalities usually nonspecific.[13] While these studies may be helpful, none are sensitive or specific for SEA, therefore further evaluation with advanced imaging is necessary.[6,10]

The imaging modality of choice is a Gadolinium-enhanced MRI as sensitivities are greater than 90% for SEA.[6,10] Unfortunately, as the case with our patient, CT scans have much lower sensitivities for epidural abscess (as low as 6% in one study[8,14] and up to 18% in a second study),[15] especially with early infection. This may explain why our patient's CT neck with contrast on 1/31 did not show any evidence of SEA. They can provide clues as to if there is adjacent discitis (osteomyelitis), which were not seen in our patient.[8,12] Overall sensitivity with CT can be improved when combined with myelogram (such as in patients who are contraindicated from MRI) but not recommended over MRI due to its invasive nature, additional risk of infection, [16] and difficulty distinguishing an SEA from other compressive lesions.[6,10] MRI with Gadolinium should be obtained if available, even if this may require transport to another facility with the capability.[6,10] The entire spine should be imaged given the possibility of noncontiguous skip lesions (some affected regions may not be tender). [17]

Initiation of broad-spectrum empiric antibiotics to cover MRSA and pseudomonal infection (often vancomycin with cefepime or meropenem) should be started as soon as SEA is suspected and later adjusted based on cultures and infectious disease consultation.[6,10] Once a diagnosis is made, the patient will need emergent neurosurgery evaluation for decompressive surgery and ICU admission. In neurologically intact patients or those with neurologic deficits > 72 hours, a CT-guided aspiration of the SEA vs. conservative antibiotic therapy can sometimes be considered by the neurosurgeon but will require ICU monitoring for decompensation that may require surgery. [18]

## V. Final Thoughts and Takeaway Points

**Lessons learned:** Diagnosis momentum is a real form of confirmation bias. When evaluating bounceback patients, consider that you now have access to more information than on the previous visit. This patient continued to receive a diagnosis of torticollis long after her head tilt resolved. The patient's penultimate diagnosis of muscle strain does not account for her headache, low grade temperature, or significant tachycardia. These new findings should prompt the clinician to broaden the differential diagnosis. At the very least, the medical decision-making should clearly lay out why the clinician did not think any further work-up was necessary. However, bounceback patients require an escalation in their work-up.

This case rests on the expert witnesses' opinions that the patient had an epidural abscess which caused her severe neck pain and ultimately septic shock. With reports of fever and several bouncebacks for intractable pain, the clinician is compelled to consider this diagnosis. An ESR may have been used as a reasonable screening test, but with progressive symptoms, she ultimately required an MRI. The clinicians in this case may have been falsely reassured by the negative CT scans, or in this case, the "Donut of Half-Truths."

Some biases that physicians can succumb to and were likely at play in this case include the following:

- **Diagnosis momentum:** Sometimes called diagnostic creep, diagnostic momentum bias occurs when an initial premature diagnosis is made and becomes perpetuated to downstream members of the patient's care team. The diagnosis gains momentum as it is passed down and eventually becomes definitive, making it less likely that other diagnostic possibilities will be considered.
- **Premature closure:** This bias occurs when there is a premature acceptance of a diagnosis early in the work-up without sufficient verification or consideration for other differentials. It has frequently been quoted, "when the diagnosis is made, the thinking stops."
- **Yin-Yang out:** Yin-yang out (also known as yin-yang bias, serum rhubarbs, or standing stool velocities) occurs when a patient has been extensively worked up ("worked up Out the Yin-Yang") without a clear diagnosis, leaving the provider to feel as if there is nothing more they can do. This can sometimes be true but may leave the diagnosis open to error. We often see this in "frequent flyers" in the ED where further work-up may feel futile or an inappropriate allocation of resources. However, it is important to consider that many disease processes have similar presentations or that a patient's disease process may have evolved providing a new opportunity for diagnosis.
- **Zebra retreat:** Zebra retreat bias occurs when a rare diagnosis ("zebras") is prominently supported in the differential diagnosis but shied away from due to a variety of reasons including its scarcity, concern for wasting limited resources, inconvenience/difficulty of testing, unfamiliarity with the diagnosis, self-consciousness/under-consciousness for entertaining rare diagnoses, and fear of judgment from other providers.

## References


1. Babic M, Simpfendorfer CS, Berbari EF. Update on spinal epidural abscess. Curr Opin Infect Dis 2019;32(3):265-71. doi: 10.1097/QCO.0000000000000544. PMID: 31021957.
2. Bhise V, Meyer AND, Singh H, et al. Errors in diagnosis of spinal epidural abscesses in the era of electronic health records. Am J Med 2017;130(8):975-81. doi: 10.1016/j.amjmed.2017.03.009. Epub 2017 Mar 31. PMID: 28366427.
3. Danner R, Hartman BJ. Update on spinal epidural abscess: 35 cases and review of the literature. Rev Infect Dis 1975;9(2):265-74.
4. Nussbaum ES, Rigamonti D, Standiford H, et al. Spinal epidural abscess: A report of 40 cases and review. Surg Neurol 1992;38(3):225-31.

5 Gellin BG, Weingarten K, Gamache FW Jr, et al. Epidural Abscess. In: Infections of the Central Nervous System, 2nd ed, Scheld WM, Whitley RJ, Durack DT (Eds), Lippincott-Raven Publishers, Philadelphia 1997. p.507.

6. Rigamonti D, Liem L, Wolf AL, et al. Epidural abscess in the cervical spine. Mt Sinai J Med 1994;61(4):357-62.
7. Kapeller P, Fazekas F, Krametter D, et al. Pyogenic infectious spondylitis: Clinical, laboratory and MRI features. Eur Neurol 1997;38(2):94-98.
8. Sampath P, Rigamonti D. Spinal epidural abscess: A review of epidemiology, diagnosis, and treatment. J Spinal Disord 1999;12(2):89-93.
9. Rosc-Bereza K, Arkuszewski M, Ciach-Wysocka E, et al. Spinal epidural abscess: Common symptoms of an emergency condition—A case report. Neuroradiol J 2013;26(4):464-68.
10. Tanski ME, Ma O. Central nervous system and spinal infections. In: Tintinalli JE, Ma O, Yealy

DM, Meckler GD, Stapczynski J, Cline DM, Thomas SH. eds. Tintinalli's Emergency Medicine: A Comprehensive Study Guide, 9e. McGraw Hill; 2020. Accessed March 20, 2023. https://accessmedicine-mhmedical-com.proxy.lib.ohio-state.edu/content.aspx?bookid=2353&sectionid=220293696

11. Urrutia J, Zamora T, Campos M: Cervical pyogenic spinal infections: Are they more severe diseases than infections in other vertebral locations? Eur Spine J 2013;22(12):2815-20.
12. Darouiche RO. Spinal epidural abscess. N Engl J Med 2006;355(19):2012-20. doi: 10.1056/NEJMra055111. PMID: 17093252.
13. Darouiche RO, Hamill RJ, Greenberg SB, et al. Bacterial spinal epidural abscess. Review of 43 cases and literature survey. Medicine (Baltimore) 1992;71(6):369-85. PMID: 1359381.
14. Rausch VH, Bannas P, Schoen G, et al. Diagnostic yield of multidetector computed tomography in patients with acute spondylodiscitis. Rofo 2017;189(4):339-46. English. doi: 10.1055/s-0043-101864. Epub 2017 Mar 1. PMID: 28249310.
15. Shroyer S, Boys G, April MD, Long B, Mehta S, Davis WT. Imaging characteristics and CT sensitivity for pyogenic spinal infections. Am J Emerg Med 2022;58:148-53. doi:10.1016/j.ajem.2022.05.050])
16. Bond A, Manian FA. Spinal epidural abscess: A review with special emphasis on earlier diagnosis. Biomed Res Int 2016;2016:1614328. doi: 10.1155/2016/1614328. Epub 2016 Dec 1. PMID: 28044125; PMCID: PMC5156786.
17. Ju, K.L., et al. Predicting patients with concurrent noncontiguous spinal epidural abscess lesions. Spine J 2005;15(1):95-101.
18. Patel AR, Alton TB, Bransford RJ, et al: Spinal epidural abscesses: Risk factors, medical versus surgical management, a retrospective review of 128 cases. Spine J 2014;14(2):326-30.

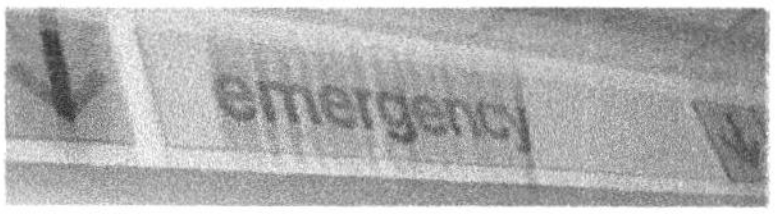


# Case 13

## A 49 Year-old Man with COPD Exacerbation: An Administrative Decision Becomes Legal Quicksand

**Primary case author:**
**Michael Weinstock**

### PART 1—MEDICAL



### PART 2—LEGAL

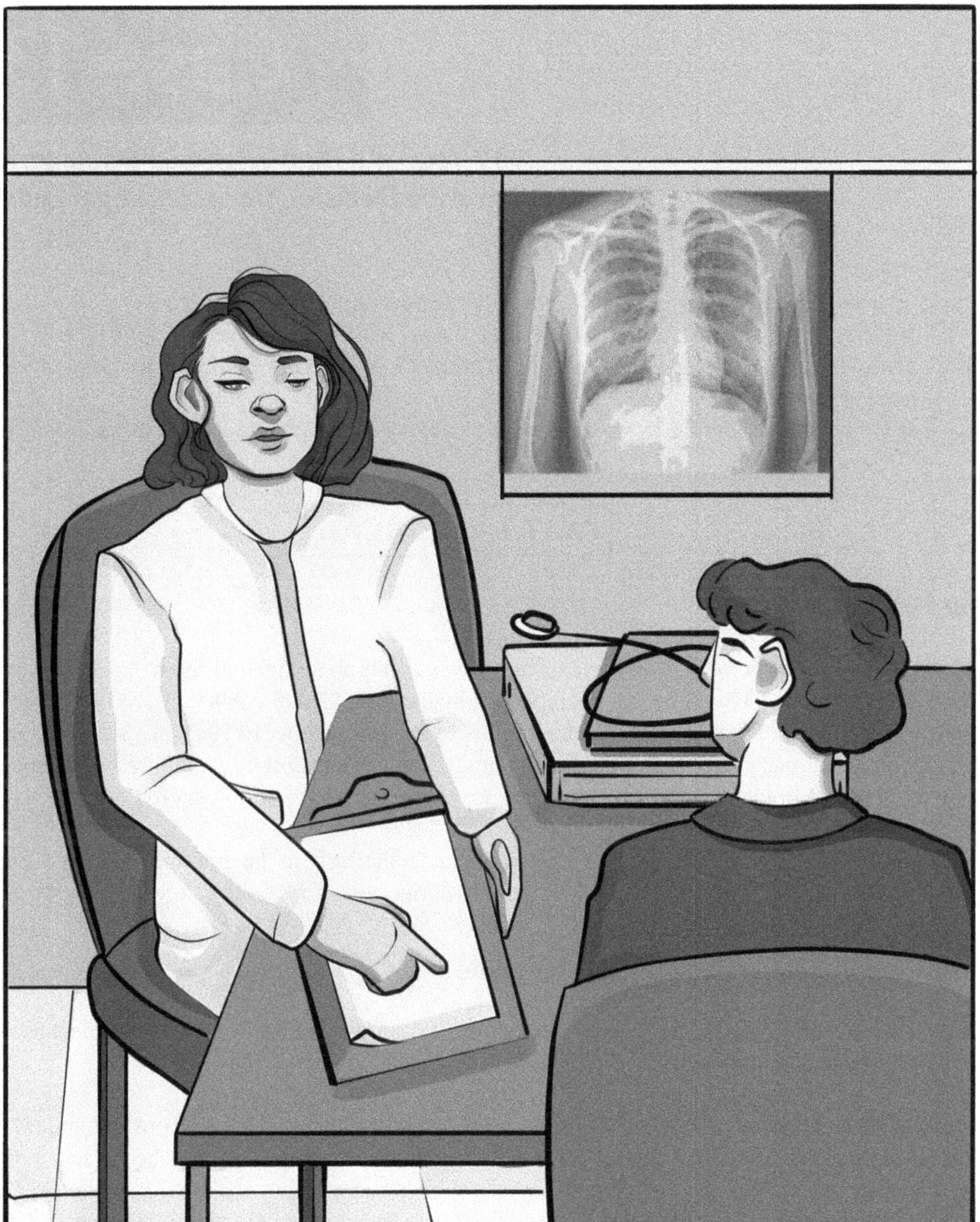

**Aftercare instructions for COPD exacerbation**

# Case 13

## A 49 Year-old Man With COPD Exacerbation: An Administrative Decision Becomes Legal Quicksand

***Deep thoughts:***

1. *How do we account for a likely diagnosis and a less likely diagnosis?*
2. *Is the emergency physician accountable for events which occur after their shift ends?*
3. *Does a signed discharge paper asking the patient to follow up with primary care absolve us of legal responsibility?*
4. *Is the emergency physician (EP) expected to double check the board-certified radiologist after a CT scan result?*

**PART 1—MEDICAL**

## I. The Patient's Story

Roger Hall has a passion for working on cars and music and is an avid fan of football. He has struggled to hold down a steady job, with recent tax returns showing only $2,000–$9,000 in yearly income for the last 3 years. Prior to that, there are no tax returns as he spent almost 10 years in a state institution due to recurrent burglary and robbery and trafficking of controlled substances; in fact, he has spent approximately half of his adult life incarcerated.

Toward the end of August, his smoker's cough worsens. In the early in the morning of August 29th, he is awoken by shortness of breath. He calls 911, and EMS transports him to the emergency department.

## II. The Doctor's Version ED visit #1—August 29th

**Chief Complaint/Nurse (04:52):** "Pt c/o a cough that is non-productive for 4–5 days and an asthma attack that started at 4AM today."

**History of Present Illness – Documentation by PA (05:09):** Patient with a PMH of asthma, HTN, and smoking presents via EMS with c/o SOB. He states that for the past 4–5 days he has had a dry nonproductive cough. He has been using his inhaler which was working well until it ran out which is why he called the squad. He admits to rhinorrhea and nasal congestion. He did try OTC cold medicine without relief. He smokes 1PPD. States this feels like an asthma exacerbation to him. Denies fever, cp, wheezing, HA, sick contacts.

I have introduced myself as the PA/CNP and informed the patient of the supervising/collaborating physician who is available upon request. I have discussed the case with the ED physician who participated in the decisions regarding any therapeutic interventions.

**PMH:** Asthma, hypertension
**PSH:** Negative

**SH:** Smoker 1 PPD

Vital Signs

| Time | Temp(F) | Pulse | Resp | Syst | Diast | $O_2$ sat (RA) |
|---|---|---|---|---|---|---|
| 04:48 | Oral | 80 | 20 | 168 | 93 | 96 |

**Constitutional:** WNWD, no conversational dyspnea
**Eyes:** PERRL, no scleral icterus
**Nose:** Turbinates are erythematous and edematous with edema present
**Lungs:** Course breath sounds in the RLL without wheeze. No use of accessory muscles
**Card:** Regular rate and rhythm, nl. S1 S2
**ABD:** Soft without r/r/g
**Skin:** Normal, warm and dry, no apparent lesions

**Emergency Department Course:**
Albuterol aerosol x 1
Azithromycin 500mg PO

**Image #1: CXR on August 29th visit:**

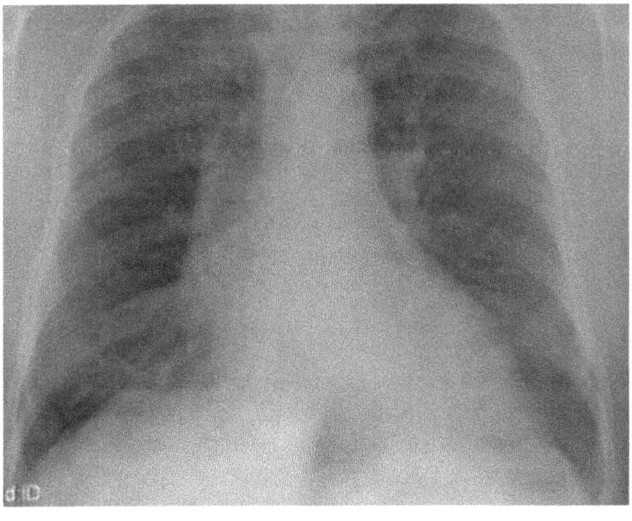

**CXR:** (physician documentation at 05:57) "infiltrate"
Note: This is the actual CXR, but the appearance of the right hilum is distorted due to some modifications of the actual film. Please concentrate on the pulmonary infiltrate/opacity in the RUL.

**Diagnosis:** COPD exacerbation

**Disposition (06:21):** Albuterol MDI – 2 puffs every 4 hours while awake for 5 days then 4x per day as needed, Azithromycin [Z pack]. Follow up with Dr [PCP] in 2–3 days.

**Author comments (Weinstock):** At 7AM the physician shift ends. Before the bounceback visit is revealed, consider if the care administered was standard. After all, what is the goal of ED care? We would all agree that it is essential to prove an imminently life-threatening process is not occurring, but, as discussed by Edlow and Pronovost in a JAMA viewpoint article, the main goal is to make a "safe disposition" and at times, the eventual diagnosis upon ED discharge might still be incomplete.[1]

In fact, what is malpractice anyway? I (Weinstock) would define it as:
1) Incomplete data gathering and
2) Poor medical decision-making
Malpractice is not simply failing to make a diagnosis

**Behind the scenes/what happened next?**
The radiologist did not see the film until about an hour after patient discharge, and their report was not formalized until mid-afternoon, long after patient discharge (at 6:21 AM), and long after the night shift physician left the ED (approx. 7AM). The report stated:

[Preliminary] Impression: "4 cm x 2.7 cm opacity right upper lobe, could be acute pneumonia, follow-up needed to be sure this resolves."

The full report expands on the preliminary report:
*[Final] Impression: "4 cm x 2.7 cm opacity right upper lobe, could be acute pneumonia, follow-up needed to be sure this resolves. If this does not resolve, the patient will need a chest CT scan."*

**Author comments (Weinstock):** In fact, this hospital did have a review process, where the "EMR coordinator" reconciled radiology reports:
The formal radiology report was reviewed in the afternoon, well after patient discharge, per hospital/ED protocol to review all radiologic studies. Review was by Paula Oliver, a former Emergency Department Nurse, now (and then) "EMR Coordinator" who documented that "no physician follow-up was necessary." (It is unclear if the "EMR coordinator" saw the preliminary report or the final report).

**Per the legal analyses (this is the report from the defense attorneys to the malpractice carrier):**
We do not presently know whether a discrepancy report was issued and there is no documentation in the ED chart that the radiologist called about this unexpected finding. Further, there is no indication that [the radiologist] made a comparison to the earlier CT scan (14 months previous when the patient had presented for an axillary boil), which is not surprising, since it was ordered and reported as a "Upper Extremity CT;" [The radiologist] would have no way to know it also imaged some lung. That is unfortunate, because had this study been reviewed, it would probably have revealed that the lesion was present earlier and enlarged in the interval between the studies, thus leading to a conclusion that this was likely not acute pneumonia.

**Author comments (Weinstock):** Whaaaat? So, the patient had an extremity CT 14 months previous which included some of the lung? This was unknown to the EP and was not compared by the radiologist (see below). So, additional information is present here which was unlikely to have been discovered at the time of the ED visit but was certainly important, both medically and legally. Here is some of the documentation from the ED visit 14 months previous.

**[Bounce] back to the future (documentation from the ED visit 14 months previous):**
Of note, the patient had been to the ED 14 months prior to ED visit #1 (The visit described above from August 29th) and had an axillary "boil" drained. The symptoms did not resolve, so the patient returned one week later and had a CT scan done. The official impression read:

*Soft tissue swelling is seen in the epidermis, but there is no subcutaneous fluid collection to suggest an abscess.*

The patient was admitted and started on IV vancomycin, seen by surgery, and discharged on oral antibiotics.

A later review of the CT images confirmed there was no abscess, but that it did catch some images of the lung. When they were reviewed, a pulmonary mass was seen in the right lung apex.

The radiologist was added to the list of defendants.

**Image #2: CT scan from visit 14 months previous when patient presented for right axillary "boil" (actual CT)**

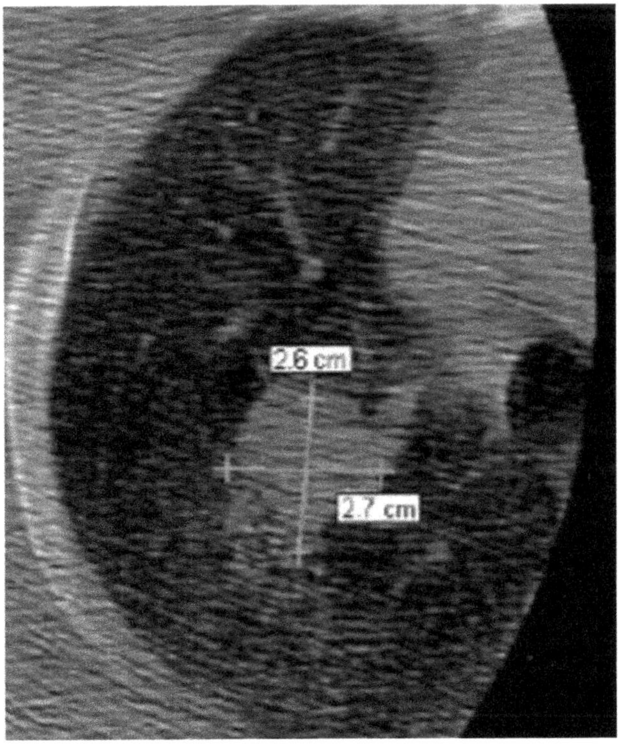


**Author comments (Weinstock):** A question which will become very germaine to this case is, "Why are all ED radiologic studies overread by a radiologist?" The answer is simple, because there are sometimes discrepancies. Tranovich, et al. looked at over 16,000 X-rays and found almost 94% agreement, with discrepancies being minimal or non-significant, with just less than 2% requiring a return to the ED or change in management.[2]

## III. Risk Management/Patient Safety Opportunities (Weinstock)

**Author comments (Weinstock):** So, now we see the diagnosis and some opportunities for improvement in care. Primary is the hospital nurse, Ms. Oliver, who was tasked with reviewing the discrepancies; this was a massive fail. But what about culpability of the emergency physician (EP)? This case did result in a legal action and to quote Greg Henry, MD, past president of ACEP, "In a legal action, no one wins; there are two losers, one loser and a bigger loser." In fact, one study estimated that EPs spend about 13% of their careers involved in a legal action, with the mean time from occurrence date and resolution of the claim being almost 44 months (all physicians). [3]

**Risk Management/Patient Safety Opportunity #1:**

**Opportunity:** Leave room for other diagnoses, even if the ED diagnosis seems obvious.
**Discussion:** We have become much more comfortable with an "acceptable miss rate" with many diseases, including pediatric head injury, [4,5] pulmonary embolism (the PERC rule still has a 1–2% false negative rate,[6]) and even a major adverse cardiac event (MACE) in patients with a negative evaluation for chest pain. In fact, The American College of Emergency Physicians (ACEP) says in the 2018 chest pain clinical policy that there is a 1–2% acceptable miss rate for MACE as trying to get lower than this number will result in patient harm from false positive tests. [7] In the same way, just about every ED diagnosis has potential for a rare cause but that is fine because we have the ability to ask the patient to return if their symptoms progress, change, or worsen. If some diagnostic uncertainty remains, ensure the patient is aware, and they agree to follow up with primary care or to return to the ED. In all fairness, in the case of our patient, though they were asked to follow up with primary care, it is unlikely the clinicians felt there was a question as to the diagnosis.
✔ **Teaching point:** Ensure the patient understands if there is "diagnostic uncertainty" remaining at ED discharge.

**Risk Management/Patient Safety Opportunity #2:**

**Opportunity:** When reading a radiological study, evaluate it first from an anatomic-specific perspective, then a diagnosis-specific perspective.
**Discussion:** Just as we evaluate a patient at the bedside first in a symptom-based fashion (onset, duration, character, exacerbators, etc.), we often then close with a diagnosis-specific evaluation (i.e., could the chest pain be from acute coronary syndrome (ACS), pulmonary embolism (PE), or thoracic aortic dissection (TAD))? We should evaluate the chest X-ray ) in the same fashion. One approach is to evaluate from an anatomic standpoint looking at the heart, bones, abdomen, then the lungs. Another approach, after the anatomic standpoint is completed, is to look again at the CXR from a diagnostic standpoint: think of the hard to find and commonly missed diagnoses and specifically look for them, including, a retrocardiac infiltrate, apical pneumothorax, bone lesion, free air, or a lung mass.
✔ **Teaching point:** Consider malignancy in smokers with lung opacities.

**Risk Management/Patient Safety Opportunity #3:**

**Opportunity:** Ensure the patient understands the importance of follow-up.
**Discussion:** This is the way we will catch that rare or atypically presenting diagnosis but only if the patient actually follows up! In this case, there was an impediment to follow-up in that the PCP refused to see the patient. While there is no way the EP could have known this, having the patient return to the

ED is always an option. In fact, while some clinicians might be reluctant to put the word cancer in their reading of "cannot exclude mass," etc., we do our patients a disservice if we refrain from telling them why they need to follow up.

✔ **Teaching point:** We are partners with the patient in their own health care; though the discharge is appropriate, we count on them to return if their symptoms worsen, progress, change, or do not resolve.

**Risk Management/Patient Safety Opportunity #4:**

**Opportunity:** Consider adding a question for patients at increased risk of cancer: "Do you have any unintentional weight loss (UWL)?"

**Discussion:** Though our patient, in the eyes of the EP, clearly had an infiltrate, there are many times when a simple question could be game changing. For example, in patients with back pain, headache, hematochezia or a dry cough, this additional information may be crucial. Though the literature is not robust on how often this question will help make the diagnosis, one study found that of those patients with unexplained weight loss (UWL) defined as 5% over the previous 6–12 months, an organic cause was found in 56% with 22% of the total being from a malignancy.[8] Another study examined over 70,000 patients with UWL finding a higher risk of nearly all serious diseases including cancer which was the most common finding in men over the age of 60.[9]

✔ **Teaching point:** Asking patients about unintentional weight loss can be game changing.

**Risk Management/Patient Safety Opportunity #5:**

**Opportunity:** Ensure there is a fail-safe way to review results which are not available to the EP.

**Discussion:** At this point in our case, this point is now obvious. Still, when this is left to the physician who arrives with patients knee deep in the lobby or already roomed, it is easy to see how an abnormal test result (lab or radiological) could slip through the cracks, which is why it is so surprising that the CXR discrepancy in our case was not flagged by the nurse doing the reviews.

✔ **Teaching point:** To keep things a bit light, we can summarize this point with a funny expression; If we pick our nose in public and get a positive result, we need to figure out what to do with it!

**Author comments (Weinstock):** During the subsequent legal encounter, the patient was questioned about the receipt of discharge instructions. He did agree that he received discharge instructions to follow up with his primary care physician.

Plaintiff agrees he signed the patient instructions form related to his ER visit, which instruct him to follow-up with his family doctor, Dr. Crumbo, in two or three days. Plaintiff states he called, but Dr. Crumbo refused to see him due to an "insurance issue." He stated [they told him that] they would try to get him into a low-cost primary care clinic, but never got back in touch with him. Plaintiff states he personally appeared in Dr. Crumbo's office 6 weeks later, but they "made [him] leave" after he "had some words" with a secretary. He admitted that he did not see any other clinician until his [bounceback] ED visit 6 months later.

## IV. The Bounceback (6 months later)

**History of Present Illness text:** The patient presents at the emergency room with a complaint of chest tightness, shortness of breath and yellow productive cough for the past 4–5 days. He states at one point it felt very tight but denied any pain though the triage note states otherwise. He states that he had taken a nebulizer treatment at home with total relief of his chest tightness. He states that his chest tightness has returned however. He states that he does smoke approximately a pack and a half of cigarettes a day. He has had pneumonia before but denies any previous hospitalizations for it. He admits to nasal congestion and states that is why he believes that has a headache. He denies any headache currently but states that he still feels congested. He also states that his family physician wants him started on a blood pressure medication but he does not want to take one at this time. He states that he did have an episode of bilateral arm tingling and heaviness. He states that he was working overhead at the time and when he relaxed his arms the sensation had resolved.

**A CTA of the chest was ordered with indications: r/o pulmonary embolism:**
**Impression:**

1. Large right upper lobe mass contiguous with the right upper mediastinum and hila with multiple enlarged lymph nodes in the mediastinum consistent with neoplasm with metastatic disease.
2. No acute pulmonary embolus.

## PART 2—LEGAL

**Author comments (Weinstock):** The legal discussion here will be a little different than in the other chapters. Though depositions were taken, we will instead focus on the Report of Counsel where the facts of the case are assessed by the insurance company, in regards to the risk of losing, which venue will be assigned and even which judge will try the case if it goes to trial (and how sympathetic they are to the defense). The patient's past income comes into play when quantifying the damages.
Of note, there were at least four experts retained by the defense, two were EPs, one was a radiologist (to weigh in on whether EPs should be held accountable for reading CTs or XRs) and one was a surgical oncologist.
The verbiage below is condensed directly from the Report of Counsel as presented to the insurance company by the defense medical malpractice team.

## I. Report of Counsel

**Insurance company asks a question to the defense attorney(s). Hypothetical question:**
*Assume that trial is one (1) week away and state whether liability against the Insured is probable, questionable, doubtful or non-existent. Outline the strengths and weaknesses of all sides of the case. Provide an opinion as to whether the case should be tried against the Insured. Provide an evaluation of the venue, judge and anticipated jury panel. Please answer this hypothetical question: the jury has just returned a verdict against the Insured, why was the case lost?*

### A. Estimate of risk for each physician:

**1. ED physician, visit #1 (August 29th with Dx of COPD exacerbation):**

**Defense attorney:** I would estimate liability as to [Dr. EP #1] as doubtful to non-existent. A chest X-ray was ordered, six months before the cancer diagnosis, because of a patient complaint of shortness of breath. It confirmed a diagnosis of pneumonia. [The physician] saw infiltrates, not a right upper lobe density.

The radiologist saw a possible right upper lobe density, noted a need for follow-up to make sure the density went away (as it ought to if it was a pneumonia artifact), did not communicate by telephone, but did put it in his preliminary and final reports which, routinely, made their way to the emergency department. Whether [Dr. EP #1] ever saw the preliminary report, which was issued an hour after patient discharge, is presently unknown, but the argument will be made that he should have, and will have, some reasonability to it. Why else get a radiology interpretation?

The discharge instructions told the patient to follow-up with his family physician. However, the importance of this follow-up (to rule out lung cancer) could not have been communicated to the patient because it was not known to the caregivers until, at the earliest, an hour after patient discharge, when the preliminary radiology report was issued. Plaintiff will argue that there is a big difference between being routinely asked to follow-up with a family physician and being asked to follow-up to rule out lung cancer. That argument will have some traction.

**Defense EP expert #1:** "Dr. [EP #1] told the patient to follow-up with his family physician, and that is within the accepted standard of care. Whether or not the family physician ever received the information regarding the need for [the patient] to follow-up with a chest CT is not the problem of your clients, because the way hospitals are now set up, that is the nurses' responsibility to do that." We do know that at least the final report was reviewed by a hospital nurse, who documented that she saw no reason to bring it to the attention of a physician.

Certainly, the hospital is open to criticism based upon the nurse's action; possibly the radiologist is to be faulted for not directly communicating an unexpected, but potentially significant clinical findings. In my judgment Dr. [EP #1] still comes in a very distant third, if at all, in this scenario.

Plaintiff will have to climb a stiff causation hurdle as of this encounter, even if he gains some ground on the standard of care with respect to follow-up. At this point, the patient was only six months from diagnosis of a locally advanced lung cancer.

**Defense EP expert #2:** In short, your clients are just fine here, and I see no reason whatsoever why they're named in the suit, and also see no way they will be pursued by the plaintiff's attorney here. They're going to be pretty hard-pressed to find an ER expert to say that your guys did anything wrong. The radiologist is in trouble, so is the nurse, and probably the hospital, too.

**Defense surgical oncology expert:** There is plenty of medical literature out there that states a delay in diagnosis of 18–24 months is significant, but anything under 18 months is not, with regards to the outcome. I believe that this is a case that should be tried, without offer, on behalf of both of these emergency physicians.

**Possible approach to defense (this is per the attorneys, not from the EP):**
The chest X-ray that I ordered was interpreted by me as showing infiltrates, secondary to an acute pneumonia. The radiologist reviewing the same X-ray noted a more subtle finding of a possible lesion in your right lung. It is commonplace for the definitive interpretation of an X-ray by the radiologist to differ from the preliminary reading by the emergency physician. That's why radiologists look at them. Had I been notified that there was a discrepancy, I would certainly have referred you for further work-up. Additionally, at this point the most that could have been achieved would have been a 6 month jump on the cancer diagnosis, which is clinically meaningless.

**2. ED physician who saw patient for axillary abscess (14 months previous to visit #1):**

**Per attorneys:**
I would estimate liability as doubtful to non-existent. This physician saw the patient 21 months before diagnosis. From a causation point of view, plaintiff will be powerfully motivated to concentrate on this encounter, because a 21 month jump on a locally advanced tumor with no evidence of distant metastases is an attractive proposition causally. As stated by [the surgical oncology expert], "There is plenty of medical literature out there that states a delay in diagnosis of 18–24 months is significant."

However, to get to causation, plaintiff must first prove a standard of care departure, and here the defense of this physician is very strong; they do not claim competence in the interpretation of CT imaging, he relies, of necessity, on the radiologist. He probably did not even look at the CT scan and the expert testimony on this issue will be that he had no obligation to do so.

**Defense emergency expert:** "Interpreting CT's of extremities is not within the accepted standard of care for emergency physicians, and so, there would be no reason whatsoever why they would or should have looked at these films."

**Defense radiology expert:** "Obviously, there's no excuse whatsoever for missing the lung mass that was on the original film but equally obvious, if not more so, your ER physicians are in no way, shape, or form responsible for looking at the X-rays. In fact, the standard of care dictates that ER physician should not try to read the X-rays. That's why radiologists are there.

Apparently, the radiologist had a bad day on the day he read that film, and bad days subsequent in which he read every X-ray regarding the chest of this patient. I honestly cannot believe that any radiologist who looked at these films could miss this. The main thing is that it's the radiologist who's in big trouble here. Your guys are just fine, because they acted appropriately, based on what they were advised by the radiologist."

**Possible approach to defense (this is per the attorneys, not from the EP):**
I ordered a CT scan of your right arm, as requested by the consulting surgeon, for your axillary abscess problem. While I sometimes look at CT scans, I do not consider myself competent to render a definitive interpretation of them. I rely on the interpretation of the radiologist. In this case, the radiologist found no evidence of a lesion in your right lung. I cannot be expected to outperform a board-certified radiologist. Further, if I did review it, I would have been looking at the area of interest, the axilla, for evidence of deep abscess extension, which was why the CT was ordered.

**3. And for the sake of completeness—assessment of liability of the hospital:**
Unknown at this point but assessed as difficult to defend. The decision of the nurse that the radiologist's finding of a new potential lesion in the right lung of a cigarette smoker did not need to be brought to physician attention is not very defensible.

**Image #3:** Initial CXR on visit #1 August 29th: Note that the image initially presented in this chapter was photoshopped to remove the ring (which is why the right hilum had a strange appearance).

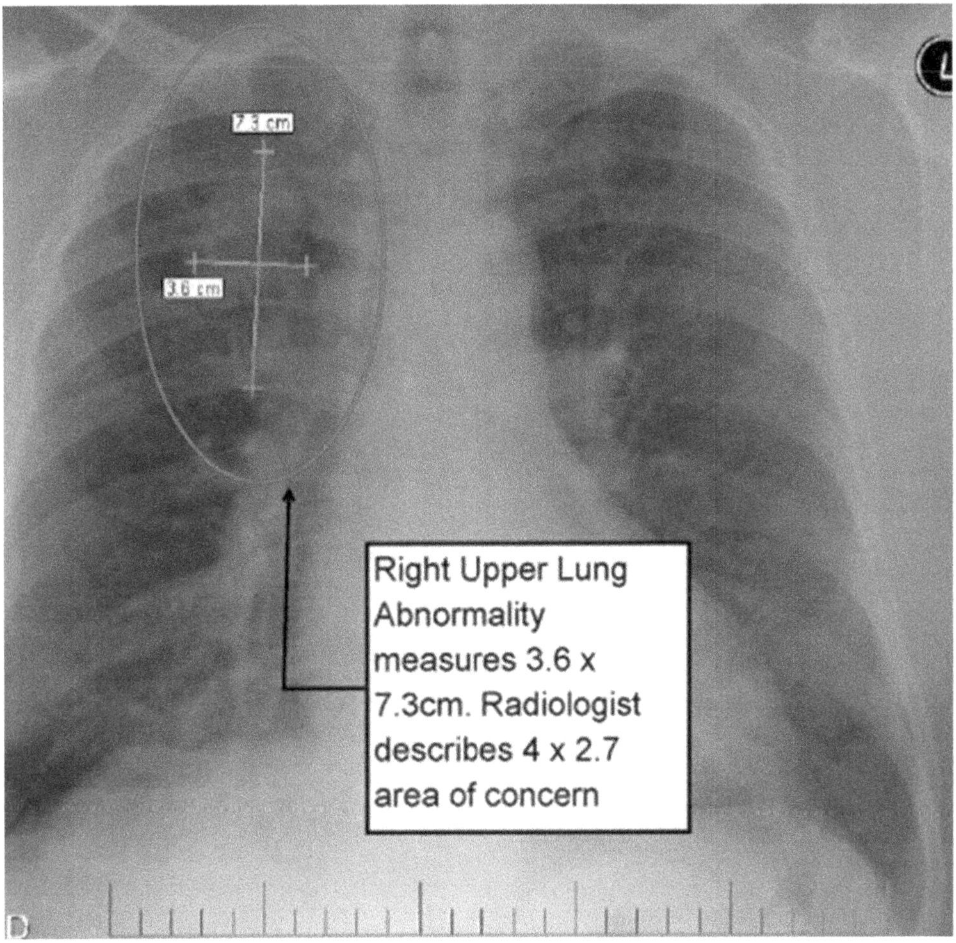


**B. Venue demographics:**

The Report of Counsel includes a description of the county with population, median income including the percentage of those below the poverty line, and even age of the population. Previous verdicts are described. The assigned judge is defined as to reputation, if they are fair and even-handed, and how they run cases. This specific judge in our case is deemed "fair and even-tempered" and that they have and excellent reputation.

**C. Answer to hypothetical question (as stated above):**

To answer your hypothetical question "The jury has just returned an adverse verdict, why was the case *lost?"* I would have to say that the jury felt very bad for [the patient] and bought the plaintiff's case hook line and sinker, painting everyone with the same broad brush. I don't think that's likely to happen.

**D. Apportionment of fault:**

List each party and assign each an estimated percentage of fault. Please note whether apportionment is permitted in this venue and applicable to this case.

1. EP who saw the patient for axillary abscess: 0%
2. EP who say the patient on visit #1 (August 29th) for COPD exacerbation: 5%

3. Radiologist: 50%
4. Hospital (which employed nurse who did the radiology discrepancies):45%

**E. Estimated verdict value:**

Provide an estimation of the adverse verdict value for this case. Include an evaluation as to whether punitive or exemplary damages are recoverable for this case in this venue.

Best case for the plaintiff, perhaps $1.8 million. The best case is not very likely, however. More likely, a plaintiff's verdict would consider his criminal history and his somewhat spotty work record and, subliminally, his cigarette habit, with a verdict range from 0.8 to 1.2 million Dollars. Punitive damages are not included in the complaint and would not be supported by the facts of this case in any event.

**F. Estimated settlement value:**

*Provide an estimated settlement range for the case globally and for the Insured individually. State the Insured's position regarding settlement—whether the Insured is opposed or agreeable to settlement. State whether this case should be mediated and, if not, why. State plaintiff's settlement demand, if any, and provide an opinion regarding settlement value. Answer the following hypothetical question: if you were the plaintiff's attorney, what is the lowest dollar amount that you would recommend to the plaintiff if offered by the Insured?*

This case might be settled for $900,000 globally, with each of the emergency physicians contributing perhaps $100,000. I do not think this is a case to be mediated. I believe this case should be tried and not settled. Neither EPs have expressed an interest in settling this case, a position with which I agree. Plaintiff has not made a demand, nor has one been solicited. To answer your question "if I were the plaintiffs' attorney what is the lowest dollar amount I would recommend to the plaintiff if offered by the insureds" I would say $100,000 a piece.

## II. The Legal Analysis

**T. Marc Calvert, JD**
Medical malpractice defense attorney with over 35 years of experience
Calvert, Leever & Ostler
Cypress, Texas

**A. How does the Report of Counsel affect a decision to proceed to trial vs. settle?**

These types of reports, though varying in form and in the specific questions, are used by every insurance carrier that I have dealt with since starting practice in 1987. Carriers make decisions, sometimes exclusively, by the representations made by defense counsel in these reports. Thus, the questions often seek answers that require an educated guess (e.g. who is going to win the game this weekend, and if our team loses—why would that be?) as well as a prediction. It is a guess because we are asked to anticipate what unknown people on a jury will decide about a complex fact situation where combatants are offering differing versions and explanations.

Knowing that the company is making million-dollar decisions based on the words of an attorney should sober us. It is also wise to avoid understating the potential problems. I do not know these players well enough to grade each comment and opinion in the report, but when you assign a 0% chance of losing, it reminds me of the Titanic being called unsinkable.

It is important to respect the variability of how information is processed by different people. In these reports, I have said plenty of times things like: "I think reasonable people on a jury will view our client as having acted properly and I believe that the evidence backs that up. We have better experts, and we have a good judge but ultimately, we will have strangers on a jury, and they will judge these facts as they digest them. They could make a decision based on sympathy, or it could be founded on something even more unfair such as a bias or dislike."

On a personal note, I write more balanced reports now than I did 25 years ago. This is true, at least in part, due to a realization that the insurance carrier is hanging their decision on what I have reported to them. So, when I let them know that one of our witnesses did well, I hope I worded the report, sent well before trial, in such a way that I did not promise infallibility by our witnesses. One trial that I recall involved an ectopic pregnancy, and we had a great expert. In the Report of Counsel, I overpromised how he would do in testifying, and I later regretted it. The expert was capable and, at trial, did well on my direct examination. He later admitted to me, he decided to give the other side a few agreeing answers on cross-examination "in order to come across as fairer." He had heard that an expert should do that, and his approach almost cost us the case. The plaintiff's attorney scored some major points in cross-examination, and in closing argument he lauded the courage of our expert to agree with him on some things. I will never forget that he then said to the jury "I am going to name my first child after this expert, that is how much I admire his honesty." OMG!

We won. However, I learned a lot from that experience. One of those things was to never overstate how a witness will do when under pressure. I have seen juries do weird things, experts make mistakes, and nervous clients stumble on a key point. There is no safety net under the high wire of testifying, and predictions must take that into account.

**B. What is the EPs liability when there is an X-ray discrepancy, and the physician has already completed their shift?**

When an X-ray is later read, by a specialist, as having different or additional findings than those identified by the ED physician, we need to return to the basics of patient care. First, did the EP reasonably read the X-ray, report the findings, and respond to those? If the EP does not learn of the later interpretation, the analysis moves to one of what did he know and when did he know it. If he knew that there would be a later read by a specialist, perhaps there is an argument that he should have let the patient know to check back later for the results.

In the case before us, I agree that the radiologist and the hospital are more in the cross-hairs. The radiologist's basic duty is to reasonably read films and to communicate the findings. When there is a misread film, and a radiologist exercising ordinary care would have not made the same miss, the radiologist is culpable. If there is a failure to properly communicate the results, culpability may also exist. Letting the ER know of the issue, with a call or some other direct communication, is a good idea. Here, the policies and procedures of the hospital come into play. These procedures are set-up for a reason, due to the benefit of having a specialist catch something that the EP does not appreciate. So, when the report of the same X-ray is significantly different, that should trigger activity, whether it is referral to primary care, return to the ED, or even having the current EP act on the findings. These responsibilities fall mostly on the radiologist and the hospital.

## C. Speak softly...

Teddy Roosevelt said "Speak softly and carry a big stick." I think defense counsel are wise to follow that approach. We usually do not trash talk or make brash promises. We try to get our team ready, fairly evaluate the evidence, obtain great experts and supportive literature, and prepare our client to show caring and competence when defending their care. The report to the insurance company should be long on reality, and its angles, and short on "unsinkable" extremes.

# III. Medical Discussion—CXR Findings, Follow-up of Abnormal Test Results, Was this Malpractice?

**Michael B. Weinstock, MD**
Emergency Medicine attending physician, Adena Health System
Director of Research and Scholarly activity, Adena Health System GME
Professor of Emergency Medicine, Adjunct, The Wexner Medical Center at The Ohio State University

**A. The practice of emergency medicine: How do we factor in the patient's story?**
The practice of an emergency clinician has been compared to that of an airline pilot but there are some very distinct differences. We are not simply obtaining data from objective instruments in the cockpit, but instead dealing with the "human condition" of people, who are subject to fears, intoxication, disability, or distraction. It is understandable that there is often a different story given to a student, resident, nurse or attendings. But shouldn't radiology results be objective?

**B. How often are there radiology discrepancies and how often does it change practice?**
When it comes to an objective test, such as a chest X-ray (CXR), shouldn't the reading be identical between clinicians? Well, not so much. It turns out that funny statement "clinical correlation required" does make sense! Even among board-certified radiologists, there is a discrepancy of 3–5%.[10] Of course, all disagreements are not the same; clinically significant differences which result in a change of management are what we really care about. How about correlation between the emergency physician and the radiologist? Tranovich, et al. evaluated over 16,000 X-rays finding 93.5% agreement between the emergency physician (EP) and the radiologist (45% of these were CXRs), with only a small percentage (1.7% of the discrepancies) requiring a return to the ED and only 0.2% (of the discrepancies) being major discrepancies representing risk of serious harm to the patient (this was 0.01% of the total).[2]

Which raises an interesting question in regard to this case; was the discrepancy between the EP and the radiologist malpractice? Even the radiologist read the CXR as a probably infiltrate, and the EP had even more reason to suspect an infectious process in a patient with COPD who arrives by EMS for acute SOB – clinical correlation was not only "required"... but actually occurred! This decision regarding malpractice will likely be left to a jury or an insurance carrier.

**C. Following up an abnormal test result after the clinician completes their shift:**
There is one plaintiff allegation that most would agree on, that the nurse administrator who was responsible for reviewing the discrepancies should have alerted the patient or their primary care clinician. In fact, Callen, et al., in a systematic review, found a significant number of radiology discrepancies were not followed up, ranging from 1% in one study to 36% in another. They also demonstrated that there were actually adverse outcomes which occurred from lack of follow-up, including missed diagnoses of cancer. [11] Two areas with significant problems included 1) critical test results and 2) patients moving across health care settings. [12]

Could the documentation have been improved? It is hard to say, as there does not seem to be much doubt in the eyes of the EP or the PA that the patient was suffering from a COPD exacerbation as a result of an infectious process. It is hard to include discharge instructions to processes (such as a new diagnosis of lung cancer) which we feel are very unlikely and could serve to confuse the patient with too much information.

**D. A possible "game changing" question:**

It would have been interesting to learn how the patient would have answered a simple question: "Have you had unintentional weight loss?" As defined by at least 5% of unintentional weight loss over the previous 6–12 months. Metalidis, et al. found that organic causes were present in 56% of the total, including malignancy in 22% of the total.[8] We are not alleging that this question should have been asked or that malpractice occurred because it was not, but consider whether it had been and answered in the affirmative, perhaps this would have moved us from "standard of care" to "excellence in care." Kuo, et al. found that there was prognostic significance of unintentional body weight loss in colon cancer patients.[13]

**E. Lung cancer stats and such:**

Lung cancer is the 2nd most common cancer in the U.S. (after prostate cancer in men and breast cancer in women) with 238,340 new cases per year and 127,070 deaths (the leading cause of cancer death) in 2023 [https://www.cancer.org/cancer/types/lung-cancer/about/key-statistics.html]. In our patient, these authors feel that it would have been appropriate, if the radiology read was available at the time of discharge, to send the patient home with the knowledge that a course of antibiotics was appropriate, but that he would need follow-up in the next few weeks to ensure resolution. In fact, there are many plain films which do not reliably show a fracture, frequently cited are hip fractures;[14, 15, 16] when these are suspected the patient either needs further imaging (MRI) or to be treated "as if" with a splint.

**F. The essence of the case: Was this malpractice?**

The essence of the case is the allegation that the PA and EP were negligent (committed malpractice) by erroneously diagnosing "COPD exacerbation" and failing to confirm a malignancy. Was this malpractice? We know that surgeons have a known complication rate for all procedures; infection from appendectomy, stroke after a carotid endarterectomy; when these rare events occur, this is not typically viewed as malpractice. How about "dropping a lung" after a central line placement? With ultrasound, this almost never happens but if it occurs less than 1% of the time, it still occurs… is it malpractice?

Most emergency clinicians would agree that the management of this patient displayed reasonable care (will need to see if the jury agrees!), but were there any ways to make this patient safer? We (the authors) feel that there were only a few things that could have been done, but it is questionable if any would have made a difference:

- Ensure that the patient understands that the CXR read was preliminary and would be overread by a radiologist.
- Discuss and document that the patient will need follow-up in a defined period of time (this was done) and that the patient should return if symptoms progress, change, or do not resolve.
- Consider further questioning as to other conditions (such as malignancy) with possible questions of weight loss (unknown if this would have been helpful), chronic or changed cough (patient reported only a 4–5 days cough which would make cancer less likely), or hemoptysis (not asked but would likely have been negative).
- The hospital needs better protocols for reconciling X-ray discrepancies, but this is not something that the bedside PA or EP would have been able to affect, especially when the final radiology read arrived hours after they completed their night shifts.

In the end, this was a tough case for the PA and EP, but we hope the discussion furthered an understanding of the legal process, defined some follow-up recommendations, and demonstrated what a "Report of Counsel" is all about.

## IV. Author Summary (Weinstock)

- All testing is not 100%; when there is a question of a subsequent "over read," ensure the patient is aware of this.
- Define follow-up in an 1) action and 2) time-specific fashion.
- Though it would not have been helpful in this case as the radiology read of the extremity CT done 14 months previously for a "boil" was incorrectly read, reviewing past records may sometimes be helpful.
- There must be a fail-safe hospital or ED protocol for recognizing and acting on radiology and laboratory findings.

## References


1. Edlow JA, Pronovost PJ. Misdiagnosis in the emergency department: Time for a system solution. JAMA 2023;329(8):631-632. doi: 10.1001/jama.2023.0577. PMID: 36705932.
2. Tranovich MJ, Gooch CM, Dougherty JM. Radiograph interpretation discrepancies in a community hospital emergency department. West J Emerg Med. 2019;20(4):626-632. doi: 10.5811/westjem.2019.1.41375. Epub 2019 Jul 2. PMID: 31316702; PMCID: PMC6625692.
3. Seabury SA, Chandra A, Lackdawalla DN, et al. On average, physicians spend nearly 11 percent of their 40-year careers with an open, unresolved malpractice claim. Health Aff (Millwood) 2013;32:111-19
4. Kuppermann N, Holmes JF, Dayan PS, et al. Identification of children at very low risk of clinically-important brain injuries after head trauma: A prospective cohort study [published correction appears in Lancet 2014;383(9914):308]. Lancet 2009;374(9696):1160-1170. doi:10.1016/S0140-6736(09)61558-0
5. Schonfeld D, Bressan S, Da Dalt L, et al. Pediatric Emergency Care Applied Research Network head injury clinical prediction rules are reliable in practice. Arch Dis Child 2014;99(5):427-431. doi:10.1136/archdischild-2013-305004],
6. Kline JA, Mitchell AM, Kabrhel C, et al. Clinical criteria to prevent unnecessary diagnostic testing in emergency department patients with suspected pulmonary embolism. J Thromb Haemost 2004;2(8):1247-55. doi: 10.1111/j.1538-7836.2004.00790.x. PMID: 15304025.
7. American College of Emergency Physicians Clinical Policies Subcommittee (Writing Committee) on Suspected Non–ST-Elevation Acute Coronary Syndromes; Tomaszewski CA, Nestler D, Shah KH, Sudhir A, Brown MD. Clinical Policy: Critical issues in the evaluation and management of emergency department patients with suspected non-st-elevation acute coronary syndromes. Ann Emerg Med 2018;72(5):e65-e106. doi: 10.1016/j.annemergmed.2018.07.045. PMID: 30342745.
8. Metalidis C, Knockaert DC, Bobbaers H, et al. Involuntary weight loss. Does a negative baseline evaluation provide adequate reassurance? Eur J Intern Med 2008;19(5):345-9. doi: 10.1016/j.ejim.2007.09.019. Epub 2007 Nov 26. PMID: 18549937
9. Withrow DR, Oke J, Friedemann Smith C, Hobbs R, Nicholson BD. Serious disease risk among patients with unexpected weight loss: A matched cohort of over 70 000 primary care presentations. J Cachexia Sarcopenia Muscle 2022;13(6):2661-2668. doi: 10.1002/jcsm.13056. Epub 2022 Sep 3. PMID: 36056750; PMCID: PMC9745555.

10. Brady AP. Error and discrepancy in radiology: Inevitable or avoidable? Insights Imaging 2017;8(1):171-182. doi: 10.1007/s13244-016-0534-1. Epub 2016 Dec 7. PMID: 27928712; PMCID: PMC5265198.].
11. Callen JL, Westbrook JI, Georgiou A, et al. Failure to follow-up test results for ambulatory patients: A systematic review. J Gen Intern Med 2012;27(10):1334-1348. doi:10.1007/s11606-011-1949-5
12. Callen J, Georgiou A, Li J, et al. The safety implications of missed test results for hospitalised patients: a systematic review. BMJ Qual Saf 2011;20(2):194-199. doi:10.1136/bmjqs.2010.044339].
13. Kuo YH, Shi C-S, Huang CY, et al. Prognostic significance of unintentional body weight loss in colon cancer patients. Mol Clin Oncol 2018;8(4):533-38.
14. Haj-Mirzaian A, Eng J, Khorasani R, et al. Use of Advanced imaging for radiographically occult hip fracture in elderly patients: A systematic review and meta-analysis. Radiology 2020;296(3):521-531. doi:10.1148/radiol.2020192167
15. Wilson MP, Nobbee D, Murad MH, et al. Diagnostic accuracy of limited mri protocols for detecting radiographically occult hip fractures: A systematic review and meta-analysis. AJR Am J Roentgenol 2020;215(3):559-567. doi:10.2214/AJR.19.22676] and scaphoid fractures
16. Bäcker HC, Wu CH, Strauch RJ. Systematic review of diagnosis of clinically suspected scaphoid fractures. J Wrist Surg 2020;9(1):81-89. doi:10.1055/s-0039-1693147

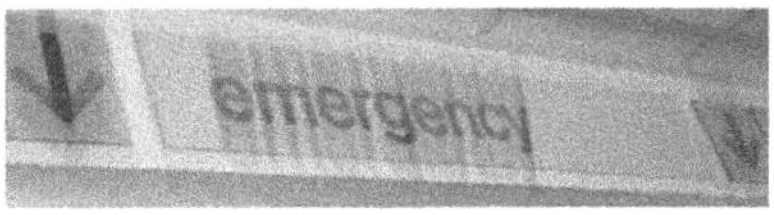


# Case 14

## A 67 Year-old Woman with Flank Pain: What is the "Rule Out" Diagnosis?

**Primary case author:**
**Eric Funk**

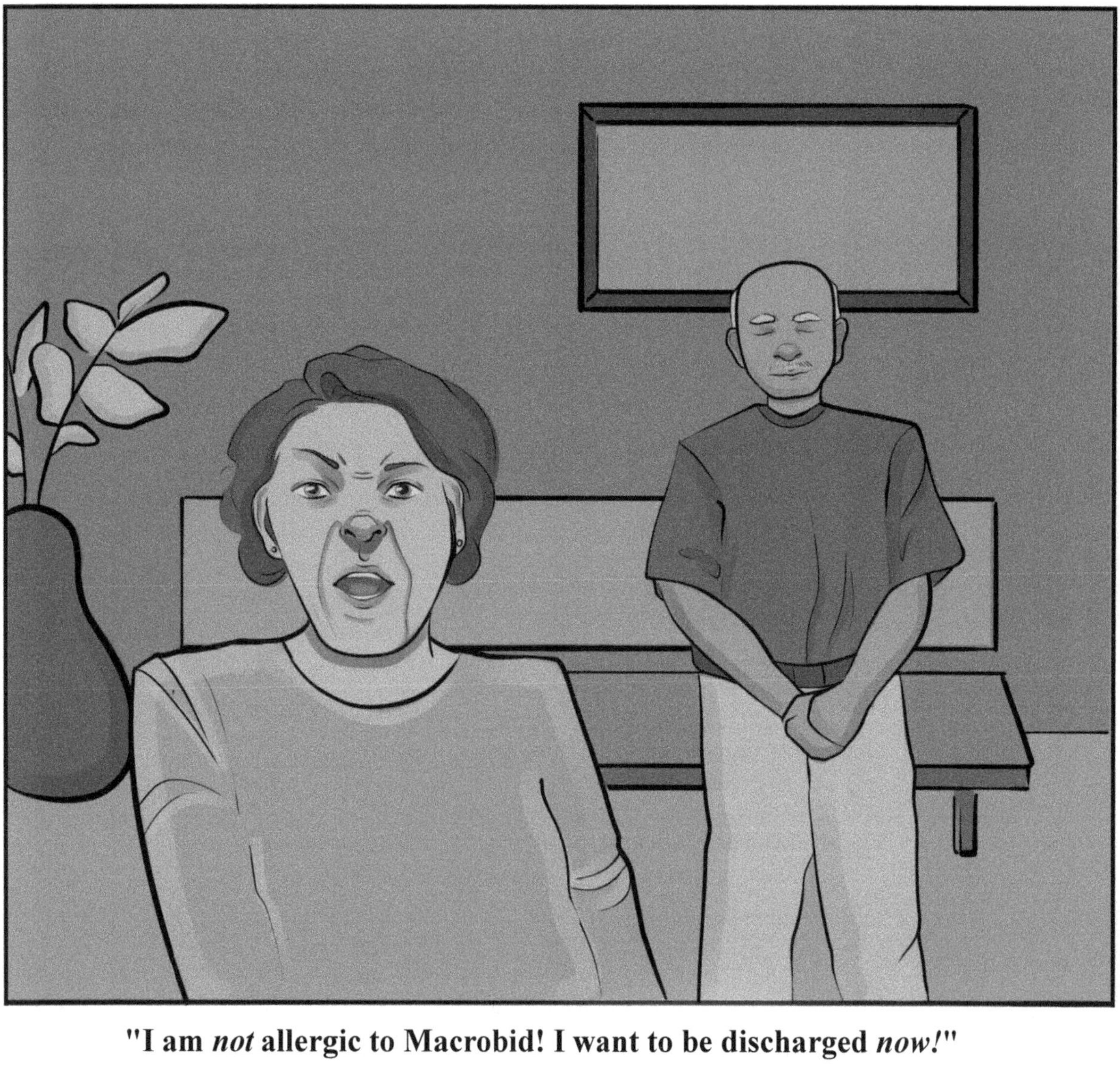

**"I am *not* allergic to Macrobid! I want to be discharged *now!*"**

# Case 14

## A 67 Year-old Woman with Flank Pain: What is the "Rule Out" Diagnosis?

**PART 1—MEDICAL**

## I. The Patient's Story

Linda Baker is a 67 year-old woman who lives in a large city in the Northeast. She is active in her synagogue and multiple philanthropic organizations. Both she and her husband had worked long careers and are now enjoying their retirements. They enjoy spending time with their children and grandchildren. Over the previous years, Linda has had medical issues; she has been treated for breast cancer, ovarian cancer, and brain cancer.

On a cool fall day in October, she is suddenly awoken with severe right flank pain. She tries to reposition herself and fall back to sleep, but the pain persists. She is particularly frustrated because it was Yom Kippur, and does not want her plans to be interrupted. She has been fasting since sunset the previous evening.

Soon, it becomes clear that the pain is not going to resolve on its own. She has a history of kidney stones and this feels similar. Her husband drives her to a nearby emergency department, hopeful that her pain can be controlled and the plans for the day would not change.

## II. The Doctor's Version (the following is the actual documentation of the provider)

**Date:** October 12

**Chief Complaint:** Flank pain

**Nurse Note (10:52am):** Patient received in stretcher with right flank x 6 AM this morning. Sudden onset with radiation to right lower abdomen. Patient denies chest pain or shortness of breath. Denies fever but complaints of chills but states "I always have chills, it's been cold." Patient denies pain or difficulty urinating. She has right CVA tenderness.

**History of Present Illness (11:35am):** 67 year-old female with PMH CVA, HTN, kidney stones, R breast Ca, L brain tumor, thyroid tumor, eczema, cataracts presenting with right flank pain since 6am this morning. Patient states the pain started in lower abdomen, radiated to the right side of her abdomen, and then went to her right flank. She states the pain is 8/10, worse with movement, and tried Tylenol and Gas-X with no relief. Had 3 episodes of vomiting this morning (non-bloody, nonbilious). Denies fever, diarrhea, constipation, dysuria, blood in urine. Patient states she has been drinking less fluids and eating less due to religious fasting for holiday today.

**Past Medical History:**
**Allergies:** PCN (rash), niacin (rash), sulfa (rash), latex (swelling), Celebrex (unable to breath), Macrobid (unknown), Levaquin (unknown), doxycycline (unknown), Biaxin (unknown)
**Meds:** Vytorin, Toprol, nizatidine, asa, Benadryl
**PMH:** Breast CA, brainstem tumor, HTN, hyperlipidemia, renal calculi, GERD
**PSH:** Breast lumpectomy, brain surgery, partial thyroidectomy, ovarian
**Social:** Married. Lives with spouse. No tobacco, alcohol, drugs

**Physical Examination:**
**Vitals (10:52am):** Temp 98.5F, HR 92bpm, BP 171/94, RR 18/min, 92% on room air.
**Constitutional:** Well appearing, well nourished, awake, oriented to person, place, time/situation, no apparent distress.
**Head:** Head atraumatic, normal cephalic shape, head shape is symmetrical.
**Cardiac:** Normal rate, regular rhythm, heart sounds S1, S2, no murmurs, rubs or gallops.
**Respiratory:** Breath sounds clear and equal bilaterally.
**Gastrointestinal:** Abdomen is soft, nondistended. Pain in the right lower quadrant, right costovertebral angle.
**Psychiatric:** Alert and oriented to person, place, time/situation, normal mood and affect, no apparent risk to self or others.

**Emergency Department Course:**
IV fluids 1L 0.9NS bolus
Morphine 4mg IVP
Ondansetron 4mg IVP

**CBC:**
WBC – 9.5
Hemoglobin – 14.0
Platelets – 266

**BMP:**
Sodium – 140
Potassium – 4.2
Chloride – 109
Bicarb – 22
Anion gap – 9
BUN – 33
Creatinine – 1.7 / GFR - 31
Glucose – 109

**Urinalysis:**
Color – Yellow
Urine appearance – Slightly Turbid
Ketones – Negative
Specific Gravity – 1.015
Protein – Negative
Urobilinogen – Negative
Nitrite – Positive

Leukocyte Esterase – Moderate
Blood – Large
Glucose – Negative
pH – 5.0

**CT Renal Stone Impression:** Mild right-sided hydroureteronephrosis secondary to a 3mm calculus within the mid-ureter. There is moderate associated perinephric fluid.

**Reassessment (15:47):** Patient feels better at this time. Patient now states is not allergic to Macrobid. Case d/w Dr. Smith (urologist) who states to start Abxs and will see in office tomorrow. Patient and family agree.

**Diagnosis:** Renal colic on right side.

**Disposition (16:14):** Pt demonstrates quick and easy understanding. Pt asked questions. Verbalized understanding. Discharged home ambulatory. Private car. Condition: Improved.

## III. Risk Management/Patient Safety Opportunities (Weinstock)

**Risk Management/Patient Safety Opportunity #1:**

**Opportunity:** Consideration of most serious diagnosis.
**Discussion:** With all of our ED patients, we "think worst first," a consideration of what could possibly end with a devastating outcome. The complaint of flank pain has more than several possibilities including an abdominal aortic aneurysm, malignancy, retroperitoneal bleed, cholecystitis, appendicitis, or even zoster. Of course, not all are serious (zoster) or emergent (malignancy), but once the CT scan finds a ureteral stone, the Ddx and the potential for decompensation significantly decrease. Perhaps, an obstructed solitary kidney could result in renal failure (unlikely), a second diagnosis could be occurring (very unusual), or an infection could be present (very much the diagnosis to rule out).
✔ **Teaching point:** With an obstructing ureteral stone, the diagnosis to rule out is an "infected stone."

**Risk Management/Patient Safety Opportunity #2:**

**Opportunity:** Picking the correct antibiotic for the likely organism and the anatomic location.
**Discussion:** There are many factors which come into consideration when selecting an antibiotic for a UTI: Suspected organism, interactions and side effects, history of allergy, and site of infection. Usually it is pretty easy but not so with multiple allergies. In this case, the selected antibiotic, Macrodantin, is more of a "urinary antiseptic" without adequate penetration into the renal parenchyma. Of note, the CT scan revealed, "there is moderate associated perinephric fluid," likely indicative of upper tract disease (pyelonephritis), not a simple cystitis.
✔ **Teaching point:** When treatment choices are limited due to an extensive allergy history, the selection still needs to meet the indication.

**Risk Management/Patient Safety Opportunity #3:**

**Opportunity:** Reassurance of a normal WBC count.
**Discussion:** The white count was normal, and we will never know if that was reassuring to the physician,

as the medical decision-making (MDM) note did not discuss this further. This might have been a factor for the urologist? We are left to wonder that also. With a urinalysis nitrite positive, in some studies suggestive of 95% specificity for a UTI, and an obstructing stone, concern for an "infected stone" should be high and if the patient is sent home, the MDM should reflect why the patient is not getting a nephrostomy tube or ureteral stent (just as we document why a stroke patient is not a thrombolytic candidate).

✔ **Teaching point:** A normal WBC count does not rule out serious infection.

**Risk Management/Patient Safety Opportunity #4:**

**Opportunity:** Poor documentation of consultation.

**Discussion:** The physician deserves kudos for consulting the urologist and arranging follow-up the next morning. But if they think that this completely absolves them of responsibility… not so fast! We have no idea what this conversation entailed, or if the urologist even knew the urine or CT results. It is easy to imagine a scenario, with an adverse outcome, where the urologist later says, "If I had known there was an obstruction and a UTI in a 67 year-old patient with cancer, I would have recommended admission for IV antibiotics, close observation, and consideration of a bypass of the obstruction." One approach to documentation might be: "I spoke with Dr. Smith and we discussed the patient's presentation, lab results, positive nitrite and leukocyte esterase and CT results. The patient currently is not septic and he recommends starting antibiotics and he will see the patient in the morning." Of course, there are many ways to do this, but the above approach certainly reflects the urologist's understanding of the clinical picture.

✔ **Teaching point:** If there is a need to speak with a consultant, it is helpful to document what was discussed.

**Risk Management/Patient Safety Opportunity #5:**

**Opportunity:** Ensure the patient understands if there is diagnostic uncertainty.

**Discussion:** Our patient decompensated so quickly after discharge from the ED and did not have an opportunity to return "if symptoms worsened." Many times the adverse event occurs more slowly. When asked at trial, "Why did you not return to the ED?"a frequent refrain is, "I was just there, they did all the tests and told me everything was fine." If there is diagnostic uncertainty upon discharge, whether for chest pain, pediatric head injury, or pulmonary embolism, ensure the patient understands and the importance of returning if symptoms progress, change or don't resolve.

✔ **Teaching point:** Our "last chance to get it right" are if the patient returns with worse symptoms.

**Author comments (Weinstock):** What do patients remember from their discharge? Following is the deposition of the patient's husband regarding his understanding of the discharge instructions. This discussion does not imply anything improper was done in the ED but instead serves to confirm what the husband's understanding was after the bounceback occurred.

**Urologist defense attorney cross-examination of the patient's husband:**

**Q.** Do you remember who discharged your wife that day?

**A .**The doctor in the ER.

**Q.** Do you remember that doctor's name?

**A.** No, I don't.

**Q.** Do you remember what time of day that doctor discharged your wife?
**A.** Late afternoon.

**Q.** Do you know if that doctor spoke to Dr. Smith [the urologist] prior to discharging your wife or after discharging your wife?
**A.** Prior.

**Q.** Do you know the sum and substance of that conversation between that doctor and Dr. Smith?
**A.** He said that he spoke to Dr. Smith, said for him — for me to call his office and make an appointment for tomorrow.

**Q.** Did you receive any discharge instructions from the hospital on that day?
**A.** Probably.

**Q.** Do you know if any doctors are named on those discharge instructions?
**A.** Probably.

## IV. The Bounceback

The patient leaves with her husband and picks up the macrodantin from the pharmacy, then takes the first dose. However, after arriving at home, she has difficulty going up the stairs to her bedroom. She falls, landing on her buttocks. Her husband helps her up, and she goes to take a bath. About 45 minutes later, when she has not left the bathroom, he goes to check on her, finding her eyes open and breathing but unresponsive. He calls 911, and she is brought back to the same ED.

**ED visit #2:**

- On arrival she has altered mental status and is febrile.
- She is started on broad-spectrum antibiotics (vancomycin, Aztreonam, Flagyl).
- Urology is consulted, and she is taken to the OR emergently for right ureteral stenting.
- She is extubated following the procedure, but begins to decline over the next few hours.
- She develops respiratory distress and is re-intubated.
- She develops hypotension from septic shock, requiring multiple vasopressors.

**Hospital Course:** The relationship between the family and hospital staff became very contentious over the course of several weeks. The daughter does not like one of the intensivists, because he "came over and he didn't examine [her] and he said she looked very bad." He goes on to say, "It's not good." She also does not like the infectious disease physician, "He was another one that would say they are trying to do this and that. We just didn't like his attitude. We didn't think he was doing enough." They ask the charge nurse that these doctors not be involved in her care. They also later fired one of the nephrologists who recommended dialysis as her kidneys failed.

During deposition, the husband relates that he did not believe the patient's pain was being adequately addressed:

**Q.** What, if anything, did you say to the ICU doctor regarding the medication that your wife was receiving for pain?
**A.** If they could give her anything stronger, probably.

**Q.** Did her pain medication ever change?
**A.** I don't believe so.

Her hands and feet become ischemic. The family is advised that she would require amputations of both forearms and both legs, and still would be unlikely to survive.

Understanding the grim prognosis, her ongoing pain, and facing the necessity of amputations of all 4 limbs, they elected to switch to comfort care. Following, is the deposition testimony from the husband regarding the decision to withdraw care as well as which family members were critical of the care received:

**A.** She wasn't responding to anything and they told us that the fingertips and her toes might fall off and we thought to speed it up might be a better idea than have her suffer like this not realizing that they were going to take off her hands and her feet and that was no way to – we weren't gonna do that.

**Q.** Who was present for this conversation other than you and the ICU doctor?
**A.** Possibly my son if it was at night. I don't remember exactly when we spoke to the doctor.

**Q.** So just you, your son and the doctor?
**A.** And my daughter, probably.

**Q.** So after the doctor represented to you that the amputation would have to go to her elbows and her knees, what was the decision that you made?
**A.** We discussed that amongst ourselves, my daughter, my son and myself, and we said that wouldn't happen. We weren't gonna do that. And she might not survive that anyway, they said. It was an option, but there was no guarantee that she was gonna survive and probably she wouldn't.

**Q.** When you approached the ICU doctor, what were you requesting be done regarding your wife's fingers and feet?
**A.** The fingertips and her toes because that's what they told us were gonna fall off. They just kept getting worse; her hands and her feet.

**Q.** So where did you anticipate the amputation taking place?
**A.** On her fingertips. I asked the doctor if she's ever gonna leave here.

**Q.** To which doctor did you ask this?
**A.** The ICU doctor.

**Q.** What was the sum and substance of that conversation?
**A.** He said no; she's not gonna survive.

**Q.** Did you ever sign a DNR?
**A.** Yes. I spoke to my kids first to tell them what was going on and they both agreed. We can't let her suffer like this.

**Q.** So your wife was removed from life support?
**A.** Yes.

**Q.** Aside from any conversations that you might have had with your attorney has anyone been critical of the care your wife received at Plainview Hospital?
**A.** Not that I know of. I shouldn't say that. My daughter-in-law, my son, my daughter.
She passed away shortly thereafter, after 2 weeks in the hospital.

# PART 2—LEGAL

Cast of characters (names changed, except where noted):
**The patient:** Linda Baker
**The patient's husband:** Mr. Baker
**The emergency medicine physician:** Dr. Oliver
**The urologist:** Dr. Smith

## I. Bird's Eye Summary

**A. The Accusation/Cause of Action:**
- Failure to initiate appropriate antibiotic therapy
- Failure to perform ureteral stenting in a timely manner
- Failure to admit at the first ED visit

**B. Deposition of the ED physician (Dr. Oliver):**
- The patient and her husband were very impatient and demanding. They were in a rush to leave.
- The ED physician recommended she be given a dose of IV ceftriaxone in the ED but she refused and wanted to be discharged.
- The ED physician spoke with the urologist on the phone about follow-up and appropriate antibiotics. He kept the urologist on hold while speaking to the patient about her various allergies.
- The plaintiff's attorney pointed out that the ED physician did not ask the urologist to come to the ED, did not consult an infectious disease specialist and did not order a urine culture.

**C. Deposition of the urologist (Dr. Smith):**
- The urologist was not in the office that day due to Yom Kippur but was covering calls for the entire urology group.
- He did not remember any part of the conversation with the ED physician.
- The urologist states that he would have immediately come to the ED if asked to do so by the ED physician.
- He would have requested a cath urine specimen for a patient like this.

**D. Deposition of the patient's husband (Mr. Baker):**
- The husband recounted her entire medical history including 4 separate kidney stones, the first treated with lithotripsy and the rest passed spontaneously.
- He recounted that she was allergic to penicillin, with the reaction being "she would break out."
- She felt better after being treated in the ED, but he was irritated they were there "forever. Five, six hours."
- She had problems giving a urine sample but her husband stated ultimately "she gave them a couple of drops of urine. I don't know if they were able to test that. I doubt that."
- The ER doctor stated he wanted to give her antibiotics, and the husband stated she was allergic to antibiotics. The ER doctor had him go out to his car where they kept a list of her allergies.
- He had no memory of the ER doctor recommending IV antibiotics.
- After she was discharged, he called the urology office, but the urologist wasn't there that day so the receptionist said to call back the next day to set up an appointment.

- He recounted multiple criticisms of her doctors and nurses, and stated that an anesthesiologist whispered "you should have gone to a different hospital" shortly after they arrived back to the ED.

**Q.** You testified that an anesthesiologist told you that you should have taken her to [other hospital] correct?
**A.** Correct.

**Q.** What did you say to that anesthesiologist once that doctor told you that?
**A.** I said why? And he didn't answer me.

## II. Deposition Testimony of Emergency Physician

**A. What does the doctor remember, after the fact?**

**Author comments (Weinstock):** There are some patients whose presentations are so unique that we remember them for years and others that we forget on the ride home. If there is an adverse outcome, often we learn about it months or years later and have only our documentation to rely on. During the deposition of this patient, Dr. Oliver related that they learned about the bounceback visit the next day. So, there is likely an anchor to remind them of the actual bedside documentation. Following is the deposition of how the plaintiff's attorney tries to learn about additional information not part of the medical record.

**Q.** Dr. Oliver, you told me a few minutes ago that you have some independent recollection of your encounter with Ms. Baker. What, if anything, is it that you can remember about Ms. Baker?
**Defense attorney.** Note my objection. Over objection, you can answer.
**A.** I recall I recall what room she was in. I recall she was with her husband. I recall the time of day. I recall that her and her husband were very demanding, they were very impatient. They were in a rush. I know it was the holidays around that time. I know – I believe, she was fasting, and she wanted to go home for the holidays. I mean, I could keep on going.

**Q.** Please do.
**A.** I recall that – I'm sure you're going to be asking these questions.

**Defense attorney.** That is okay. If he wants, he can follow up. He wants to know what you recall. If something comes to you afterwards, you can tell him.

**A.** I recall – I believe, it was her son that was there. It may have been her son and daughter. I'm trying to – once again, trying to recall things that may not have been you asked me not in the chart, correct?

**Q.** The last question that you are answering right now was, what is it that you remember?

**Defense attorney.** Do not worry whether it is in the chart. Tell him everything that you remember and we will take it from there.

**A.** I remember having discussions with the patient and family regarding how she was feeling, and I know that midday she was feeling a lot better, and was urging to go home. I remember wanting to give her antibiotics, and she was in a rush, did not want to receive any intravenous dose of antibiotics, because that would take an extra hour. I remember wanting to make sure that the electronic prescription for a medication, I wanted to make sure it went through the pharmacy, and they didn't want to wait, and I urged them to wait, to make sure that it was – it was transferred appropriately.

**B. A "demanding" patient who wanted to leave:**

**Author comments (Weinstock):** Food for thought: Would documenting that the patient is demanding be helpful if there is an adverse outcome? Maybe just demanding of good medical care, which we know did not occur (says a plaintiff's attorney, as evidenced by the fact that there was an adverse outcome). On the other hand, if an intervention is refused, such as administration of IV antibiotics or admission, then certainly the documentation will reflect that the patient refused care. How does this play out in our case? Here is an initial exchange:

**Q.** You told me, among other things, that you recall Ms. Baker was a demanding patient and that she was impatient. Doctor, did you document that information anywhere in the chart?
**A.** I did not.

**Q.** You told me that Ms. Baker wanted to get home due to the holidays, correct?
**A.** Correct.

**Q.** Did you document that in the chart?
**A.** I did not.

**C. Antibiotic selection:**

**Q.** As of the time that you got the information about the results of the CT scan, was there any plan, at that point in time, to put this patient on any antibiotics?
**A.** I don't remember the exact time, but the decision for antibiotics or no antibiotics would not be based only upon the radiographic finding.

**Q.** Did the discussion with Dr. Smith take place before or after the CT scan was done?
**A.** It would have been after.

**Q.** Was a discussion with Dr. Smith done before or after you became aware of the results of the urinalysis?
**A.** The discussion with Dr. Smith, I know was after I had the results of the urinalysis.

**A.** Two ways; one, I know I have an independent recollection, but also in my note, ED provider note, [it reads] "Patient now states is not allergic to Macrobid. Case discussed with Dr. Smith who states to start antibiotics and will see in office tomorrow."

**Q.** Macrobid is a medication that is often prescribed for UTIs, correct?
**A.** Macrobid is an antibiotic used for UTIs, correct.

**Q.** Prior to getting the results of the urinalysis, did you have a suspicion that the patient had a UTI?
**A.** No.

**Q.** Dr. Oliver, did the results of the urinalysis evidence that there might be a UTI?
**A.** That there may be a UTI.

**Q.** As opposed to-might?
**A.** Might be a UTI.

**Q.** Dr. Oliver, in terms of effectiveness as a medication, not on the route of delivery, did you think that there was a difference between the Ceftriaxone and the Macrobid?

**Defense attorney.** Note my objection to the form of the question. Over objection, you can answer.

**A.** Ceftriaxone is better.

**Q.** Why is it better?
**A.** Well, Ceftriaxone has to be administered intravenously. The second reason is, most of the time, it is a little bit better, in terms of spectrum, to cover *E. Coli, Klebsiella* and *Proteus*.

**Q.** Had you made a determination that Ceftriaxone was not one of those antibiotics that this patient had an allergy to?
**A.** Well, she had a problem with Ceftin, which is in the same class as the Ceftriaxone. I know she had a problem with gastrointestinal problems with what I think she was trying to describe as pseudomembranous colitis, which is usually – when it happens is usually due to, I'll use the word prolonged, you know, antibiotics use. Rarely does it occur after one dose. So, I wanted to get, at least, one dose, you know, in her system. If the allergies to Ceftin would have been anaphylaxis, shortness of breath or wheezing, I wouldn't have even recommended that.

**Author comments (Weinstock):** Well this is a little confusing. If the patient had a GI side effect from the antibiotic, then they were not in fact allergic. However, did Dr. Smith actually recommend it to the patient, and she refused it because she was anxious to leave or was it not actually recommended? It would have been nice if this part of the encounter (arguably the most important part of the encounter) was documented.

**D. Discussion with the consultant:**

**Q.** I am going to ask you a number of very specific questions about your discussion with Dr. Smith [the urologist]. I ask you to listen to the question and try to answer that question that I ask. Did you advise Dr. Smith that this was a patient in the emergency department?
**A.** Yes.

**Q.** Did you advise Dr. Smith that, on physical examination, you noted that there was tenderness in the costovertebral angle?
**A.** I don't recall if I – specifically for that.

**Q.** That is my question. Did you advise Dr. Smith of the initial results from the oxygen saturation of 92 percent?
**A.** No.

**Q.** Did you advise Dr. Smith, when the patient came into the ER, that her pulse was 92 beats per minute as documented by the nurses?
**A.** Specifically for that and not the reassessment.

**Q.** Did you tell Dr. Smith what the patient's pulse was?
**A.** I would have told Dr. Smith the the … entire day what happened over a five-hour period of time.

**Author comments (Weinstock):** This line of questioning is curious; why is it prefaced by the plaintiff's attorney with, "I am going to ask you a number of very specific questions, and I ask you to listen to the question and answer that question that I ask." I will tell you right now, this doctor is in fact not answering the questions from his recollection, but from his usual and customary practice. Does the attorney know this? Seems like it to me! Remember that it is not only the emergency physician who is named but also the urologist.

**Q.** I am asking you specific questions. Did you advise Dr. Smith that there had been three episodes of vomiting, prior to the patient coming into the hospital?
**A.** Yes.

**Q.** Did you advise Dr. Smith that Ms. Baker had been on Morphine and on Zofran?
**A.** Yes.

**Q.** Did you advise Dr. Smith that she had, among the documented complaints, a complaint of chills?
**A.** That, I'm not sure.

**Q.** Did you advise him of the BUN and creatinine?
**A.** Yes.

**Q.** Did you advise Dr. Smith of the GFR?
**A.** No.

**Q.** Dr. Smith is a urologist. Would the GFR be something that you normally would discuss with him?
**A.** No.

**Q.** Did you advise Dr. Smith of the results of the urinalysis –
**A.** Yes.

**Q.** – including the protein?
**A.** Yes.

**Q.** The nitrites?
**A.** Yes.

**Q.** The leukocyte?
**A.** Yes.

**Q.** – esterase?
**A.** Yes.

**Q.** Did you advise him of the microscopic findings?
**A.** Yes.

**Q.** Did you advise him that on the there was noted to be a 3 millimeter the right ureter?
**A.** Yes.

**Q.** Did you advise him that the radiologist had told you that there was perinephric fluid seen on the scan?
**A.** Yes.

**Q.** Did you advise Dr. Smith that there was a thought to be hydroureteronephrosis?
**A.** Yes.

**Q.** Did you advise Dr. Smith that there was thought to be atrophic left kidney?
**A.** No, because I'm not even sure I knew it at that time.

**Q.** You just answered a lot of very detailed questions. Do you have an independent recollection of all the answers to the questions that I just posed to you or are you talking about what your custom and practice would have been?
**A.** My custom and practice would be to let the consultant – in this case, he would be the consultant – to let him know all the abnormalities, and anything that was – all the abnormalities. In addition, anything that was pertinent to the case. I'm practicing medicine a long time. I can tell you, no one has ever reported that on a renal stone hunt, verbal report to me. So, I wouldn't have told that to Dr. Smith.

**Q.** Was there a discussion about antibiotics with Dr. Smith?
**A.** Yes.

**Q.** Why was there a discussion about antibiotics?
**A.** Patients – patients with kidney stones, in general, are at – at least, the potential for higher risk for infections, and we very often like to – like to prophylax patients that are at a higher risk for infection. So, that the discussion took place. That' s why.

**Q.** Was there a discussion between you and Dr. Smith about which antibiotics to choose for this patient?
**A.** Yes.

**Q.** Who had initiated that discussion?
**A.** I do not remember exactly who initiated it.

**Q.** We know from the note that Macrobid was discussed. Were any other antibiotic agents discussed?
**A.** There were a number of agents discussed.

**Q.** How do you know that?
**A.** I know that, because it's my custom and practice to – especially for any potential urinary issues that Ceftin is an antibiotic that is used very often. Bactrim is used very often, and because this patient had so many allergies I know even the husband got involved in what she's potentially allergic to, and Ms. Baker got involved in it. I remember trying to get one of the most appropriate antibiotics, you know, prescribed for her along with, you know, obviously, the recommendations of Dr. Smith Dr. Smith concerning a plan going forward; for example, a plan for stenting or some other therapy?

**Q.** Was there any discussion with Dr. Smith about whether the patient should be discharged from the hospital or kept in the hospital?
**A.** Yes.

**Q.** What was the discussion?
**A.** The discussion was to since she was feeling better, and her vital signs were all normal, and antibiotics were to be started, and that she was to see him the following morning, and if any of her symptoms – if any of her symptoms worsened, in any way, to return back immediately.

**Q.** Did Dr. Smith say something about seeing this patient in his office in the morning?
**A.** Correct.

**Q.** That is what you documented in the notes?
**Q.** Did you ask Dr. Smith to come to the hospital?
**A.** No.

**Q.** Dr. Oliver, other than advising Dr. Smith about the perinephric fluid did you have any further discussion with the urologist, Dr. Smith, about the finding of the perinephric fluid?
**A.** No.

**Q.** Did Dr. Smith suggest to you that the urine sample be cultured to determine what the organisms were?
**A.** I don't – I don't recall that conversation.

### E. Who has ultimate responsibility, the EP or the consultant?

**Q.** Whose decision was it to discharge the patient?
**A.** Ultimately, the decision to discharge the patient is my – is my decision, but it's – clearly, in this case, it's in consultation with, you know, a specialist.

**Q.** Did you determine that Ms. Baker should be discharged?
**A.** In consultation you're asking?

**Q.** I am asking, did you decide to discharge her?
**A.** It was decided to discharge the patient.

**Author comments (Weinstock):** This line of questioning gets to the heart of what we do and who has the ultimate responsibility. What if a consultant tells us something wrong or if they tell us something right but we disagree (despite not being a specialist in that field)? Or what if they agree to come in, but don't do it in a timely fashion (for example, a STEMI). In the end, as this plaintiff's attorney confirms, we do have the ultimate responsibility. This applies also in another uncomfortable situation, when the consultant or hospitalist refuses to care for a patient.

### F. Examination of the emergency physician (EP) from urologist's attorney (who was present for the EPs deposition as the urologist was also a defendant):

**Q.** My name is [plaintiff's attorney], I represent Dr. Smith. I am with the law firm of defense and defense. I just want to follow up on a couple of things. I will not be too long. I want to refer you back to your phone conversation with Dr. Smith that we were speaking about earlier. Do you recall how long that telephone conversation was?
**A.** Definitely, under 10 minutes.

**Q.** Aside from what you told plaintiff's counsel about that phone call, do you recall telling Dr. Smith anything else?
**A.** No.

**Q.** To your understanding, would Dr. Smith have the authority to discharge the patient? I know you talked earlier about how you worked—
**A.** Together.

**Q.** —together. If you know, would Dr. Smith, himself, be able to discharge the patient from the hospital?
**Emergency physician's defense attorney.** The patient was in the ED. So, the patient was not actually admitted. Do you want to rephrase your question?

**Q.** Would Dr. Smith have authority, on his own to – admitted to the ED. You want to know on discharge from what?
**Urologist attorney.** He said they worked together to discharge the patient or allow the patient to go home.
**EP's attorney.** Over objection, you can answer.
**Urologist's attorney.** I will rephrase the question.

**Q.** Would Dr. Smith, himself, have the authority not to admit the patient to the hospital?
**Emergency physician defense's attorney.** Note my objection. Over objection, you can answer.
**A.** Not to admit?

**EP's attorney.** Discharge from the ED is what he is getting at.
**A.** No.

**Q.** Dr. Oliver, did you tell Dr. Smith that you wanted the patient to be on IV antibiotics?
**A.** I – I remember having a conversation with Dr. Smith that ideally one dose of the appropriate antibiotics, which was Ceftriaxone, would be the best thing for this patient.

**Q.** That was during the conversation that you had with Dr. Smith over the phone, correct?
**A.** Correct.

**Q.** What did Dr. Smith say to you?
**A.** He agreed that, that would be the ideal thing.

**Q.** What did you say?
**A.** I would try to talk the patient into staying for a period of time to allow me to give that one dose of intravenous antibiotics.

**Q.** Who was it that recommended Macrobid as the antibiotic?
**A.** The two of us went back and forth on – based upon all the allergies, and I remember I remember putting Dr. Smith on hold, because there was so many allergies. We were, sort of, at a loss, at that point, what other antibiotic can be given orally, because she really was in quite a rush to leave the department, and the husband was in quite a rush to leave the department. So, we wanted to choose an antibiotic that she was wasn't going to have a serious reaction to. So, I remember going back. We saw the Macrobid she was allergic to, and I remember going back and speaking to her husband. I know I – I didn't document

on there, but we had – we had agreed that it was not an allergy to the Macrobid. So, I spoke to Dr. Smith, again, and relayed to him that the patient was – safe to give the patient Macrobid and that's how it was chosen.

## III. The Outcome

Almost exactly 1 year after the ED visit, the lawsuit was initiated. Almost 7 years later, the case was closed per court records as both the plaintiff and defendants jointly filed to discontinue the lawsuit. It does not include any reasoning, but this almost certainly means that they reached a confidential settlement.

## IV. The Legal Analysis—An Interview

**T. Marc Calvert, JD**
Medical malpractice defense attorney with over 35 years of experience
Calvert, Leever & Ostler
Cypress, Texas

### A. How could documentation have been improved?

**Discussion with the family:**
Although everything cannot be recorded, as if we had a court reporter in the ED, it is important to note what is important. For example, the discussion where the patient and her husband declined therapy; the failure to have an adequate discussion, or note about it, will allow the plaintiff's attorney to raise the question of whether or not it truly happened (especially if the husband later denies that it occurred) as well as questioning if the patient and her husband understood the implications of declining therapy. To lay people on a jury, it could seem convenient and contrived to claim a discussion happened when there is inadequate documentation, a perception that could be hard to overcome with the jury.

**Discussion with the consultant:**
Another crucial area for documentation is the conversation with the urologist. This happens to be a fairly common situation in cases that I have handled. The emergency medicine doctor reaches out to a consultant, documents a cryptic note in the chart, and later there are significant questions about what was conveyed to the consultant, and when. This section of notes does not have to be long, but noting the time the discussion occurred, and a highlight of the contents, including the key information provided to the consultant, and what the plan is, should be included. If it is detailed, it can be brief and take only seconds to do.

Many of these conversations occur during inconvenient times, such as in the middle of the night, or on the weekends, when covering doctors might be reluctant to weigh in. There are obvious pressures in this case. The consultant does not want to come in at 2 AM if they don't have to. Sometimes the ED doctor desires to accommodate the consultant, and the question of what is in the best interest of the patient collides with the schedule of the consultant. The better course is to shoot straight if there is reason for the patient to be seen by a specialist sooner rather than later, make that request, without fear or favor, and note it in the chart. If indicated, admit the patient and request a consult in the appropriate medical specialty. You may have to live with a frustrated consultant, and some personal or political fallout, but looking out for what is best for the patient is the obvious higher path.

**B. Would you have taken this case for the defense?**

Yes, I would take this case. I would want to have a detailed conference with my client and determine their specific thought processes, and how they will respond to cross-examination. We would then take the important steps of securing expert reviews, assessing the literature, and realistically evaluating the chances in front of a jury.

**C. Should the physician settle or go to trial?**

The path forward is dependent on several variables.

How does the emergency medicine doctor come across? I cannot overstate how important this factor is. To be well received, the doctor has to come across as smart, compassionate, and reasonable. It is critical to avoid arrogance before the jury, and to be aware of the areas of vulnerability in order to provide understandable context, and to properly explain the care process.

Doctors who come across as passionate rescuers, who are trying their best to help other people, are hard to beat. Those who come across as if working on an assembly line, checking boxes, and moving patients through, are much more likely to lose at trial.

I am not saying we would automatically go to trial or that we would win, but we would defend this doctor and give it our best shot!

**D. How can emergency physicians decrease the chance that this will happen to them?**

There is a formula that minimizes the chance of a claim even in the face of a bad outcome.

1. The first variable is the bedside manner. Does the doctor connect with the patient and their family in a caring and compassionate manner? This makes it less likely a lawsuit would be initiated, and harder to testify aggressively against such a doctor. I have seen plaintiffs on the stand acknowledge the sincere effort, and kindness, of the doctor they are suing and essentially apologize for having sued them.

2. Next, do the entries in the records reflect the bedside caring and compassion? It is not reasonable for every chart to be the length of a Russian novel, but it is necessary for every chart to be precise and as thorough as necessary to show that appropriate care is being provided.

3. Finally, having a sharp antenna of judgment, almost a sixth sense, allows the provider to think outside the box and go the extra mile when warranted. Everyone understands that emergency departments can get busy, but those who dance through the raindrops of claims and litigation are able to sense which situations require more time, and they are able to divide up their energy and hours appropriately. Patients who are upset about long waits, have unanswered questions, were sent in from a concerned primary care clinician, or are leaving in pain often require extra time and explanation.

## V. Medical Discussion

**Eric Funk, MD**
Emergency Medicine Physician
Springfield, Missouri
MedMalReviewer, LLC (owner)

**Introduction:**
A competent EM physician has a strong understanding of the appropriate treatment for any medical emergency. However, applying this knowledge can become challenging when faced with numerous obstacles. In this case, there were two key obstacles: The patient's allergy list and a rush to leave the ED. These issues, combined with poor antibiotic selection and a risky discharge, ultimately ended up in a fatal outcome for the patient.

1. **Antibiotic selection:** As you might imagine, the choice of antibiotics in this case was the key medical issue. Due to numerous related issues (allergies, refusal of IV antibiotics, and the rush to discharge), macrodantin was selected to treat her infected kidney stone. Macrobid is often a safe choice to treat a lower urinary tract infection, especially in young woman. However, it does not reach effective concentrations in the upper urinary tract, which was required in this case; it would not be expected to adequately cover pyelonephritis or an infected kidney stone.

2. **Multiple allergies:** The patient's numerous allergies significantly limited her treatment options. Her reported penicillin allergy is noteworthy in light of the fact that about 90% of people with reported penicillin allergy are not actually penicillin allergic.[1] Further complicating this was the fact that she had C. diff after previously being treated with a cephalosporin, and unknown reactions to levofloxacin, doxycycline, and macrodantin. Consultation with an ED pharmacist or infectious disease (ID) may be helpful in complicated cases.

   Ultimately, the ED physician decided that he was willing to prescribe an antibiotic regardless of its presence on the allergy list. The question is why macrodantin was selected, rather than one of the other options that theoretically could have treated her infection. It seems that the physician was guided more strongly by the fact that the patient changed her mind about the macrodantin allergy, rather than which antibiotic would be truly effective.

   In the end, it seems doubtful that any oral antibiotic would have prevented this outcome. By the time she made it home (less than 60 minutes after discharge) she was already falling and becoming altered. She was likely discharged during the unfortunate window in which she was on an irreversible path to becoming septic, but before it was clinically apparent.[7]

3. **Disposition decision:** The patient and her family's rush to be discharged is apparent from the husband's deposition. Even when discussing the situation several years later, he freely admits the thought they were in the ED "forever" and just wanted to get home. Their desire to leave is understandable but it is incumbent on the physician to push back against this discharge momentum and educate patients on the appropriate medical treatment. It's easy to fall into hindsight bias when reviewing medical malpractice lawsuits but the risk here is obvious to the point of being predictable. Elderly patients with infected kidney stones and worsening kidney function are simply not good candidates for outpatient treatment.

IV antibiotics, urology consult, and admission to the hospital is the standard of care in this case. If the patient had been advised of the risks and still was refusing admission, she should have been signed out against medical advice. AMA discharges do not make physicians immune from lawsuits, but it may have offered a significant layer of protection. The nature of AMAs qualifies them all as high-risk cases.

4. **Consulting specialists:** A urologist was consulted but the resulting recommendations are suspicious. It seems likely that he simply agreed with what the ED physician wanted to do (oral antibiotics and outpatient follow-up), especially because it meant that he wouldn't have to come back to the hospital and do a procedure on a holiday.

   Recommendations from specialists sometimes need to be considered with respectful skepticism, especially if they haven't seen the patient. I have no doubt that the urologist was an excellent surgeon but it raises red flags that he did not flatly recommend against macrodantin. A urologist isn't expected to know the complexities of every single antibiotic but they should know the basics of treating urinary tract infections.

   The urologist's attorney attempted to have him dismissed from the lawsuit by claiming that he wasn't consulted, and therefore, there was no doctor-patient relationship. They claimed that a phone call from an ED physician does not constitute a consult and was simply a courtesy call, primarily for scheduling purposes. This is a common tactic used in cases in which a consultant and an ED physician are both named in a lawsuit. This line of thinking is almost universally rejected by courts. It is well-established that taking a phone call from an ED physician to discuss a specific patient's care and provide recommendations does in fact qualify as a consult and establishes a patient-doctor relationship.

5. **Documentation:** The ED physician stated at his deposition that he recommended IV ceftriaxone, but the patient and her husband refused. This is a critical piece of information that should have been documented. A plaintiff's attorney always has an expert witness review the chart before filing a lawsuit. If the expert witness had any sense of ethics, seeing this in the record may have significantly changed their recommendations of the merits of the case. The old adage, "If it's not documented, it didn't happen," comes to mind. It's impossible to document every tiny detail but a patient refusing a recommended treatment is a critical piece of information that should be documented. Documenting a discussion with a consultant is also critical. It's tempting to just write down the consultant's name and time stamp but having a more detailed note about the substance of a conversation can be extremely beneficial during a lawsuit. It is preferrable to maintain a collaborative relationship between consultants and ED physicians (in the medical record, during discussions while working, and in the court room) but documenting what the consultant was told and what they recommended is always advisable should an adverse outcome occur.

6. **Management:** As with all forms of sepsis, the mainstays of treatment focus on antibiotics, fluids, vasopressors (as the clinical situation dictates), and source control (i.e., treating the underlying source). In the case of obstructive pyelonephritis, source control consists of emergency decompression. This is accomplished with either the use of a ureteral stent or placement of a percutaneous nephrostomy tube; the 2016 American Urologic Association (AUA) and the Canadian Urologic Association (CUA) recommend use of either a nephrostomy tube or ureteral stent.[2,3] If septic shock accompanies an infected stone, mortality approaches 30%.[4] Mortality is significantly increased if decompression is not performed.[5] The presence (or absence) of a particular specialist may

influence the decision, as stents are generally placed by urologists and nephrostomy tubes are usually placed by interventional radiologists.[6] Prior studies have not shown any significant differences in clinical outcomes between stent placement and percutaneous nephrostomy tube use.[7]

**Author comments:** I expect this lawsuit to end in a settlement. The facts are in the plaintiff's favor. Many malpractice cases come down to a difference of opinion, but in this case, there is very clear evidence that the selected antibiotic was simply insufficient to treat an infected kidney stone. There is a significant risk of sudden and drastic decompensation from infected kidney stones.

**Key learning points:**

1. Macrodantin is not appropriate for upper urinary tract infections.
2. Though it can be frustrating to face a long list of allergies that are of dubious veracity, clarifying which are allergies and not side effects can improve patient care.
3. Recommend the appropriate treatment and explain the risk of deviating; if the patient is not willing to stay, document and have them sign AMA papers.
4. Document details of discussions with consultants.

## References


1. Joint Task Force on Practice Parameters representing the American Academy of Allergy, Asthma and Immunology; American College of Allergy, Asthma and Immunology; Joint Council of Allergy, Asthma and Immunology. Drug allergy: An updated practice parameter. Ann Allergy Asthma Immunol 2010 Oct;105(4):259-273y
2. Assimos D, Krambeck A, Miller NL et al: Surgical management of stones: American Urological Association/Endourological Society Guideline, part II. J Urol 2016; 196: 1161
3. Ordon M, Andonian S, Blew B, et al. CUA Guideline: Management of ureteral calculi. Can Urol Assoc J 2015;9(11-12):E837-51. doi: 10.5489/cuaj.3483. Epub 2015 Dec 14. PMID: 26788233; PMCID: PMC4707902.
4. Reyner K, Heffner AC, Karvetski CH. Urinary obstruction is an important complicating factor in patients with septic shock due to urinary infection. Am J Emerg Med 2016;34(4):694–6.
5. Borofsky MS, Walter D, Shah O, et al: Surgical decompression is associated with decreased mortality in patients with sepsis and ureteral calculi. J Urol 2013; 189: 946
6. Marien T, Miller NL. Treatment of the Infected Stone. Urol Clin North Am 2015;42(4):459-472. doi:10.1016/j.ucl.2015.05.009
7. Thomas B, Tolley D. Concurrent urinary tract infection and stone disease: pathogenesis, diagnosis and management. Nat Clin Pract Urol 2008;5(12):668-675. doi:10.1038/ncpuro1254

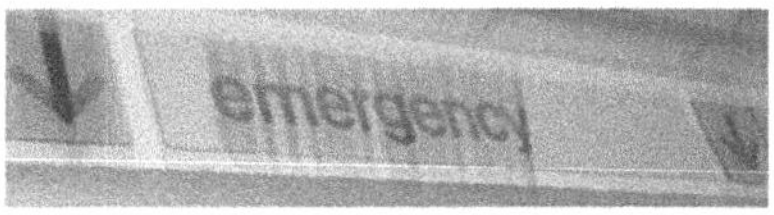


# Case 15

## A 57 Year-old Man with Chest Pain: Documenting the Conversation with a Consultant

**Primary case authors:**
**Cody McCoy**
**Michael Weinstock**
**Susy Demeester**

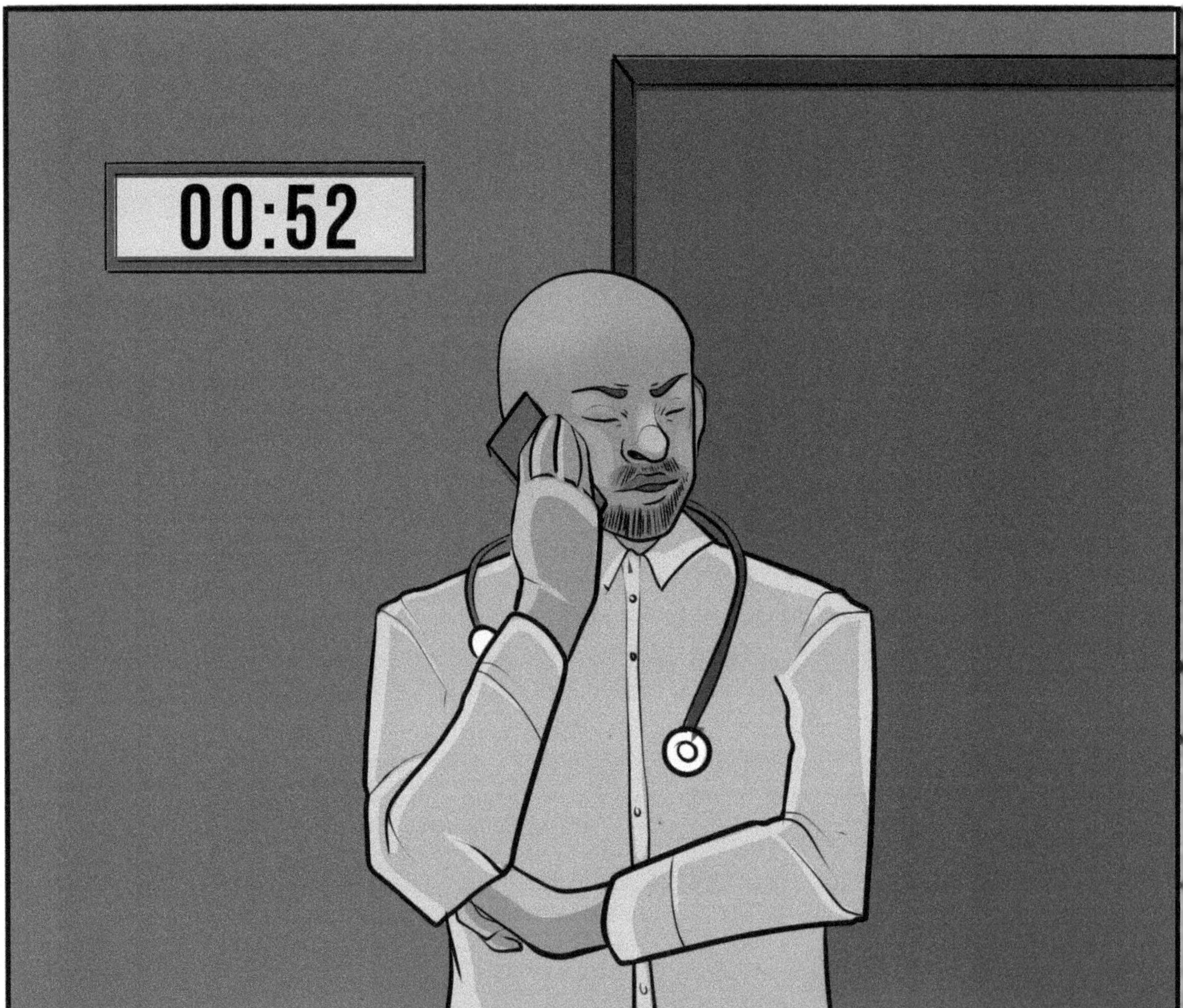


"...but Dr. Cardio..."

# Case 15

## A 57 Year-old Man with Chest Pain: Documenting the Conversation with a Consultant

***Deep thoughts:***

1. *Which ECG findings qualify to activate the cath lab?*
2. *Who should call the STEMI alert, EM or cardiologist?*
3. *What is the best way to document the interaction with a consultant?*
4. *Is it wise to have a family in the waiting room in the ICU, who are advocating for a cardiology consultation, removed by security?*

**Author comments (Weinstock):** This case is not really a "bounceback" but more of a "bounce-up;" the patient was seen in the ED then admitted to the ICU. Progressing through this case, it is easy to imagine ourselves in the footsteps of the emergency physician. The care was pretty well done.

The documentation reflects a conversation with the cardiologist and then with the hospitalist but there is no reflection of the actual discussion which took place. When the patient was admitted, it turned out that the hospitalist was taking a call from home. So, there was not a physician to physically receive the patient in the ICU. In a cynical twist, when the family became disruptive later that night by repeatedly asking for more "intensive care," they were removed by security. However, when the cardiologist ultimately arrived early the next morning, they found the patient in bad shape, with an ECG indicating STEMI, a significantly elevated troponin, and a very unstable patient.

A word of caution: This case, and the lawsuit that ensued, is upsetting, because the emergency physician recognized the seriousness of the situation right off the bat, saw the patient immediately, and then contacted the interventional cardiologist. Would you do anything differently medically or with the documentation? This case was the subject of a mock trial which can be viewed at: www.atls2020.com/atls2020

After the mock trial we conducted and published the largest survey of participants that had ever been done finding that 72% would change or consider changing their practice, and 92% would change or consider changing their documentation. After reading this chapter, see if you agree![1]

Was this standard of care? Probably. Was it excellence in care? You be the judge! Though it is not a true bounceback case, we thought it was important to include as there are some very important patient safety and risk management themes including timeliness of care, interactions with consultants, documentation, and transition of care.

## PART 1—MEDICAL

## I. The Patient's Story

On April 4th at around 11pm, Bobby Freeze, with a history of well-treated HTN, starts to experience sharp chest pain which radiates to his back and is associated with diaphoresis and shortness of breath; 911 is called by a family member who reports "he is having a heart attack." En route to the emergency department two ECGs are completed which indicate a possible ST elevation MI but with no evolving changes. He is placed on a cardiac monitor and receives 2 SL nitroglycerin and oxygen and an 18g hep lock to the right AC. Aspirin 324mg is given PO.

The ED doctor sees the patient immediately upon arrival at 11:54. (Below are the 2 ECGs done by EMS)

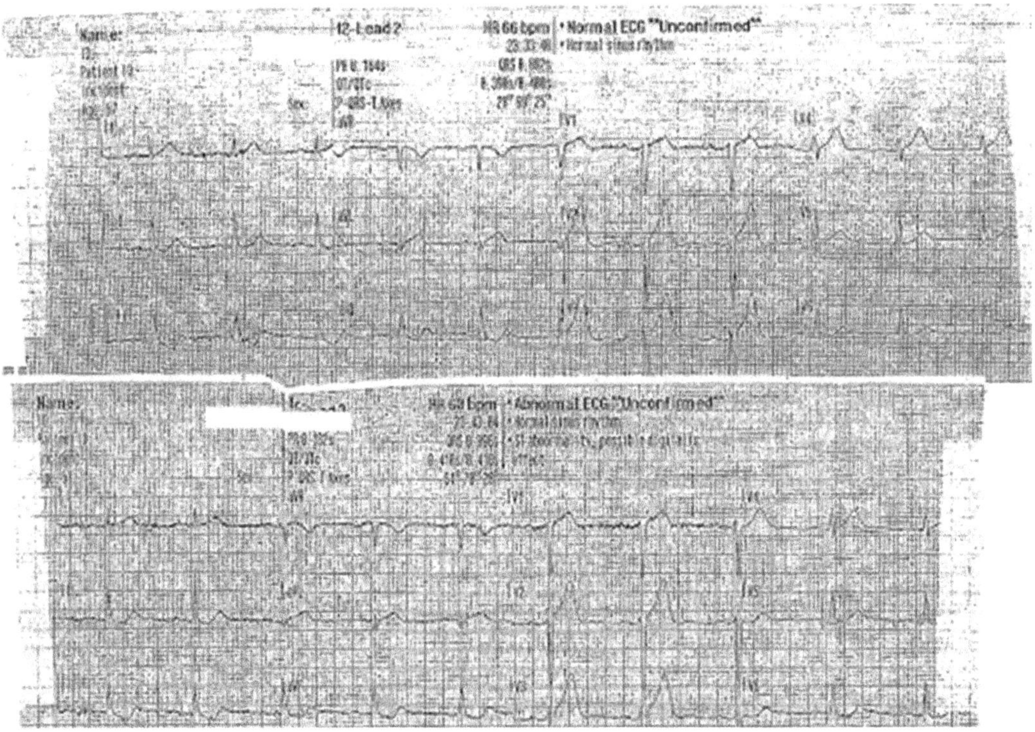


ECG #1— 23:33:48
ECG #2—23:43:0

## II. The Doctor's Version (the following is the actual documentation of the provider)

**Chief Complaint: April 5th (00:07):** "Chest pain"
**Triage (nurse):** Patient said he is having midsternal chest pain, sharp, constant, non-radiating since 2300, also with left upper back pain, sharp, constant. no dyspnea, patient given 1 NTG 0.4 mg sl en route, pain from 6/10 drop to 4/10.

**History of Present Illness text (physician) (00:12):** Patient presents for the evaluation of ongoing chest pain. History obtained from patient. History obtained from EMS. Onset of symptoms reported as gradual. Onset was 11pm, just prior to presentation. Patient currently has symptoms. Symptoms are improved. Pain most severe in left chest. Radiation to arm. Pain moved from anterior chest to back. Associated with nausea, no vomiting, diaphoresis present, shortness of breath [present]. Maximum severity is moderate. Currently symptoms are mild. Patient's condition exacerbated by nothing. Patient's condition relieved by nothing.

**Past Medical History:**
**Allergies:** PCN
**Medical History:** Flu vaccine is up to date, Tetanus is up to date, History of hypertension, which has been treated, Pneumococcal vaccine is not up to date.
**Surgical History:** Patient has had no previous surgical history.
**Social History:** Denies alcohol abuse. Denies tobacco abuse. Denies drug abuse. Lives with others. Nurse's notes reviewed. Agree with nurse's notes.

Vital Signs

| BP | PULSE | RESP | TEMP | PAIN | $O_2$ | SAT |
|---|---|---|---|---|---|---|
| 00:01 | 107/65 | 64 | 18 | 96.5 | 4 | 100 on ra |
| 00:35 | 104/67 | 58 | 18 | | 4 | 100 on 21 nc |
| 00:48 | 91/55 | 56 | 17 | | 4 | 100 on 21 nc |
| 00:56 | 102/56 | 56 | 17 | | 4 | 100 on 21 nc |
| 01:09 | 87/55 | 59 | 59 | | 4 | 100 on 21 nc |
| 01:48 | 95/53 | 59 | 59 | | 3–4 | 100 on 21 nc |

**Physical Examination (00:14):**
**Constitutional:** Vital Signs Reviewed.
**Head:** Atraumatic, Normocephalic.
**Eyes:** Eyes are normal to inspection, Pupils equal, round and reactive to light, No discharge from eyes, Extraocular muscles intact, sclera are normal. Conjunctiva are normal.
**ENT:** Ears, normal to inspection, Nose examination normal. Posterior pharynx normal. Mouth normal to inspection.
**Neck:** Normal ROM, No jugular venous distention, No meningeal signs, Cervical spine nontender, Normal thyroid.
**Respiratory Chest:** Chest is nontender, Breath sounds normal, No respiratory distress.
**Cardiovascular:** RRR, Heart sounds normal, No murmurs, normal S1S2, PMI normal to palpation, BP normal in both arms, Femoral pulses normal, pedal pulses normal.
**Abdomen:** Abdomen is nontender, No masses, Bowel sounds normal, No distension, No peritoneal signs.
**Back:** There is no CVA Tenderness, There is no tenderness to palpation, Normal inspection.
**Upper Extremity:** Inspection normal, No cyanosis, No clubbing, No edema, Normal range of motion, Normal pulses.
**Lower Extremity:** Inspection normal. No cyanosis, No clubbing, No edema, Normal range of motion, No calf tenderness, Normal pulses.
**Neuro:** GCS is 15, No focal motor deficits, No focal sensory deficits, No cerebellar deficits, Speech normal, Gait normal, Memory normal.
**Skin:** Skin is warm, Skin is dry, Skin is normal color.

**Lymphatic:** No adenopathy in neck, No adenopathy in axillae, No adenopathy in groin.
**Psychiatric:** Oriented x 3, Normal affect, Nom lal insight, Normal concentration.

**Initial Emergency Department ECG (00:03):**

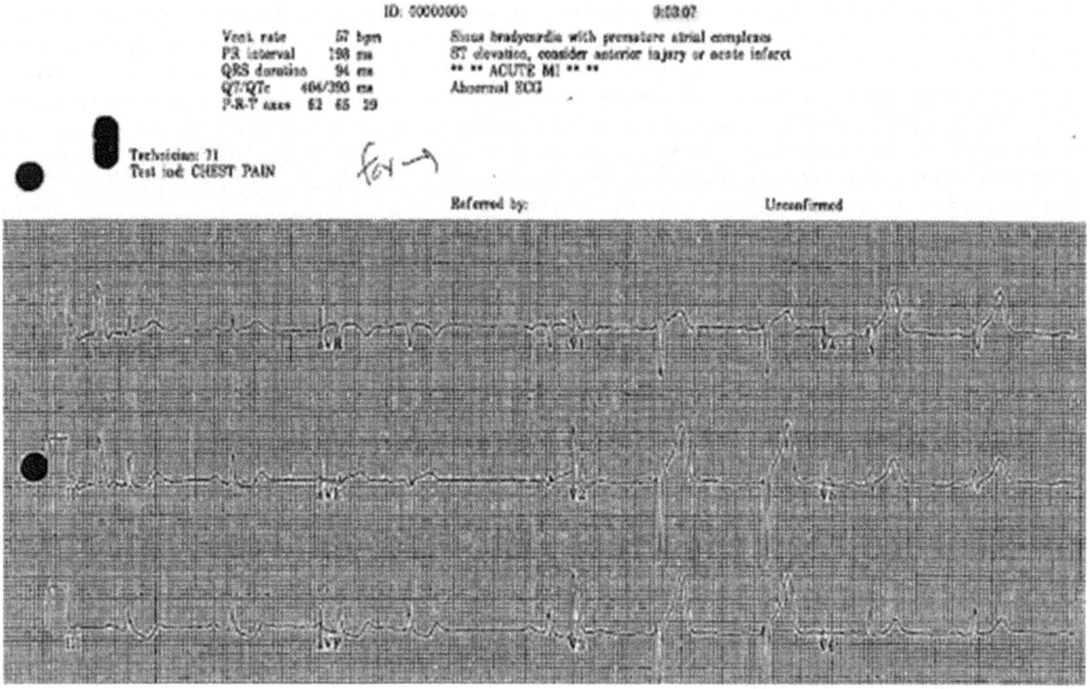

**PCXR:** The lungs and the cardio mediastinal silhouette are normal. The skeleton and soft tissues are normal. **Impression (per radiology):** Normal chest X-ray.

**Timeline:**
**00:03:** Initial ECG done (12:03) in the ED and handed to emergency physician. The ED Nurse documents inquiry "asked Dr. ER if we should activate STEMI protocol." and "Dr. ER to consult with Dr. interventional cardiologist (IC)." The initial call to cardiologist reached a cardiologist who was not on call, and the ED then called for the second cardiologist who was reached at:
**00:29 (EM Physician)** – "Discussed this case with Dr. On-call interventional cardiologist, called him stat as ECG has concave st elev vl thru v4 with nonspec st dep inferiorly." The interventional cardiologist asks the ER doctor to fax him the ECG (note the hand-written word "fax" on the above ECG. Also, note that the personal phone number of the cardiologist was hand-written just after the arrow and has been deleted) and to repeat the ECG. The repeat ECG was done at 00:36.

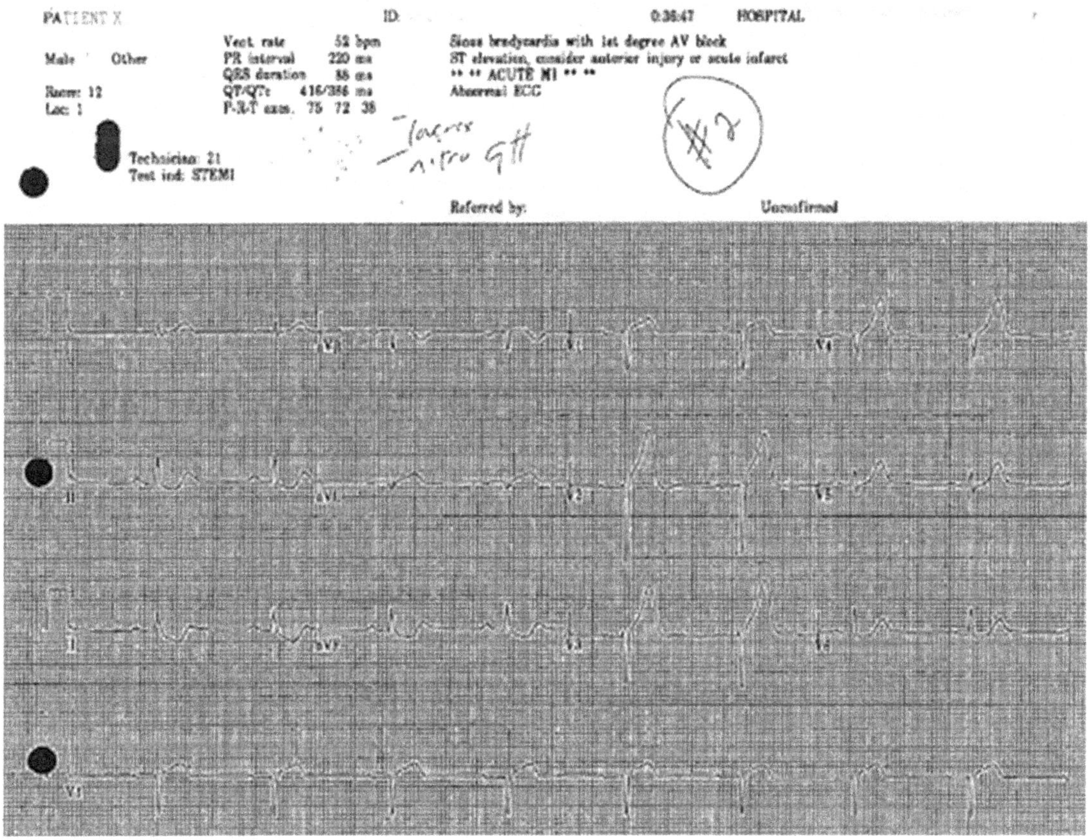


**00:52** – Patient has improved since arrival to emergency department. Discussed this case with Dr. Interventional cardiologist. The patient will be admitted to the hospital, The patient requires intensive care, and will be placed in ICU.

Per information obtained later, the interventional cardiologist felt that the patient was suffering from unstable angina and that he needed to be admitted to the ICU so that he could be carefully monitored and any changes observed. He also instructed Dr. ER to change the patient's heparin to Lovenox. He indicated he would come and see the patient later.

**00:54** – No beta blockers as heart rate is 55. Total number of minutes (30 minutes) spent in direct and indirect care of this critically ill patient excluding procedure time.

**00:54** – CORE MEASURES: This patient meets criteria for consideration of acute myocardial infarction core measures, smoking history within past year assessed, Aspirin was given within 24 hours of patient arrival in ED, Beta blocker was not given within 24 hours of patient arrival in ED, Beta blocker contraindicated due to bradycardia, Thrombolytics were not given within 30 minutes of patient arrival in ED.

**01:00 (RN)** - bp= 87/55, Dr [ER doctor] notified, VVO by [ER doctor] to give another 500ml 0.9 ns bolus.

**Below is the actual documentation from the emergency physician** (note that the first on call doctor at 00:29 was the diagnostic cardiologist (who was not on call) and the second on call doctor at 00:52 was the hospitalist):

**Testing (results at 00:53):**

| Test | Flag | Value | Units | Ref. range |
|---|---|---|---|---|
| WBC | | 9.0 | K/uL | 4.6-10.2 |
| HGB | | 14.1 | G/DL | 13.5-17.5 |
| PLT | | 240 | K/uL | 142-424 |
| NA | | 137 | MMOL/L | 135-144 |
| K | | 3.2 | MMOL/L | 3.5-5.1 |
| CL | | 95 | MMOL/L | 98-107 |
| $CO_2$ | | 28 | MMOL/L | 22-29 |
| GLU | | 129 | | 70-119 |
| BUN | | 11 | MG/DL | 7-18 |
| CREAT | | 1.1 | MG/DL | 0.6-1.3 |
| LFTs - WNL | | | | |
| Troponin | | 0.08 | NG/ML | 0.00–0.15 |
| BNP | | 8 | PG/ML | 0–100 |

**Medications:**

| **Drug Name** | **Dose** | **Route** | **Status** | **Time** |
|---|---|---|---|---|
| Sodium Chloride 0.9%, Intravenous | 500 mL | IV Fluids | Given | 01:10 |
| Sodium Chloride 0.9%, Intravenous | 500 mL | IV Fluids | Given | 00:58 |
| Morphine Sulfate | 4 mg | IV Meds | Given | 00:56 |
| Morphine Sulfate | 4 mg | IV Meds | Given | 00:34 |
| heparin 4,000 units i.v. bolus | | IV Meds | Given | 00:31 |
| heparin 800 units/hour i.v. drip | | IV Meds | Given | 00:30 |
| nitroglycerin 5 mcg/minute i.v. drip | | IV Meds | Given | 00:29 |

**Diagnosis (00:54):** Unstable angina
**Disposition:** Admission to the ICU

*Dr. Waidley*

## III. Risk Management/Patient Safety Opportunities (Weinstock)

**Risk Management/Patient Safety Opportunity #1:**

**Opportunity:** Calling a STEMI alert.
**Discussion:** Though this will be debated (a lot!) in the legal section below, with a 57 year-old man and new onset of chest pain and with anterior ST elevation, it all makes sense for STEMI. In EM, we often default to the more serious diagnosis. There are other causes of ST elevation such as early repolarization, aneurysm, pericarditis, or LBBB, but in a patient with concerning symptoms, if we cannot definitively exclude STEMI (for example an identical old ECG), we will often still call the alert. In fact, the EM physician recognized the concern, was right at the bedside, and contacted cardiology immediately. Then how did things go so wrong?

An explanation made by the defendant EM physician was that, per hospital protocol, all STEMI alerts were to go first through the cardiologist, as this was a new hospital with a new cath lab. A response to this could be to call the alert and, if the patient needed transfer, it would facilitate everything being done more quickly. Another response might have been that if you disagree with the cardiologist, ask them to come to the bedside, call a different cardiologist, or consider transfer. The EM plaintiff's expert has much more to say about this later.

✔ **Teaching point:** Defaulting to the more serious diagnosis when there is a strong clinical concern, will enable more timely care.

**Risk Management/Patient Safety Opportunity #2:**

**Opportunity:** Documentation.
**Discussion:** Arguably, the most important part of this chart is the interaction with the specialist. If in fact, per issue #1 above, the cardiologist did not want to call the STEMI alert, let's get that in writing (our own documentation of the fact)! From the EPs testimony, there were at least two discussions with the interventional cardiologist: First just after presentation (initially documented as a discussion with the diagnostic cardiologist at 00:29 and then within a few minutes with the interventional cardiologist) and at least once or twice again including when they gave instructions on admission orders (undocumented). However, we know nothing more than the discussions occurred as nothing about them was documented.

One way to document a conversation with a consultant is: "I spoke with Dr _____, and we discussed the patient's presentation, test results and my concern for STEMI. They have viewed the ECGs and recommend ______and will come in to see the patient within the next ____ period of time."

In fact, at the deposition, the EP needed to refer the attorney to the ECG with the fax number of the cardiologist written on the ECG itself (see the handwritten words on the 00:03 ECG above). Though we have deleted the names in the "Doctor Notes," the first doctor was the cardiologist (at 00:29) and the second call was to the hospitalist (at 00:52). A follow-up call to cardio was not documented. This also came up during the deposition (See Legal Section below).
✔ **Teaching point:** Documentation of the nature and specifics of a conversation with a consultant, the name and time of discussion, will be helpful if there is an adverse outcome.

**Risk Management/Patient Safety Opportunity #3:**

**Opportunity:** Address changes in hemodynamics.
**Discussion:** The blood pressure on presentation at 0001 was 107/65 but when the patient was getting admitted and just after the conversation with the hospitalist, it dropped to 87/55 (at 01:09). Now, we have a patient in his 50s with new onset chest pain, a concerning ECG (diagnostic or not diagnostic of STEMI?), and significant hypotension. Would a repeat ECG now have shown a definitive STEMI? Would a repeat call to interventional cardiology have prompted an emergent cath? Would a repeat call to the hospitalist have prompted a bedside evaluation?
✔ **Teaching point:** When there is a change in hemodynamics, a reassessment of the patient and an update of the receiving doctors can help ensure best care.

**Risk Management/Patient Safety Opportunity #4:**

**Opportunity:** Documentation of improvement is not clear.
**Discussion:** The EP documented that the patient was "improved" but it is a little unclear how they had "improved." Was it in relation to his symptoms of chest pain or with his ECG? Perhaps, he was no longer sweating? Though it might sound like nit-picking, just saying, "improved," actually does not say that much, especially when a blood pressure obtained 17 minutes later was 87/55. Especially with a patient whom the physician was obviously concerned about (see deposition testimony below noting the physician maintained almost constant bedside attendance), spending time to describe what is happening in the MDM note is medically and legally vitally important!

✔ **Teaching point:** Be precise in the documentation with words such as "Sudden onset." "Severe," or "Improved."

**Risk Management/Patient Safety Opportunity #5:**

**Opportunity:** Answering a question.
**Discussion:** The documentation reflected that the patient's pain radiated to the back. It is interesting that this would be included, as the insinuation is that thoracic aortic dissection (TAD) was still in play. As it turns out, which we will soon see, that was not the diagnosis, but if that is documented, (just like "sudden onset headache" or "a lethargic child" or "painless hematuria"), the onus is on the doctor to rule out the more serious diagnosis or to document why we don't think it is occurring.
✔ **Teaching point:** When a buzz word is documented, explain in an MDM note why you don't think that diagnosis is occurring.

## IV. The Bounce-up (To the ICU)

The patient is admitted to the ICU by the hospitalist with a diagnosis of unstable angina and orders for oxygen and cardiac monitoring, cardiac enzymes every 6 hours, fluids, a consult to interventional cardiology, aspirin, Lovenox, nitro titrated to chest pain relief with blood pressure parameters, morphine every 2 hours as needed, Zofran, and vitals every hour. Note the that orders are written by the EM physician, as instructed by the interventional cardiologist. There was no documentation of a discussion about the patient's hypotension prior to arrival to the ICU, except for in the vitals flow sheet. It is unclear if this information was passed along to the hospitalist. The patient was transferred to the ICU at 01:20, just over an hour after arrival at the ED.

02:48 – The ICU nurse notes a left bundle branch block on monitor. The hospitalist is called who orders hydrocodone and dopamine via telephone. An ECG is performed but not read by a physician:

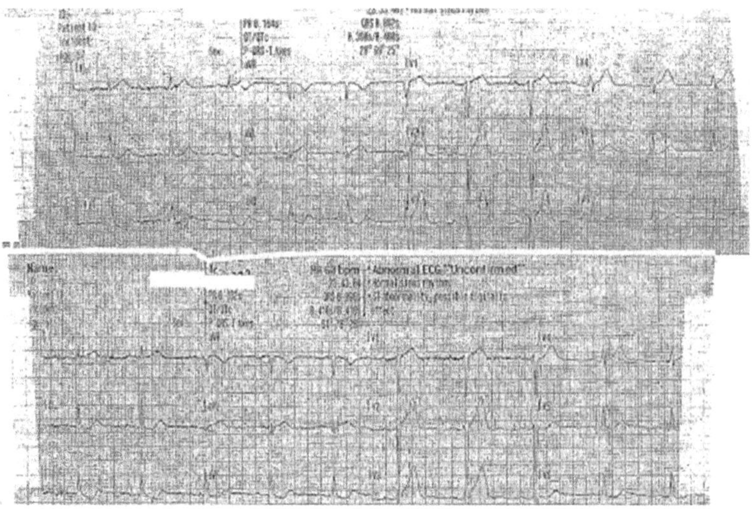

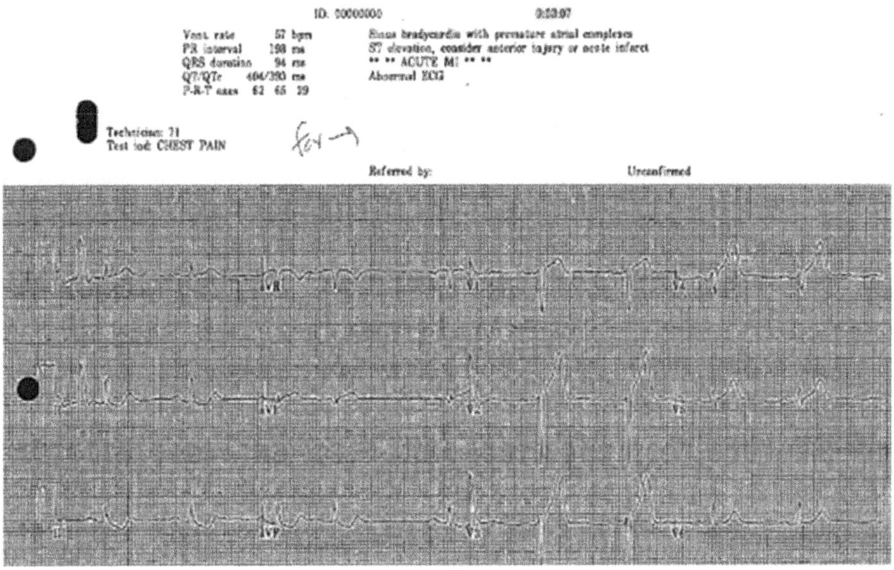


**05:15** – The patient starts vomiting and ICU nurse calls the interventional cardiologist and hospitalist. Another ECG is performed and faxed to the interventional cardiologist.

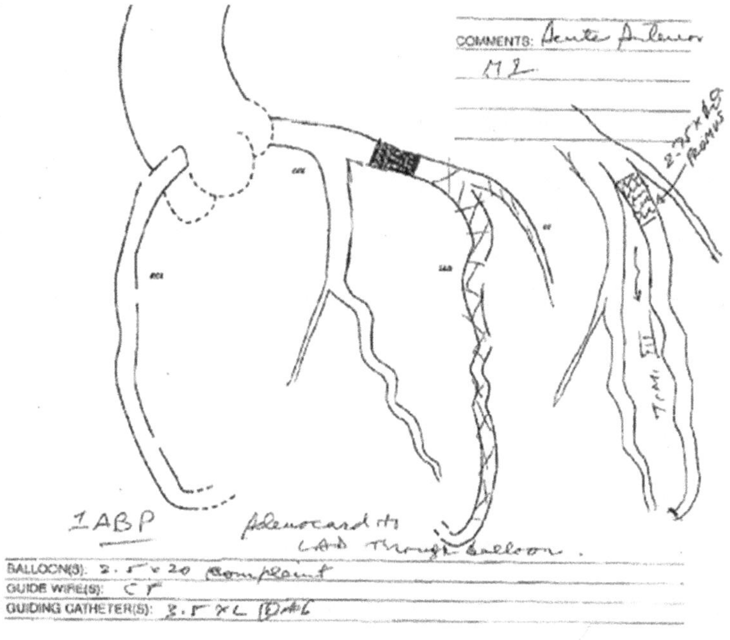


The interventional cardiologist notes an anterolateral STEMI. Cath lab is activated. Troponin trended up to 4.5 (H). Cardiac catheterization shows 100% occlusion of the LAD and could not be successfully recanalized. An intra-aortic balloon pump and temporary pacemaker are placed, and the patient is transferred to a different hospital for further care.

**Outcome:** Patient is left with irreversible myocardial damage.

**Author comments (Weinstock):** A lawsuit ensues…

## PART 2—LEGAL

**Author comments (Weinstock):** Before deposition and trial, a medical malpractice case starts with discovery, which includes obtaining opinions from plaintiff and defense experts. Below is the shortened opinion of the plaintiff's expert with predictable allegations: The MI should have been diagnosed and if it had, the patient would still be alive. Opinions generally start with the experts' qualifications (I went to the best school ever and I am totally awesome) and with which documents have been reviewed (ED charts, hospital records, autopsy, photos, police/EMS reports, etc.)

### I. The Accusation/Cause of Action

- Failure to diagnose
- Failure to activate STEMI protocol
- Failure to provide thrombolytic therapy or emergency cardiac catheterization

Cast of characters (names changed, except as noted):
**The patient:** Bobby Freeze
**ED physician defendant:** Dr. Waidley
**Dr. Hospitalist physician**
**Dr. Interventional cardiologist**
**Dr. Diagnostic cardiologist**
**Plaintiff's attorney**
Defense attorney: T. Marc Calvert JD (actual attorney for this case)

### II. Affidavit of EM Plaintiff's Expert, MD, FACEP

I am residency trained and board-certified in emergency medicine with 30 years of clinical experience and have evaluated and cared for hundreds of patients with symptoms similar to [the] plaintiff. I have read the complete medical records in this case, and I have reviewed other records including hospital policies procedures and on-call schedules. I have also read several depositions taken in this case including those of the plaintiff [the patient] and his family, [the interventional cardiologists] as well as the ICU nurse who later cared for the patient. All of the above, plus other materials including affidavits supplied for [the] summary judgment motion, as well as my education, training and experience are the basis for my opinions.

[The defendant's] major defense in this case is that he was simply an emergency medicine physician, and his management was under the control of the consulting cardiologist (by phone). This is quite simply an incorrect position and counter to the training and skill set that is expected, per the standard of care, for an emergency medicine physician. Emergency physicians do not simply serve as conduits of care from consultants to patients. Rather, emergency physicians are and must be, per the standard of care, independent thinkers and treaters, as well as patient advocates. Unfortunately, there are times in the practice of emergency medicine that we receive poor advice or lack of support from a consultant.

The standard of care in this case mandated that [the emergency physician] independently diagnose and arrange appropriate investigations and treatment for the (STEMI – ST elevation myocardial infarction) regardless of the incorrect input from a cardiologist over the phone. The standard of care in this case required [him] to immediately recognize the need to activate the hospital STEMI protocol which would have led to timely evaluation and treatment of [the patient's] heart attack. This independent act is not contingent upon a cardiologist consultation. Such consultations are not needed or appropriate in such a circumstance and in fact the American Heart Association has specifically recommended against consulting cardiology prior to activating a STEMI protocol. It matters not what the hospital "politics" were at the time of this incident. If the staff cardiologists insisted on being notified prior to activating the catheterization lab, then the standard of care mandated that [the emergency physician] find a cardiologist who would do so immediately. Alternatively, there was the option to provide thrombolytic therapy in the emergency department (ED), and/or transfer the patient to a facility that would appropriately provide the much-needed catheterization procedure. A refusal to activate the cath lab by a cardiologist reviewing ECG's at home does not excuse [the emergency physician's] central role in diagnosing, treating and managing [the patient's] STEMI.

The medical records reflect that on two occasions the emergency department nursing staff urged [the emergency physician] to activate the hospital STEMI protocol (once at 0003 and a second time at 0036). Both times this recommendation was rejected by [the emergency physician].

There were several ECGs obtained both pre-hospital (by the EMS crew that transported Mr. Freeze to the hospital) and in the ED that revealed an acute MI. These ECG's, coupled with the patient's history (age 57, past medical history of hypertension, brother with MI), presentation ("pressure" chest pain, shortness of breath, radiation of pain to the arm and back, shortness of breath, nausea, sweating), positive laboratory findings (positive CKMB – indicative of heart damage), response to treatment (decrease of pain with nitroglycerine by EMS) are diagnostic of acute MI and demand timely and appropriate actions on the part of the emergency physician. These actions are well known to all emergency physicians and include: 1) Emergent cardiac catheterization on site; 2) Transfer to another medical facility where emergent cardiac catheterization is available; or 3) Administration of IV thrombolytics in the ED.

I have reviewed all of the ECG's in this case. The two obtained in the ED actually state "ACUTE MI" on them as interpreted by the ECG computer. In this case I agree with this interpretation. Additionally, it is not only the ECG that makes a diagnosis in the case of acute MI. The emergency physician must obtain historical, physical and laboratory information that will support or contradict the diagnosis in each patient. In this case, all of the above was actually done, and as noted above the information obtained was diagnostic for acute MI that required emergent further evaluation and treatment that must be organized and arranged by the treating emergency physician. This is NOT a subtle or questionable case. As noted above, Mr. Freeze had a presentation, history, examination, laboratory and ECG findings that when taken together were conclusive for STEMI. Therefore, it was incumbent upon [the emergency physician] and in fact the standard of care demanded that he activate the STEMI protocol and arrange for the patient to be taken to the cath lab in an expeditious fashion. If the consulting cardiologist refused to cooperate with this plan, then it was required of [the emergency physician] to arrange for an alternative form of consultation, treatment and/or transfer. His duty to the patient did not end with the incorrect consultation with a cardiologist who was not at bedside.

The records and testimony in this case indicate that [the emergency physician] spoke to Dr. Diagnostic Cardiologist, a non-interventional cardiologist. Evidently, this physician did not recommend emergent cardiac catheterization. Dr. Diagnostic Cardiologist has testified that it was his understanding that he was being consulted to read the ECG, and it was the responsibility of the emergency physician to initiate the STEMI protocol as he did not "have the benefit of being in front of the patient" as [the emergency physician] was. It is indeed the responsibility of the emergency physician to initiate the STEMI protocol as he/she is with the patient and has undertaken to obtain a history, perform a physical examination and interact with the patient. It was [the emergency physician's] job to tell (not ask) the cardiologist that he was activating the STEMI protocol and it was now the cardiologist's obligation to present him/herself to the hospital to evaluate the patient and expedite a diagnostic and therapeutic cardiac catheterization.

If Dr. Interventional Cardiologist unreasonably did not or could not fulfill his responsibilities as noted above, then Dr. ER doctor had three options per the standard of care: 1) contact another cardiologist with staff privileges at this hospital (and in fact there was an interventional cardiologist on-call that night); 2) transfer the patient to another hospital with cardiac catheterization capabilities; or 3) administer thrombolytic therapy.

Due to the breach of the standard of care by [the emergency physician], the STEMI protocol was not activated for Mr. Freeze. Because of this, a timely cardiac catheterization was not performed and the blood supply to Mr. Freeze's heart was not restored for many hours. This delay in reperfusion resulted in severe and permanent heart damage. This extensive damage was directly and proximately caused by the breach in the standard of care by [the emergency physician]. I have been provided with the definition of willful and wanton negligence under Texas law, as follows:

"Willful or wanton negligence means an act or omission when viewed objectively from the standpoint of the defendant at the time of its occurrence involves an extreme degree of risk, considering the probability and magnitude of the potential harm to others AND of which the defendant has actual, subjective awareness of the risk involved, but nevertheless proceeds with conscious indifference to the rights, safety, or welfare of others."

In my opinion, based on my review of the available materials and my experience in this area, [the emergency physician] committed willful and wanton negligence in his care and treatment. On April 4–5, [the patient] faced an extreme degree of risk, namely injury to his heart and/or death. [The emergency physician] was well aware of this risk and the need to have [the patient] undergo emergent cardiac catheterization. Unfortunately, [the emergency physician] proceeded with conscious indifference by failing to activate the hospital STEMI protocol in light of compelling and obvious symptoms, findings and results that were diagnostic of STEMI. Additionally, he openly rejected the nursing staffs repeated requests to appropriately activate the STEMI protocol and failed to exercise any other available options to appropriately care for his patient with a life-threatening emergency. These acts and omissions constitute willful and wanton negligence.

Further, affiant says not.____________________________________________

Plaintiff EM expert, M.D., FACEP

SWORN TO AND SUBSCRIBED before me on the______________ day of ___________________

to certify which witness my hand and official seal. ________________________________________

Notary Public in and for The State of Texas

**Author comments (Weinstock):** There are some very specific allegations, and the plaintiff has decided that there is a possible case here. They are paying for this expense "out of pocket" and often they get the opinion of an expert who does not suggest malpractice and decide not to take the case. However, with this situation, they proceed. Following is the deposition of the attending emergency physician, Dr. Waidley.

## III. Deposition Testimony of Defendant EM Attending Physician

### 1. What happens when a STEMI patient presents to the ED?

**Q.** I'd like to direct your attention to the time period that included April 4th and April 5th at Sundowners Hospital. And we'll talk about the treatment of Mr. Freeze here in a moment. But first of all, if you could explain to the ladies and gentlemen of the jury, what was the setup in the emergency room at Sundowners Hospital with respect to referring patients to the catheterization lab?
**A.** At the time, Sundowners was a new hospital. In addition to this, obviously, the cardiac catheter lab was new. So were the emergency room doctors, and my understanding, that if we had any concern about a possible STEMI, that we would immediately call the interventional cardiologist on call and have them make the ultimate decision as to whether or not to catheterize the patient, and if so, where?

**Q.** And why at that hospital did the cardiologist have that arrangement with you?
**A.** That was a unique situation. And the primary reason was that at – Sundowners at the time, again, was a community hospital. And it had a relatively new and inexperienced catheter lab. In addition, it didn't have CV surgery backup.

**Q.** Okay.
**A.** So it was made clear to us at the time that if we had any concern for an ST Elevation MI, that we'd involve and consult with the interventional cardiologist immediately.

**Q.** Did they make the decision whether or not the catheterization lab would be activated?
**Mr. Plaintiff's Attorney.** Leading.

**Q. (By Mr. Defense Attorney):** You can answer.
**A.** Yes.

**Q.** And if they decided that a catheterization may be indicated, you're saying sometimes they would transfer the patient to the Medical Center?
**Mr. Plaintiff's Attorney.** Leading.
**A.** Yes.

**Q. (By Mr. Defense Attorney):** To the Medical Center?
**Mr. Plaintiff's Attorney.** Leading.
**A.** Yes.

**Q. (By Mr. Defense Attorney).** What was your understanding of why the cardiologist would sometimes transfer patients who may need catheterization to the Medical Center?
**A.** Mr. Defense Attorney, as you know, the Medical Center a world-renowned heart institute, and a lot more experience and backup that we could provide at Sundowners. And one of the big differences, again, was that they had CV surgery backup if they anticipated any — or if there were any complications.

**Q.** So is it true that before the catheterization team would be activated and come to Sundowners, that the interventional cardiologist would make the determination if a catheterization was going to be done, and if it was going to be done in Sundowners, or it was actually going to be done in the Medical Center —
**Mr. Plaintiff's Attorney.** Leading.

**Q. (By Mr. Defense Attorney).** — is that true?
**A.** Yes.

**Author comments (Weinstock):** One of the main allegations (and perhaps the only allegation from the plaintiff EM expert witness' opinion) was that the defendant should have activated the cath lab himself. The preceding testimony certainly flies in the face of this expert. Care is sometimes different depending on resource availability; after all, non-trauma ED's often stabilize then transfer, sick pediatric patients will not be admitted to an adult hospital, and cardiac patients will sometimes receive systemic thrombolytics if they are not able to receive an interventional catheterization in a timely manner. Should this EP have called the STEMI alert despite a hospital protocol to first notify the interventional cardiologist? More to come...

**2. Do you remember this patient?**

**Q.** Okay. Do you remember if there were other emergency room doctors that were working with you at that time?
**A.** No. I do remember, and there were not.

**Q.** Okay. Did this patient become a priority to you — Mr. Freeze?
**Mr. Plaintiff's Attorney.** Leading.
**A.** Yes, he did.

**Q.** [What do you remember about his presentation]?
**A.** Due to his age and his reporting symptom of chest pain, I was concerned that Mr. Freeze might be suffering from a heart attack, so I instituted the chest pain protocol, which included putting the patient on a cardiac monitor and oxygen, giving heparin, morphine, nitroglycerin, aspirin, and fluids, ordering lab work including cardiac enzymes, ordering a chest X-ray, and ordering a 12-leak ECG. The first ECGin the ER was completed at 12:03 AM on April 5th, 2009, and the ECG showed some ST elevation, but it was in the non-inferior leads. Also, the ECG was not significantly different from those done by EMS, so was not showing evolving changes. In my opinion, the 12:03 ECG did not show a clear-cut STEMI, but I thought it was a possible STEMI and that catheterization was a possibility for this patient, so promptly contacted the cardiologist listed as on call for the catheterization lab. This specialist, or a colleague, would be performing the catheterization and would ultimately make the decision if the patient should undergo catheterization and, if so, whether it was going to occur at Sundowners or at the Medical Center.

**Q.** So you gave information to the cardiologist, and he would make this decision that we talked about earlier: Should the patient be transferred, should the patient be kept at Sundowners —
**Mr. Plaintiff's Attorney.** Leading.

**Q. (By Mr. Defense Attorney):** — correct?
**A.** Yes.

**3. Conversation with the consultant:**

**Q. (By Mr. Defense Attorney):** So, what happened here with Mr. Freeze; what was — what was the result of your request to obtain the interventional cardiologist on call?

**A.** The cardiac cath lab at Sundowners Hospital had just recently opened. At that time, the cardiologists were making the decision whether to activate the cath lab at Sundowners or to transfer the patient to the Medical Center. The first person I spoke to was Dr. Diagnostic Cardiologist, and our conversation was very brief. I may have gotten two sentences out to him. I knew – he knew what I was calling for, and he told me immediately before I discussed the case with him in detail that he wasn't on call, that Dr. Interventional Cardiologist his partner was on call for interventional cardiology that night.

**Mr. Plaintiff's Attorney.** Hearsay.

**Author comments (Weinstock):** We will be seeing this word a lot. The plaintiff's attorney is essentially trying to keep the focus on the emergency physician (EP) and not the interventional cardiologist. When the EP deflects onto the cardiologist without documentation that a conversation occurred, the plaintiff alleges that this is hearsay!

**Q. (By Mr. Defense Attorney).** What did you do next after that conversation with Dr. Diagnostic Cardiologist?

**A.** Right after that, I called — asked the unit clerk to page Dr. Interventional Cardiologist, who paged back quickly. I spoke with Dr. Interventional Cardiologist, told him about the patient's presentation, condition, and my concerns about the 12:03 ECG. Dr. Interventional Cardiologist asked me to fax him the 12:03 ECGand to do a repeat ECG. I instructed the nurse to fax the ECG to Dr. Interventional Cardiologist's fax number, which I had written on the 12:03 ECG, and I ordered a repeat ECG, which was completed at 12:36. This ECG was also sent to Dr. Interventional Cardiologist at approximately 12:40. I spoke with Dr. Interventional Cardiologist shortly thereafter and we discussed the two ECGs, the cardiac enzyme results, which were all within normal limits, and the patient's condition. I reiterated my concern about the patient's status and I inquired whether the patient needed to go to the cath lab. Dr. Interventional Cardiologist felt that the patient was suffering from unstable angina and that he needed to be admitted to the ICU so that he could be carefully monitored and any changes observed. He also instructed me to change the patient's heparin to Lovenox. He indicated to me that he would come and see the patient later. I had worked with Dr. Interventional Cardiologist on other prior occasions, and know him to be a very experienced and well-trained interventional cardiologist. I trusted his judgment on Mr. Freeze and had no reason to second guess his analysis, diagnosis, and treatment decisions. I followed his instructions, contacted Dr. Hospitalist, a specialist in internal medicine, and arranged to admit the patient to her care. I told her of the patient's condition, presentation, the consultation with the cardiologist, and his assessment, diagnosis, and plan. I wrote the admitting orders as instructed by Dr. Interventional Cardiologist and the patient was transferred to the ICU and out of my care at 1:20 AM.

**Mr. Plaintiff's Attorney.** Objection; hearsay, and form.

**4. The differential diagnosis:**

**Q. (By Mr. Defense Attorney):** Dr. Waidley, let me ask you a few questions about that time — time period and that event. Now, have you encountered possible STEMIs before?

**A.** Many.

**Q.** All right. When you saw Mr. Freeze after talking to him and examining him, what did you think was going on with him?

**A.** My first reaction is to go through the chest pain differential diagnosis. But one of the first things and probably the highest on my list was an acute coronary syndrome, the non-STEMI, the STEMI, or unstable angina.

**5. What were you doing during your shift?**

**Q. (By Mr. Defense Attorney).** I would like to — to talk to you about your exposure to Mr. Freeze that evening. How often were you with Mr. Freeze on April 4th and April 5th, 2009?
**A.** On that night, I was immediately at his bedside when the EMS came in. And they were still there, because I got the history initially from them. And then I was there pretty continuously at his bedside. Occasionally, I would have to go out and take care of other stuff, but I was there regularly.

**Q.** Why; why were you there so much?
**A.** Because I was concerned about him. He was complaining of chest pain, and I believe he's 57 years old. So, we wanted to make sure he was okay and that he was stable.

**Q.** Did you notice any improvement?
**A.** I did.

**Q.** How did he improve?
**A.** According to my recollection, his pain subjectively improved before he was admitted to the ICU. His blood pressure trended and began to improve before he went to the intensive care unit. And his pain scale went from 4 out of 10, according to Bernard, the nurse, to 3 to 4 out of 10.

**6. The second call with the interventional cardiologist:**

**Q.** Okay. Now, did you have a second phone call with Dr. Interventional Cardiologist?
**Mr. Plaintiff's Attorney.** Leading.
**A.** Yes.

**Q. (By Mr. Defense Attorney).** And what to the best of your recollection occurred in that conversation with Dr. Interventional Cardiologist?
**Mr. Plaintiff's Attorney.** Hearsay.
**A.** My second conversation happened approximately 12:40. We got our second ECG at 12:36. I read it. It looked the exact same as the first ECG. I called Dr. Interventional Cardiologist. He called back promptly. I faxed him the second ECG while I was still on the phone with him. Right about that time, 12:40, we got his labs back. By that time, I already looked at the chest X-ray. And then I waited for further instructions from Interventional Cardiologist.
**Mr. Plaintiff's Attorney.** Hearsay.

**Q. (By Mr. Defense Attorney).** And what — what did Dr. Interventional Cardiologist tell you in that second conversation?
**Mr. Plaintiff's Attorney.** Objection; hearsay.
**A.** Dr. Interventional Cardiologist's expert opinion, being the interventional cardiologist on call, he told me that he didn't think the patient was experiencing the ST elevation MI. He thought the patient was having an acute coronary syndrome, specifically unstable angina. That he wanted to admit the patient to the ICU for close monitoring, and that he'd be in promptly to see the patient.

**Mr. Plaintiff's Attorney.** Hearsay; facts not in evidence.

**Q. (By Mr. Defense Attorney).** Okay. Dr. Waidley, if you would, look at your affidavit, No. 6. And if you would, read to us No. 6.
**A.** "Dr. Interventional Cardiologist took over the management of this patient from a cardiac perspective, and as a highly trained and very experienced interventional cardiologist, he was in the best position to evaluate the ECGs and to decide what treatment this patient needed. His instruction to send the patient to ICU seemed reasonable to me. I expected that the ICU staff, Dr. Hospitalist, and Dr. Interventional Cardiologist would then closely monitor the patient's unstable angina and provide indicated care as needed. If Dr. Interventional Cardiologist had ordered that the patient be sent to the catheterization lab rather than the ICU, I would have complied with that order. I deferred to Dr. Interventional Cardiologist on his assessment of what he wanted to do to treat Mr. Freeze because he was an experienced expert on cardiac issues and was going to be the one to provide the treatment he felt was necessary. I felt that promptly heeding the orders of the cardiology expert was in the best interest of a patient who I felt was having cardiac issues, and I felt it offered Mr. Freeze the best chance for successful treatment."

**Q.** Okay.
**Mr. Plaintiff's Attorney.** Objection; hearsay, and form.

**7. Transition of care to hospitalist:**

**Q. (By Mr. Defense Attorney).** I want to ask you about what happened after your second conversation with Dr. Interventional Cardiologist. What did you do after Dr. Interventional Cardiologist gave you the instructions in the second phone call?
**Mr. Plaintiff's Attorney.** Objection; form, and hearsay.
**A.** What did I do?

**Q. (By Mr. Defense Attorney).** Right.
**A.** I wrote the orders. I called Dr. Hospitalist and discussed the entire case and all the findings that we had at that time, and she agreed to admit the patient. We went back in and would have continuously reassessed Mr. Freeze, gotten any further history, and seen if anything changed significantly, and prepared the patient to go up to the ICU.
**Mr. Plaintiff's Attorney.** Objection; hearsay.

**Q. (By Mr. Defense Attorney).** Now, your role as the emergency medicine doctor, do you provide treatment of Mr. Freeze in the ICU?
**A.** I do not.

**Q.** What did you envision would happen for him in the ICU?
**A.** Well, it — it would be reasonable for us to expect that the patient would be taken care of in a — in a very sound manner. That he would have been attempted to be stabilized, and that the physicians would come and see him in a reasonable time frame.
**Mr. Plaintiff's Attorney.** Objection; form.

**Q. (By Mr. Defense Attorney).** Did you hear anything further that morning, April 5th, 2009, about Mr. Freeze or his status?
**A.** No.

**Q.** You never saw any of Mr. Freeze's family members?
**Mr. Plaintiff's Attorney.** Leading.
**A.** No.

**Q. (By Mr. Defense Attorney).** Did you see anyone in the emergency room with Mr. Freeze, other than Mr. Freeze?
**A.** No, I don't believe so.

**Q.** Now, do you remember Mr. Freeze?
**A.** I do.

**Q.** Do you remember the treatment that you provided to him from shortly before midnight, April 4th, 2009, until he was transferred to the ICU around 1:20 AM on April 5th, 2009?
**A.** I remember it very well.

**Q.** All right. How is it that you remember it today, years later?

**8. A subsequent meeting… is it protected?**

**A.** This was a unique case. And after – after the fact, the emergency room and hospital had a meeting to discuss the patient's care, how it could have been changed, how it was appropriate, things like that.

**Q.** When did that meeting occur?
**A.** Two months, approximately, after.

**Q.** And did you have any indication that there were any questions about Mr. Freeze's care prior to that meeting?
**A.** I did not.

**Q.** When you went to the meeting, were you informed that the family had questions about the care provided by the hospital?
**Mr. Plaintiff's Attorney.** Leading.
**A.** It was one of the things that was discussed.

**Q. (By Mr. Defense Attorney).** And who do you recall being in attendance at the meeting?
**A.** The ER nurse manager, ER nurse involved, the case manager, myself, Dr. Interventional Cardiologist, were the primary people that attended that.
**Mr. Plaintiff's Attorney.** Objection; peer review violation.

**Q. (By Mr. Defense Attorney).** Do you remember Dr. Hospitalist being present?
**A.** She was.

**Q.** And what do you remember about that meeting with respect to what Dr. Interventional Cardiologist said?
**Mr. Plaintiff's Attorney.** Objection; hearsay, and peer review violation.
**A.** Go ahead and answer it?

**Q. (By Mr. Defense Attorney).** Yes.
**A.** I remember exactly what happened at that meeting. And our primary concern was to figure out what could have been done different, if anything, and how to fix it so it doesn't happen again. And the primary —

**Q.** Now, let me ask you this before you tell us what Dr. Interventional Cardiologist said. Did you know that Mr. Freeze had gone to the ICU after seeing you in the emergency room, and that neither Dr. Hospitalist nor Dr. Interventional Cardiologist came in to see him for several hours? Did you —
**Mr. Plaintiff's Attorney.** Leading.

**Q. (By Mr. Defense Attorney).** — know until that meeting occurred?
**Mr. Plaintiff's Attorney.** Leading.
**A.** No.

**Q. (By Mr. Defense Attorney).** What do you remember Dr. Interventional Cardiologist saying?
**A.** Doctor —
**Mr. Plaintiff's Attorney.** Hearsay.
**A.** Dr. Interventional Cardiologist took the blame on his shoulders.

**Q. (By Mr. Defense Attorney).** What did he say?
**A.** He looked down and said that he should have come in and seen the patient sooner.

**9. Back to the documentation:**

**Q. (By Mr. Plaintiff's Attorney)**
**Q.** Dr. Waidley, the only evidence that the jury has right now that you actually called Dr. Interventional Cardiologist contrary to his — contrary to his testimony is your statement today, correct?
**Mr. Defense Attorney.** Object to the form.

**Q. (By Mr. Plaintiff's Attorney).** Do you understand my question?
**A.** Can you repeat it, please?

**Q.** The only evidence — the only evidence under the sun that the jury has that you claim that you called Dr. Interventional Cardiologist at 12:10, the only evidence they have is your testimony, correct?
**Mr. Defense Attorney.** Object to the form.
**A.** Yes, and I noted his phone number, I believe, on the first ECG, his fax —
**Mr. Plaintiff's Attorney.** Objection; nonresponsive.

**Q. (By Mr. Plaintiff's Attorney).** Did you understand my question?
**A.** I believe so, yes.

**Q.** What's the answer?
**A.** I believe, yes.

**Q.** You can't show us any entry in the record that a 12:10 phone call to Dr. Interventional Cardiologist was truthfully made, correct?
**A.** Looking at the record, it does not document 12:03 or 12:10; however, the way we document in the emergency room is electronically, so the —
**Mr. Plaintiff's Attorney.** Objection; nonresponsive.
**Mr. Defense Attorney.** Hang on. He's not done yet. Please let him finish.
**A.** So the only and the best way we can do it is to document when we think it's reasonable and appropriate. Looking back at this case, could I have documented more accurately? Yes. We do our best, and I'm testifying what happened in this case. I remember, because I was there.

**Mr. Plaintiff's Attorney.** Objection; nonresponsive.
**Q. (By Mr. Plaintiff's Attorney).** It's not in the record, is it?
**A.** Not at 12:03.

## IV. Opinion from the EM Defense Expert i.e., How is the Case Defended?

**Affidavit of EM Defense Expert, M.D.**
Before me, the undersigned authority, on this day personally appeared EM DEFENSE EXPERT, M.D. and who, after first being sworn according to law, upon his oath, did state as follows:

I am over the age of 18 years and am fully competent to make this affidavit. The facts contained herein are within my personal knowledge and are true and correct.

My attached C.V. outlines my qualifications, which includes being Board Certified in Emergency Medicine and a Fellow of the American College of Emergency Physicians. I currently practice as an Emergency Medicine Physician at ______ Hospital in the ______Medical Center, am a Professor of Emergency Medicine. I have been practicing as an emergency department physician for [almost 20] years. I have had hundreds of patients such as Mr. Freeze who have presented to the emergency department ("ED"): with the same or similar symptoms as experienced by Mr. Freeze on April 4 and 5, and have had to evaluate ECGs and consult with specialists in cardiology. I am very familiar with the decision-making process in an ED when treating patients such as Mr. Freeze.

I have reviewed the attached medical records. According to my review of the attached records, a brief summary of the facts is that Mr. Freeze began experiencing chest pain and some back pain at around 11:00 PM on April 4, 2009. It is documented several times in the ED record that this pain was non-radiating. EMS transported Mr. Freeze to the hospital, arriving at approximately 11:54 PM. Two ECGs were performed by EMS personnel en-route. The nurses' notes indicate that the EMS personnel reported that initially the patient had ST changes but that they had resolved. Dr. Waidley was at the bedside at 11:54 to perform a physical exam and started the patient on vital signs monitoring, morphine, heparin, aspirin, nitroglycerin, oxygen, and fluids. He also ordered a chest X-ray and two ECGs. He contacted the cardiac interventionalist on call, faxed the ECGs, and was instructed to admit the patient to the ICU with a diagnosis of unstable angina. The patient was admitted to the ICU at about 1:20 AM.

The standard of care for a reasonably prudent emergency department physician when a patient like Bobby Freeze, a 57 year-old male with hypertension, presents to the emergency department via EMS with the symptoms that Mr. Freeze had, including chest pain, is to take the following actions: Take a history and conduct a physical exam and evaluate what the patient's condition is at the time while considering the history of the present illness. The doctor would then consider taking steps that address the condition, including putting the patient on a cardiac monitor, starting an IV, giving aspirin, morphine, nitroglycerin, and heparin, performing an ECG, and ordering cardiac enzymes and other lab work.

The attached records show that Dr. Waidley met the standard of care in his treatment of Mr. Freeze because he did take a history and conduct a physical exam, instituted the chest pain protocol which included putting the patient on a cardiac monitor and oxygen, giving the patient IV fluids, aspirin, morphine, nitroglycerin, and heparin, ordering a chest X-ray, ordering two ECGs, one at 12:03 and one at 12:36, and ordering cardiac enzymes and other lab work.

Based upon my experience as an emergency department physician who has reviewed hundreds of ECGs of similarly situated patients, the initial ECGs by themselves were not diagnostic for STEMI (ST elevated Myocardial Infarction). There are ST abnormalities, but the ST segments were concave and so there were other possibilities on the differential diagnosis.

The standard of care for a reasonably prudent emergency department physician with a patient such as this is to consult with a specialist such as an interventional cardiologist for his evaluation of the ECGs and to follow his recommendations.

Dr. Waidley met the standard of care by sending the ECGs to the cardiologist, Dr. Interventional Cardiologist, consulting with him, and following his instructions to change the patient's heparin to Lovenox and to send the patient to the ICU.

If the consulting cardiologist determines that the patient does not need to be sent to the cardiac catheterization lab for an interventional procedure, a reasonably prudent emergency department physician will rely on and defer to the cardiologist's expert opinion and treatment decision. There is no compelling reason in this case why the ED physician should override the recommendations of the specialist. The cardiologist is the expert and is the one who will ultimately determine if a catheterization is indicated and if there is another treatment approach to take. Dr. Waidley met the standard of care because, according to the attached medical records, he followed the consulting cardiologist's instructions, contacted the Internal Medicine specialist Dr. Hospitalist, who agreed to admit the patient to the ICU under her care, and Dr. Waidley ordered that the Heparin be changed to Lovenox, per the cardiologist's instructions.

The standard of care for an emergency physician is to administer thrombolytics to patients who meet all inclusion and exclusion criteria if the patient will not be able to be in a cardiac cath lab and have the culprit artery repaired within ninety minutes of arrival. If, however, the consulting cardiologist determines that the likelihood of STEMI is too low to warrant emergent intervention then there is no expectation that the ED physician administer thrombolytics. Because the consulting cardiologist concluded this was not an Acute MI situation, thrombolytics were not indicated and it would not have been appropriate for Dr. Waidley to administer them at that time. There are risks to thrombolytics, and the cardiologist's opinions in this regard should be deferred to by the ED doctor. Dr. Waidley met the standard of care by not administering thrombolytics, and by following the instructions of the cardiologist and admitting the patient to the ICU as he was instructed to do.

According to the attached medical records, Dr. Waidley took specific documented actions to care for this patient: physical exam, put the patient on a cardiac monitor and oxygen, gave the patient IV fluids, aspirin, morphine, nitroglycerin, and Heparin, ordered two ECGs, chest X-ray, cardiac enzymes and other lab work, sent the ECGs to the cardiologist, consulted with the cardiologist, consulted with the admitting physician, wrote admitting orders per the cardiologist, and sent the patient to the ICU. All of these actions provide clear indications to me and evidence that Dr. Waidley was attentive to the rights, health, and welfare of the patient, Mr. Freeze. He acted within the standard of care and met it in all respects in the caring for this patient. Based upon the actions taken by Dr. Waidley, as outlined in the attached medical records, it is my opinion that they are evidence that Dr. Waidley did not create an extreme degree of risk in harming Mr. Freeze. In my opinion the actions taken are evidence that Dr. Waidley did not act with conscious indifference to the health and welfare of Mr. Freeze. In my opinion the actions taken are evidence that Dr. Waidley did not act with any intent to harm this patient. Indeed, he acted in a manner indicating his desire to care for and to help this patient.

Based upon the attached medical records, my education training and experience as outlined in my attached CV, and based upon the attached affidavit of Dr. Waidley wherein he explains and highlights his care of Mr. Freeze, it is my opinion that Dr. Waidley's care and treatment of Mr. Bobby Freeze on April 4–5, was not negligent or grossly negligent and that he met the standard of care in all respects of a reasonably prudent emergency department physician in the same or similar circumstances.

*Signed: EM Defense Expert, MD*

## V. The Verdict (decision by jury)

This case was quite hard fought. The plaintiff's lawyer was a very successful and highly aggressive specialist in medical cases. At every deposition and hearing, he brought his two partners, one of whom was also a physician. Every portion of the case was contested, usually in an acrimonious way.

The case underwent early mediation. Mediation is a form of alternative dispute resolution, and it is routinely used in most states to determine if the case can be resolved prior to trial. In this case, the other side's demands were so exorbitant that the mediation was adjourned. More discovery ensued, including deposing several experts, and this occupied several months. Because we had stout experts, we could sense that we were gaining leverage in our defense. As we approached trial, the court encouraged the re-opening of negotiations and, somewhat to my surprise, the plaintiff's attorney said that they would be willing to take what we had offered at mediation many months earlier. The exact figure of settlement is confidential, but it was in the mid five figures and less than the costs of continuing through a trial. It was a good resolution for my young client and sealed off the risks of an adverse verdict at trial.

## VI. The Legal Analysis—An Interview

**T. Marc Calvert, JD**
Medical malpractice defense attorney with over 35 years of experience
Calvert, Leever & Ostler
Cypress, Texas
(Actual defense attorney in this case)

*1. You were the actual attorney for this case – any colorful insights?*

This was a memorable case! I have great respect for the skills of the plaintiff's lawyer, and he utilized every stratagem in the book. One example is when one of the cardiologists was deposed, the one whose name was in the chart but who did not provide care. It was early in the case, and the plaintiff's attorney walked in with a giant enlargement of some cardiac guidelines. It was maybe 4 feet by 8 feet, and in color. He put it right near the witness and just blitzed him with questions, applying the American Heart Association guidelines to the facts of the case. He used him as an unwitting expert and the testimony hurt all of the defendants, as this cardiologist nervously agreed to pretty much everything he was asked.

Another example is how personal the other side approached the questioning, including digging for skeletons in the closet. It underscores the psychological warfare that is often utilized, and the "shock and awe" tactics employed. This was intended to weaken the will of the defendants. I fought back, and later in the case, I brought the dirty tricks of the other side to the attention of the judge in a motion for sanctions. We prevailed on that motion, and it was shortly after that decision that the case resolved.

2. *Did you take this to trial? Why were you confident on prevailing at trial instead of settling?*

My feeling is that we would have ultimately prevailed if the case had gone to trial, and this was based on the strength of our experts but it was a close call. This is not uncommon. Vulnerabilities were evident, however, ranging from errors in the records, to a defendant who would have struggled on the witness stand in front of the jury. The patient's outcome of being a "cardiac cripple" (a phrase his attorney used repeatedly) would likely evoke sympathy and the image of the patient "falling through the cracks" of the medical system would have put gas on the fire.

My job is to look out for my client and protect their interests. The willingness to settle for what amounted to "cost of defense" money made the decision easy. The jury verdict could have been astronomical, and unless my client was impassioned about going to court on principle, the risks were too high to pass up a relatively nominal settlement.

3. *What do you wish the defendants had done differently when they saw the patient in the ED (that would have made the defense easier)?*

I wish my client had been more assertive with the on-call cardiologist and had clearly noted that effort in the records. The cardiologist who was on call was an older doctor, and my client explained to me how resistant he was to coming in. It is a sad truth; the on-call consultant is awakened with a call after midnight, and grumpily wants to evade coming in. For the patient's sake, and for the ED doctor's sake, this hurdle needs to be cleared. The ED doctor needs to press forward and provide the information and then advise them that the patient needs to be seen. Next, a note to that effect needs to be documented. This is the formula that is not only medically proper, but it is also the best route from a legal perspective.

While admitting this patient was a great move, the question is going to be when the patient will be seen by a specialist. Activating the STEMI protocol may not be indicated, but there could be expectations on the ED doctor to take other steps to trigger a prompt in-person visit by the specialist. Appreciating how this could unfold can be a catalyst to proactive steps being taken. If the on-call doctor is mad for having to get up and come in, so be it!

4. *What did they do well?*

Reaching out to the on-call cardiologist and faxing him the ECGs was a big help. It showed the effort to consult and it handed the baton of care, at least somewhat, to that specialist. Getting the patient admitted made the case more defensible and began a sharing of responsibility. The patient worsened in the ICU, and the nurse did not convey that information in a timely manner. So, other providers being involved relieved some pressure on my client.

5. *When coordinating care with a consultant, what are important factors to record in the documentation?*

The note does not have to be lengthy but it needs to be substantive and meaty; that is, it needs to document that the important information (history, complaints, findings, test results, etc.) was communicated to the consultant and that it was requested that the patient be seen soon by the consultant. If a STAT consult is indicated, then that is what should be requested and noted. If the patient can be admitted, and the consultant can reasonably evaluate them remotely, the note should set out the plan, the justification, and that the patient will be seen in person asap if any changes occur. If discharge is the reasonable route, the reasons why should be noted and so should the fact that the consultant agreed with this plan.

The bottom line is that the ED doctor must proceed, without fear or favor, and reasonably involve consultants at a level that is warranted based on the medical indications. The note needs to be pointed, complete, and accurate, addressing the key facts and details and making sure to note that these things have been communicated to the consultant.

6. *Was there culpability of the cardiologist as well as the emergency physician?*

The cardiologist was arguably the culprit in this case. However, the twist is that the wrong name was entered into the record, and then, the statute of limitations expired. Thus, the wrong cardiologist got sued and he was eventually dismissed when he could show that he never saw the patient nor spoke to the ED doctor. It was too late to add the correct cardiologist to the lawsuit!

7. *How did the removal of the family from the ICU for being "disruptive" possibly factor in their decision to initiate a lawsuit?*

I think the overall care provided by the hospital nurse when the patient was admitted was subpar and was the catalyst for the lawsuit. Her scolding of the family, as they expressed their deep concern at the deterioration of the patient, was the cherry on top. The hospital was forced to settle early because of the layers of issues created by one nurse.

8. *Final thoughts*

In some ways, the care was well done: The patient was seen quickly, ECGs and labs were done soon, and a specialist was consulted promptly. However, the checklist starts to fall apart as the records are not thorough enough, and at times inaccurate (e.g., listing the wrong cardiologist as the on-call doctor), and the consultant is a reluctant participant given the late hour. A young ED doctor dealing with an older cardiologist has some potential political ramifications, as the ED doctor balances whether the patient really needs to be seen in the ED immediately. In hindsight, he should have made that request, or instituted the STEMI protocol to get the wheels in motion and then lived with the political drama if it came his way. Instead, he lived with a lawsuit for over 2 years.

## VII. Medical Discussion—Evaluation of Chest Pain and Management of STEMI

**Cody McCoy, DO**
Internal Medicine
Adena Regional Medical Center

**Michael Weinstock, MD**
Emergency Medicine Physician and Director of Research, Adena Regional Medical Center
Professor of Emergency Medicine, adjunct, The Ohio State University Wexner Medical Center

**Susy DeMeester, MD**
Emergency Medicine Physician
Central Oregon Emergency Physicians

**Why can't patients just present *typically?***
It would be nice if our patients presented like we learned in medical school, but they don't always read the textbook. Complicating our assessment of acute coronary syndrome (ACS) is that fact that the heart has a visceral innervation, with angina manifesting sometimes as shoulder pain, jaw pain, or even dyspnea or diaphoresis (this is discussed in greater detail and referenced in chapter 1). However, this case is different. The physician did suspect ACS/STEMI from the initial assessment and immediately involved interventional cardiology. The problem was that not only do patients present differently than the textbook, but so do ECGs!

The incidence of a STEMI presentation in the ED is 7.3 per 10,000 individuals.[2] The ECG which prompted a call to the cardiologist in our case suggests an anterolateral MI, with ST segment elevations in V2, V3, V5 and V6 from what turns out to be a 100% LAD occlusion.

With ongoing discomfort, ECGs should be repeated at 15 to 30-minute intervals to assess for progression and compared to previous ECGs.[3,4,5] In this case, the ECG was repeated and continued to show concerning findings, but not diagnostic of STEMI, per the opinion of the interventional cardiologist who reviewed a FAX'd copy. It would have been prudent to repeat the ECG and document re-evaluation of the patient when he became hypotensive at 1:03 am.

**STEMI equivalents:**
In addition to ST elevation in anatomically contiguous leads, several additional findings are concerning for coronary occlusion, collectively, referred to as STEMI equivalents[5] doi:10.1016/j.jacc.2022.08.750]:

1. Posterior STEMI –ST segment depression in V1 through V3 and confirmed with a posterior ECG
2. Smith-modified Sgarbossa Criteria – applied to an ECG showing ventricular pacing or left bundle branch block.
   - Concordant ST segment elevation (≥1mm) in leads with a positive QRS
   - Concordant ST segment depression (≥1mm) in leads V1–V3, or
   - ST Discordant ST segment elevation at the J point at least 1mm and amplitude at least 25% of the preceding S-wave
   - (≥5mm) in leads with negative QRS complexes
3. Hyperacute T waves – Broad, asymmetric peaked T waves – sometimes seen in early MI
4. De Winter sign – Precordial leads containing prominent and symmetrical T waves following upsloping ST depression at the J point.

**Acute occlusion MI (not STEMI…):**
The evolving terminology of occlusion myocardial infarction over classic dichotomy of STEMI vs. NSTEMI has also shifted focus to the underlying pathophysiology (acute coronary occlusion).[6, 7] The basis of this nomenclature change is grounded in the evidence that STEMI criteria are neither sensitive or specific and that up to 25% of patients labeled as NSTEMI actually have an acute coronary occlusion.[8,9] These patients benefit from emergency PCI and have increased morbidity and mortality when compared to those without obstructive lesions.[8] Occlusion myocardial infarction includes the previously outlined STEMI equivalents as well as numerous other patterns and requires a significant degree of ECG interpretation practice and skill. In this particular case, it could be argued that the presenting ECG showed hyperacute T waves.[10] Additionally, the validated subtle anterior STEMI calculator suggests that the ECG in question is consistent with "likely anterior STEMI" (Ref– ecg blog, stemi calculator in med calc). Both are considered representative of an occlusion myocardial infarction.

Once the diagnosis of STEMI is made, actions are dependent upon availability of percutaneous coronary intervention (PCI). PCI is recommended within 12 hours of symptom onset and current ACC/AHA guidelines recommend a door-to-balloon time of 90 minutes after patient presentation to the ED.[11] Patients who will undergo primary PCI should additionally receive a P2Y12 inhibitor in addition to aspirin 325mg. Even with a provisional diagnosis of NSTEMI, ACC/AHA guidelines recommend immediate PCI for patients with active ACS and hemodynamic or electrical instability, as well as patients with "refractory angina."[12] The patient in this case, certainly appears to have met these conditions.

Patients presenting to hospitals that are not PCI-capable should be considered for fibrinolytic therapy within 12 hours of symptom onset if PCI is unable to be performed within 120 minutes.[11] Transfer to a PCI capable facility is associated with a significant reduction in mortality and reinfarction rate [13] (Our patient did not receive PCI or fibrinolytic therapy). As the cardiologist thought the presentation represented unstable angina and not STEMI, the number needed to treat with PCI to prevent short-term mortality and long-term mortality are 45 and 29, respectively.[14] Certainly, with a diagnosis of STEMI and patient should undergo prompt PCI or fibrinolysis.

So, the "elephant in the room" remains: Could the emergency physician have done anything to avoid the adverse patient outcome? The documentation could have been better but this would not have changed the outcome. The initial call to the wrong cardiologist would have saved a few minutes but not changed the outcome. Activating the STEMI protocol could have helped, but in the end, this was essentially done with the call to the cardiologist. As cardiologist did not feel this was a STEMI, the protocol would likely have been canceled and would not have changed the outcome. Unfortunately, the EP was significantly constrained by inadequate hospital policy for the management of STEMI. While a prosecuting attorney may argue that the physician should have overridden hospital policy, readers know that this is not realistic or feasible as, the EP cannot do the PCI themselves.

Here are some suggestions from these authors on how care could have possibly been improved (though we do not know if this would have changed the ultimate outcome):

- As there was ongoing pain and a change in the patient's condition (developing hypotension), repeat the ECG (a third time).
- When the patient became hypotensive (BP 87/55) at 01:09 AM with ongoing pain, a repeat call could have been made to the interventional cardiologist to request bedside assessment and consideration of emergent cath lab activation. Perhaps, more forceful statements by the EP to the effect of "this patient needs to go to the cath lab or the cath lab must be activated" may have advocated for more prompt interventions. Clearly, a multitude of factors go into our conversations with consultants, including previous relationship, seniority, time of day/night, and the specific practice patterns of the EP and the consultant.
- Ensure that the accepting physician took ownership of the patient. Though this is not really a job of the EP, we certainly do practice differently based on institutional capabilities and culture. We would not admit a traumatic aortic dissection to a non-trauma center. We would not admit a patient with a necrotizing soft tissue infection (NSTI) to a center which is not able to provide timely assessment and surgical intervention. This hospital was a cath capable facility but was this hospitalist (who was taking ICU call from home and did not see this patient at the bedside) able to provide ongoing care to activate the cath lab from the ICU if necessary?
- Consideration of repeating a troponin within 2–3 hours: Though this would have been more of a hospitalist order, with significant concern from the EP about ongoing care, perhaps, a subsequently rising troponin would have tipped the scales for repeat conversation with the cardiologist.

This case is a great reminder that we must advocate for our patients and sometimes that fight is hard. In this case, the EP knew this patient had ACS but could not convince ("sell") the need for emergency cath lab activation.

## VIII. Additional information (Weinstock)

This case was played out as a mock trial (with T. Marc Calvert, JD playing himself as in the actual trial as the defense attorney and Amal Mattu playing himself as defense expert in the actual trial + Mark Kitrick JD as the plaintiff's attorney and Matt Delaney as plaintiff's expert.) The trial can be seen at: https://www.atls2020.com/atls2020

The trial was viewed live by 682 clinicians around the world. After completion of the trial, a survey was administered to the participants to answer 2 main questions:

1. Based on what you know now, would you change your documentation practices?
2. Based on what you know now, would you change your clinical practice?

Findings were that a significant number of participants 290 (72%) stated they would change or consider changing their practice and 374 (92%) stated they would change or consider changing their documentation after watching the mock trial. Conclusions were that a mock trial appears to be an effective teaching modality to create practice change and documentation change. This was the largest study ever performed of responses to the educational value of a mock trial.

**The full article can be accessed here:**
Weinstock M, Frost K, Jolliff H, Mattu A, McIntire S, Calvert M, Kitrick M, Delaney M. See you in court: practice and documentation change from a mock trial. J Urgent Care Med. 2022;16(5):23-27.

Further discussion can be heard on the podcast EM RAP in May and June 2016; "Is it or isn't it a STEMI" with Michael Weinstock, Anand Swaminathan, Amal Mattu and T. Marc Calvert, JD

## References


1. Weinstock M, Frost K, Jolliff H, et al. See you in court: practice and documentation change from a mock trial. J Urgent Care Med 2022;16(5):23-27.
2. Ward MJ, Kripalani S, Zhu Y, et al. Incidence of emergency department visits for ST-elevation myocardial infarction in a recent six-year period in the United States. Am J Cardiol 2015;115(2):167-70. doi: 10.1016/j.amjcard.2014.10.020. Epub 2014 Oct 29. PMID: 25465931; PMCID: PMC4276502.)
3. Thygesen K, Alpert JS, Jaffe AS, et al. fourth universal definition of myocardial infarction (2018) [published correction appears in Circulation. 2018;138(20):e652]. Circulation 2018;138(20):e618-e651. doi:10.1161/CIR.0000000000000617
4. Gulati M, Levy PD, Mukherjee D, et al. AHA/ACC/ASE/CHEST/SAEM/SCCT/SCMR Guideline for the evaluation and diagnosis of chest pain: A report of the American College of Cardiology/ American Heart Association Joint Committee on Clinical Practice Guidelines [published correction appears in Circulation 2021;144(22):e455]. Circulation. 2021;144(22):e368-e454. doi:10.1161/ CIR.0000000000001029
5. Writing Committee, Kontos MC, de Lemos JA, et al. 2022 ACC expert consensus decision pathway on the evaluation and disposition of acute chest pain in the emergency department: A report

of the American College of Cardiology Solution Set Oversight Committee. J Am Coll Cardiol 2022;80(20):1925-60. doi:10.1016/j.jacc.2022.08.750).

6. Sankardas MA, Ramakumar V, Farooqui FA. Of occlusions, inclusions, and exclusions: Time to reclassify infarctions? Circulation 2021;144(5):333-35. doi:10.1161/CIRCULATIONAHA.121.055827
7. Aslanger EK, Meyers HP, Bracey A, et al. The STEMI/NonSTEMI dichotomy needs to be replaced by occlusion MI vs. non-occlusion MI. Int J Cardiol 2021;330:15. doi:10.1016/j.ijcard.2021.02.015
8. Khan AR, Golwala H, Tripathi A, et al. Impact of total occlusion of culprit artery in acute non-ST elevation myocardial infarction: A systematic review and meta-analysis. Eur Heart J 2017;38(41):3082-89. doi:10.1093/eurheartj/ehx418
9. Koyama Y, Hansen PS, Hanratty CG, et al. Prevalence of coronary occlusion and outcome of an immediate invasive strategy in suspected acute myocardial infarction with and without ST-segment elevation. Am J Cardiol 2002;90(6):579-84. doi:10.1016/s0002-9149(02)02559-6
10. Smith SW, Meyers HP. Hyperacute T-waves can be a useful sign of occlusion myocardial infarction if appropriately defined. Ann Emerg Med 2023;82(2):203-06. doi:10.1016/j.annemergmed.2023.01.011
11. O'Gara PT, Kushner FG, Ascheim DD, et al. 2013 ACCF/AHA guideline for the management of ST-elevation myocardial infarction: executive summary: A report of the American College of Cardiology Foundation/American Heart Association Task Force on Practice Guidelines [published correction appears in J Am Coll Cardiol 2013;62(11):1039]. J Am Coll Cardiol 2013;61(4):485-10. doi:10.1016/j.jacc.2012.11.018)
12. Writing Committee Members, Brindis RG, Casey Jr. DE, Ganiats TG, et al. 2014 AHA/ACC NSTE-ACS guideline. JACC 2014;64(24). https://www.jacc.org/doi/pdf/10.1016/j.jacc.2014.09.017
13. De Luca G, Biondi-Zoccai G, Marino P. Transferring patients with ST-segment elevation myocardial infarction for mechanical reperfusion: A meta-regression analysis of randomized trials. Ann Emerg Med 2008;52(6):665-76. doi:10.1016/j.annemergmed.2008.08.033
14. Huynh T, Perron S, O'Loughlin J, et al. Comparison of primary percutaneous coronary intervention and fibrinolytic therapy in ST-segment-elevation myocardial infarction: Bayesian hierarchical meta-analyses of randomized controlled trials and observational studies. Circulation 2009;119(24):3101-09. doi:10.1161/CIRCULATIONAHA.108.793745

# Bonus Case: Case 16 is Case 3 from the *Bouncebacks! Critical Care* book

In this fourth book in the *Bouncebacks!* series, we employ a fresh approach by focusing on the bounceback visit, putting the reader in the footsteps of the clinician as the patient deteriorates. The story pauses at important decision points as possible management strategies are considered in a literature-based fashion, followed by a revelation of the path chosen by the actual provider and the subsequent patient outcome. Expert whisperers, including, 7 all-star section editors, and critical care expert Scott Weingart, MD provide context and commentary along the way... buckle up for the ride!

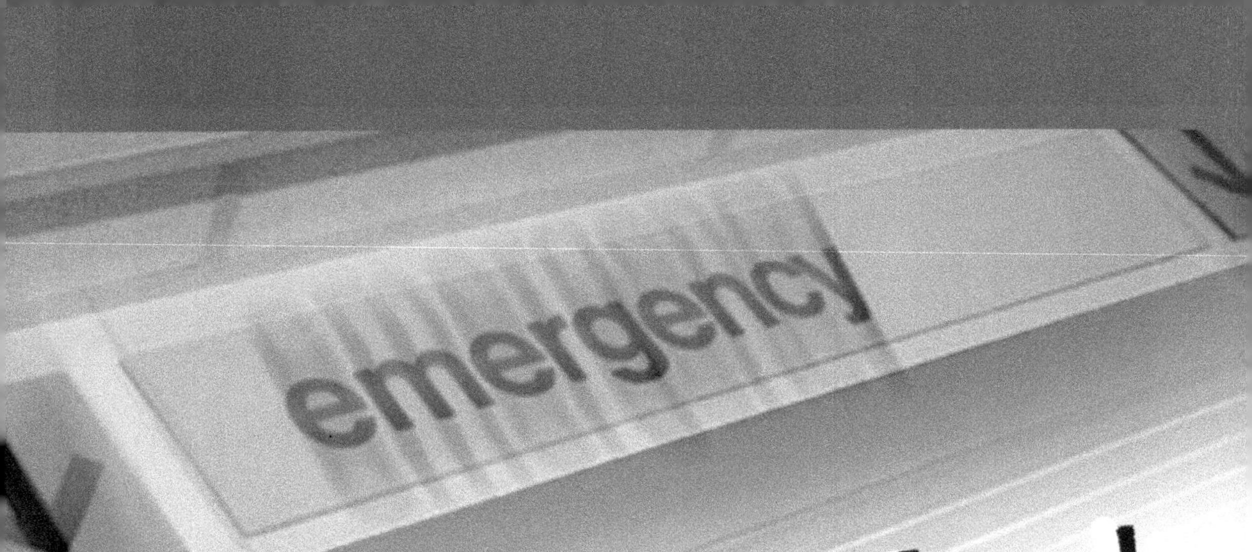


# Bouncebacks! Critical Care


Michael B. Weinstock

Kevin M. Klauer

Consulting editor:

Scott D. Weingart

Legal commentary:

Gregory L. Henry



Anadem Publishing

1.800.633.0055

anadem@anadem.com m

Anadem, Inc

Ohio ACEP

American College of Emergency Physicians

Advocacy | Education | Leadership

# CASE 16

## Chapter 3: A 41 Year-old Woman with Chest Pain

Note: The final case is provided from the *Bouncebacks! Critical Care* book.

It is a fascinating case with a lot of trial tesimony included.

**David A. Farcy, MD, FAAEM, FACEP, FCCM**

Chairman, Department of Emergency Medicine
Director, Emergency Medicine Critical Care
Mount Sinai Medical Center, Miami Beach, FL
Clinical Associate Professor
Department of Emergency Medicine & Critical Care
Herbert Wertheim College of Medicine
Florida International University, Miami, FL
Immediate past President, American Academy of Emergency Medicine

**Ramin Vejdani, DO**

Emergency Medicine Attending Physician
Director, Informatics
Mount Sinai Medical Center

Section editor:

**Lillian L. Emlet, MD, MS, FACEP, FCCM**

Clinical Associate Professor
Depts. of Critical Care Medicine & Emergency Medicine
Associate Program Director, IMCCM Fellowship of the MCCTP
Interim Associate Chief of Staff of Education, VA
Pittsburgh, PA

Legal commentary:

**Gregory L. Henry, MD**

Former president of The American College of Emergency Physicians (ACEP)
Former Professor of Emergency Medicine at the University of Michigan
Former CEO of Medical Practice Risk Assessment

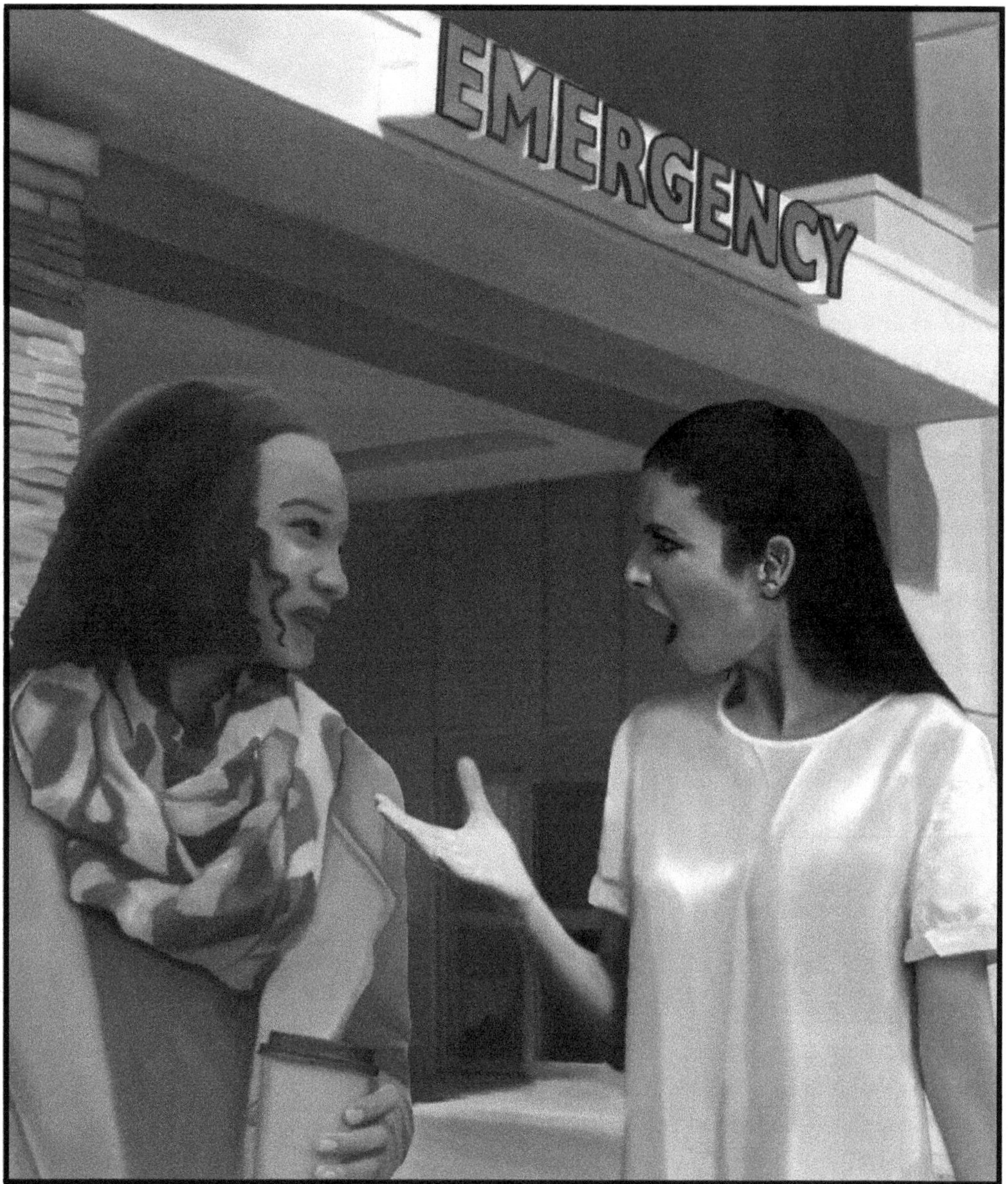


**"THEY *NEVER* ANSWERED MY QUESTION!"**

# CASE 16

## A 41 Year-old Woman with Chest Pain

In the United States, 130.4 million patients visited an emergency department in 2013 and chest pain was the second most common chief complaint, accounting for about 6% of all visits. Chest pain is a complaint with a wide array of differential etiologies, ranging from benign, such as muscle strain, to life threatening, such as Acute Myocardial Infarction (AMI), Pulmonary Embolism (PE) and Thoracic Aortic Dissection (TAD). If missed or not diagnosed in a timely fashion, there may be catastrophic outcomes. The highest frequency of malpractice cases are missed AMI, acute appendicitis, and missed fracture, while missed AMI is the diagnosis associated with the highest paid verdicts.[1,2,3]

Diagnostic errors may occur from cognitive errors, perception, failure in fact finding, and/or bias. Thus, performing a good history of present illness (HPI), family history, risk factor stratification, physical exam, and then proceeding to appropriate usage of diagnostic testing will be essential to properly diagnosing patients with chest pain.

Lifetime risk factors include:

- Age
- Gender
- Hyperlipidemia
- Hypertension (HTN)
- Diabetes
- Smoking
- Race

While recognition of presence of these risk factors is important, they have little value in predicting acute disease. When none of these risk factors are present, the lifetime risk of CAD for a 45-year-old is estimated to be < 5%, whereas with ≥ 2 major risk factors, it is 50% for men and 31% for women respectively."[4]

To make the evaluation even more difficult, patients do not read textbooks and commonly present with atypical ischemic complaints. Whereas the most typical complaints with ischemia are chest pain, chest pressure radiating down the left upper extremities, to the shoulders or jaw, associated with shortness of breath (SOB) and diaphoresis, atypical complaints, also referred to as "anginal equivalents," are dyspnea followed by nausea, dizziness, diaphoresis, malaise, back pain and/or unexplained weakness. Atypical presentations occur more commonly in elderly, female, African-American, Hispanic and diabetics patients.

**Author comments (Weinstock):** This case has another dimension; after her bounceback and adverse outcome, the case proceeds to legal action. Actual trial testimony, as well as commentary by medical-legal emergency physician expert Greg Henry, follows. Before we just go to the conclusion, please meet Stacy:

## PART 1—MEDICAL

**A 41-year-old woman with pain from her waist to her head.**
(extracted and summarized from trial testimony)

## I. The Patient's Story

Stacy is a hard worker, at one point working 3 jobs: cleaning the credit union and Mr. Payroll during the day and working at UPS at night. According to her mother, "She never stopped working. She did whatever anybody needed her to do."

At the age of 26, Stacy delivers a healthy baby girl, Celina. During the delivery, Stacy suffered a "diabetic stroke" and is told to have a tubal ligation. At this time, she is married to Leo, but the marriage ended badly, and she was left to raise Celina on her own—Leo does not provide assistance. Though she does not have much money, Stacy is a wonderful mother, supporting her daughter's interest in gymnastics and taking her to the beach. Through the years, Celina becomes her "best friend."

When Stacy sees others in need, she rises to the occasion; opening her home to two children of a father who hung himself after the mother disappeared, as well as taking in a little girl who is having problems with her stepmother.

In her early 30's Stacy starts dating a man named Robert. At one point, she walks upstairs after doing laundry and overhears Robert saying, "I don't want the baby. You might as well do something with it. I don't want it." When confronted he denies the conversation, so Stacy calls the woman back and says, "I'll take the baby. I'll raise him as my own." She borrows money for the adoption papers and brings the baby home from the hospital, calling him Matthew.

On the evening of October 2, Stacy calls her mother and tells her she is having pains in her chest. "Do you think its indigestion?" her mother asks.

"No." Stacy replies. "I've been taking something for indigestion and it's not working."

Stacy decides to go to the emergency department.

## II. INITIAL ED VISIT

**CC (RN AT 18:13):** Chest pain - pain from above waist to head, neck and arms

**Vitals:**

| Time | Temp (F) Rt. | Pulse | Resp | Syst | Diast | O2% | Pain |
|---|---|---|---|---|---|---|---|
| 18:28 | 97.9 | 97 | 20 | 186 | 96 | nl | 8/10 |

**NKDA**

**PMH:** HTN, CVA, DM
**PSH:** Choly
**SH:** Smoker
**Meds:** Glucophage, Avandia, Norvasc, Accupril – pt out of meds last 3 months

**HPI (18:55 - MD note):** Pt is a 46-year-old woman with chief complaint of chest pain for the last 1 day or so. Pain is a tightness across the chest and upper arms which is worsened by deep breaths. Radiates to the left arm. PMH of high blood pressure and diabetes. No nausea and vomiting, coughing blood, syncope, feeling of doom, shortness of breath, sweating and palpitations. Nursing notes reviewed. SH Smoker. FH: Hx cardiac disease after the age of 55.

**PE:**
**GENERAL:** A&OX3, appears very uncomfortable
**EYES:** PERRL
**CV:** RRR without m/r/g. Normal heart sounds. Good capillary refill. No peripheral edema
**RESP:** No resp distress. Prolonged splinting and decreased air movement and wheezing.
**ABD:** Soft and NT throughout, without r/r/g
**BACK:** No CVAT
**SKIN:** Normal without petechiae, vesicles, erythema

**CXR (19:11):** WNL. Fingerstick BS= 255

**Vitals:**

| Time | Temp (F) Rt. | Pulse | Resp | Syst | Diast | O2% | Pain |
|---|---|---|---|---|---|---|---|
| 19:20 | | 87 | 16 | | | 97 | |

**Exam (15:25)**

**Constitutional:** Chronically ill-appearing male who appears much older than his stated age; in no acute respiratory distress-- he is on blow by oxygen with a respiratory rate of 22 per minute; no retractions or labored respirations.

**ECG#1 @ 19:20**

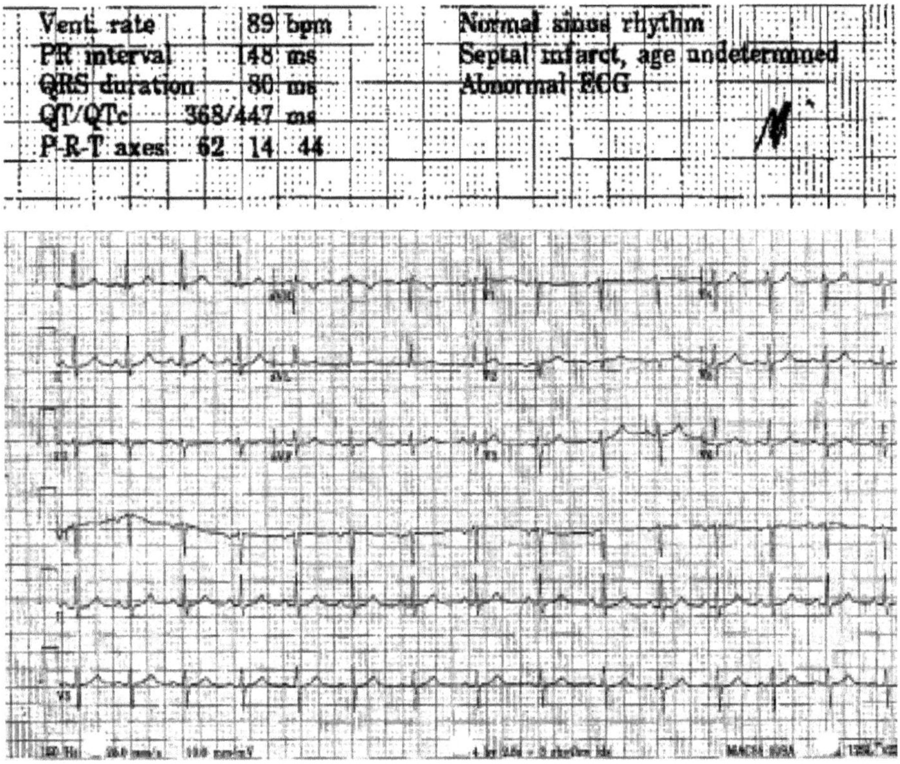


**MDM:**

Albuterol aerosol #1 (19:20)
Albuterol aerosol#2 (19:31)

**Vitals:**

| Time | Temp (F) Rt. | Pulse | Resp | Syst | Diast | O2% | Pain |
|---|---|---|---|---|---|---|---|
| 20:25 | | 71 | 16 | 130 | 82 | 100 | 3/10 |

**ECG#2 @20:55**

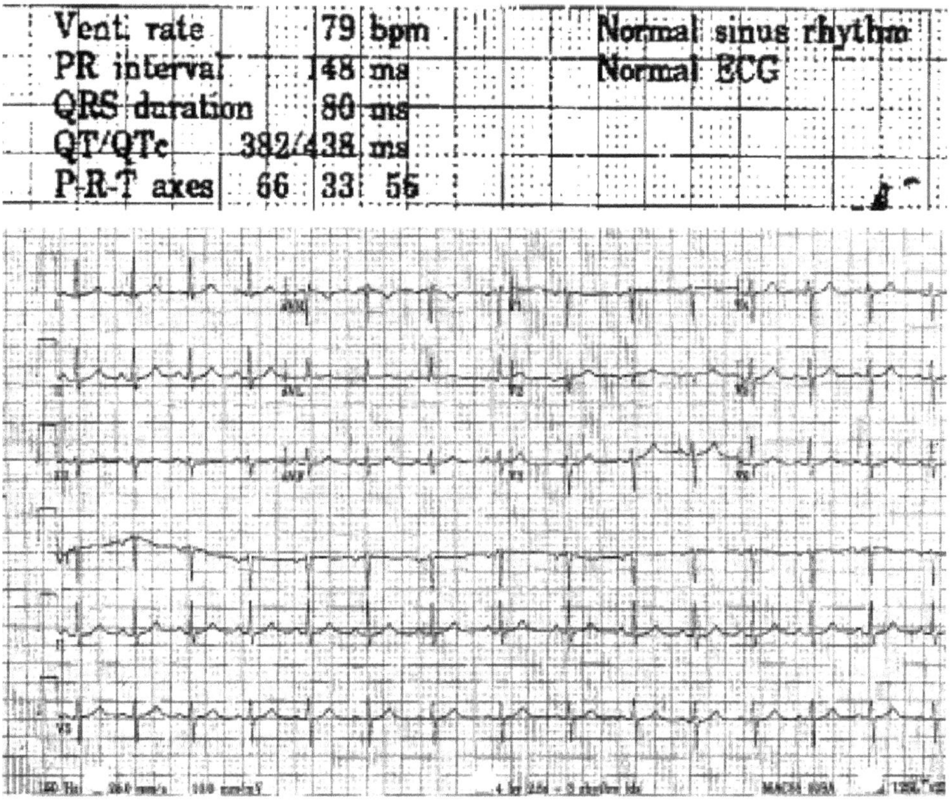


**MDM/ED course:** "CXR and ECG's reviewed. Albuterol aerosol, captopril 25mg PO"

**Diagnosis:** HTN, bronchospasm

**Condition:** Stable
**Disposition**: Home
**RN:** d/c home with driver. Pt states pain much better. Verbalizes understanding

**Discussion of the initial visit—evaluation of chest pain, medical decision-making, documentation and patient safety:**

Seems a straightforward case of "typical" angina with risk factors that include, DM (non-compliant), smoker, history of coagulopathy with TIA, and a potential positive family history. Certainly, a more thorough history and work-up could have been performed, as well as better documentation of the medical decision-making process. We believe the initial physician on the diagnosis of "bronchospasm," even though the patient did not have a history of asthma or COPD, but she is a smoker.

**1. Lack of correlation between chief complaint and final diagnosis:**

Let's start with the biggest problem with this evaluation; the final diagnosis of HTN, bronchospasm; this has no correlation with the presenting chief complaint (chest pain)! Bronchospasm typically presents with an intractable cough and wheezing, though as the bronchospasm worsens, an increased obstruction to air entry might limit the auscultation of audible wheezing secondary to lack of poor air exchange. The patient's chief complaint is chest pain with a respiratory rate of 20 and normal oxygen saturation, a focused review of systems stated no shortness of breath and the physical exam showed: *"no respiratory distress. Prolonged splinting and decreased air movement and wheezing."*

In short, nothing in the history or physical exam supports a diagnosis of bronchospasm. There is no cough, accessory muscle use, tachypnea, hx of asthma or COPD, or previous history of respiratory problems. The chart does point out chest pain: "Pain is a tightness across the chest and upper arms which is worsened by deep breaths. Radiates to the left arm." In a prospective analysis of 893 patients, investigators performed a multivariant analysis in AMI and Acute Coronary Syndrome (ACS) patients, finding that the most commonly associated symptom for both entities was chest pain that radiated to the shoulder or radiates to both arms.[5] Is a physician's gestalt good at predicting the diagnosis and outcome in patients with ACS? Several trials showed that gestalt alone had little to moderate diagnostic value compared to gestalt plus electrocardiogram (ECG) and troponin.[5]

**2. The ECG:**

Can an ECG aid in ruling out ACS? The initial ECG has a sensitivity of 20–60% for AMI, similar to flipping a coin.[6] If the ECG has ST-segment depressions greater than 0.05 mV with or without T-wave inversions, sensitivity increases to about 75%.[7] Unfortunately, the 12-lead has geography limitation, leaving the right ventricle and posterior wall untraced. Is there an approach to improving sensitivity? Though not commonly done, the addition of leads V3r, V4r, V5r, V7, V8, and V9, increases diagnostic sensitivity for ACS by 18%. The use of a 15-lead ECG containing V4r, V8, and V9 leads in addition to the 12 standard leads increases the diagnostic rate of AMI by 22% compared to standard 12-lead ECG.[8]

**3. Risk factors:**

Since gestalt combined with an ECG is not much help in ruling out ACS, what should we do? An assessment of risk factors originally came from the Framingham study group, which looked at the risk of developing cardiovascular disease over 10 years. Although they predict the long-term probability of a coronary event, cardiac risk factors are usually not helpful in identification of ACS in patients presenting with *acute* chest pain. A patient with no risk factors does not eliminate the possibility of ACS but does bring it to less than 5%. However, in patients less than 40 years of age, one study showed that in patients with a very high risk factor burden (4 to 5 risk factors) the likelihood of ACS was increased by > 20-fold.[9] Risk stratification tools have been developed, such as the HEART score and the Thrombolysis in Myocardial Infarction (TIMI) score; both incorporate risk factors.[10]

Now let's go back and look at our patient; just her age and past medical history gives her 4 factors, which puts her in a high-risk category. To add to the complexity, women experience significant differences in their presentation of ACS, leading to higher morbidity and delay in diagnosis of ischemic heart disease compared to men.[11,]

**Author comments (Weinstock):** Spoiler alert— the actual diagnosis was not: "HTN, bronchospasm." Something big was missed. At trial, the plaintiff's attorney focused on inadequate gathering of data, specifically risk factors. Though there is some controversy as to the utility of risk factors in the assessment of acute chest pain, we can all agree that it would be uncomfortable to sit on the stand and answer the following questions. The plaintiff's attorney was clever, not leaving anything to chance; there is only one way to answer these questions:

**Plaintiff's attorney questioning physician testifying for the defense:**

**Q.** Let's count the risk factors. One, diabetes, right?

**A.** Yes, sir.

**Q.** Two, smoking, correct?

**A.** Yes, sir.

**Q.** Three, hypertension or blood pressure, correct?

**A.** Yes, sir.

**Q.** Four, stroke?

**A.** Yes, sir.

**Q.** Correct? Five, age over 40, correct?

**A.** Yes, sir.

**Q.** Six, family history?

**A.** Yes, sir.

**Q.** It's a bunch, isn't it?

**A.** Yes, sir.

**Poor history:**

History taking is an art. We are asking questions not just to meet the billing standard but to also show consideration of "worst first." All non-traumatic chest pain patients need to be risk stratified as either low or high risk. In a 46-year-woman with chest pain; our differential includes:

- Acute coronary syndrome (ACS)
- Pulmonary embolism (PE)
- Thoracic aortic dissection (TAD)
- Pneumothorax

Because there is essentially no medical decision-making (MDM) section, we need to default to the history, exam and evaluation to determine what this provider actually considered in the differential. Unfortunately, the chart points only to consideration of ACS (2 ECGs were done). One could argue that pneumothorax was considered because a chest X-ray was ordered, though there was not a preliminary EP interpretation specifically addressing pneumothorax. It would have been nice to see an interpretation which stated that "there is no evidence of PTX or a widened mediastinum." Even during the cross-examination, the physician cannot defend his own actions.

**Author comments (Weinstock):** The plaintiff's attorney hammers it home about the poor data gathering (history of present illness) obtained on this patient:

**Plaintiff's attorney questioning physician testifying for the defense:**
**The importance of history:**

**Q.** Now, in order to put the pieces of the puzzle together for what is causing chest pain, you need to get an accurate history, don't you?
**A.** Yes, sir.

**Q.** You don't just take the patient's words for it. There are criteria for doctors to probe into what exactly the nature of the pain is, isn't that correct? Those questions should have been asked, correct?
**A.** Yes, sir, they typically would be asked.

**Q.** And the reason they need to be asked is because we're dealing with something that could be missed and you need as much information to put the puzzle together?
**A.** Yes sir.

**4. Tips for evaluating a multiple-complaint patient:**

Unfortunately, multiple-complaint patients take longer, but it is essential to maintain an appropriate differential and that our evaluation is logical. Instead of viewing the patient as difficult, try to determine their underlying reason for presentation. This approach will provide insight into their *main* concern. Our patient had a chief complaint and many associated complaints. There was a poorly obtained history and an inadequate attempt to correlate the complaints into a cohesive story. Just considering her history of non-compliance puts her in a higher risk category.

**Author comments (Weinstock):** Even if their concern seems unlikely to us, patient anxiety over a serious perceived diagnosis can be disabling. Though not as "emergent" as resuscitating an unrestrained MVA victim, understanding the reason for the patient's visit can focus the evaluation and guide the management and provide an opportunity; reassurance that a serious illness is not occurring is also a part of healing.

**5. Poor documentation of MDM:**

This is where everything should come together. Historically, EM physicians will over-document the catastrophic case, thinking they may be involved in a lawsuit; however, it is rarely those cases that come back to haunt us, but rather the cursory evaluation and discharge. In our case, there is no MDM, just a statement "CXR and ECG's reviewed. Albuterol aerosol, captopril 25mg PO."

The MDM is also a chance to address the key points on your initial differential. An example of a better MDM might have been to explain that the X-ray AP/Lat showed no pneumothorax, widen mediastinum, or aortic knob blunting. We all know that an X-ray lacks sensitivity but this screams to anyone reading your chart that you considered pneumothorax and aortic dissection.

A common error is ignoring or not following through on abnormal test results. In our patient, chest pain is referenced twice, 2 ECGs are done, but there is no mention of ACS. Imagine how things may have played out differently at trial if the documentation contained this discussion; "46 y/o with CP, TIMI score of 1 due to risk factors, initial ECG and repeat ECG without ST changes, no T wave inversion, no ischemic patterns. Pain is reproducible and more likely musculoskeletal. Follow-up care discussed with her PCP." Now this is only an example, since a troponin was not done, and in this case a TIMI score is not applicable, but this is an example of a reasonable discussion of consideration of ACS. We may disagree on the disposition, but this "example" MDM is clear, you considered ACS, you looked at the ECG, and you planned close follow-up. "Experts" can argue at your disposition, but not against your *thinking*; even if there is a bad outcome, your decision-making process is well-described and sound, which is defensible.

Of note, the considerations of PE (in a patient with pleuritic pain who is over the age of 35 and who is a smoker on oral contraceptives) and TAD (in a patient where there is no specific exclusion of pain radiating to the back) have still not been appropriately explored or excluded. Unfortunately, during the initial visit, the physician seems to have come to premature closure and anchored on a diagnosis of bronchospasm.

**Author comments (Weinstock):** "Hard stop" your MDM! Before the patient leaves, ask if you would be comfortable explaining your care to the patient's family or friends; if not, reassess and obtain additional data.

## III. The Story Continues

(information extracted from trial testimony):

When Stacy returns home from the hospital, she tells her daughter she is feeling better. As everything seems fine, Celina goes to bed around 10:00, but she is awoken around 2:00 with the sounds of her mother moving around the kitchen. According to Celina, "I went in there to see what was going on and [my mom] went outside to smoke a cigarette, so I went out there and sat [down on the front steps] with her. She told me that she loved me and that everything was going to be OK and she was sorry if she ever did anything to hurt me or my brother, [Matthew]."

"I told her I loved her too and that it was OK. She gave me a hug and kiss and then I went back to bed. [The next thing I remember] my mother's boyfriend Steve waking me up screaming and crying because my mom is on the floor and she is not talking to him. I called 911 and they told me to give CPR. I tried it but nothing helped."

## ED RETURN
**(early the next morning)**

**CC:** Cardiac arrest

**EMS (summary-time of arrival on scene 4:21):** 41 yo F apneic and pulseless according to family. Pt was up making coffee and collapsed. They stated she has been c/o chest pain for a couple of days. Pt unresponsive CPR and BVM assist with 100% $O_2$. ET tube 7.5 25cm @ lip. Tube secured. BX X4 clear. IV. Epi 1:10000 1mg ivp. Pt rhythm changed to v-fib. Pt shocked 200 biphasic. Vasopressin 40 units IVP. Rhythm still v-fib. 300J shock biphasic. Amiodarone 300mg ivp. No change. CPR continues. Pt transported to hospital without incident or change. Report given to staff. Pt placed in hospital bed. The actual EMS sheet is reproduced below:

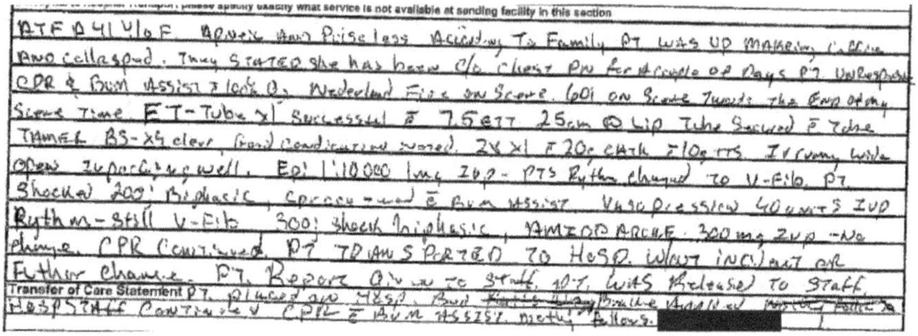
…please specify exactly what service is not available at sending facility in this section

ATF A 41 Y/O F Apneic And Pulseless According To Family PT WAS UP MAKEING Coffee And collasped. They STATED she has been c/o chest Pn for A couple of Days PT UnRespon. CPR & BVM ASSIST c 100% $O_2$. Wederland Fire on Scene. 601 on Scene Towards the End of my Scene Time. ET-Tube x1 Successful c 7.5 ETT 25cm @ Lip Tube Secured c Tube TAMER BS-X4 clear, Good conditions noted. 2X x1 c 20g CATH c 10g TTS. IV running wide open infusing well. Epi 1:10000 1mg IVP - PTS Rythm changed to V-Fib. PT Shocked 200: Biphasic, CPR continued c BVM ASSIST. Vasopressin 40 units IVP Rythm - still V-Fib 300: shock biphasic, AMIODARONE 300mg IVP - No change. CPR Continued. PT TRANSPORTED TO HOSP. W/OUT INCIDENT OR Futher change. PT. Report Given to staff. PT. WAS Released TO STAFF.

Transfer of Care Statement PT. placed on HOSP. Bed ~~[illegible]~~ Breathe Applied ~~[illegible]~~ HOSP STAFF Continued CPR c BVM ASSIST. [illegible] follows. [redacted]

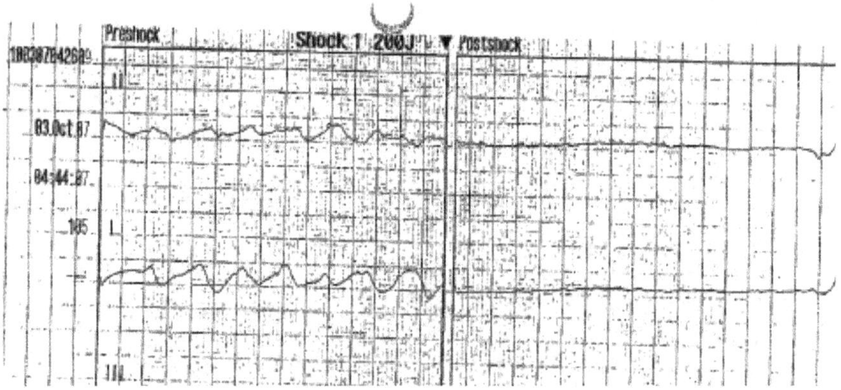


**ED documentation:**

**HPI (physician):** Presents via EMS w witnessed arrest by husband. Pt had complained of chest pain prior to arrival. EMS information reviewed. Pt is unable to give additional information secondary to medical condition of cardiac arrest.

**PE:**
**GA:** Unresponsive, CPR in progress
**EYES:** Pupils dilated and unresponsive
**Neck:** Normal
**CV:** No spontaneous heart tones
**LUNGS:** Clear with equal breath sounds with bagging
**ABD:** Slightly distended
**Ext:** Normal

**ED course:**
EMS arrival on scene 04:21
Pt arrives in ED @ 0500 in full arrest:

**Author comments (Weinstock):** You are at the bedside of a patient seen and discharged less than 24 hours ago, now in cardiac arrest. You are at decision point A:

## IV. DECISION POINT A—YOU ARE FACED WITH 4 QUESTIONS

1. **What are the important actions to take prior to a patient in full arrest arriving in the ED?**
2. **What are the important actions to take when a patient in full arrest arrives in the ED?**
3. **Are mechanical compressions better than CPR?**
4. **What is the role off end tidal $CO_2$ monitoring during CPR?**

**Q#1: What are the important actions to take prior to a patient in full arrest arriving in the ED?**
EMS pre-arrival notification serves one main purpose; it is to give you time to prepare and anticipate what resources and equipment will be needed. In the case of impending arrival of cardiac arrest, ensure:

- The availability of end tidal $CO_2$, intubation equipment including difficult airway supplies, suction, IO and code cart.
- Review and establish each team member's specific roles including specifying the team leader, the procedure and airway person, and chest compression team as well as pharmacy and radiology and a unit clerk who will be able to contact additional help, such as a vascular surgeon for diagnosis of a ruptured abdominal aortic aneurysm (AAA) or interventional cardiology for a STEMI.

**Q#2: What are the important actions to take *when* a patient in full arrest arrives in the ED?**
EMS personnel provide invaluable information, including:

- Circumstances/discussions with family or bystanders
- Down time
- Location
- Initial rhythm
- Interventions
- Impending arrival of family/friends

Ask EMS to stick around if possible, should further questions arise. An initial rhythm of ventricular fibrillation or ventricular tachycardia points more to a cardiac origin, most commonly associated with a coronary artery obstruction. In contrast, an initial rhythm of Pulseless Electrical Activity (PEA) warrants a review of potentially reversible causes including:

1. Hypovolemia
2. Hypoxia
3. Hydrogen ion (acidosis)
4. Hypo-/hyperkalemia
5. Hypothermia
6. Tension pneumothorax
7. Cardiac tamponade
8. Toxins
9. Pulmonary or coronary thrombosis

For example, getting a history that a patient was found down in a park known to be frequented by "drug users" points to overdose with emergent oxygenation and naloxone. A history of mental illness or an empty pill bottle found near the patient points to a suicide attempt.

**Q#3: Are mechanical compressions better than CPR?**

Chest compression is the most important procedure in cardiopulmonary resuscitation. The rate should be 100–120 compressions per minute. Depth of chest compressions should be between 2in (5cm) and 2.4in (6cm), allowing full chest recoil after each compression with minimized interruptions. Over the years, several commercial mechanical devices have surfaced with the impetus being that rescuer fatigue is directly proportional to the quality of chest compression. One study found that during the first minutes of a resuscitation, CPR was performed correctly 92% of the time, but that number dropped to 39.2% after 3 minutes of chest compressions.[13] With limited pre-hospital personnel, mechanical chest compression makes, but does it improve survival in the ED? In two systematic reviews and meta-analysis, looking at survival to hospital discharged with Cerebral Performance Category score of 1 and 2 (both considered a good neurologic outcome), neither trial provided sufficient evidence of an advantage of mechanical chest compressions. They concluded that mechanical chest compression should not replace high quality manual chest compression, but rather serve as a supplemental therapy in the overall care off cardiac arrest patients.[14,15]

**Q#4: What is the role off end tidal $CO_2$ monitoring during CPR?**

The end tidal $CO_2$ ($ETCO_2$) monitor can serve as a surrogate for cardiac output during chest compressions, with the 2015 AHA guidelines stating that $ETCO_2$ should be maintained above 10mmHg after the patient is successfully intubated but does not recommend a specific cutoff value as a predictor of mortality or as a decision to stop resuscitation efforts. If there is a drop, this may suggest inadequate chest compressions, most likely related to fatigue, with an indication for replacement. Conversely, an abrupt increase in $ETCO_2$ could suggest return of spontaneous circulation (ROSC) even before a pulse check. Lack of an increase in $ETCO_2$ could help to limit interruptions for pulse checks. An $ETCO_2$ of 20mmHg has some correlation with a better outcomes, but the opposite is not true.[16]

**DECISION POINT A –** ***What did the actual provider do?***

Below is an image of the actual document in the ED recorded on the code sheet:

EMS stated they arrived and found pt pulseless and apneic @ 0421.
EMS arrived at ER at 0500.
0500 Arrival and attached to cardiac monitor
    BS checked and confirmed
    ETT 7.5 @ 22cm lip
0502 CPR continued
    Epi 1mg
    Atropine 1mg
    Bicarbonate 50mEq
0508 Shock 150J
    PEA, CPR continued
    Lidocaine 100mg
0509 Epi 1mg
    CPR held, Wide complex Bradycardia
    2nd IV initiated at R AC (20ga), blood drawn
    Dopamine @ 20mcg/kg/min (pt weight - 80kg)
    BG - 343

**Chapter author comments: Were the provider's actions appropriate?**
It is difficult to know what rhythm and specific algorithm was followed, as the patient received epinephrine and then atropine by the ED physician. Currently, atropine is only recommended for brady-arrhythmias that are symptomatic (altered mental status, ischemic pain, heart failure, shock) in nature and not for PEA or asystole. This recommendation was not reviewed or revised in the 2015 guidelines. The 2010 ACLS guidelines state that "Routine use of sodium bicarbonate (SB) is not recommended for patients in cardiac arrest;" however, ACLS guidelines recommend administration of SB for QRS widening in cases of severe cardiotoxicity or cardiac arrest from hyperkalemia or tricyclic antidepressant overdose. Bicarbonate has been de-emphasized as it makes the intracellular compartment more acidotic, resulting in cells which are more resistant to medication and electricity. Thus, SB is only indicated for a pH below 7.1 and in a prolonged arrest over 20 minutes.

Due to the prolonged down time, with our patient severely acidotic, the physician likely thought that would improve the pH… or it may have fallen under the "makes us feel better" doctrine—why not give it? It is understandable that we want to do more during a cardiac arrest, especially with previous ACLS protocols involving complex algorithms; however, there are serious limitations to our medications. Emphasizing high quality CPR, decreasing pulse checks, and consideration of underlying causes will provide the best chance for a positive outcome.

**ED course: Vital signs are checked, showing:**

**Vitals:**

| Time | Temp (F) Rt. | Pulse | Resp | Syst | Diast | Sat |
|---|---|---|---|---|---|---|
| 05:09 | | 77 | bagged | 82 | 18 | 82% vent |

**Author comments (Weinstock):** We have achieved ROSC, but our patient is still unconscious with an unknown etiology for her arrest and a sat of only 82% with100% vent oxygen. We are at decision point B:

## V. DECISION POINT B—YOU ARE FACED WITH 4 QUESTIONS:

1. **The patient has a pulse—what are the initial steps after ROSC?**
2. **Was the initiation and choice of vasopressors appropriate?**
3. **Is rapid cooling indicated?**
4. **What are the best initial ventilator settings?**

***What does the literature say?***

**Q#1: The patient has a pulse—what are the initial steps after ROSC?**

Once a patient has ROSC, the highest priority should be (in this specific order):

1. Obtain a 12-lead ECG
2. Maintain perfusion by increasing the blood pressure
3. Address the respiratory status to prevent severe hypoxemia

In this case, at 5:09, the attending documented a wide complex bradycardia, so the differential diagnosis is fairly simple including an electrolyte abnormality including hyperkalemia, hypokalemia, and hypomagnesemia. Initiate suspected hyperkalemia management by administration of calcium chloride to stabilize the cardiac membrane. Calcium chloride is preferred, but if not available, then calcium gluconate is acceptable; however, a higher dose of gluconate will need to be administered as the dose of calcium chloride is 3 times the strength of gluconate.

ACLS guidelines have removed trans-venous and transthoracic pacing from their pulseless algorithm for complete AV dissociation. In a symptomatic bradycardia, such as hypotension in this case, one may consider transcutaneous pacing to see if capture is obtained and if the hemodynamic status is improved? Atropine in complete third-degree block has not been shown to improve outcome, but it often given since it has not been shown to cause harm.

Hypoxemia can also be a cause of bradycardia. In this case, the patient is saturating at 82%, while being ventilated by BVM. A patient who suffered complete cardiac arrest has lost their functional residual capacity. During daily activities, our lung volume never collapses to 0 thus making it easier to breath, but in cardiac arrest or trauma, patients lose those residual volumes. Bagging during the initial resuscitation causes inflation and deflation to a pressure of 0 and does not provide any recruitment of alveoli, thus providing a VQ mismatch.

There have been no studies that have shown any benefit of using BVM with a peep valve vs. no peep valve; however, those studies were conducted with animals and no human trials have been performed. It is the authors belief that adding a Peep valve to BVM at a minimum PEEP of 5, causes alveolar recruitment, thereby decreasing VQ mismatch and increasing alveolar oxygenation. The exact amount of PEEP is at the provider's discretion; however, a minimum of 5 is recommended.

It seems a common belief of EM physicians is that PEEP causes hypotension due to an increase in intrathoracic pressure resulting in decreased preload. This oftentimes results in the removal of PEEP in hypotensive patients. In an already hypovolemic patient, one would believe that the BP would drop; however, by providing fluids to a depleted tank and a vasopressor, preload will be increased.

**Q#2: Was the initiation and choice of vasopressors appropriate?**

What is the vasopressor "du jour?" There are two trials which help to clear up years of controversy. The first, published in 2010, which is a randomized double-blind controlled trial, demonstrated the superiority of norepinephrine over dopamine. Specifically, this trial demonstrated an increase in 28-day mortality among patients with cardiogenic shock who received dopamine as the first line agent when compared to those receiving norepinephrine. Also in this trial, the dopamine group was associated with a greater frequency of tachyarrhythmias including A-fib with RVR, V-tach and V-fib.[17] In the second trial, published in 2012, dopamine compared to norepinephrine had an increased mortality rate in septic shock, thus making norepinephrine the preferred initial pressor of choice. Now, one might argue, that in a symptomatic bradycardia, dopamine may be the preferred agent, secondary to the potential for tachyarrhythmia events. However, since it might increase mortality in cardiogenic shock, it is our belief at this time that norepinephrine is the preferred agent.[18]

**Q#3: Is rapid cooling indicated?**

To cool or not to cool—that is the question? Even after achieving ROSC, the chance of a full neurologic recovery is dismal. Nothing had been shown to either prevent or reverse anoxic encephalopathy associated with prolonged cardiac arrest until a landmark trial published in 2002 on targeted temperature management (TTM) as a neuroprotective therapy in post-arrest resuscitation. This trial was conducted in out of hospital V-tach/V-fib cardiac arrest patients. Patients were cooled within 6 hours post-ROSC if they were comatose, defined by a GCS or 8 or less for a period of 12–24 hours. Both groups who were cooled had a significant decrease in anoxic encephalopathy and better neurologic outcome based on a cerebral perfusion pressure (CPP) of 1–2. Several other trials have confirmed these neuroprotective benefits, but the optimal cooling temperature has varied. A 2013 prospective double-blind study, compared a cooling goal of 33° vs. 36° C, but there was no benefit in morbidity or mortality. The AHA 2015 guidelines strongly recommends TTM to be performed as soon as possible if no contraindications exist.

It is the belief of these authors that TTM should be an essential part of post-cardiac arrest resuscitation, since keeping a patient at 35°–36° C is only mild hypothermia and has few complications. It is our belief that the potential neurologic benefits far outweigh the minimal risks. We have noted that physician resistance to TTM is mainly due to a lack of understanding of that therapy and/or familiarity of its use. Some physicians mistakenly believe that 36° C is normothermic, thereby precluding the need to initiate cooling. However, the benefit of TTM may actually lie in the prevention of hyperthermia, which stimulates the inflammatory cascade that contributes to cell death. The exact understanding of this pathophysiology is still in its early understanding. TTM should be started immediately, even during the acute phase of resuscitation, with a goal of 36°C or less to be obtained as quickly as possible, but caution should be used to prevent a temperature < 35° C.[19,20,21]

**Q#4: What are the best initial ventilator settings?**

Patients in cardiac arrest will have complete collapse of their alveoli (de-recruitment), thus, the ventilator settings should be set to promote recruitment and decrease potential barotrauma which may be associated with high tidal volumes, as well as rapid opening and closing of alveoli. A tidal volume of 6–8mm of $H_2O$ should be used as a lung protective strategy. Plateau pressures should be used to guide our tidal volume and should remain < 30mmHg. There has been much debate on the initial tidal volume secondary to the ARDS NDS net. In 2000, a decreased morbidity was shown with patients ventilated with a TV of 4–6mm to obtain a PP of < 30, but no benefit in non-ARDS has been reported in the literature. Thus, the exact tidal volume remains controversial, which is why we recommend 6–8mL per kg as the initial tidal volume.

The respiratory rate should be started anywhere between 12–16 and titrated to accommodate minute ventilation (a lower tidal volume would therefore require a higher respiratory rate since MV = TV x RR). The ventilator needs to be adjusted either by following oxygen saturation with a goal to maintain sat > 92% and/or based on an ABG.

$FiO_2$ should be started at 50–100%, based upon an understanding of the potential cause of the cardiac arrest. The AHA recommends starting at 100% $FiO_2$; however, recent data shows that hyperoxemia, defined as a $PaO_2$ > 300 is associated with increased cerebrotoxic effects. It is not clear if this hyperoxygenation injury is related to a prolonged vent setting at the higher $FiO_2$. We recommend starting the $FiO_2$ at 100% with a rapid titration of $FiO_2$ to maintain an oxygen sat of 92–95% by lowering $FiO_2$ by 10% in the first 1–2 hours post-resuscitation. If you are able to achieve normotension, then titration of the $FiO_2$ can be maintained by following end tidal $CO_2$ (titrating to 35–42mmHG) or by ABG $PaO_2$ < 300mmHg, but higher maintaining $PaO_2$ than 60mmHg.

Lastly, no mode of ventilation has been shown to be superior to another. Volume vs. pressure has also not been shown to be beneficial. We recommend using the mode with which you have greatest familiarity.

**The ED course continues:**

The patient is placed on the vent but with 4 minutes, again loses her pulse. The resus continues:
0512–CPR is resumed and an additional epinephrine 1mg IVP is given. NS IVF bolus 500mg is started
0514 – Rhythm is PEA. Bicarb 50mEq IVP
0516 – Rhythm check shows wide complex PEA. Epi 1mg IVP
0518 – Rhythm check = V-fib
Shock 150J

Pulses present (femoral) – BP check recorded as 176/142. Pulse = 91. Pulse ox = 74%
V-fib
Shock 150J

**The labs begin to return:**
WBC = 14.5 (H)
Hb = 13.1gm/dL
Plt = 233thou/mcL (L)
Sodium = 141 mmol/L
Potassium = 3.0 mmol/L (L)
Chloride = 100 mmol/L
$CO_2$ = 17 mmol/L (L)
BUN = 10 mg/dL
Creatinine = 1.2 mg/dL
LFTs = WNL

Troponin = 1.09 ng/ml (H)
BNP = 53 pq/ml

**The resus continues:**
0519 – Pulse check reveals no pulses. CPR is continued
0520 – V-fib
    Shock 150J
    Atropine 1mg
0522 – CPR held – no pulse
0523 – CPR started
Epi 1mg IVP
Shock 150J
0526 – Epi 1mg IPV
0527 – Bicarbonate 50mEq
0531 – CPR held, pulses present.
0532 - Rhythm strip shows:

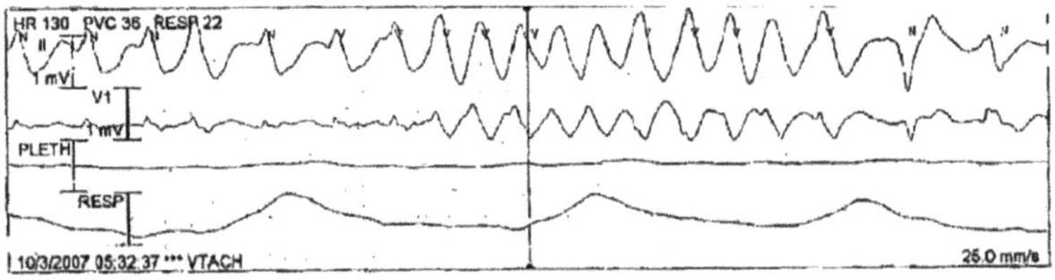


Shock 150J
Shock 150J
Wide complex sinus rhythm – heart rate is 143. Pulse ox 72%
0537 – Amiodarone 150mg
    Shock 150J
0538 – Levophed 4mg/250ml wide open

The patient is now is refractory vs. tach with a pulse. How did the provider do?

## VI. DECISION POINT C—YOU ARE FACED WITH 5 QUESTIONS:

1. **How is refractory V-fib and V-tach managed?**
2. **Our patient remains hypoxic, what can be done to optimize the oxygenation? Should the patient receive lytics for a suspected diagnosis of PE?**
3. **What is the role of cardiac US during a code?**
4. **When should the code be called?**
5. **What about ECMO?**

***What does the literature say?***

**Q#1: How is refractory V-fib and V-tach managed?**

Meds: Refractory V-fib/V-tach is defined as persistence or re-occurrence of V-fib and or V-tach after 1 shock. The role of antiarrhythmics is to pharmacologically convert these non-perfusing rhythms into a perfusing one. Unfortunately, the evidence is troublesome; when amiodarone vs. lidocaine was used there was a trend for increase ROSC in the amiodarone group but no mortality difference. Similar trials with Procainamide showed some conversion and return of spontaneous circulation, but overall data did not show improved mortality. The AHA recommends the choice of antiarrhythmic agents be based on the morphology of the ventricular arrhythmia, with the 2015 AHA guidelines recommending amiodarone use initially.

**Cutting edge defibrillation (single/multiple sequential):** Let's first review the principles of defibrillation, specifically, the type of equipment available and their limitations. Monophasic uses a unidirectional form of electricity, while biphasic are bidirectional. Biphasic devices use one of 3 different designs: biphasic truncated exponential (BTE), rectilinear biphasic (RLB), and pulsed biphasic waveforms. They each have set joule protocols that are manufacturer directed, ranging from 120 joules to 200 joules, thus familiarity is critical.

In patients with refractory V-fib and V-tach, an emerging concept is double sequential defibrillation, performed by using 2 defibrillators by placing 1 set of pads posteriorly and anteriorly, while placing the other set at the apex and the sternum. Both defibrillators are charged at their maximum delivery of joules, while CPR is continued. When both defibrillators have fully charged, on the count of 3 (and after verifying that everyone is clear), both defibrillators are discharged together or within a second apart. The original data came from electrophysiologists who performed defibrillation and employed double sequential technique in the conversion of their patient and obtained conversion on their first defibrillation. Each shock was delivered between 0.4.–0.5 sec. None of these patients received pharmacological agents. The theory was that the sequential shock decreased the relative refractory period of the cardiac muscle and potentially decreased the transthoracic impedance by leading to more electrical delivery. Until recently, most of the trials were retrospective or case reports. Unfortunately, due to the patient population and conditions, it is very difficult to perform a double-blind, placebo-controlled trial. At this time, we can only say that adequate performance of CPR and delivery of early defibrillation is the standard. If the rhythm conversion is not successfully achieved after 3 defibrillations, double sequential defibrillation may be attempted. There is minimal potential for harm, falling into the category of a Hail Mary pass.

Whichever path is chosen, the primary emphasis is to only minimally interrupt chest compression.[19,20,21]

**Q#2: Our patient remains hypoxic, what can be done to optimize the oxygenation? Should the patient receive lytics for a suspected diagnosis of PE?**

Our patient had several episodes of PEA as well as ROSC but continued with severe hypoxemia. After careful consideration of the potential etiologies of the cardiac arrest, we must ask ourselves, what is the cause of this hypoxemia? Could it be a tension pneumothorax or PE? We can either intervene or do further diagnostic testing, such as performing a bedside ultrasound (which will be discussed in the next section) to evaluate for pneumothorax. If the suspicion of a PE remains high on the differential due to the clinical presentation, the use of TPA has shown some modest clinical benefit, without increased evidence of decreased morbidity and mortality, but the AHA in 2015 stated that no evidence is available to support or refute the effectiveness of empiric thrombolysis in suspected but unconfirmed PE.[21]

How about thrombolysis in ACS? The use of TPA in potential ACS as the etiology of the cardiac arrest is classified as not effective and potentially harmful. In summary, fibrinolytic therapy should not be routinely used in cardiac arrest. There have been multiple case reports where TPA was administered with a successful return of circulation and survival, but caution is warranted; these authors believe that it might be associated with timing of the thrombolytic. Currently, it is usually used as a last-ditch effort in prolonged arrest, but if administered early, could yield different results. Note that this is based on no evidence, but a single case study; no formal recommendations can be made at this time.

Our patient had 3 episodes of ROSC, lasting anywhere between 1 to 4 minutes, but no ECG was obtained—this should have been a priority. Placing ECG pads on the chest while CPR is performed, in the hope of ROSC, could have facilitated rapidly obtaining and ECG when ROSC was achieved; this could have been diagnostic and potentially lifesaving. In this case, from the initial visit to the second visit, this patient is screaming ACS.

**Consulting editor comments (Weingart):**

If you have a place that does not have ECMO and you highly suspect acute myocardial infarction, unless you're in that like one in a hundred place where they'll actually take the patient to the Cath lab with a mechanical CPR device (and those places are vanishingly small), then you pretty much have no chance except to push lytics. If I don't suspect PE or MI, then I will not empirically give lytics.

**Q#3: What is the role of cardiac US during a code?**

0POCUS can be utilized during a code to evaluate for pneumothorax, cardiac tamponade, estimated cardiac EF, cardiac standstill, and to estimate the patient's volume status by looking at the IVC. Standstill is defined as no cardiac activity and can be used to terminate resuscitation efforts. Use caution as a prospective cohort study during cardiac arrest resuscitation comparing times between pulse check with ultrasound vs. pulse check alone found that the use of ultrasound was associated with nearly double the 10 second maximum duration recommended in 2015 current guideline.[19, 22]

**Q#4: When should the code be called?**

There are only several predictors in cardiac arrest including time from arrest to time of CPR initiation and a prolonged resuscitative effort. Much has been said on when to stop, but little is known. We recommend that family members or loved ones be given the opportunity to be present in the resuscitation efforts, as this serves multiple purposes.

- It will bring closure. They witness all the efforts that the team puts toward saving their loved one.
- There is opportunity for a discussion about advanced directives and quality of life while the resuscitation is being conducted.

We personally have experienced on several occasions family members asking to stop because of the futility of continuing the resuscitation. Note that patients in asystole or prolonged PEA over 30 minutes have little to no chance of a meaningful recovery.

**Consulting editor comments (Weingart):**

We have a tendency to run codes for a long time. Now that we are using ECMO, we begin to realize that our conceptions of how long we can perform CPR and still have neurologically intact survival are wrong. We've had ECMO patients an hour and 20 minutes with perfect neurologic outcome, and we've had patients without ECMO who had a code continue till the 45 minute mark who had a full recovery and walked out of the hospital. I have a tendency on young patients to run the codes a long time. After I've taken everything out of my arsenal and I have nothing at the 45 minute mark, what are you going to do? We don't have an end game at that point.

**Q#5: What about ECMO?**

E-CPR has recently had made a re-emergence in the medical literature. Even though the AHA in the 2015 guidelines does not recommend the use of E-CPR, several retrospective studies performed in Korea, Taiwan, and one in San Diego found an increased rate of survival with good neurological outcome defined by a CPP of 1 or 2. E-CPR is a costly, time-consuming maneuver that is best left to centers that are experienced and have dedicated ECMO resources. While we are excited about the future of E-CPR, it currently enjoys only limited availability; there is much to come from future research.[19]

***What did the actual provider do?***

**ED course:**

0538 – Vitals: Heart rate is 90. Sat is 72%. Summary: Dopamine and Levophed are running
0539 - Pulse check = no pulses. CPR is continued
0540 – V fib
Shock 150J
Shock 150J
0541 – CPR held. The rhythm strip shows:

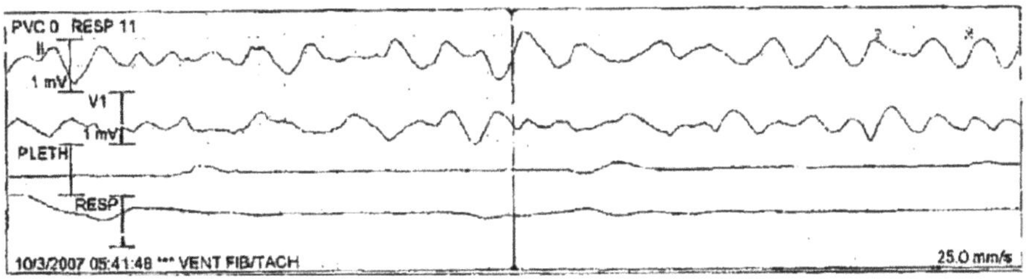

0542 – Pt apneic and pulseless
0543 – Code called
0619 - Numerous family and friends arrive and are taken into the room by the chaplain to view the body

An autopsy reveals:

**Outcomes**
Time CPR Stopped: 0543
Expired: 0543

PATHOLOGICAL FINDINGS

1. Acute myocardial infarction.
2. Severe atherosclerotic involvement of the circumflex and the right coronary artery.
3. Patchy fibrosis of the myocardium.
4. Medical history of hypertension, diabetes mellitis and prior cerebrovascular accident.

CAUSE OF DEATH: Acute myocardial infarction due to severe atherosclerotic heart disease.

**Summary:** Patients in cardiac arrest benefit from:
- Early initiation of CPR.
- Adequate compressions at a rate of 100–120, and depth of 2–2.4 inches.
- Early defibrillation for V-fib/V-tach.
- Early ECG after ROSC to identify STEMI.
- Target Temperature Management should be obtained at 35–36° C for patients with ROSC and GCS of less than 8 without other contraindications.

## PART 2—LEGAL

Shortly after Stacy's untimely death, a malpractice action was entered, proceeding to discovery, depositions and eventually a trial. Allegations of malpractice were entered not only against the initial treating physician, but against the hospital and nursing staff. As it turns out, the hospital had recently rewritten its procedure for triage with a recommendation to assign a triage category of 2 for chest pain patients, but Stacy had only been assigned a category of 3, in direct contradiction of the hospital's own policy.

This is one of the three cases in this book where we explore the legal issues. Following the testimony are comments by **Greg Henry, MD**, past president of ACEP and an expert in many legal cases.

**The Plaintiff's strategy:**
Stacy collapsed at her home just over seven hours after ED discharge. The pathologist who performed the autopsy testified that Stacy had severe atherosclerosis of the circumflex coronary artery and the right coronary artery. The left anterior descending artery had moderate atherosclerosis. A discolored region along the lateral side of the left ventricle indicated an acute

MI. The plaintiff's expert on emergency medicine testified that St. Mary's nurses contributed to Stacy's death, partly because they assigned an incorrect triage category. They further opined that the proper treatment for unstable angina is to first make the diagnosis by assessing myocardial function, performing a cardiac perfusion study, or taking the patient directly to cardiac catheterization or CT angiography. Based on these findings, a decision would be made as to angioplasty and stenting or a bypass. The experts did not think that either the doctor or the nurses intentionally harmed Stacy, but Stacy presented with symptoms that were very consistent with unstable angina and myocardial infarction. In their opinion, with her significant risk factors of hypertension, smoking, and diabetes, the possibilities of myocardial infarction and unstable angina were not adequately evaluated.

**The Defense's strategy:**
Though there was a delay in obtaining the ECG, there was no reason to believe that an earlier ECG would have changed the management. The chart reflects the presence of multiple risk factors for coronary artery disease, however, Stacy exhibited no associated symptoms—nausea and vomiting, coughing blood, syncope, feeling of doom, shortness of breath, sweating and palpitations—and a physical examination of her cardiovascular system—regular rate/rhythm, no murmur, no gallop, no friction rub, pulses full/equal—presented in normal range. She was not cyanotic, diaphoretic, or pallid. There were two "ECGs with a whole day of pain, not having acute changes." Because his impression was that Stacy's chest pain was of non-cardiac origin, the doctor did not order cardiac enzyme tests. According to the doctor, the level 3 triage assigned to Stacy provided more than enough time for him to make the correct decision.

The discharge nurse told Stacy to return to the emergency room if the pain returned or worsened. The doctor instructed Stacy to set up an appointment the following day with her doctor to address her high blood pressure. The nurse took Stacy's vital signs and assessed her pain. At 8:25 Stacy's blood pressure was "130/82," her pulse was "71," and her respirations were "16." Stacy would not have been discharged if those vital signs had been abnormal. The nurse acknowledged that a patient may have stable vital signs and still have unstable angina. The hospital's emergency admission record states that the doctor diagnosed Stacy with high blood pressure and prescribed lisinopril. Stacy was discharged at 8:45 p.m. The discharge instructions informed Stacy to call sooner if she thought it was necessary, and to return immediately if her symptoms worsened.

## I. The Trial

**Plaintiff's opening statement:** Good morning, everybody. One of the major reasons people come to ED's in the U.S. is because of chest pain. Not all of it is fatal. And it's not always easy to diagnose. And the rule in ED's is that you treat chest pain as a heart attack until you rule it out. That's the rule. The evidence is going to show that when Stacy left the hospital with her friend Doreen, they were in shock. Doreen regrets to this day that she did not bar the door and say, "No, we're not leaving. We're not leaving." But they did.

It's going to be up to you to figure out whether the discharge of Stacy was wrong, was negligent —the failure to even get a basic history was a violation of the standard. We strongly believe that had these things been done, Stacy would be here today and she would be raising her children. Thank you.

**1. Triage category:**

**Q.** I want to get some clarity for the jury's sake. Your position is she shouldn't have been triage one.
**A.** Yes, sir.

**Q.** And you are going to stand by this statement?
**A.** Yes, sir.

**Q.** I want you to look at Exhibit #30, please. It says departmental procedure, correct?
**A.** Yes, sir.

**Q.** It was revised June of '07, that is 4 months prior to Stacy's presentation, correct?
**A.** Yes, sir.

**Q.** It is the emergency department policy. The purpose is to describe the steps to be taken when caring for patients over 18 with chest pain, correct?
**A.** Yes, sir.

**Q.** It says the SOC for all patients who present to the ED with a complaint of chest pain should be evaluated as soon as possible by the triage nurse to initiate appropriate steps to minimize mortality and morbidity, correct?
**A.** Yes sir.

**Q.** First, obtain a patient assessment. Next obtain a history including precipitating factors, duration of pain, quality, intensity of pain. She had at least 1, 2, 3, 4, 5, 6 risk factors. Read the department procedure to me.
**A.** Assign a triage category one or two.

**Q.** Didn't say 3, did it?
**A.** It does not.

**2. Should the provider document that it is busy?**

**Author comments (Weinstock):**

The physician alleged that it was very busy when Stacy presented… is this a good idea? Sounds like it… until, the attorney subpoenas the hospital for the patient logs for the day. They are reproduced below. Was it really too busy for good care? You be the judge…

**Q.** Now we agreed yesterday, doctor, that the most severe patient, the patient that was most urgent was triaged as a level one, correct?
**A.** Yes, sir.

**Q.** All right. Look on the log for October 2nd, is there a single triage 1 on there?
**A.** There does not appear to be.

**Q.** Okay. And we'll just go through it. What time did you come on duty that day?
**A.** Generally 6 p.m.

**Q.** Okay. And this is military time, so 6 p.m. would be?
**A.** That would be 1800.

The actual log from the chart is reproduced below:

| Time In | LOS (Length of Stay) | Physician Time | Chief Complaint - Triage Level |
|---|---|---|---|
| 13:29 | 6:05 | 15:04 | right side flank pain-Level 4 |
| 16:42 | 5:59 | 16:45 | Pneumonia Level 3 |
| 17:30 | 2:09 | 18:07 | Fatigue Sore throat headache Level 3 |
| 17:35 | 3:21 | 17:59 | Abdominal pain vomiting Level 3 |
| 17:58 | 1:25 | 18:22 | Eye complaints (laceration) Level 3 |
| 18:01 | 1:42 | 18:15 | leg hurts, chills, left leg giving out Level 3 |
| 18:13 | 2:37 | 18:28 | [redacted] chest pain - Level 3 |
| 18:53 | 1:01 | 19:32 | finger hurts - Level 4 |
| 19:27 | 3:32 | 19:34 | attempted suicide - Level 3 |
| 19:59 | 1:32 | 20:52 | shoulder pain - level 3 |
| 20:09 | 2:31 | 20:21 | abdominal pain, chest pain - Level 3 (nurse practitioner) |
| 20:17 | 1:36 | 20:37 | Pediatric fever - Level 4 |
| 20:39 | 5:40 | 20:47 | abdominal pain - Level 3 (nurse practitioner |
| 20:45 | 1:10 | 21:09 | fell at Walmart, cut lip - Level 3 |
| 20:50 | 1:06 | 21:03 | Left side hurts, Flank pain- Level 4 |

**3. Plaintiff goes a bit too far:**

**Q.** Wouldn't it be nice to learn from a traumatic experience? Wouldn't it be nice to learn from somebody's death and be willing to say, "You know what? Maybe let's go back and let's retrace our steps, highlight

granted, but do we want this to happen again?"
**A.** No sir, I think about this every day, I do not want it to happen again. This is very emotional for me. Do you know why I am a doctor? When I was 16—

**Q.** Your honor, can I have the witness instructed to...

**A.** I'm answering your question.

**Q.** Your honor, can I have the witness instructed to—
**A.** It's important for me to let this out. You asked me a question

**Q.** Your honor—

**The Court:**
"Just a minute everybody, listen very carefully. Doctor, you will have a full opportunity to give your side of the story when counsel questions you. At the juncture, please answer the plaintiff's questions. I understand it's emotional for you and you want the jury to understand. You will have your opportunity, at this juncture, simply answer his question."

**4. Emotional response: Defense attorney to physician:**
**Q.** Doctor, you've been on the stand for a few hours. While you were giving testimony a few moments ago, you started to say something about why you became a physician and the plaintiff's counsel stopped you. Would you like to share that with the jury?
**A.** Yes sir, he had asked if I understand what they're going through. When I was 16 I took a chemistry test and the secretary came and told me, "You're to go right home." I drove home. My mother had died of a heart attack at age 42. I understand what they're going through. This is a horrendous case for me. When they subpoenaed the documents, I mean, I literally sat down and sobbed, that—that I—all of those risk factors and everything is on there. And if the nurses mis-triaged it, it's my job to do that. And even there is enough information there, that I missed this. I don't know how I missed this. But I understand very well what they're going through. I go through it every day, I think about this case because it's almost an ironic mirror image of what happened. My mom had had some chest pains. Her doctor thought she was just an anxious housewife that drank too much sherry and it turns out she dropped dead of a heart attack at 42. So I'm very much aware of what they're going through. This is a very emotional case. And, again, I'm—I'm sorry that I am reacting this way, but this is—I understand what they're going through.

**Q.** Thank you for sharing that, doctor.

**Author comments (Weinstock):**

What follows next is truly astounding, the physician, besieged by genuine guilt and self-doubt, admits that they were wrong. One a side note, there were 2 legal actions, one against the physician, and the other against the hospital... read on....

**5. I was wrong (Plaintiff's attorney to physician):**

**Q.** You know what I'm getting at. At the hospital, worst case scenario, her chances are tremendously better than in a trailer park? You checked that she was stable when she left the hospital, correct?

**A.** I appear to be in error about her being stable.

**Q.** Whoa. Wait, wait. What did you just say?

**A.** I appear to be in error in checking she's stable. History has shown the fullness of time, she apparently had unstable angina, and so was not stable at discharge.

**Q.** So, you –

**A.** I was in error. I made a mistake. The nursing staff didn't make a mistake. The hospital didn't make a mistake. I made a mistake. I had a lady that had many risk factors. I thought I had answered her complaint with her BP and her bronchospasm and the 2 ECG's that didn't have evolving change. I thought she was stable. I was wrong. I failed her.

**6. So, what happened?**

The defense now starts calling witnesses, with the cardiologist undergoing direct examination by the defense counsel. He is being questioned about testimony we have just heard; that the doctor admitted wrongdoing to the jury. Then the [not adequately prepped] cardiologist admits that he knows the physician defendant has already settled his case. *At this point in the trial, this is *not* known by the jury:

**Q.** Did you learn that the doctor confessed to the jury that unstable angina caused her death?

**A.** When I did my report?

**Q.** No. Did you learn before you got on the witness stand?

**A.** I know that he—he has—he already settled his case with them and that he admitted he probably shouldn't have sent her home.

**Q.** He—he told the jury—and—

**COURT:** Why don't y'all approach [the bench].

**Q.** (Plaintiff): The cardiologist just blurted out that the [ED] doctor had settled. We have all been told by the court to instruct the witnesses not to mention that there was a settlement.

**Author comments (Weinstock):**

This is a major twist in our story. Why is it important? Because this trial was actually against the hospital, and in this trial, the physician was a witness for the defense! The concern for the plaintiff's attorney was that if the jury thought there was a big settlement which gave money to the family, they would be less likely to award additional money from the hospital to the family. Here is the plaintiff's attorney appealing to the judge:

**Plaintiff's attorney:** In my life, your honor, I have never moved for a mistrial, ever, in a civil case. But I think it is warranted here because you can't un-ring this bell. "Well the guilty party has already paid, and so, you know, the hospital should be exonerated." In this case, your honor, we are faced with a very high burden of willful and wanton behavior. The settlement amount [already paid] was $200,000, for a 46-year-old woman with 2 minor children, is insignificant and paltry.

The motion for mistrial is denied.

## II. Trial Outcome

Jury sides with plaintiff, according to the newspaper report "the jury hit the hospital with a $1.4 million verdict Thursday, concluding that the hospital nurses were negligent in their treatment of the late Stacy."

The hospital appeals, as in Texas there is a very high standard of malpractice saying the physician's actions need to be "Willful and Wanton."

## III. Vote On Appeal

"We hold that the evidence of deviation from the standard of care by St. Mary's nursing staff is legally insufficient to support the jury's finding that the willful and wanton negligence of the hospital was a proximate cause of Stacy's death," the opinion states.

"Accordingly, we reverse the trial court's judgment and render a take-nothing judgment."

### JURORS HEAR EMOTIONAL TESTIMONY FROM DOCTOR IN MALPRACTICE TRIAL!

January 13, 2010 1:43 PM
By David Yates
*Reporter with the Southeast Texas Record, reprinted with permission.*

The doctor who treated the late Stacy [_______], recently testified during a malpractice trial that he could have done more to prevent her fatal heart attack.

Her family claims the nursing staff at Hospital violated nursing standards because they failed to assess her condition, failed to inquire and determine the nature of the chest pain and failed to discuss the case with the emergency room attending physician.

Nurses also failed to trigger the chain of command with a call to the nursing supervisor when no satisfactory resolution could be reached and failed to ask for orders from the ER physician for biochemical marker studies, according to the complaint.

## MED-MAL TRIAL AGAINST LOCAL HOSPITAL ENDS WITH $1.4 M VERDICT

October 17, 2011 2:00 PM
By David Yates
*Reporter with the Southeast Texas Record, reprinted with permission.*

Last Thursday, the Texas Ninth Court of Appeals found the evidence "legally insufficient" for jurors to levy a $1.2 million verdict against the hospital
As previously reported, on Jan. 21, 2010, a Jefferson County jury concluded that nurses were negligent in their treatment of the late _____, levying a $1.4 million verdict against the hospital.
Her mother, sued the hospital in November 2008, alleging nurses and [the initial doctor] incorrectly diagnosed and treated the patient.
Court records show she died of a heart attack a day after receiving treatment.
[The initial doctor] settled for $150,000 in August 2009, while the hospital opted to take its chances in court.
According to the charge of the court, jurors found [the initial doctor] was 20 percent responsible in his treatment and diagnosis, pushing the remaining 80 percent of the blame upon the hospital.
After the application of settlement credits, statutory damage caps and medical expenses, the judgment was reduced from $1,215,075 to $331,390, court papers say.
The following month, Christus filed an appeal questioning whether there was sufficient evidence of wanton negligence.
On Oct. 13 the Ninth Court issued an opinion, authored by Justice Charles Kreger, finding in favor of the hospital.
"We hold that the evidence of deviation from the standard of care by the nursing staff is legally insufficient to support the jury's finding that the willful and wanton negligence of the hospital was a proximate cause of death," the opinion states.
"Accordingly, we reverse the trial court's judgment and render a take-nothing judgment."

**Gregory L. Henry, MD – Legal commentary**
Past president of The American College of Emergency Physicians (ACEP)
Former Professor of Emergency Medicine at the University of Michigan
Former CEO of Medical Practice Risk Assessment
He has been an expert witness in over 2,000 malpractice cases

*"First, there is no relationship in the documentation between the chief complaint and the diagnosis; this is a mountain which is difficult to climb."*

**Documentation and evaluation:**
The approach to finding negligence with the initial doctor and hospital is simple, as our patient was a walking disaster when she entered the hospital. First, there is no relationship in the documentation between the chief complaint and the diagnosis; this is a mountain which is difficult to climb. Second, she is high-risk. She did not have a normal life expectancy. She a diabetic, she's a smoker, she's a this, she's a that. None of it is good. Third, the ECG was not normal. Exactly when her infarct took place is difficult to determine but considering all factors, this woman should be considered to have acute coronary syndrome. Confusing a jury with whether she should have been a category 1 or a category 2 is useless. She was in the department,

she got her ECG, and she had a concerning presentation; that's enough! The triage category would not have changed the work-up. But the larger picture is clear. She has just about every risk factor, and we do not have another explanation for her chest pain. Defense of the first visit is difficult, and I would advise an insurance company to consider a reasonable settlement.

**Insurance company payout:**

The monetary expense from the insurance company falls into two parts:

1. The allocated loss adjustments which are the cost of running the case. This includes paying the attorneys, paying for analysis, paying the experts, etc. etc.
2. The second part is the award. This is then divided by the patient and the attorneys.

It is the combination of these two costs which determine the risk to the insurance company. Sometimes it is better when there are multiple problems to cap losses before a runaway jury does something untoward. I have been involved in discussion of settlements and believe the amount paid in this case was reasonable and probably could have been arrived at with early negotiations.

**Defending the physician(s):**

There is no question that being a defense expert for the first treating physician would be extremely difficult. It is a much different situation for the second physician. When a patient comes back and there had been a return of spontaneous circulation from an arrest, but no return of consciousness the prognosis of the patient is terrible. Comments are made about multiple defibrillations, using norepinephrine to support both heart rate and pressure, and when you're at this level, you're talking about minute numbers of patients saved. The real question is, are we saving patients who have a reasonable life? It is extremely rare that a patient who has gone down in the field without immediate ROSC is going to have a good outcome. The plaintiff would have been wise to strictly concentrate on the first visit. Juries like cases which are simple and easy to understand. They don't want to have to balance multiple people who have made multiple errors. Emphasis on the second visit would only serve to confuse the jury.

**Hospital liability:**

It is interesting to note that the 9th Circuit Court of Appeals found the evidence legally insufficient for juries to find against the hospital. This usually means the hospital personnel i.e. the nurses. Although the initial verdict included everyone, the court was essentially also focused on the first visit. It is also interesting that the initial EM doctor settled for $150, 000, while the hospital opted to take its chances in court. The attorney for the initial physician was very wise. The fact that the initial judgment was reduced from $1.2 million to $330,000 does say something about the legal system. It is also noted that the 9th Circuit Court issued an opinion finding in favor of the hospital, saying "We hold the evidence of deviation from the standard of care by nursing is legally insufficient to support the jury's finding that willful and wanton negligence of the hospital was a proximate cause of this death." The court therefore gave to the hospital essentially a "take nothing" judgment, meaning they got themselves out of the case.

**Was it fair?**

Is this fair? Well, it's difficult to say. The "willful and wanton" negligence standard in the state of Texas certainly had an impact on the results. Instead of coming away with $1.4 million the patient's family comes away with $150,000, a small amount to provide for parentless children, especially after attorney fees are deducted. Fairness is difficult to judge.

## References


1. Rui P, Kang K, Albert M. National hospital ambulatory medical care survey: 2013 emergency department summary tables. Available at: http://www.cdc.gov/nchs/data/ahcd/nhamcs_emergency/2013_ed_web_tables.pdf. Accessed on Sept 20, 2017.
2. Heart Disease Facts, Centers for Disease Control and Prevention. Available at: https://www.cdc.gov/heartdisease/facts.htm. Accessed on Sept 20, 2017.
3. Brown TW, McCarthy ML, Kelen GD, et al. An epidemiologic study of closed emergency department malpractice claims in a national database of physician malpractice insurers. Acad Emerg Med 2010;17(5):553-60.
4. Berry JD, Dyer A, Cai X, et al. Lifetime risks of cardiovascular disease. N Engl J Med 2012;366(4):321-9.
5. Goodacre S, Locker T, Morris F, et al. How useful are clinical features in the diagnosis of acute, undifferentiated chest pain? Acad Emerg Med 2002;9(3):203-8.
6. Speake D, Terry P. Best evidence topic report: First ECG in chest pain. Emerg Med J 2001;18:61-62.
7. Forberg JL, Green M, Björk J, et al. In search of the best method to predict acute coronary syndrome using only the electrocardiogram from the emergency department. J Electrocardiol 2009;42(1):58-63.
8. Ashida T, Tani S, Nagao K, et al. Usefulness of synthesized 18-lead electrocardiography in the diagnosis of ST-elevation myocardial infarction: A pilot study. Am J Emerg Med 2017;35(3):448-57.
9. Han JH, Lindsell CJ, Storrow AB, et al. The role of cardiac risk factor burden in diagnosing acute coronary syndromes in the emergency department setting. Ann Emerg Med 2007;49(2):145-52, 152.e1.
10. Backus BE, Six AJ, Kelder JC, et al. A prospective validation of the HEART score for chest pain patients at the emergency department. Int J Cardiol 2013;168(3):2153-58.
11. Pollack CV Jr, Sites FD, Shofer FS, et al. Application of the TIMI risk score for unstable angina and non-ST elevation acute coronary syndrome to an unselected emergency department chest pain population. Acad Emerg Med 2006;13(1):13-8.
12. Amsterdam EA, Wenger NK, Brindis RG, et al. 2014 AHA/ACC Guideline For The Management of Patients with Non ST-elevation Acute Coronary Syndrome: A Report of the American College of Cardiology/American Heart Association Task Force on Practice Guidelines. Circulation 2014;130:e344-426.
13. Crea F, Battipaglia I , Andreotti F. Sex differences in mechanisms, presentation and management of ischaemic heart disease. Atherosclerosis 2015;241(1):157-68. doi: 10.1016/j.atherosclerosis.2015.04.802. Epub 2015 Apr 27.
14. Li H, Wang D, Yu Y, Zhao X, et al. Mechanical versus manual chest compressions for cardiac arrest: a systematic review and meta-analysis. Scand J Trauma Resusc Emerg Med 2016;24:10. doi:10.1186/s13049-016-0202-y.
15. Bonnes JL, Brouwer MA, Navarese EP, et al. Manual cardiopulmonary resuscitation versus CPR including a mechanical chest compression device in out-of hospital cardiac arrest: A comprehensive meta-analysis from randomized and observational studies. Ann Emerg Med 2016; 67(3):349-60. doi:10.1016/j.annemergmed.2015.09.023.
16. Hazinski MF, Nolan JP, Aickin R, et al. Part 1: Executive Summary 2015 International Consensus on Cardiopulmonary Resuscitation and Emergency Cardiovascular Care Science With Treatment

Recommendations. Circulation 2015;132:S2-S39, originally published October 14, 2015.

17. Heradstveit BE, Sunde K, Sunde GA, et.al. Factors complicating interpretation of capnography during advanced life support in cardiac arrest–a clinical retrospective study in 575 patients. Resuscitation 2012;83(7):813-8.
18. De Backer D, Biston P, Devriendt J, et al. Comparison of dopamine and norepinephrine in the treatment of shock. N Engl J Med 2010;362(9):779-89.
19. De Backer D, Aldecoa C, Njimi H, et al. Dopamine versus norepinephrine in the treatment of septic shock: A meta-analysis. Crit Care Med 2012;40(3):725-30.
20. Link MS, Berkow LC, Kudenchuk PJ, et al. Part 7: Adult Advanced Cardiovascular Life Support 2015 American Heart Association Guidelines Update for Cardiopulmonary Resuscitation and Emergency Cardiovascular Care. Circulation 2015(18 Suppl 2);132:S444-S464.
21. Callaway CW, Donnino MW, Fink EL, et al. Part 8: Post–cardiac Arrest Care 2015 American Heart Association Guidelines Update for Cardiopulmonary Resuscitation and Emergency Cardiovascular Care. Circulation 2015(18 Suppl 2);132:S465-S482.
22. Lavonas EJ, Drennan IR, Gabrielli A, et al. Part 10: Special Circumstances of Resuscitation 2015 American Heart Association Guidelines Update for Cardiopulmonary Resuscitation and Emergency Cardiovascular Care. Circulation 2015(18 Suppl 2);132:S501-S518.
23. Huis In 't Veld MA, Allison MG, Bostick DS, et al. Ultrasound use during cardiopulmonary resuscitation is associated with delays in chest compressions. Resuscitation 2017;119:95-98. PMID: 28754527.

**Epilogue: The End of Your Shift**

So there you have it. You just finished a relatively light 12-hour shift – you only saw 15 patients and sent them all home; bronchitis, gastroenteritis, benign abdominal pain, a few headaches, a COPD exacerbation, anxiety, and a homeless woman with a diagnosis of substance abuse who refused acetaminophen and was made to sign an AMA form when she complained of pain from her IV.

The day went fast; you caught up on email and met your SO for a drink on the way home. In the span of a career, this should be a completely forgettable day…

Kevin and Marc and I have been touched by the stories within these pages and enlightened by the commentary of the national medical and legal experts who have contributed.

Interestingly, when I presented these cases at conferences, the participants have surprised me by overwhelmingly voting malpractice had occurred and guessing (usually incorrectly) that the jury decided for the plaintiff; turns out we are tougher on ourselves than a jury of our "peers."

We would be interested in your thoughts on these cases, subtleties and criticisms, insights and commiserations. To read more detailed information including full opening and closing statements and trial testimony (for some cases) as well as links to videos of the Bouncebacks! book clubs and mock trials, visit my website at: www.embouncebacks.com

**In the words of Bob Dylan:**
May your thoughts always be joyful,
May your song always be sung,
And ~~may you stay… forever young~~
And may you never have a light 15-patient day in the ED…

Michael and Kevin and Marc
May 2024